D0642418

Promoting Health

Intervention Strategies from Social and Behavioral Research

Brian D. Smedley and S. Leonard Syme, *Editors*

Committee on Capitalizing on Social Science and Behavioral Research to Improve the Public's Health

Division of Health Promotion and Disease Prevention

INSTITUTE OF MEDICINE

NATIONAL ACADEMY PRESS
Washington, D.C.

NATIONAL ACADEMY PRESS • 2101 Constitution Avenue, N.W. • Washington, DC 20418

NOTICE: The project that is the subject of this report was approved by the Governing Board of the National Research Council, whose members are drawn from the councils of the National Academy of Sciences, the National Academy of Engineering, and the Institute of Medicine. The members of the committee responsible for the report were chosen for their special competences and with regard for appropriate balance.

Support for this project was provided by The Robert W. Woodruff Foundation. The views presented in this report are those of the Institute of Medicine Committee on Capitalizing on Social Science and Behavioral Research to Improve the Public's Health and are not necessarily those of the sponsor.

International Standard Book Number 0-309-07175-5

Additional copies of this report are available for sale from the National Academy Press, 2101 Constitution Avenue, N.W., Box 285, Washington, D.C. 20055. Call (800) 624-6242 or (202) 334-3313 (in the Washington metropolitan area), or visit the NAP's home page at **www.nap.edu.** The full text of this report is available at **www.nap.edu.**

For more information about the Institute of Medicine, visit the IOM home page at **www.iom.edu.**

The serpent has been a symbol of long life, healing, and knowledge among almost all cultures and religions since the beginning of recorded history. The serpent adopted as a logotype by the Institute of Medicine is a relief carving from ancient Greece, now held by the Staatliche Museen in Berlin.

First Printing, February 2001
Second Printing, June 2001
Third Printing, March 2002

"Knowing is not enough; we must apply.
Willing is not enough; we must do."
—Goethe

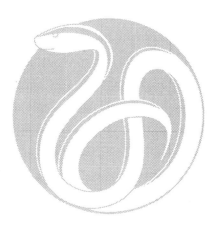

INSTITUTE OF MEDICINE

Shaping the Future for Health

THE NATIONAL ACADEMIES

National Academy of Sciences
National Academy of Engineering
Institute of Medicine
National Research Council

The **National Academy of Sciences** is a private, nonprofit, self-perpetuating society of distinguished scholars engaged in scientific and engineering research, dedicated to the furtherance of science and technology and to their use for the general welfare. Upon the authority of the charter granted to it by the Congress in 1863, the Academy has a mandate that requires it to advise the federal government on scientific and technical matters. Dr. Bruce M. Alberts is president of the National Academy of Sciences.

The **National Academy of Engineering** was established in 1964, under the charter of the National Academy of Sciences, as a parallel organization of outstanding engineers. It is autonomous in its administration and in the selection of its members, sharing with the National Academy of Sciences the responsibility for advising the federal government. The National Academy of Engineering also sponsors engineering programs aimed at meeting national needs, encourages education and research, and recognizes the superior achievements of engineers. Dr. William A. Wulf is president of the National Academy of Engineering.

The **Institute of Medicine** was established in 1970 by the National Academy of Sciences to secure the services of eminent members of appropriate professions in the examination of policy matters pertaining to the health of the public. The Institute acts under the responsibility given to the National Academy of Sciences by its congressional charter to be an adviser to the federal government and, upon its own initiative, to identify issues of medical care, research, and education. Dr. Kenneth I. Shine is president of the Institute of Medicine.

The **National Research Council** was organized by the National Academy of Sciences in 1916 to associate the broad community of science and technology with the Academy's purposes of furthering knowledge and advising the federal government. Functioning in accordance with general policies determined by the Academy, the Council has become the principal operating agency of both the National Academy of Sciences and the National Academy of Engineering in providing services to the government, the public, and the scientific and engineering communities. The Council is administered jointly by both Academies and the Institute of Medicine. Dr. Bruce M. Alberts and Dr. William A. Wulf are chairman and vice chairman, respectively, of the National Research Council.

Preface

Participating in the development of this Institute of Medicine report has been of special importance to me. I have worked for over 40 years to identify social and behavioral factors that could be useful in improving health and well-being and it is especially satisfying to now work with colleagues to assess the progress that has been made in this effort. My first exposure to this field took place in 1957 when I entered the first graduate training program at Yale University in what was then called Medical Sociology. The Commonwealth Fund supported four students in that first class. Other people were already at work on these issues, notably David Mechanic who was a member of the committee for this report, but the program at Yale was the first, formal institutionalized recognition of the existence of the field.

Ten years later, Professor Leo Reeder and I convened a conference in Phoenix, Arizona, to review the work that was being done in the social and behavioral sciences with special reference to the most vigorously studied disease at the time: coronary heart disease. A group of distinguished scholars spent several days assessing the evidence. In our report of the conference,[*] we concluded that progress was being made (but not enough to warrant interventions) and that more research was needed. Progress since then has been made but there have been at least as many false starts and dead ends as successes. But the field has grown enormously and it is entirely reasonable that we now pause again to assess the state of the field.

---

[*] S. Leonard Syme and Leo G. Reeder (eds.), Social stress and cardiovascular disease. *Milbank Memorial Fund Quarterly,* Vol. XLV, April 1967.

The charge to our committee was both clear and challenging: to identify promising areas of social science and behavioral research that could improve the public's health. The committee met for the first time in the spring of 1999 to consider this charge and to think about ways to best address it. That first meeting was a difficult one and it was not until after our second meeting that we finally were able to reach our first two decisions: one of these decisions—by far the easiest one—was to focus attention not only on the behavior of individuals but also on the social forces in the environment that shape and support such behavior. The second decision was more difficult and controversial: we decided not to focus our work on such clinical disease categories as coronary heart disease, arthritis, and cancer, because most behavioral and social factors affect many diseases. For the same reason, we decided not to organize our work around such disease risk factors as smoking, overeating, and physical inactivity. We decided instead to emphasize the role of social and behavioral factors as they influence health and disease at various stages of the life cycle.

This was a difficult decision because almost everything we do in the health field is organized around clinical diseases. While this way of thinking about health may be appropriate for the diagnosis and treatment of disease in individuals, it may not be as useful in thinking about the prevention of disease. Our success in preventing most infectious diseases involved classifying them not on the basis of their clinical characteristics but on their modes of transmission. Thus, by considering diseases as being water, food, air, or vector borne, one could more effectively target prevention efforts. We thought we could adopt this conceptual model in thinking about the diseases of concern today.

Our next decision was to invite some of the most thoughtful scholars in the nation to prepare papers that addressed this model in their particular area of expertise. The papers they wrote provide a valuable and unique resource that we hope will stimulate new thinking regarding social and behavioral interventions. These papers were of great help to the committee but to further enhance their value, the committee invited an additional group of 33 distinguished researchers and practitioners to provide their assessments of these papers. All of these experts were carefully chosen because they brought a diversity of opinion about and experience with intervention programs. The committee's final recommendations are based therefore not only on its own deliberations but also on the considered judgement of a larger group of outstanding thinkers with diverse backgrounds and experience. I hope this report will stimulate a dialogue about its importance for health in our society.

S. Leonard Syme, Ph.D.
Chair

Acknowledgments

Many individuals contributed directly and indirectly to the information contained in this report. In addition, several others assisted greatly in the February 2–3, 2000, symposium that the committee staged at the Emory Conference Center in Atlanta, Georgia. The committee expresses its appreciation to Emory University, the U.S. Centers for Disease Control and Prevention (CDC), and the Morehouse School of Medicine for their cosponsorship of the symposium. In particular, the committee wishes to thank individuals representing these institutions, including Drs. Michael M.E. Johns and David Blake of the Robert W. Woodruff Health Sciences Center at Emory University; Drs. Louis Sullivan and Peter MacLeish of the Morehouse School of Medicine; and Drs. Lynda Doll, Lynda Anderson, Ruth Berkelman, and Dixie Snyder of CDC. Renee Brown-Bryant of CDC was particularly helpful in securing Internet access for the symposium, so that the event could be viewed worldwide by individuals unable to attend in person. In addition, the committee wishes to thank Barbara and Jerome Grossman, M.D., whose generous gift supported the symposium.

The committee also extends its thanks to several of the above individuals for their thoughtful comments provided during the symposium. Dr. Johns, Dr. Snyder, and Dr. James Curran of the Rollins School of Public Health provided introductions for keynote speakers. These speakers included Dr. Sullivan, Dr. Berkelman, and Dr. William Foege of Emory University.

The symposium featured paper presentations by several authorities; versions of these papers are included in this volume. The committee wishes to express its gratitude to these authors (in order of appearance at the symposium and in this volume): Drs. George Kaplan, Susan Everson, and John Lynch of the

University of Michigan; Drs. James House and David Williams of the University of Michigan; Dr. Carol Korenbrot of the University of California, San Francisco and Dr. Nancy Moss of the Pacific Institute for Women's Health; Drs. Allison Fuligni and Jeanne Brooks-Gunn of Columbia University; Dr. Cheryl Perry of the University of Minnesota; Dr. Karen Emmons of the Harvard School of Public Health; Dr. George Maddox of Duke University; Dr. Lawrence Wallack of Portland State University; Dr. Robert Sampson of the University of Chicago and Dr. Jeffrey Morenoff of the University of Michigan; Lawrence Gostin of the Georgetown University Law Center; Dr. Kenneth Warner of the University of Michigan; and Dr. Andrew Baum of the University of Pittsburgh.

Several equally distinguished authorities reviewed these papers and provided thoughtful commentary during the symposium. Much of this commentary is reflected in the committee's findings and recommendations. Discussants included (in order of appearance at the symposium): Dr. Bruce Link of Columbia University; Dr. David Takeuchi of Indiana University; Dr. Thomas LaVeist of the Johns Hopkins University; Dr. Ruth Zambrana of the University of Maryland; Dr. Carol Hogue of the Rollins School of Public Health at Emory University; Dr. Margaret Heagarty of the Harlem Hospital Center and College of Physicians and Surgeons, Columbia University; Dr. Amado Padilla of Stanford University; Dr. Penny Hauser-Cram of Boston College; Dr. Deborah Coates of the City University of New York; Dr. William Vega of the Robert Wood Johnson Medical School; Dr. Dennis Gorman of Texas A&M University; Dr. Ralph DiClemente of the Rollins School of Public Health, Emory University; Dr. Louise Russell of Rutgers University; Dr. Fernando Trevino of the University of North Texas Health Sciences Center; Dr. Sherry Mills of the National Cancer Institute; Dr. Robert Kahn of the University of Michigan; Dr. Manuel Miranda of California State University, Los Angeles; Dr. Elaine Leventhal of the Robert Wood Johnson Medical School; Dr. Howard Leventhal of Rutgers University; Dr. Rima Rudd of the Harvard School of Public Health; Dr. William Smith of the Academy for Educational Development; Dr. Nina Wallerstein of the University of New Mexico; Dr. Ichiro Kawachi of Harvard Medical School; Dr. Marshall Kreuter of CDC; Patricia King of the Georgetown University Law Center; Dr. Ralph Hingson of the Boston University School of Public Health; Jon Vernick of the Johns Hopkins University; Dr. Judith Auerbach of the Office of AIDS Research, National Institutes of Health; Dr. J. Michael McGinnis of the Robert Wood Johnson Foundation; Dr. Carol Runyan of the University of North Carolina; Dr. Neil Schneiderman of the University of Miami; Dr. Vicki Hegelson of Carnegie-Mellon University; and Dr. Ann O'Leary of CDC.

The committee also expresses gratitude to Dr. Kathleen Toomey of the Georgia Department of Human Resources for her help in planning and moderating a panel during the symposium on public health needs of Georgia, featuring committee members Drs. Eugene Emory, Arthur Kellermann, and Claire Sterk.

REVIEWERS

The report was reviewed by individuals chosen for their diverse perspectives and technical expertise in accordance with procedures approved by the National Research Council's Report Review Committee. The purpose of this independent review is to provide candid and critical comments to assist the authors and the Institute of Medicine in making the published report as sound as possible and to ensure that the report meets institutional standards for objectivity, evidence, and responsiveness to the study charge. The contents of the review comments and the draft manuscript remain confidential to protect the integrity of the deliberative process. The committee wishes to thank the following individuals for their participation in the report review process:

Nancy E. Adler, Ph.D., Professor of Medical Psychology and Director, Health Psychology Program, Center for Social, Behavioral, and Policy Studies, University of California at San Francisco School of Medicine

Lisa Berkman, Ph.D., Professor of Health and Social Behavior and Epidemiology, Harvard School of Public Health

Richard J. Bonnie, L.L.B., Battle Professor of Law and Director, Institute of Law, Psychiatry, and Public Policy, University of Virginia

Susan Scrimshaw, Ph.D., Dean, University of Illinois at Chicago School of Public Health

Although the reviewers listed above have provided many constructive comments and suggestions, they were not asked to endorse the conclusions or recommendations nor did they see the final draft of the report before its release. The review of this report was overseen by Elaine Larson, R.N., Ph.D., Professor of Pharmaceutical and Therapeutic Research, Columbia University School of Nursing, appointed by the Institute of Medicine and Lee N. Robins, Ph.D., Professor of Social Science, Department of Psychiatry, Washington University School of Medicine, appointed by the NRC's Report Review Committee, who were responsible for making certain that an independent examination of this report was carried out in accordance with institutional procedures and that all review comments were carefully considered. Responsibility for the final content of this report rests entirely with the authoring committee and the institution.

Contents

Promoting Health: Intervention Strategies from Social and Behavioral Research

INTRODUCTION

At the dawn of the twenty-first century, Americans enjoyed better overall health than at any other time in the nation's history. Rapid advancements in medical technologies, breakthroughs in understanding some of the genetic underpinnings of health and ill health, improvements in the effectiveness and variety of pharmaceutical interventions, and other developments in biomedical research have helped to develop cures for many illnesses and to extend and improve the lives of those with chronic diseases. In support of these efforts, the vast majority of the nation's health research resources have been directed toward biomedical research endeavors. By itself, however, biomedical research cannot address the most significant challenges to improving the public's health in the new century. Approximately half of all causes of mortality in the United States are linked to social and behavioral factors such as smoking, diet, alcohol use, sedentary life-style, and accidents (McGinnis and Foege, 1993). Yet less than 5% of the approximately $1 trillion spent annually on health care in the United States is devoted to reducing risks posed by these preventable conditions (Centers for Disease Control and Prevention, 1992; Health Care Financing Administration, 2000). Behavioral and social interventions therefore offer great promise to reduce disease morbidity and mortality, but as yet their potential to improve the public's health has been relatively poorly tapped.

Within this context, the Institute of Medicine (IOM) Committee on Capitalizing on Social Science and Behavioral Research to Improve the Public's Health (hereafter referred to as "the committee") was charged to help identify promising areas of social science and behavioral research that may address public health needs. Although this report is not intended as an encyclopedic review

1

of the growing literature on social and behavioral interventions that may improve health, it serves to assess whether this knowledge base has been useful, or could be useful, in the development of broader public health interventions.

To aid the committee, 12 papers were commissioned from some of the nation's leading experts to review these issues in detail (see paper contributions). The first of these papers provides a descriptive overview of the challenges posed in understanding the role of behavioral and social factors in health and the distribution of disease. The second paper considers how social and behavioral factors contribute to socioeconomic and racial/ethnic health disparities. Five papers then discuss what has been learned in behavioral and social research that is of value in improving health at different stages of life. Three papers examine specific "levers" for public health intervention: media and public health marketing; legislation and public policy; and efforts to enhance the social capital of communities. In addition, one paper was commissioned to provide a review of psychosocial and biobehavioral interventions in disease processes, an area of research that offers promise to uncover specific mechanisms linking social and behavioral forces to health. Of necessity, all of these papers deal with one or another particular aspect of the problem. For this reason, one paper was commissioned to consider all of these issues simultaneously in a multilevel, multidisciplinary approach. The case of tobacco control is used to illustrate this type of multifaceted intervention program.

When these papers were completed, the committee invited the authors to attend a symposium held at the Emory Conference Center in Atlanta, Georgia. In addition, 33 discussants were invited to comment on the papers. These discussants were specifically chosen not only because of their expertise in the subject matter, but also because they brought to the discussion a diversity of opinions and experience with intervention efforts. The committee's report reflects a careful consideration of information presented in these papers, as well as in the symposium discussion.

A Social Environmental Approach to Health and Health Interventions

The committee examined a wide range of social and behavioral research that was intended to promote the health and well-being of individuals, their families, and their communities, and found an emerging consensus that research and intervention efforts should be based on an ecological model. This model assumes that differences in levels of health and well-being are affected by a dynamic interaction among biology, behavior, and the environment, an interaction that unfolds over the life course of individuals, families, and communities (Satariano, in press). This model also assumes that age, gender, race, ethnicity, and socioeconomic differences shape the context in which individuals function, and therefore directly and indirectly influence health risks and resources. These demographic factors are critical determinants of health and well-being and should receive careful consideration in the design, implementation, and interpretation of the results of interventions.

This ecological model is best operationalized by a social environmental approach to health and health interventions. This approach places emphasis on how the health of individuals is influenced not only by biological and genetic functioning and predisposition, but also by social and familial relationships, environmental contingencies, and broader social and economic trends. The model also suggests that intervention efforts should address not only "downstream" individual-level phenomena (e.g., physiologic pathways to disease, individual and lifestyle factors) and "mainstream" factors (e.g., population-based interventions), but also "upstream," societal-level phenomena (e.g., public policies).

The latter two sets of health influences, however, have not received the same degree of scientific attention as individual-level phenomena, due in part to their inherent challenges. One challenge posed by population or societal-level research is that it is methodologically complex and requires different methods than individual-level research. As a result, some population-level research has been less conclusive because it is at an earlier stage of scientific development and sophistication. In addition, population-level interventions may raise social, political, and ethical questions regarding attempts to change social conditions, as changes may produce unintended effects. Further, individuals subject to change efforts rarely have an opportunity to offer consent to the intervention.

Evidence is emerging, however, that societal-level phenomena are critical determinants of health, and not just for those at the lower rungs of the socioeconomic hierarchy. Greater scientific attention must be given to the development of upstream interventions, for several reasons. First, many of the risks for disease and poor health functioning are shared by large numbers of people. Stress, insufficient financial and social supports, poor diet, environmental exposures, community factors and characteristics, and many other health risks may be addressed by one-to-one intervention efforts, but such efforts do little to address the broader social and economic forces that influence these risks. Further, one-to-one interventions do little to alter the distribution of disease and injury in populations because new people continue to be afflicted even as sick and injured people are cured. It therefore may be more cost-effective to prevent many diseases and injuries at the community and environmental levels than to address them at the individual level.

Second, a social environmental approach is useful because many population groups have a characteristic pattern of disease and injury over time, even though individuals come and go from these groups. This suggests that there may be something about the group or the broader social and environmental conditions in which they live that either promotes or discourages injury and disease among individuals in these groups. This patterned consistency of disease rates among various social and cultural groups emphasizes the importance of social and other environmental factors in disease etiology. The identification of these factors is important in order to develop intervention programs to prevent or control disease.

Third, there is impressive evidence from previous work in infectious diseases and injury control that an environmental approach can be successful. There is strong evidence (McKeown, 1976; McKinlay and McKinlay, 1977; Fogel, 1994) that the dramatic decline since 1900 in overall mortality in both Britain and the United States cannot be explained by the introduction and use of medical interventions. Indeed, many medical measures against disease (both chemotherapeutic and prophylactic) were introduced several decades after a marked decline in mortality from these diseases already had taken place. In fact, it has been argued that most of the decline in mortality during the second half of the nineteenth century was primarily due to improvements in hygiene and to rising standards of living, especially improved nutrition. Likewise, the marked reduction in motor vehicle crash deaths and injuries that has been achieved over the past 50 years is due largely to improvements in the design of crashworthy automobiles, the construction of safer roadways, and to recent changes in social norms regarding alcohol use and seat-belt use (Institute of Medicine, 1998; Centers for Disease Control and Prevention, 1999).

A fourth reason for an environmental approach to disease prevention and health promotion is that while some behavioral interventions have succeeded in improving health behaviors, many narrow, individually focused models of behavior change have proven insufficient in helping people to change high-risk behavior. The importance of this problem is illustrated by interventions such as the Multiple Risk Factor Intervention Trial. In this study, 6,000 men who were in the top 10%–15% risk group in the nation because of their high rates of cigarette smoking, hypertension, and hypercholesterol levels were enrolled in a 6-year intervention program. They knew ahead of time of their risk status, the behavioral changes they would be required to make, the difficulties they faced, and the time they would need to invest to improve their health. The intervention was well-funded, well-staffed, and used the best behavior change techniques available at the time. The results were disappointing: 62% of these men continued to smoke after 6 years of effort, 50% still had hypertension, and very few men had changed their eating patterns (Multiple Risk Factor Intervention Trial Research Group, 1981, 1982).

To prevent disease, we increasingly ask people to do things that they have not done previously, to stop doing things they have been doing for years, and to do more of some things and less of other things. Although there certainly are examples of successful programs to change behavior, it is clear that behavior change is a difficult and complex challenge. It is unreasonable to expect that people will change their behavior easily when so many forces in the social, cultural, and physical environment conspire against such change. If successful programs are to be developed to prevent disease and improve health, attention must be given not only to the behavior of individuals, but also to the environmental context within which people live.

For all of these reasons, the committee decided to focus attention not only on individual behavior, but also on the social forces that shape and support such behavior. In addition, the committee decided not to organize its work around clinical disease categories such as coronary heart disease, arthritis, or cancer, because most behavioral and social factors transcend particular diseases, and instead influence susceptibility to disease in general. Thus, for example, people in lower social class positions have higher morbidity and mortality rates for diseases involving many body systems, including the digestive, genitourinary, respiratory, circulatory, nervous, blood, and endocrine systems. They also experience higher rates of most malignancies, infectious and parasitic diseases, unintentional injuries, poisoning and violence, perinatal mortality, diabetes, and musculoskeletal impairments. A similarly broad range of diseases has been observed in relation to smoking, poor diet, stress, physical inactivity, inadequate social support, and other psychological and social factors. Not only do people in these high-risk groups have higher rates of diseases, they also are at higher risk for multiple, comorbid conditions (Syme and Balfour, 1998). An exclusive focus on the presence or absence of single disease categories does not provide the best characterization of the health of individuals, and certainly not the best characterization of the health of communities.

Summary of Findings and Recommendations

The recommendations developed by the committee are based on papers presented by the commissioned authors, the views of discussants who reviewed these papers, and the committee's deliberations. These recommendations are organized below in terms of promising intervention strategies, important research gaps, the needed partnerships between researchers and community members, and funding priorities.

The committee's review of the prepared papers and study of the discussants' opinions reinforced the view that assessing the promise of social and behavioral research for improving the public's health is a complex task. There are several reasons for this. First, of course, is the recognition that health, disease, and well-being are complex states that develop and change over the entire life course. No single intervention, or set of interventions, is likely to address the wide range of factors that influence health, disability, and longevity. It is also apparent from the committee's work that the most effective interventions have involved research evidence that transcends the boundaries of a single scientific discipline. Because health is a complex issue and because interventions need to be similarly complex, the science underpinning this work must integrate the work of many disciplines and professions. These include medicine, nursing, psychology, sociology, anthropology, engineering, economics, political science, biology, history, law, and demography, among others.

A review of successful and unsuccessful interventions also reveals that communities must be involved as partners in the design, implementation, and evaluation of interventions. The best intervention results have been achieved when people who benefit from interventions work closely with researchers and public health practitioners. This phenomenon emphasizes the fact that those in the health community have "messages," while individuals in target communities have "lives." A partnership between these two groups offers the best chance to bridge this divide.

Further, it is clear that children should be a major focus of intervention efforts. Many of the risk factors observed in adults can be detected in childhood, such as high blood pressure, overweight, and poor respiratory function. The evidence is that interventions in early life can change the trajectory of these risk factors. A compelling case can be made for focusing attention on ensuring that children get a strong start by providing, for example, appropriate early education, immunization, injury prevention, nutrition, and opportunities for physical activity.

Opportunities for public health intervention do not end at childhood; evidence indicates that intervention efforts with adolescents, adults, and older adults can be successful if these efforts address major developmental tasks at each stage and address major sources of health risk at multiple levels. Adolescents, for example, are heavily influenced by their peers' conduct and attitudes, yet peer group norms can be influenced to improve health behaviors and attitudes, as long as these efforts are supported by consistent and complementary efforts in schools and communities.

The committee's review of all of these materials strongly suggests that interventions need to:

1. focus on generic social and behavioral determinants of disease, injury, and disability;

2. use multiple approaches (e.g., education, social support, laws, incentives, behavior change programs) and address multiple levels of influence simultaneously (i.e., individuals, families, communities, nations);

3. take account of the special needs of target groups (i.e., based on age, gender, race, ethnicity, social class);

4. take the "long view" of health outcomes, as changes often take many years to become established; and

5. involve a variety of sectors in our society that have not traditionally been associated with health promotion efforts, including law, business, education, social services, and the media.

FINDINGS AND RECOMMENDATIONS

Overarching Recommendations

The committee finds that two fundamental issues must be addressed in developing interventions based on social and behavioral research. These include the need to address generic social and behavioral determinants of health, and the need to intervene at multiple sources of health influences (see Box 1).

BOX 1. Overarching Recommendations

Recommendation 1: Social and behavioral factors have a broad and profound impact on health across a wide range of conditions and disabilities. A better balance is needed between the clinical approach to disease, presently the dominant public health model for most risk factors, and research and intervention efforts that address generic social and behavioral determinants of disease, injury, and disability.

Recommendation 2: Rather than focusing interventions on a single or limited number of health determinants, interventions on social and behavioral factors should link multiple levels of influence (i.e., individual, interpersonal, institutional, community, and policy levels).

Addressing Generic Determinants of Health

As noted above, risk behaviors account for approximately half of preventable deaths in the United States. In addition, health care expenditures on chronic and preventable diseases and injury account for nearly 70% of all medical care spending (Fries et al., 1993). These data illustrate the tremendous toll, in both economic and human costs, of poor health behaviors and suggest strongly that initiatives to develop and implement effective interventions to reduce risk behaviors are an important component of efforts to improve the nation's health and to lower health care costs. Further, as illustrated above, risk behaviors are closely linked to social and economic conditions, such as economic inequality, social norms, and other forces (Kaplan, Everson, and Lynch, Paper Contribution A). Interventions are therefore needed to address these generic factors, and to broadly reduce risks across large segments of the population.

As yet, however, this need has not been met. The Robert Wood Johnson Foundation recently conducted an assessment of progress in population-based health promotion in six areas of behavioral risk (tobacco use, sedentary lifestyle, alcohol abuse, drug abuse, unhealthy diet, and sexual risk behavior), and concluded that more progress has been made in developing and implementing individually oriented interventions than in developing and implementing more environmentally focused interventions, even though the latter are necessary for greatest population impact (Orleans et al., 1999). Broad intervention strategies that address generic social and behavioral determinants of health must therefore receive greater attention.

Recommendation 1: Social and behavioral factors have a broad and profound impact on health across a wide range of conditions and disabilities. A better balance is needed between the clinical approach to disease, presently the dominant public health model for most risk factors, and research and intervention efforts that ad-

dress generic social and behavioral determinants of disease, injury, and disability.

Intervention at Multiple Levels

As the preceding discussion illustrates, there is substantial heterogeneity in health outcomes by social factors such as place, race and ethnicity, gender, and socioeconomic position. These findings indicate that it is not realistic to think that one might identify a single set of explanatory determinants, and thereby identify a single focus for interventions. Rather, as is pointed out across the reports in this volume, a multilevel approach to interventions is needed.

The framework for this approach is not new. A social ecological model provides a structure for intervening at multiple levels of influence, including the individual, interpersonal, institutional, community, and policy levels, as articulated in the paper by Emmons (see Paper Contribution F). This model assumes that health outcomes are the result of a dynamic interplay between multiple factors such as individuals' physiological processes; behavioral patterns and personality structures; physical, social, and economic contexts; and larger social processes that broadly influence health risks. However, interventions targeting health behavior change have a tradition of focusing first on individual factors, such as increasing knowledge, motivation, or skills related to health behavior change.

On the other hand, a multilevel approach is not meant to emphasize population- or societal-level interventions to the exclusion of individual-level approaches; rather, there is a need for integration of interventions across levels. By linking interventions, consistent intervention messages, support, and follow-up can be provided over time. Support for a multilevel approach is provided in this volume by Perry, Emmons, and Warner (see Paper Contributions E, F, and K). Perry, for example, observes that the effects of school-based smoking prevention programs are sustained when changes in the larger community are also present and when there is reinforcement of the intervention over time. Maintenance of health behavior change appears to be limited when behaviors promoted by school-based programs are inconsistent with larger community norms, so that healthy behavior change is not supported and reinforced after the program is completed.

Another excellent example of the promise offered by multilevel interventions is tobacco control, reviewed in this volume by Warner (see Paper Contribution K). The case of tobacco control is a major success story for public health. The prevalence of smoking in the United States dropped to 25% in 1997, down from about 45% in 1963, the year prior to the first publication of the Surgeon General's report on smoking and health[*] (U.S. Department of Health, Education,

---

[*]A major exception to this trend has occurred among adolescents, whose use of tobacco increased steadily through the first half of the 1990s before declining slightly in the latter half of the decade. In 1999, over one-third of high school students and one in eight

and Welfare, 1964). Extensive efforts to intervene exclusively at the individual level, using behavioral and pharmacological interventions, have yielded only marginal success. However, Warner, Gostin, and House and Williams (see Paper Contributions K, J, and B) all conclude that major progress in reducing the prevalence of smoking has resulted from population-wide interventions, including economic disincentives (e.g., increases in the cigarette excise tax), and laws and regulations (e.g., clean indoor air laws, minimum age of purchase laws, and regulation of advertising). These interventions are most effective at the population level when applied concurrently with individual-level interventions. The committee finds the evidence compelling that coordinated, multilevel interventions offer the greatest promise to address most public health needs.

Recommendation 2: Rather than focusing interventions on a single or limited number of health determinants, interventions on social and behavioral factors should link multiple levels of influence (i.e., individual, interpersonal, institutional, community, and policy levels).

Promising Intervention Strategies

Defining "Promising Interventions"

The literature on behavioral and social interventions that purport to reduce injury and disease and promote health is large and growing. Perhaps the most significant contribution of behavioral and social sciences to health research is the development of strong theoretical models for interventions. Not all such research, however, has been guided by sound theory. In some cases, empirical findings suggest that interventions may be effective, but without sound theoretical underpinnings, the mechanisms through which interventions operate remain unclear. The committee defines promising interventions as those that have both a theoretical basis for efficacy and empirical evidence supporting at least some parts of the theoretical model. Promising interventions can be identified by studies showing beneficial effects on select populations, accompanied by a theoretical model for supporting expansion of the intervention to other populations. Alternatively, similar promise can be demonstrated by studies that reveal only modest effects of an intervention on wider application, but where a strong theoretical basis is present for expecting improved efficacy by changing the intervention in some way. The committee notes, however, that "promising" is not the same as "proven"—proven interventions would be those already known to be efficacious on wide-scale application. The promising strategies identified by the committee are listed in Box 2.

---

middle school students reported using some form of tobacco in the past month (Centers for Disease Control and Prevention, 2000).

BOX 2. Recommendations for Intervention Strategies

Recommendation 3: Intervention strategies must attend to aspects of the social context that may hinder or promote efforts at behavioral change and health risk reduction. Modifying the social capital of communities and neighborhoods offers promise to enhance social contexts. These interventions should therefore be developed, implemented, and evaluated.

Recommendation 4: Research consistently indicates that life circumstances associated with low socioeconomic status, gender, race, and ethnic disadvantage and other high-risk circumstances are strongly associated with a wide range of poor health outcomes. Policies that take account of and enhance positive health outcomes among subgroups at high risk of poor health outcomes need to be designed and implemented.

Recommendation 5: Improvements in reproductive outcomes will require addressing social and behavioral influences on the health of women well prior to conception, in addition to the perinatal and postnatal periods.

Recommendation 6: High-quality, center-based early education programs should be more widely implemented. Future interventions directed at infants and young children should focus on strengthening other processes affecting child outcomes such as the home environment, school and neighborhood influences, and physical health and growth.

Recommendation 7: Multi-level interventions should address aspects of adolescents' social environment as they affect health outcomes, including peer norms, role models, performance expectations, social and neighborhood supports, and ties to community institutions.

Recommendation 8: Community and work site interventions and evaluations are needed to promote behavioral change, prevent injuries, reduce exposure to occupational risks, and increase healthy environments. Such interventions should include multiple points of leverage, such as individual-level attributes, social supports and social norms, family and neighborhood factors, and environmental and social policies.

Recommendation 9: Interventions to improve the health of older adults should focus on the social, environmental, and behavioral conditions that minimize disability and promote continuing independence and productive activity. Interventions that enhance the social support and self-efficacy of older adults are particularly promising. Community senior centers and community-assisted housing are two examples of interventions that are especially promising for the frail elderly.

Interventions Directed at the Social Context

The preceding discussion of multilevel interventions offers examples of the importance of attending to the social context in which people live and work in the development of health interventions. The social context is comprised of socioeconomic conditions and factors in one's physical, social, and cultural environment that influence access to health information, social support, social networks, social norms, and cultural beliefs and attitudes regarding health. Because these factors directly and indirectly influence health and health risks, interventions must address the social context as a critical element of intervention design. For example, Syme's (1978) study of people with hypertension illustrates that addressing underlying social and economic conditions appears to enhance the management of hypertension and improve the effectiveness of antihypertensive therapy. In a randomized controlled study, blood pressure was most likely to be controlled among patients receiving visits from community health workers who not only provided information about hypertension, but also discussed family difficulties, financial strain, employment opportunities, and, when appropriate, provided support and assistance.

Beyond adapting to differences in social contexts, interventions must also directly influence attributes of the social context that promote health. Sampson and Morenoff and Wallack (see Paper Contributions I and H) discuss one attribute of social contexts—social capital—that holds promise for improving population health. Social capital is defined as a characteristic of communities stemming from the structure of social relationships that facilitates the achievement of individuals' shared goals. This includes the quality of social networks, as well as the by-products of these networks—such as shared norms and mutual trust—that facilitate cooperation. Social capital is therefore an attribute of social structures (e.g., organizations, communities, neighborhoods, extended families) rather than individuals.

The importance of social capital is best illustrated by research that demonstrates an association between neighborhood cohesiveness, stability, and measures of mutual "trust" and a range of public health outcomes, including the health and mental health status of community residents and levels of crime and violence. Communities characterized by high poverty, low residential stability, and a high percentage of single-parent households often possess low levels of social capital, and are linked to poor individual health outcomes such as coronary risk factors and heart disease mortality, low birthweight, smoking, and other negative outcomes, even when individual attributes and behaviors are taken into account. Analyses of the Alameda County Health Study reveal, for example, that self-reported fair/poor health was 70% higher for residents of concentrated poverty areas than for residents of nonpoverty areas, independent of age, sex, income, education, smoking status, body mass index, and alcohol consumption (Sampson and Morenoff, Paper Contribution I). In addition, Kawachi (1999) has found that measures of distrust correlate strongly with age-adjusted mortality at the state level, even while controlling for individual risk factors.

Further, experimental and quasi-experimental studies lend strength to the hypothesis that improvements in community socioeconomic environments lead to better individual health and behavioral outcomes. Sampson and Morenoff (see Paper Contribution I), for example, cite a study of housing project residents in Boston indicating that children of mothers randomly assigned to an experimental group that received housing subsidies allowing them to move into low-poverty neighborhoods had a significantly lower prevalence of injuries, asthma attacks, and personal victimization than children of mothers who received no special housing assistance or conventional housing assistance. Because the experimental design of this study controlled for individual-level risk factors, the study lends support to the view that changes in community socioeconomic conditions can lead to improvements in individual health.

Questions remain as to why these associations persist. Sampson and Morenoff suggest that benefits stem from social processes involved in collective aspects of neighborhood life, such as information exchange, reciprocal assistance, voluntary associations, and parental support. Perhaps more importantly, the collective efficacy of communities—that is, the trust shared among residents and willingness to intervene in support of public order—reflects the potential of communities to mobilize to improve community conditions. Sampson and his colleagues have found a strong association between collective efficacy and rates of neighborhood violence, controlling for concentrations of poverty, residential stability, and other individual-level characteristics (Sampson and Morenoff, Paper Contribution I).

Wallack (see Paper Contribution H) suggests that a "lever" to enhance social capital is presented by media and marketing strategies. He notes that traditional behaviorally oriented media campaigns, while useful, have been of limited effectiveness in creating and sustaining significant behavior change. Media campaigns have the potential, he argues, to address more fundamental aspects of the social context in which health behaviors occur, most significantly by enhancing involvement in civic life and encouraging social justice, participation, and social change. While experimental evidence for this approach is scant, Wallack discusses findings from three areas of research—civic journalism, media advocacy, and photo voice—that encourage community mobilization to advance public policies that promote health. Civic journalism involves efforts by the media to engage the community in civic life by providing information and other support to increase community debate and public participation in problem-solving. Media advocacy is commonly used in combination with community organizing to advocate and draw attention to the need for improvements in public policies. Photo voice is a tool used by community members to enhance awareness of social and economic conditions in their communities that are detrimental to health. Rigorous evaluation and refinement of these strategies is very much needed.

Recommendation 3: Intervention strategies must attend to aspects of the social context that may hinder or promote efforts at behavioral change and health risk reduction. Modifying the social capital of communities and neighborhoods offers promise to enhance social contexts. These interventions should therefore be developed, implemented, and evaluated.

Understanding and Reducing Socioeconomic, Racial/Ethnic, and Gender Disparities in Health

The preceding discussion consistently notes that important health disparities exist among population groups. In particular, socioeconomic disparities in health are large, persistent, and increasing (House and Williams, Paper Contribution B). Racial and ethnic disparities are generally consistent, in that African Americans, Hispanics, and Native Americans face higher rates of age-adjusted morbidity and mortality from a number of diseases associated with behavioral and social factors. A number of important exceptions to this pattern exist; many foreign-born Hispanics and individuals of African descent enjoy better birth outcomes than American-born Hispanics and African Americans (House and Williams, Paper Contribution B). The implications of these exceptions are discussed below (see "Research Needs"). In addition, while women in the United States live 7 years longer on average than men, these additional life-years are characterized by greater levels of impairment in functional status and morbidity (Rogers et al., 1989).

As House and Williams illustrate (see Paper Contribution B), understanding these disparities requires further research and intervention into psychosocial and physiologic pathways that translate disparities into poor health, and into the broader social, cultural, economic, and political processes that determine the nature and extent of disparities. Socioeconomic status, for example, is commonly thought to exert its effects on health through discrete risk factors such as individuals' coping skills, health knowledge, health behaviors, and access to health-enhancing resources. House and Williams present compelling evidence, however, that disadvantaged socioeconomic status exerts its effects by shaping the experience of and exposure to virtually all known behavioral, psychosocial, and environmental risk factors for health. Thus, the effects of socioeconomic status on health are multiply determined, exerting its effects across all of the developmental stages, social contexts, and community attributes discussed above.

Further, House and Williams note that while racial and ethnic disparities in health are to a great extent the result of socioeconomic disparities among these groups, minority racial and ethnic status are associated with adverse health outcomes beyond those explainable by socioeconomic differences. This disparity is best illustrated by data indicating that for most causes of death and disability, ethnic minorities suffer from poorer outcomes relative to whites, even at equivalent education and income levels. House and Williams note that these disparities may result from racism and discrimination, including racism inherent in the health care system, and the ways in which racism and discrimination restrict socioeconomic and housing opportunities and elevate stress among their victims. The authors note further that because of the pervasive and insidious fashion in which low socioeconomic status, racism, and discrimination shape virtually all risks for poor health and poor health outcomes, interventions to improve access to medical care and reduce behavioral or psychosocial risks have only limited potential to reduce health disparities among these groups. Rather, they argue, broader efforts to reduce socioeconomic and racial/ethnic disadvantage remain the single most powerful tool for alleviating health disparities. House and Williams cite evidence that socioeconomic change and policies that improve the status and life circumstances of socioeconomically and racially/ethnically disadvantaged populations have the most significant effects on reducing health disparities. For example, they cite research indicating that policies adopted at the height of the civil rights movement successfully removed barriers to occupational and educational integration. As a result, the socioeconomic status of blacks relative to whites improved, and concurrently, between 1968 and 1978 blacks experienced a larger decline in mortality rates (on both a percentage and an absolute basis) than whites.

Although basic biological differences by sex clearly influence health outcomes, potent health consequences emerge from the social construction of gender. Gender differences in health spring from many aspects of the social context, including differences in economic, political, and social power (Sorensen, 2000). Research is needed to better understand factors that contribute to gender inequalities in health, including stress related to gender roles, the types of jobs men and women hold, the amounts of money they are paid, and the patterning of household responsibilities. For example, men earn more than women, despite women's higher educational levels relative to men in similar occupations. While gender roles may be associated with poor health effects for both men and women, women continue to carry primary responsibility for household duties, in addition to work-related demands. Women's socioeconomic disadvantages and their irregular career trajectories, generally related to family responsibilities, limit the availability of pensions and savings in later life. Given that employed women may be balancing job roles and family responsibilities, it is not surprising that most studies find that employed women experience more stress and distress relative to employed men (Williams and Umberson, 2000). And as noted by Korenbrot and Moss (see paper contributions), social constructions of gender roles shape the views and experiences women have of sex, contraception, and pregnancy, as well as their health behaviors and interactions with the health care system. These structural factors may also have long-term and often unforeseen consequences. For example, Kaplan (see paper contributions) points out that economic policies that alter work force participation by women may depress and delay reproduction, thereby increasing the risk of breast cancer.

It is critical to address socioeconomic, racial/ethnic, and gender disadvantages, not only to improve the health of individuals in disadvantaged groups, but also because the greatest opportunity for improvement of the nation's health as a whole lies in improving the health of these groups.

Recommendation 4: Research consistently indicates that life circumstances associated with low socioeconomic status, gender, race and ethnic disadvantage, and other high-risk circumstances are strongly associated with a wide range of poor health outcomes. Policies that take account of and enhance positive health outcomes

among subgroups at high risk of poor health outcomes need to be designed and implemented.

Opportunities for Intervention Across the Life Span

Preconception, Prenatal, and Postnatal Influences on Health. An implicit yet often unstated assumption in public health is that early intervention programs offer promise for improving health, with the potential benefit of reducing long-term costs to individuals, communities, and the larger society. Perhaps the most significant of such efforts are interventions to improve the health of very young children, starting at birth. Poor birth outcomes (e.g., low birthweight) are related to a range of poor cognitive and physical health indicators as infants grow and develop (Korenbrot and Moss, see Paper Contribution C). Substantial public health resources have therefore been devoted to improving birth outcomes, ranging from improved prenatal care, to health education and outreach, nutrition and psychosocial services, and other efforts. Some successes have been achieved; infant mortality, for example, has declined dramatically, due in large part to improvements in medical technologies that improve survival among preterm and low-birthweight infants.

Korenbrot and Moss (see Paper Contribution C), however, note that little progress has been made in improving other birth outcomes, despite major policy and program efforts. Improvements in the use of and access to prenatal care generally have not resulted in reductions in low birthweight and other poor birth outcomes, although prenatal and perinatal medical interventions may reduce morbidity substantially in those born with complications. In particular, racial/ethnic and socioeconomic disparities have not been reduced, suggesting strongly that overall rates of poor birth outcomes are less related to reductions in risk behaviors (e.g., smoking, adolescent childbearing) or improvements in prenatal health care in individuals, and are more likely the direct consequence of disparities between socioeconomic and racial/ethnic groups.

Factors that mediate this relationship are poorly understood. For example, African-American women are more likely to have low-birthweight infants than white women at all levels of educational attainment, suggesting that factors other than socioeconomic status influence pregnancy outcomes (Kaplan, Everson, and Lynch, Paper Contribution A). Another highly suggestive piece of evidence is that in mixed-race couples, the risk of adverse pregnancy outcomes is increased when the woman is African American but not the man (Collins and David, 1993). Other evidence suggests that early influences on women's health may play an important role. This evidence includes the fact that women who were born at lower birthweights are more likely to have low-birthweight infants (Korenbrot and Moss, Paper Contribution C). Thus, interventions to enhance reproductive outcomes must begin well prior to conception, and must attend to social and economic conditions that confer and moderate risk. This broader focus on women's health would also reinforce the importance of implementing interventions during pregnancy to enhance the health of the woman, as well as that of the fetus. Finally, to ensure that women are able to undertake their roles as parents and to prepare for subsequent children, increased attention is needed to postnatal health and health habits of new mothers.

> **Recommendation 5: Improvements in reproductive outcomes will require addressing social and behavioral influences on the health of women well prior to conception, in addition to the perinatal and postnatal periods.**

Infancy and Early Childhood. Fuligni and Brooks-Gunn (see Paper Contribution D) discuss social and behavioral influences on the healthy development of young children, noting that various domains that can be considered to define school readiness, including cognitive, emotional, and physical health outcomes, are closely correlated and should be considered simultaneously in intervention efforts. As with birth outcomes, socioeconomic status remains a key predictor of school readiness. Low socioeconomic status is associated with low cognitive test scores, behavioral problems, and a range of physical health indicators including growth stunting, low rates of childhood immunizations, high blood-lead levels, and other health outcomes. Fuligni and Brooks-Gunn explore possible pathways by which socioeconomic indicators, such as parental education and income, operate to affect young children's development, and suggest that family processes (including parental emotional and physical health, parental childrearing styles, and the quality of educational experiences in the home), the quality of child care (e.g., as reflected in home-based versus center-based care), and neighborhood influences (e.g., racial and economic segregation, inadequate social support, hazardous and unsafe living conditions, and limited access to resources such as high-quality schools) underlie these disparities.

These multiple sources of influence on young children's development suggest a number of targets for intervention, including those directed at children and their caregivers, family-level interventions, social supports, and broader social and economic policies that influence neighborhood characteristics. Research data on the effectiveness of these interventions, however, are mixed, and much of the research has focused on the cognitive and social-emotional development needed for school readiness. Comprehensive, high-quality, center-based early education for infants and children has been demonstrated to improve a range of child educational outcomes. These effects may extend to reduce socioeconomic disadvantage. The implementation and evaluation of future programs should focus on planned variations in elements and intensity of such approaches to identify the most appropriate and least costly interventions for specific communities.

Although the efficacy of center-based programs is well established, home visitation programs, larger-scale school-based programs, and family support programs have not consistently produced positive outcomes. Other interventions, such as comprehensive community initiatives, attempt to address neighborhood characteristics that influence child outcomes by promoting antipoverty programs and enhancing community-building strategies. Few of these interventions, however, have focused directly on improving child developmental outcomes, and little evidence supports the effectiveness of these approaches. However, the strong theoretical and empirical evidence linking family, neighborhood, and child care processes to child outcomes would suggest that these approaches can be strengthened to be more consistently effective.

> **Recommendation 6: High-quality, center-based early education programs should be more widely implemented. Future interventions directed at infants and young children should focus on strengthening other processes affecting child outcomes such as the home environment, school and neighborhood influences, and physical health and growth.**

Adolescence. Adolescence, as noted by Perry (see Paper Contribution E), is a time of significant developmental transition influenced by dynamic interactions between social forces and important biological changes. These forces interact to influence health outcomes for adolescents, but perhaps most significantly, they set the stage for later adult educational, vocational, and health outcomes.

Perry notes that while adolescence is generally the period of greatest health for most individuals—having outgrown the risks for childhood infectious diseases but not having reached the age of risk for chronic diseases more common to adults—it is also a period of risk for poor health. Because young adolescents typically have not fully developed abstract cognitive abilities, cannot judge the implications of their behavior for future consequences, and are particularly vulnerable to peer influences, they are susceptible to influences in the social environment that encourage risk behaviors such as smoking, violence, alcohol and drug use, and risky sexual behavior. For this reason, health messages directed to adolescents that focus on long-term consequences of behavior or that fail to provide concrete examples of health risks often fail to achieve desired results.

Because many health risks to adolescents are socially determined, research indicates that characteristics of the social environment can also serve to confer protective or health-enhancing effects. As Perry notes, the way in which the environment "fits" the needs of adolescents is a critical determinant of adolescent health behavior. Social contexts that provide positive social norms, offer appropriate role models, set appropriate expectations, provide useful information, and provide social and neighborhood supports are strongly associated with positive health outcomes for adolescents. Perry and her colleagues, for example, have found that community norms and role models accounted for nearly half of the variance in eighth grade children's alcohol use. Further, these attributes may mediate the relationship between poverty and adolescent health outcomes. Other health influences include media exposure (e.g., high exposure to violent television content is associated with subsequent aggressive behavior among adolescents), "family capital" (e.g., parents' own educational attainment, parent–child activities and time spent together), and connectedness to school.

These findings illustrate that intervention efforts must focus on adolescents' social environment, and address multiple sources of influence in these environments. In addition, these efforts are most effective when applied early (e.g., in primary school years) and sustained through adolescence. Perry presents data demonstrating that longitudinal, multicomponent interventions, such as the Seattle School Development Project, can reduce adolescent involvement in risk behaviors (e.g., violence, risky sexual behavior, heavy alcohol use). This intervention, which consisted of annual in-service teacher training, social competence training for students, and parent training classes, demonstrated long-term positive effects at age 18 for students who were exposed to the intervention in first through sixth grades.

Recommendation 7: Multilevel interventions should address aspects of adolescents' social environment as they affect health outcomes, including peer norms, role models, performance expectations, social and neighborhood supports, and ties to community institutions.

Adults. As noted earlier, behavioral and environmental factors contribute significantly to most major causes of adult physical and mental disorders and mortality. These factors are largely modifiable, and include those health risks due primarily to individual behavior (e.g., physical inactivity, smoking, diet, alcohol and drug use), to environmental or organizational-level exposures (e.g., occupational exposures and work practices, motor vehicle and other product design), and to social class (see discussion below).

As noted by Emmons (see Paper Contribution F), intervention strategies have typically focused on individuals, often addressing the needs of highly motivated volunteers. Individually based interventions may be effective for individual participants, particularly those at high risk, but may also miss important segments of the population who are not interested in participating in intensive programs. The potential population-wide impact of programs targeting individuals is further limited because these efforts often fail to consider the social and environmental attributes that support poor individual health behaviors. The population effects of interventions to improve the health of adults can be enhanced when interventions address multiple levels of influence, including individual factors (e.g., health knowledge and attitudes, motivation for behavior change), interpersonal processes (e.g., social support, social norms), institutional or organizational factors (e.g., workplace policies), community factors (e.g., neighborhood characteristics associated with poor health outcomes), and public policy (e.g., regulations and laws directed at reducing health risks). In addition, it is important that interventions be linked across multiple locations, such as work sites or communities, in order to provide consistent messages, support, and follow-up in support of healthful changes.

Again, the example of tobacco control provides evidence for the efficacy of a multilevel approach (Warner, Paper Contribution K). Individual-level behaviorally or pharmaceutically based approaches are most effective when linked with interventions that address social contextual factors that support or discourage tobacco use. These include community- and work site-based tobacco reduction programs that influence social norms and other social contingencies, and broader societal interventions, such as laws and regulations that limit access to tobacco products. Social supports and social networks can also serve to reinforce prevention and smoking cessation messages.

> **Recommendation 8: Community and work site interventions and evaluations are needed to promote behavioral change, prevent injuries, reduce exposure to occupational risks, and increase healthy environments. Such interventions should include multiple points of leverage, such as individual-level attributes, social supports and social norms, family and neighborhood factors, and environmental and social policies.**

Older Adults. Social and behavioral research increasingly demonstrates that the effectiveness of interventions does not decline with older adults; rather, social and behavioral interventions offer promise to reduce functional disability and mortality among older adults. As Maddox illustrates (Paper Contribution G), while risk for chronic diseases and physical and cognitive impairment increases with age, behavioral and social factors predict substantial differences in morbidity and mortality among older adults. Further, behavioral and social interventions can modify trajectories of functional disability and the experience of aging in ways that reduce the high costs of health and social services and promote "healthy aging."

Maddox's review of successful psychosocial interventions for older adults indicates that these interventions can improve the management of chronic conditions (e.g., osteoporosis and diabetes), and can reduce excessive dependence on the part of frail nursing home residents. Common elements of these interventions are that they enhance social supports and social network integration for health and well-being, and enhance the self-efficacy of older individuals, which is an important predictor of successful intervention outcomes. For example, an intervention to reduce excessive behavioral dependence among older adults in nursing home settings revealed that both patients and caregivers could be trained to change behavioral patterns to promote a greater sense of autonomy and self-efficacy among patients. Moreover, Maddox presents theoretical evidence that an intervention focused on addressing the structural environment of frail older adults—assisted living housing—can increase social support resources and personal choice and control among residents. Assisted living housing allows residents to purchase housing and services appropriate to their assessed needs, but encourages shared responsibility among caretakers, family, and residents, and seeks to promote maximum autonomy and participation in decisions about the community.

Recommendation 9: Interventions to improve the health of older adults should focus on the social, environmental, and behavioral conditions that minimize disability and promote continuing independence and productive activity. Interventions that enhance the social support and self-efficacy of older adults are particularly promising. Community senior centers and community-assisted housing are two examples of interventions that are especially promising for the frail elderly.

Research Needs

The committee's review of opportunities for intervention at specific developmental stages and "levers" for public health intervention yielded a great deal of information regarding promising intervention strategies. Significantly, however, this review also prompts several findings and recommendations regarding future research needs. These recommendations are summarized in Box 3.

Research on Physiologic Pathways

As noted above, there are multiple pathways through which psychosocial factors affect health outcomes; these influences occur indirectly, through behaviors such as alcohol and tobacco use, and directly, through alterations in the functioning of the cardiovascular, endocrine, and immune systems. However, relatively few of the interventions referenced above include physiological measures. Research that addresses biobehavioral mechanisms is therefore needed to understand pathways through which psychosocial factors affect disease processes (Baum, Paper Contribution L).

Evidence of the relationship between psychosocial and behavioral factors and health is large and growing. Research demonstrates that risk factors such as chronic psychological stress can lead to exacerbation of coronary artery atherosclerosis, likely via a mechanism involving excessive sympathetic nervous system activation. Furthermore, acute stress can serve as a trigger for myocardial ischemia, promote arrhythmogenesis, stimulate platelet function, and increase blood viscosity; among patients with underlying atherosclerosis, acute stress also enhances coronary vasoconstriction (Rozanski et al., 1999). The endocrine system serves as one important gateway across a spectrum of diseases because stressors can provoke the release of pituitary and adrenal hormones that have multiple effects, including alterations in cardiovascular and immune function. For example, social stressors can substantially elevate key stress hormones including the catecholamines and cortisol, and these hormones have multiple effects (e.g., chronic stimulation of cortisol and catecholamine secretion at lower levels has been linked to cardiovascular pathology).

Psychosocial factors such as depression can intensify a variety of health threats. Some of the strongest evidence comes from the cardiovascular realm, with convergent data from a number of well-controlled prospective studies: depressive

---

BOX 3. Recommendations for Research

Recommendation 10: Understanding psychosocial and biobehavioral mechanisms that influence health is critical to better understand and tailor intervention efforts. Research in this area should be encouraged.

Recommendation 11: A substantial new research effort is needed to understand the pathways through which behavioral and social factors affect pregnancy outcomes, and to address the issues of women's health across the life span and across generations.

Recommendation 12: Research on early childhood interventions needs to be extended to provide information useful to tailoring such interventions to ensure the least costly, most effective strategies for a variety of populations. Both the theory and the research must be expanded and integrated to include a full array of child outcomes (e.g., physical health as well as social, cognitive, and emotional outcomes) and the effect of interventions on these outcomes.

Recommendation 13: Research should identify sources of health strengths and resilience, as well as health risks, among individuals, families, and communities of low socioeconomic status and racial and ethnic minority groups.

Recommendation 14: Research is needed to identify pathways through which social contexts directly and indirectly affect disease pathogenesis and outcomes.

Recommendation 15: Legal and regulatory interventions represent a powerful tool for promoting public health. However, evaluations are needed to ensure that these interventions achieve their intended effects without imposing undue burdens on individuals or society.

Recommendation 16: Expansions of research methodologies are needed to address a broad range of research questions, to ensure that methods are appropriate to the research questions being asked, and to respond to the complexities of multilevel interventions. This includes the need to integrate both qualitative and quantitative research.

Recommendation 17: Cost-effectiveness analyses are necessary to assess the public health utility of interventions. Assessments are needed of the incremental effects of each component of multilevel, comprehensive interventions, and of the incremental effects of interventions over time. Such analyses should consider the broad influence and costs of interventions to target individuals, their families, and the broader social systems in which they operate.

Recommendation 18: Efforts to develop the next generation of prevention interventions must focus on building relationships with communities, and develop interventions that derive from the communities' assessments of their needs and priorities. Models should be developed that encourage members of the community and researchers to work together to design, train for, and conduct such programs.

symptoms were associated with the development of ischemic disease, as well as poorer outcome among patients who had preexisting cardiovascular disease (Glassman and Shapiro, 1998). In addition to cardiovascular risks, depressive symptoms have been linked with higher morbidity and mortality in a number of other arenas, such as cancer risk in older persons (Penninx et al., 1998), all-cause mortality in medical inpatients (Herrmann et al., 1998), risk for osteoporosis (Michelson et al., 1996), and lessened physical, social, and role function, worse perceived current health, and greater bodily pain (Wells et al., 1989).

Evidence indicates that many social and behavioral interventions have biological consequences, rather than acting primarily indirectly through such channels as health behaviors. For example, stress management-oriented interventions clearly alter a number of aspects of cardiovascular, immune, and endocrine function; some smaller studies provide encouraging results for the alteration of disease progression as well, particularly in the cardiovascular realm. Social and behavioral interventions may enhance health because they decrease psychological stress, improve mental health, alter chronic life strains, improve health behaviors, and/or enhance social support or social connectedness; indeed, the most successful interventions have positive benefits across this spectrum, rather than within any single sphere.

Within the past two decades, ample evidence has accumulated that documents diverse psychosocial influences on morbidity and mortality. Interventions that modify psychosocial risks should also alter physiology, and a better understanding of these pathways will aid in the design of more effective interventions.

Recommendation 10: Understanding psychosocial and biobehavioral mechanisms that influence health is critical to better understand and tailor intervention efforts. Research in this area should be encouraged.

Research on Pregnancy

Abundant and continuing evidence exists for socioeconomic and racial/ethnic gradients in perinatal outcomes as measured by birthweight and gestational age, yet research is still a long way from illuminating how these gradients emerge (Kaplan, Everson, and Lynch; Korenbrot and Moss, Paper Contributions A and C). Moreover, evidence is accumulating that documents intergenerational risks (e.g., women who were themselves of low birthweight as infants are more likely to give birth to low-birthweight infants). Current knowledge of the complications of pregnancy, however, does not offer immediate opportunities to alter pregnancy outcomes; new approaches are needed. Korenbrot and Moss postulate that one potential mechanism increasing the risk of poor pregnancy outcomes might be stress-inducing characteristics of disadvantageous environments. Adaptation to such stress is affected by other factors such as the process of cultural adaptation and social support. While some evidence links stress and poor pregnancy outcomes, knowledge of the pathways by which this effect occurs is very incomplete. For example, self-medication to deal with stress might include smoking or alcohol use, which in turn results in lower birthweights or congenital malformations. Research on pathways must also elucidate linkages between social and psychological variables and some of the well-established biological antecedents of poor pregnancy outcomes, such as bacterial vaginosis and pregnancy-induced hypertension. Moreover, elucidation of the pathways to poor pregnancy outcomes should include consideration of gender-based issues in reproduction and family roles (as noted earlier), and should address intergenerational risks.

> **Recommendation 11: A substantial new research effort is needed to understand the pathways through which behavioral and social factors affect pregnancy outcomes, and to address the issues of women's health across the life span and across generations.**

Research on Interventions in Infancy and Early Childhood

A strong body of evidence supports the effects of family, neighborhood, and child care processes on child cognitive and social-emotional development, and has led to effective interventions (Fuligni and Brooks-Gunn, Paper Contribution D). However, as noted above, many of the most successful center-based interventions are single-site, relatively small programs conducted in populations homogeneous for socioeconomic status or race. Many questions remain about extending these approaches to more heterogeneous groups, taking the programs to a larger scale, and comparing curricula and the intensity of participation. For example, to what extent do such programs enhance child outcomes among children of middle- and upper-income families? In addition, more research is required to identify the successful elements of other modalities such as home-visiting or family support programs when center-based interventions may not be appropriate. Finally, we are just beginning to learn about strategies at the neighborhood level to enhance collective efficacy, and the effect of these strategies on child development must be assessed.

However, a larger issue looms. The most well established body of evidence deals with child cognitive and social-emotional development. As Fuligni and Brooks-Gunn note, these are but two of the components of complete child development. The evidence about socioeconomic and racial/ethnic gradients in physical health and growth, the processes leading to such gradients, and the impact of serious child health problems on child development is much less systematically developed, although certainly some literature exists. Information on child health outcomes needs to be expanded and integrated with that for cognitive and social-emotional development to provide a more complete picture of effects of early childhood interventions. We must also understand the effect of interventions proposed to enhance cognitive and social-emotional development on the physical health and growth of children and on their parents. For example, the cognitive, social, and emotional benefits of center-based early childhood interventions may involve a trade-off between increased risk of infectious disease for the child and increased time lost from work for the parent.

Recommendation 12: Research on early childhood interventions needs to be extended to provide information useful to tailoring such interventions to ensure the least costly, most effective strategies for a variety of populations. Both the theory and the research must be expanded and integrated to include a full array of child outcomes (e.g., physical health as well as social, cognitive, and emotional outcomes) and the effect of interventions on these outcomes.

Research on Health Resources and Strengths of Low Socioeconomic and Ethnic Minority Groups

As noted in the discussion of racial and ethnic health disparities, in some cases ethnic minorities experience *lower* rates of illness and mortality than whites. For example, foreign-born mothers of African and Hispanic descent experience generally better birth outcomes than American-born black and Hispanic women. In addition, lower rates of some psychiatric problems are found among African Americans, despite their relatively greater risk for poorer health outcomes. This suggests that cultural attributes protect against negative social and economic conditions, and should be studied to identify new intervention methods. Further, despite evidence that societal-level interventions are needed to assist communities in solving many of the problems that label them as "disadvantaged," there remains a subset of children and families that succeed in these environments. Efforts should be expended to find out what qualities exist in these children and families that can be developed in others who share the same risk status.

Recommendation 13: Research should identify sources of health strengths and resilience, as well as health risks, among individuals, families, and communities of low socioeconomic status and racial and ethnic minority groups.

Research on Social Contexts and Social Capital

Research is needed to identify ways in which social context influences health behaviors, environmental exposures, psychosocial responses, and health outcomes and mediates the influence of interventions. Fuligni and Brooks-Gunn provide an important example in their discussion of the need to specify processes through which neighborhoods influence children's outcomes. Neighborhoods may include a variety of resources, such as availability of and access to quality schools or day care; relationships, such as social support networks available to parents; and norms or collective efficacy, such as the presence of physical risk to residents. The effects of these are likely to be both direct and indirect. Research that helps to elucidate these causal pathways may provide other important points for interventions.

> **Recommendation 14: Research is needed to identify pathways through which social contexts directly and indirectly affect disease pathogenesis and outcomes.**

Research on Legal and Regulatory Interventions

Governments frequently enact laws and regulations to promote public health by discouraging unhealthy behavior (e.g., indoor smoking ordinances, outlawing nonprescription use of mood-altering drugs), encouraging and mandating healthy behavior (e.g., childhood immunizations, mandatory use of safety belts), and encouraging and mandating companies to produce safe products and protect the environment. In addition to direct community appeals through public education, governments can influence individual choices through taxing and spending powers, and can penalize harmful activities through the imposition of civil and criminal penalties. Within the constitutional limits on free speech, governments regulate advertising and product labeling to ensure that the public receives accurate information about food, drugs, and other products. Finally, governments enact consumer product safety regulations, occupational health and safety laws, environmental ordinances, and building codes to reduce the likelihood of harm from hazardous products or environments (Gostin, Paper Contribution J).

Despite the magnitude and scope of government efforts to promote health, the effectiveness of legal and regulatory strategies is poorly understood, with a few exceptions such as motor vehicle safety. Few initiatives have been subjected to rigorous evaluation. In light of the cost of these interventions, and the legal and moral implications of using government power to influence individual behavior, the effects and public acceptance of interventions of this type should be studied.

The best evaluations of legal and regulatory interventions, however, provide compelling evidence that such strategies can have a profound impact on the incidence of injury and disease. For example, the decline in heart disease deaths that has occurred over the past 40 years can be attributed, at least in part, to significant reductions in the rate of cigarette smoking. This was due in no small part to the Surgeon General's report on smoking (U.S. Department of Health, Education, and Welfare, 1964) and subsequent government efforts to bring the health risks of smoking to the attention of the public (Gostin, Paper Contribution J). In addition, the rate of motor vehicle crash deaths per million miles driven has decreased dramatically since 1950. This is not due to greater skill on the part of American drivers, but rather to government-mandated improvements in the crashworthiness of automobiles, mandatory use of safety belts, and improvements in road design (Centers for Disease Control and Prevention, 1999). Further, laws that require parents to produce proof that their children have been vaccinated against measles, rubella, and diphtheria before they can be enrolled in school have dramatically increased rates of childhood immunization (Briss et al., 2000). This has resulted, in turn, in a marked reduction in morbidity and mortality from these communicable diseases.

Clearly, the force of law can be a powerful tool for public health. However, the anticipated benefits of using legal and regulatory strategies to promote public health must be balanced against the costs, including the loss of personal freedom and the potential for unintended consequences. When the benefits of the intervention are great and widely appreciated (e.g., fluoridation of water) and the burden of the intervention is slight, legal and regulatory interventions generally enjoy widespread support. When an intervention is perceived as producing limited benefit, or is viewed as unnecessarily burdensome by a substantial segment of the population, it is likely to be much more controversial. In general, individuals are much more willing to support laws that protect them from the actions of others and from involuntary exposure than from risks voluntarily assumed.

Enactment of public health laws and regulations involves political calculus and trade-offs between various interest groups. Since society devotes substantial resources to regulation, policymakers need high-quality evaluation data to determine which strategies work and which do not. They also need accurate and objective data on the cost and potential consequences of various policies. Policy cannot be entirely divorced from the political environment in which it is made, but it is essential that those involved in the process of government have access to objective information.

> **Recommendation 15: Legal and regulatory interventions represent a powerful tool for promoting public health. However, evaluations are needed to ensure that these interventions achieve their intended effects without imposing undue burdens on individuals or society.**

Research Methodologies

Because multilevel intervention approaches are a relatively new area of inquiry, a range of research questions must be addressed. Research is needed that will contribute to our understanding of how best to create linkages between levels of influence, and how to sequence or coordinate interventions across levels. While there are empirical examples of successful multilevel interventions and theoretical reasons to expect that multilevel interventions will be more successful than single-level interventions, research is also needed on the incremental cost-effectiveness of intervening on additional levels in order to establish the most efficient intervention methods (see discussion below).

Interpretation of the results of population-wide interventions should be based on different criteria from those used for trials targeting high-risk individuals. As Emmons (Paper Contribution F) points out, community intervention trials are likely to observe smaller changes in individual health behaviors than are clinic-based interventions with motivated volunteers. Indeed, the work of Geoffrey Rose (1992) provides a clear rationale for the expectation that small changes at the population level can lead to large effects on disease risk. Rose argues that when risks are widely distributed in the population, small changes in the behavior of many individuals in the population are likely to have a greater impact on risk reduction than large changes among a smaller group of high-risk individuals. Interpretation of the impact of community-based interventions must therefore be judged as a function of the intervention's efficacy in terms of producing community-level changes, as well as its reach, or penetration within the population.

Interpretation of the effects of population-wide interventions must also address problems inherent in establishing causality and time effects. Many studies of population-wide interventions are cross-sectional, and may therefore miss intervention effects that occur beyond the evaluation time frame, or may overestimate intervention effects by capitalizing on population changes not due to the intervention. As noted above, interpretation of findings must be guided by sound theory to anticipate the magnitude and timing of intervention effects. It is important to have explicit models of change and to predict in advance when results should be observed. Also, because multilevel interventions require assessments at multiple levels of influence and change—for individuals, organizations, and communities—methods for measuring change across time in these various settings are needed. In addition, it is important to identify methods for assessing factors mediating change at these multiple levels, in order to understand the pathways through which change occurs.

Finally, it is clear from the above discussion that it is necessary to study the social and cultural context in which behaviors occur. The qualitative research paradigm allows for such a detailed inquiry of the social context. In addition, it allows for the identification of various segments in a community, including hard-to-reach populations, and the impact of changes in the social context on individual behaviors. Qualitative data collection includes participant observation, open-ended questions, in-depth interviewing, and focus groups. Participant observation allows investigators to observe behaviors in the natural setting. By linking observational data to information from in-depth interviews, researchers can triangulate information on what people do versus what they say they do. In addition, the dialogue among participants in focus groups allows for a rapid assessment of themes. The triangulation of qualitative data sources complements the information provided by quantitative data.

Further, qualitative interviewing often allows greater access to information regarding sensitive behaviors (e.g., health risk behaviors or illegal activities), and allows for a better understanding of the meaning of specific behaviors. Qualitative research can therefore illuminate why individuals engage in risk behaviors, despite their knowledge of risks and an intent to change their behavior. Also implicit in qualitative research is the recognition that local circumstances vary from a street block to a neighborhood, metropolitan area, state, or country. Qualitative research is also a useful tool for conducting systematic and comprehensive needs assessments and program evaluations.

Recommendation 16: Expansions of research methodologies are needed to address a broad range of research questions, to ensure that methods are appropriate to the research questions being asked, and to respond to the complexities of multilevel interventions. This includes the need to integrate both qualitative and quantitative research.

Cost-Effectiveness Analyses

In the preceding sections, the committee has highlighted a number of promising approaches to public health intervention that draw upon important directions in behavioral and social science research. These interventions incorporate and integrate a range of approaches, spanning the continuum between traditional downstream approaches (i.e., interventions directed toward individuals to address health behaviors, attitudes, and/or knowledge) and upstream approaches (i.e., interventions directed toward public policies to address social and economic structures that influence health outcomes). While the scientific evidence base for these approaches is growing, these intervention strategies would prove impracticable for broader public health application should they fail to deliver significant gains relative to their cost and ease of implementation.

The relatively modest resources directed toward public health efforts must be carefully allocated, often while weighing alternative intervention strategies, and prioritized to yield the greatest benefit to target populations. Cost-effectiveness analyses (CEA) are therefore needed to help public health officials, foundations, and community leaders to establish priorities and assess the utility of interventions. (CEA is an umbrella term that includes other methodologies such as cost-utility analysis.) Such analyses compare alternate interventions, often using measures such as potential years of life gained or quality-adjusted life years that include changes in the quality of health as well as in the length of life, to assess the kinds of interventions that should be done, for whom, and how often. CEA therefore yields a ratio that expresses the value of an intervention relative to its cost.

In the context of the longitudinal, multilevel, comprehensive intervention strategies that are advocated in this report, CEA is critical to help assess which components of such interventions are most useful, for how long they must be applied, and with which populations they are most cost-effective. The incremental benefits of each component of multilevel intervention strategies must therefore be assessed. Further, the costs and benefits of interventions should be assessed at levels beyond that of the target individual(s). As Russell (2000) illustrates, interventions deliver effects not only on the target individuals, but also on their families, friends, social networks, communities, and so on. Interventions not only require the time and resources of providers of health care and health interventions, but also use the time and resources of individuals, as well as the social systems within which they operate. Interventions that tackle multiple levels of influence and multiple risk factors must therefore make the best use of resources at each level. Such a societal perspective of CEA considers the impacts of interventions on all persons and systems significantly affected by the intervention.

Recommendation 17: Cost-effectiveness analyses are necessary to assess the public health utility of interventions. Assessments are needed of the incremental effects of each component of multilevel, comprehensive interventions, and of the incremental effects of interventions over time. Such analyses should consider the broad influence and costs of interventions to target individuals, their families, and the broader social systems in which they operate.

Community as Partners

A consistent theme across the papers included in this volume is a call for interventions and research conducted in *partnership* with communities—that is, research efforts that are conducted *by* communities rather than *on* communities, and interventions that are not strictly message-driven but rather are guided by the voice of the community. Historically, community intervention trials have relied on community organizing principles as a means of involving communities in program planning and implementation (Sorensen et al., 1998). This model may fall short of the partnership needed to engage communities fully in health issues. Partnership with the community implies that the community has a voice in problem definition, data collection and the interpretation of results, and application of the results to address community concerns. Although further evidence is still needed to establish the effectiveness of this approach, the papers included in this volume note that community partnerships are likely to influence community priorities in the direction of health and foster social norms supportive of healthy outcomes. In addition, community-level participation and buy-in are likely to enhance the sustainability of interventions. Further, by providing an infrastructure that remains in a community after a research project ends, interventions may be more likely to be maintained beyond the funded period.

Recommendation 18: Efforts to develop the next generation of prevention interventions must focus on building relationships with communities, and develop interventions that derive from the communities' assessments of their needs and priorities. Models should be developed that encourage members of the community and researchers to work together to design, train for, and conduct such programs.

Funding

Full implementation of the above recommendations regarding intervention strategies and needed research requires significant changes in the manner in

---

BOX 4. Recommendations for Funding

Recommendation 19: Payers of health care should experiment with reimbursement structures to support programs that promote health and prevent disease.

Recommendation 20: Government and other funding agencies and universities should promote the development of interdisciplinary, collaborative research and training. Among the mechanisms that should be encouraged are interdisciplinary research centers, special program project awards, fellowships, and other postgraduate training programs.

Recommendation 21: Greater attention should be paid to funding research on social determinants of health and on behavioral and social science intervention research addressing generic social determinants of disease.

---

which health services and research funding are allocated. The committee's recommendations for funding are described below and summarized in Box 4.

Need for Health Care Funding to Place Greater Emphasis on Prevention

The United States expends more than a trillion dollars annually on health care. This vast expenditure provides considerable leverage for motivating health professionals and patients to pursue behaviors that result in preventing illness and reducing disability.

Payers for services, especially Medicare and Medicaid, have significant potential influence in encouraging widespread improvements in health behavior through the structure of their programs. For example, by benefit design decisions payers can encourage individuals to take advantage of preventive services that have been demonstrated to be cost-effective, such as immunizations and cancer screening services. Similarly, reimbursement systems can be designed so providers will be encouraged to give attention to ways of organizing preventive and care services that promote effective health behavior and contribute to the prevention of disability. One example of such action is the "healthy aging" project. For this project, the Health Care Financing Administration (HCFA) has commissioned both systematic reviews and demonstration projects to assess how changing the Medicare benefit structure can encourage the use of screening and preventive services and risk reduction behavior such as smoking cessation, increased physical activity, and chronic disease self-management.

HCFA has also developed programs to integrate acute medical care and long-term-care services to improve function among older persons. Such demonstrations include social health maintenance organizations (social HMOs) and PACE (Program for All-Inclusive Care of the Elderly). PACE, for example, integrates funding under the Medicare and Medicaid programs to develop more comprehensive service systems that seek to maintain community residence and function among older adults with substantial functional limitations.

Evaluation studies of social HMOs and PACE are continuing, but it is clear that these large reimbursement programs provide opportunities to develop and test programs of many kinds that encourage preventive health behavior, reduce risks of adverse events such as falls and malnutrition, and promote the recognition of such disabling conditions.

Recommendation 19: Payers of health care should experiment with reimbursement structures to support programs that promote health and prevent disease.

Need for Interdisciplinary Collaboration

The committee was impressed by evidence that the most successful interventions were those aimed not only at the behavior of individuals but also at the families, neighborhoods, and communities in which people live. Interventions worked best when they were supported also by legislative, media, and marketing efforts. Warner (Paper Contribution K) shows that the most successful tobacco control programs are those that include a combination of elements, including higher prices on tobacco products, laws regarding indoor air quality and restricting the use of vending machines, the development of media messages, and the establishment of smoking cessation programs.

Given the complexity required for effective interventions, it becomes increasingly important that social and behavioral scientists work closely with scientists representing other disciplines. The list of such disciplines is broad and includes genetics and human biology, clinical medicine, urban geography, law, journalism, nutrition, and education. Unfortunately, current training programs tend to focus on one or two disciplines at a time. Effective interdisciplinary collaboration is difficult because of important differences among experts in each discipline in vocabulary, history, and perspective. These experts attend different professional society meetings, train in different programs, read different journals, and rarely work together. There are now examples of programs, however, that have succeeded in developing truly interdisciplinary collaboration. One example is provided by the MacArthur Foundation Research Networks, and another by the programs of the Canadian Institute for Advanced Research. Emphasis needs to be given to developing and supporting similar programs on a broader scale. This should be done by government bodies as well as by private foundations.

Recommendation 20: Government and other funding agencies and universities should promote the development of interdisciplinary, collaborative research and training. Among the mechanisms that should be encouraged are interdisciplinary research centers, special program project awards, fellowships, and other postgraduate training programs.

*Refocusing of Research Efforts to Address Fundamental
Determinants of Health*

Most government agency and private foundation support for health research and interventions is organized in terms of particular diseases. The largest such funders, the National Institutes of Health (NIH) and the Agency for Health Care Research and Quality, are organized primarily by disease categories, although some institutes and centers of NIH support cross-cutting basic research that may inform interventions for several diseases. The predominant organization of research funding based on a clinical classification of disease may be of value for the treatment of sick individuals, but it is not as useful for studies of disease etiology and prevention. Because social and behavioral research demonstrates that several clinical entities have one or more risk factors in common, it is more useful to consider a new disease classification that unifies these different clinical entities based on the social and behavioral features they have in common. This is not a new idea. For many years, infectious disease epidemiologists grouped together different clinical diseases based on their similarities in modes of transmission (e.g., whether they are water-borne, air-borne, vector-borne, or food-borne). This way of classifying disease may not be of direct value in the treatment of sick people, but it certainly is of value in identifying those aspects of the environment to which interventions could be directed. A comparable set of social and behavioral categories for many of the diseases of concern today, for the most part, does not exist. The reasons for this are not clear. It may be that diseases such as coronary heart disease, cancer, AIDS, and arthritis are viewed as diseases of the "individual," and not as diseases influenced by social and environmental factors. Whatever the reasons, it is difficult for social and behavioral scientists to obtain funding for research and programs focused on generic determinants.

There already exist several examples of more appropriate funding arrangements to fit this model. The Centers for Disease Control and Prevention funds prevention centers, but nevertheless encourages proposals that focus on the prevention of specific diseases and conditions. The National Institute of Occupational Safety and Health deals with diseases associated with work, but a specific disease focus is often called for here as well. The National Institute on Aging and National Institute of Child Health and Human Development perhaps come closest to what is needed because their mission allows for the simultaneous consideration of several related diseases associated with human development and aging. Similarly, the Substance Abuse and Mental Health Services Administration's initiatives to fund research on the integration of prevention and treatment of comorbid substance abuse and psychiatric conditions is another example of moving the field toward integrated research and public health practice efforts.

The committee's findings demonstrate the importance of prevention efforts that are based on the reality that many diseases have numerous risk factors in common and that intervention programs are most effective when they deal with this commonality.

Recommendation 21: Greater attention should be paid to funding research on social determinants of health and on behavioral and social science intervention research addressing generic social determinants of disease.

CONCLUSION

Behavioral and social science research has provided many new advancements in the effort to improve population health, and offers promise for the development of new interventions with even greater utility and efficiency in the years to come. As summarized below, the committee finds that social and behavioral interventions can improve health outcomes across a range of developmental stages and levels of analysis (e.g., individual, interpersonal, and community levels). Further, coordination of intervention efforts across these levels may efficiently and effectively promote healthy individuals and environments.

The committee found compelling evidence that expectant mothers can deliver healthier children as we improve our understanding of the social, economic, and intrapersonal conditions that influence the mother's health status over her life course, not just in the period prior to conception and birth. The physical, cognitive, and emotional health of infants can be improved with comprehensive, high-quality services that address basic needs of children and families. These same interventions assist children to enter school ready to learn. Similarly, adolescents can enjoy healthier life-styles as researchers and public health officials pay greater attention to the social and environmental contexts in which youth operate. These interventions pay great dividends for later health, as poor health habits can be avoided and developmental risks averted.

The evidence also suggests that adolescents and adults can benefit from coordinated health promotion efforts that address the many sources of health influences (e.g., family, school, work settings). Opportunities for behavioral and social interventions to improve health do not end during adulthood, however; compelling data indicate that older adults can age more successfully as policies and institutions attend to their social, cognitive, and psychological needs, as well as their physical health needs.

While further research is needed, evidence is developing that elucidates the pathways through which behavioral and social interventions may mediate physiological processes and disease states. This evidence indicates that behavioral and social interventions can directly impact physiological functioning, and do not merely correlate with positive health outcomes due to improvements in health behavior or knowledge. Further refinements of this research will aid in the development of more efficient and effective interventions.

As interventions are developed, special consideration must be given to gender as well as to the needs of individuals of different socioeconomic, racial, and ethnic backgrounds. These attributes powerfully shape the contexts in which individuals gain access to health-promoting resources (e.g., education, income, social supports), the barriers that restrict more healthful life-styles (e.g., demands of gender roles), and the ways in which individuals in these groups interpret and respond to interventions. Because socioeconomic status exerts direct effects on health, intervention efforts must attend to the broader social, economic, cultural, and political processes that determine and maintain these disparities.

Efforts to improve the health of communities can benefit from specific levers for public health intervention, such as enhancing social capital and enacting public policies that promote healthful environments. While further research is needed to better understand means of manipulating these levers, it is clear that these interventions are most effective when members of target communities participate in their planning, design, and implementation. Communities that are fully engaged as partners in this process are more likely to develop public health messages that are relevant, are more likely to fully "buy in" and commit to community change, and are more likely to sustain community change efforts after research and/or demonstration programs end.

All such interventions are likely to be more successful when applied in coordinated fashion across multiple levels of influence (i.e., at the individual level; within families and social support networks; within schools, work sites, churches, and other community settings; and at broader public policy levels). While more research is needed to ascertain how coordination is best achieved and the cost-effectiveness of each component of a multilevel intervention strategy, the evidence from the tobacco control effort suggests that such a multilevel strategy can reap benefits for broad segments of the public. This success can extend both to those individuals at greatest risk for poor health by virtue of their unhealthful behaviors or disadvantaged social, political, or economic status, as well as those at relatively low risk. Such efforts require, however, that funders, public health officials, and community leaders are patient and persist with intervention efforts over a longer period than the 3 to 5 years typically allotted for most demonstration or research efforts.

To best accomplish these goals, researchers must learn to work across traditional disciplinary boundaries, and adopt new methodologies to evaluate intervention efforts. A range of social, behavioral, and life scientists must collaborate to fully engage a biopsychosocial model of human health and development. Further, these researchers must be open to adopting less traditional evaluation approaches, such as qualitative methodologies, and combining these approaches with quantitative methodologies.

In summary, the committee concludes that serious effort to apply behavioral and social science research to improve health requires that we transcend perspectives that have, to this point, resulted in public health problems being defined in relatively narrow terms. Efforts to design and implement multipronged interventions will require the cooperation of public health officials, funding agencies, researchers, and community members. Evaluation efforts must transcend traditional models of randomized control trials and incorporate both quantitative and qualitative methodologies. Models of intervention must consider individual behavior in a broader social context, with greater attention to the social construction of gender, race, and ethnicity, and to ways in which social and economic inequities result in health risks. Finally, efforts to address the fundamental social and behavioral causes of illness will require broad thinking that goes beyond traditional disease categories, developmental stages, focal points of interventions, and disciplinary lines. Transcending these perspectives is a critical step toward capitalizing on the promise of behavioral and social science research as a means of improving the public's health.

REFERENCES

Briss PA, Rodewald LE, Hinman AR, et al. (2000). Reviews and evidence regarding interventions to improve vaccination coverage in children, adolescents, and adults. *American Journal of Preventive Medicine*, 18(1S):97–140.

Centers for Disease Control and Prevention. (1992). Estimated national spending on prevention—United States, 1988. *Morbidity and Mortality Weekly Report*, 41:529–31.

Centers for Disease Control and Prevention. (1999). Achievements in public health, 1900–1999: Changes in the public health system. *Morbidity and Mortality Weekly Report*, 48(50):1141–7.

Centers for Disease Control and Prevention. (2000). Tobacco use among middle and high school students—United States, 1999. *Morbidity and Mortality Weekly Report*, 49: 49–53.

Collins JW, and David RJ. (1993). Race and birth weight in biracial infants. *American Journal of Public Health*, 83(8):1125–9.

Fogel RW. (1994). Economic Growth, Population Theory, and Physiology: The Bearing of Long-Term Process in the Making of Economic Policy. Working Paper No. 4638. Cambridge: National Bureau of Economic Research.

Fries JF, Koop CE, Beadle CE, et al. (1993). Reducing health care costs by reducing the need and demand for medical services. The Health Project Consortium. *New England Journal of Medicine*, 329:321–5.

Glassman AH, and Shapiro PA. (1998). Depression and the course of coronary artery disease. *American Journal of Psychiatry*, 155:4–11.

Health Care Financing Administration. (2000). Highlights—National health expenditures, 1998. From internet site http://hcfa.hss.gov/stats/nhe-oact/hilites.htm. Posted January 10, 2000.

Herrmann C, Brand-Driehorst S, Kaminsky B, Leibing E, Staats H, and Ruger U. (1998). Diagnostic groups and depressed mood as predictors of 22-month mortality in medical inpatients. *Psychosomatic Medicine*, 60:570–7.

Institute of Medicine. (1998). Reducing the Burden of Injury: Advancing Prevention and Treatment. RJ Bonnie, CE Fulco, CT Liverman (Eds.). Washington, DC. National Academy Press.

Kawachi I. (1999). Social capital and community effects on population and individual health. *Annals of the New York Academy of Sciences*, 896:120–30.

McGinnis JM, and Foege WH. (1993). Actual causes of death in the United States. *Journal of the American Medical Association*, 270(18):2207–11.

McKeown T.J. (1976). *The Role of Medicine: Dream, Mirage, or Nemesis?* London: Nuffield Provincial Hospitals Trust.

McKinlay JB, and McKinlay SM. (1977). The questionable contribution of medical measures to the decline of mortality in the United States in the twentieth century. *Milbank Memorial Fund Quarterly*, 55(3):405–28.

Michelson D, Stratakis C, Hill L, Reynolds J, Galliven E, Chrousos G, and Gold P. (1996). Bone mineral density in women with depression. *New England Journal of Medicine*, 335:1176–81.

Multiple Risk Factor Intervention Trial Research Group. (1981). The Multiple Risk Factor Intervention Trial. *Preventive Medicine*, 10:387–553.

Multiple Risk Factor Intervention Trial Research Group. (1982). The Multiple Risk Factor Intervention Trial: Risk factor changes and mortality results. *Journal of the American Medical Association* 248:1465–76.

Orleans CT, Gruman J, Ulmer C, Emont SL, Hollendonner JK. (1999). Rating our progress in population health promotion: Report card on six behaviors. *American Journal of Health Promotion*, 14(2):75–82.

Penninx BWJH, Guralnik JM, Pahor M, Ferrucci L, Cerhan JR, Wallace RB, and Havlik RJ. (1998). Chronically depressed mood and cancer risk in older persons. *Journal of the National Cancer Institute*, 90:1888–93.

Rogers RG, Rogers A, and Belanger A. (1989). Active life among the elderly in the United States: Multistate life-table estimates and population projections. *Milbank Quarterly*, 67:370–411.

Rose G. (1992). *The Strategy of Preventive Medicine.* New York: Oxford University Press.

Rozanski A, Blumenthal JA, and Kaplan J. (1999). Impact of psychological factors on the pathogenesis of cardiovascular diseases. *Circulation*, 99:2192–217.

Russell L. (2000). Presentation at Institute of Medicine symposium, "Capitalizing on Social Science and Behavioral Research to Improve the Public's Health," February 3, 2000, Atlanta.

Satariano WA. (In press). *Aging, Health and the Environment: An Epidemiological View.* Gaithersburg: Aspen Publishers.

Sorensen G. (2000). Social determinants of health. In: Goldman MB, and Hatch MC (Eds.), *Women and Health,* Pp. 523–7. San Diego: Academic Press.

Sorensen G, Emmons K, Hunt MK, and Johnston D. (1998). Implications of the results of community intervention trials. *Annual Review of Public Health,* 19:379–416.

Syme SL. Drug treatment of mild hypertension: Social and psychological considerations. *Annals New York Academy of Science,* 1978; 304:99–106.

Syme SL and Balfour JL. (1998). Social determinants of disease. In Wallace RB, and Doebbeling BH (Eds.), *Public Health and Preventive Medicine.* Stanford, CT: Appleton and Lange.

U.S. Department of Health, Education, and Welfare. (1964). *Smoking and Health: Report of the Advisory Committee to the Surgeon General of the Public Health Service.* Washington, D.C.: U.S. Department of Health, Education, and Welfare, Public Health Service, Center for Disease Control. PHS Publication No. 1103.

Wells KB, Stewart A, Hays RD, Burnam A, Rogers W, Daniels M, Berry S, Greenfield S, and Ware J. (1989). The functioning and well-being of depressed patients. *Journal of the American Medical Association*, 262:914–9.

Williams K and Umberson D. (2000). Women, stress and health. In: Goldman MB, and Hatch MC (Eds). *Women and Health,* Pp. 553–62. San Diego: Academic Press.

The Contribution of Social and Behavioral Research to an Understanding of the Distribution of Disease: A Multilevel Approach

George A. Kaplan, Ph.D.; Susan A. Everson, Ph.D., M.P.H.; and
John W. Lynch, Ph.D., M.P.H

INTRODUCTION

The popular and scientific press are replete with articles that eagerly herald great breakthroughs in public health, medicine, and biology that will arise from our expanding knowledge in genomics, bioinformatics, and biomedicine. The coming description of the human genome married with rapid advances in biotechnology is thought by many to presage an era in which many of the major sources of disease and disabilities in world populations will be prevented, delayed, or cured. Without a doubt, the increased knowledge of the molecular basis of the pathobiology of disease portends tremendous advances in our understanding and treatment of disease. However, the premise of this paper is that these advances, in and of themselves, will not be able to accomplish these goals. Instead, we argue for a public health-based approach that incorporates knowledge across a multitude of levels, ranging from the pathobiology of disease to the social and economic policies that result in differential patterns of exposure of individuals and populations to risk factors and pathogenic environments. Central

Dr. Kaplan is professor and chair, Department of Epidemiology, School of Public Health, and senior research scientist, Institute for Social Research, University of Michigan; Dr. Everson is assistant research scientist, Department of Epidemiology, School of Public Health, University of Michigan; and Dr. Lynch is assistant professor, School of Public Health, and faculty associate, Institute for Social Research, University of Michigan. This paper was prepared for the symposium "Capitalizing on Social Science and Behavioral Research to Improve the Public's Health," the Institute of Medicine and the Commission on Behavioral and Social Sciences and Education of the National Research Council, Atlanta, Georgia, February 2–3, 2000.

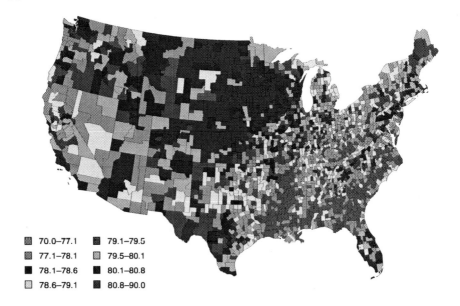

▨ 70.0–77.1	▨ 79.1–79.5
▨ 77.1–78.1	▨ 79.5–80.1
▪ 78.1–78.6	▪ 80.1–80.8
▢ 78.6–79.1	▪ 80.8–90.0

FIGURE 1 Geographic distribution of female life expectancy at birth by county and county clusters, United States, 1990.

to such a focus is an important role for economic, behavioral, and social factors, whether manifested at the individual or population level. For it is to these factors that we will largely have to look to develop a complete explanation of core epidemiologic observations concerning group and geographic differentials in the prevalence and incidence of disease and time trends in disease. In what follows we will review selected information on variations in life expectancy and the occurrence of a number of major public health problems and discuss how such a multilevel approach provides critical perspectives on the causes of these variations and on opportunities to reduce them.

Life Expectancy and Death Rates from All Causes

Overall life expectancy at birth reached 76.5 years in the United States in 1997, with almost steady increases since 1950 (NCHS, 1999). Since 1980, life expectancy at birth increased by 5.1% for males to 73.6 years, and by 2.6% for females to 79.4 years, and life expectancy at age 65 increased by 12.8% to 80.9 years, and by 4.9% to 84.2 years, for males and females, respectively. Despite these increases the United States still compares poorly to many countries— ranking twenty-fifth for males and nineteenth for females on a list of 36 countries compiled by the National Center for Health Statistics (NCHS, 1999).

Within the United States there is considerable variation in life expectancy. For example, Figure 1 presents variations in female life expectancy at birth for counties and county clusters in the United States in 1990 (Murray et al., 1998). Life expectancy at birth differs between areas by as much as 16.5 years for males and 13.3 years for females. In these analyses, the largest difference in life expectancy is between American Indian or Alaskan Native males in the cluster of Bennett, Jackson, Mellette, Shannon, Todd, and Washabaugh counties in South Dakota (56.5 years) and Asian Pacific Islander females in Bergen County in New Jersey (97.7 years). As Murray et al. (1998, p. 9) point out, this 41-year range in life expectancy within the United States is ". . . equal to 90 percent of the global range from the population with the lowest life expectancy, males in Sierra Leone, to the population with the highest, females in Japan."

There also is substantial geographic variation in life expectancy at birth within race/ethnicity and sex subgroups. For example, while American Indian and Alaskan Native males have a life expectancy of 56.5 in the six-county area in South Dakota previously mentioned, this group has a life expectancy of 92.3 years in Los Angeles County. Life expectancy for white males and females also varies considerably by county—with ranges of 9.9 years and 7.6 years, respectively.

As might be expected from trends and differences in life expectancy, consideration of age-adjusted mortality rates from all causes also indicates substantial variation by gender, race/ethnicity, and time. Figure 2 (Hoyert et al., 1999)

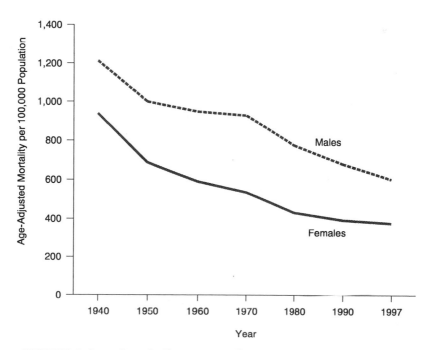

FIGURE 2 Age-adjusted, all cause mortality rates by sex, United States, 1940–1997.

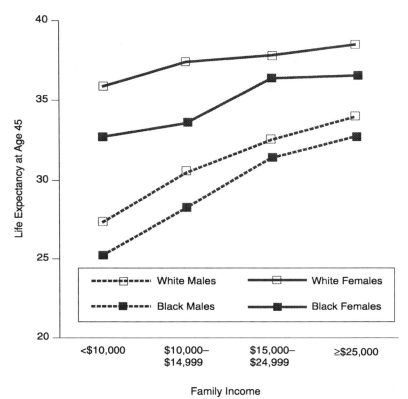

FIGURE 3 Life expectancy at age 45 by family income, race, and sex, United States, 1979–1989.

shows the decline in age-adjusted mortality rates from all causes for males and females between 1940 and 1997. During this period, rates declined by 50% for males and 60% for females. However, these declines were not experienced equally by all groups. For example, during the period from 1950 to 1997, age-adjusted mortality rates from all causes declined by 40.4% for white males, 33.6% for black males, 44.5% for white females, and 50.7% for black females. Thus, during this period, mortality differentials between white and black males increased, while for females they decreased. Detailed information for other race and ethnicity groups is not available for this period.

There is considerable variation between states in overall mortality rates. For example, in 1997, the state with the lowest age-adjusted (1990 standard) mortality rate was Hawaii (572.5 per 100,000 population), and the highest rate (exclusive of the District of Columbia) was found in West Virginia (865.1 per 100,000). This level of geographic variation in age-adjusted mortality, a difference of almost 300 deaths per 100,000 population, is very significant given that

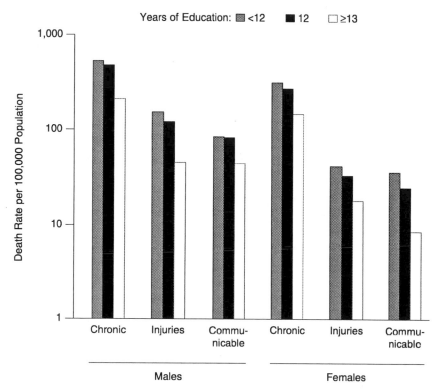

FIGURE 4 Age-Adjusted death rates among adults, age 25-65, by cause of death, sex and education, United States, 1995.

it is 40% of the overall rate for the United States (742.7 deaths per 100,000 population using the 1990 U.S. standard population).

Socioeconomic variations in mortality have been widely noted (Kaplan et al., 1987). For most diseases and health status indicators and for most measures of socioeconomic position there is an inverse relationship (Haan et al., 1987). Figure 3 shows the relationship between family income and life expectancy (1979–1989) at age 45 for white and black men and women (all ethnicities) in the United States (NCHS, 1998). The gradient between socioeconomic position and death rates is clearly seen for broad classes of causes of death, as shown in Figure 4 (NCHS, 1998).

The strong effects of socioeconomic position on mortality, coupled with substantial heterogeneity by race/ethnicity and geographic place in mortality rates and strong secular trends can lead to phenomena of major public health significance. In analyses of 1984–1993 trends in coronary heart disease (CHD) mortality in North Carolina, Barnett et al. (1999) found that declines in mortality were experienced by white men of *all* social classes, with the greatest benefit among those in the highest social class, while *only* the highest social class of black men showed any decline at all. For example, black men in social classes III and IV (e.g., occupations such as mechanic, butcher, janitor, welder, truck driver, laborer, animal caretaker) had average annual changes in Coronary Heart Disease (CHD) mortality of +0.8% and 0.0%, respectively, whereas white men in the same social classes had average annual changes of -2.1% and -6%. Over the 10-year period, black men in the lowest social class experienced an 8.0% *increase* in CHD mortality, and white men in the same social class experienced a 16% *decline.*

UNDERSTANDING VARIATIONS IN HEALTH

These large variations in life expectancy and mortality, and similar variations in other health outcomes, present fundamental challenges to our understanding of the determinants of health in individuals and populations and of how we can reduce the burdens of disease and disability. We propose that there is no single or simple explanation for such heterogeneity, and that it is highly unlikely that the triad of genomics, bioinformatics, and biomedicine, with their focus on molecular etiologic forces located within the individual, will help explain very much of the heterogeneity in health and disease among social groups, places, and times. While such an individualistic focus can help us explain events within individuals it is unlikely to be very successful in explaining the patterning of disease by subgroups, places, or eras (Rose, 1992). However, we do not argue that we should completely dismiss such pursuits and replace them solely with a focus on macrolevel determinants of health. Such an ecologic or macrolevel focus is likely to miss many opportunities for increased understanding of disease mechanisms and intervention opportunities and suffers from its own version of tunnel vision.

Observations of the complex patterning of disease, the "lens" of epidemiology, leads instead to a new approach that attempts to bridge various levels of explanation and intervention, bringing together theory and empirical work that tie together observations of causal influence and mechanism at multiple levels. It thus represents an explanatory enterprise that does not exclusively privilege the proximal, but seeks opportunities for understanding and intervention at both upstream and downstream vantage points (Figure 5). Such a pursuit is in its infancy and represents a major challenge that will succeed only with a broad interdisciplinary vision accompanied by state-of-the-art thinking in multiple domains.

In what follows we describe some general epidemiologic and demographic features of six major public health problems: low birthweight, childhood asthma, firearm-related deaths in adolescents and young adults, coronary heart disease, breast cancer, and osteoporosis. After describing the general patterns with which these problems appear, we then sketch out some examples of the type of multilevel approach that is suggested in Figure 5.

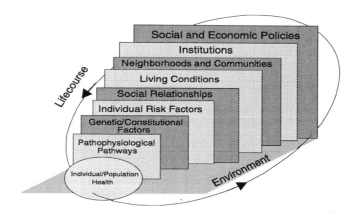

FIGURE 5 Multilevel approach to epidemiology.

THE DISTRIBUTION OF DISEASE—
SOME ILLUSTRATIVE EXAMPLES

Low Birthweight

Overall

Low birthweight, defined as a live birth less than 2,500 grams, is one of the most vexing problems facing the public health community in the United States. Low birthweight can result from babies being born prematurely and/or being born too small, and it is the major underlying cause of infant mortality and early childhood morbidity. The United States has significantly higher rates of low birthweight than other comparably developed nations. For instance, the average rate of low birthweight in the United States between 1990 and 1994 was 7 births per 1,000, while in countries like Norway, Sweden, and Finland, rates were as low 4–5 per 1,000 (UNICEF, 1998). Within some U.S. population subgroups these rates of low birthweight exceed 12 per 1,000 and match the very high levels found in some Sub-Saharan African and other developing countries. Infant mortality has declined significantly over the last 30 years, in large part due to the effects of neonatal intensive care and drug therapies that have helped to increase the survival of low-birthweight infants. In stark contrast, rates of low birthweight have remained stubbornly high (NCHS, 1998). Thus, the United States has a serious and persistent problem of low birthweight, which so far seems intractable to advances in medical care and technology.

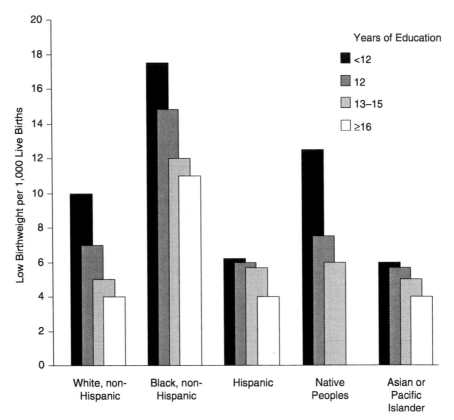

FIGURE 6 Low birthweight by education and race/ethnicity, United States, 1996.

Distribution by Race and Socioeconomic Position

As alluded to above, the problem of low birthweight is not distributed randomly across population subgroups. Figure 6 shows rates of low birthweight in 1996, according to the education and race/ethnic group of mothers aged 20 or older (NCHS, 1998). These data show both educational and race/ethnicity differences in low birthweight.

The highest levels of low birthweight, around 18 per 1,000, were among the least educated black, non-Hispanic women. The lowest rates, around 4 per 1,000, were among the most educated Hispanic, Asian Pacific Islander, and white, non-Hispanic women. While there are important educational gradients in almost every race/ethnic group, the largest differences are between race/ethnic groups (NCHS, 1998). This fact is further emphasized in a 1992 study in the *New England Journal of Medicine* showing that even among babies born to college-educated mothers, infant mortality was significantly higher among black babies. This difference in infant mortality was entirely attributable to the higher proportion of low birth-

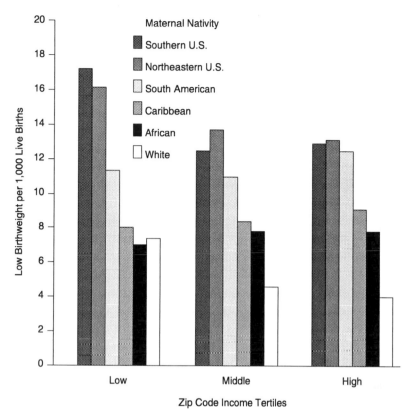

FIGURE 7 Low birthweight by zip code income tertiles and maternal nativity among "Blacks, " New York City, 1988-1994.

weight black infants (Schoendorf et al., 1992). In making any comparison between race/ethnic groups in seemingly equal socioeconomic strata, such as those with a college education, it is important to remember that the social meaning and economic value of a college education may be quite different for different race/ethnic groups. Health differences between race/ethnic groups largely reflect a wide array of accumulated social exposures, so it would be naive to expect that we can capture all of these social exposures in one socioeconomic factor such as education. We must be aware of the problems of incommensurability of socioeconomic indicators in comparing across race/ethnic groups (Krieger et al., 1993; Kaufman et al., 1997). Nevertheless, the differences in low birthweight across race/ethnic groups cannot be ignored and deserve more intensive investigation. Adding to the complexity of this picture is recent research showing that birthweights of African-born black women are more closely related to those of U.S.-born white women than to U.S.-born black women (David and Collins, 1997). (See Figure 7.) Additionally, Fang et al. (1999) have shown that rates of low birthweight among "black" women vary considerably across all income levels, according to the country of birth of the mother.

Trends

Low birthweight continues to be a stubborn public health problem, with little or no decline in rates over the last 20 years (See Figure 8.). In fact, between 1985 and 1996, New Hampshire was the only state that did not record an increase in the percentage of low-birthweight babies. For the United States, overall rates rose by an average of 9%, but in some midwestern states such as Minnesota, Iowa, Nebraska, and Indiana, low birthweight increased by as much as 20% (Annie E. Casey Foundation, 1999).

Geographic Distribution

Not unexpectedly, there also is considerable geographic variation in low birthweight across the United States. As Figure 9 shows, low birthweight is particularly concentrated in the southeastern states. These geographic differences may reflect both compositional and contextual influences on low birthweight. Compositional influences relate to characteristics of the individuals who reside

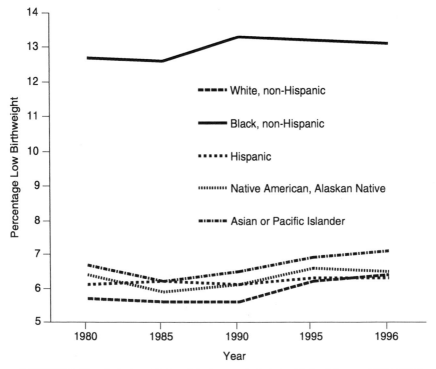

FIGURE 8 Trends in low birthweight by race/ethnicity, United States, 1980–1996.

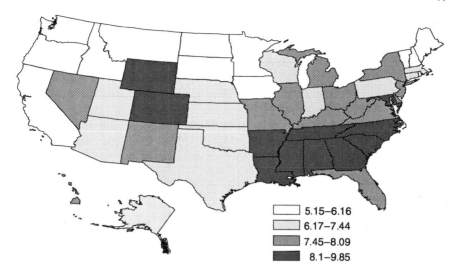

	5.15–6.16
	6.17–7.44
	7.45–8.09
	8.1–9.85

FIGURE 9 Geographic distribution of percent of live births under 2500 grams by state, United States.

in a certain area, while contextual influences refer to nonindividual aspects of the environment that also may affect rates of low birthweight. For instance, Kaplan and colleagues (1996) have shown how the extent of income inequality within a state is correlated with rates of low birthweight even after adjustment for the average incomes in the state ($r = -065$, $p < .001$). As Paneth has argued, "The effects of poverty at the level of the individual, the family and the community need all to be taken account of; the context in which pregnancy occurs is larger than the womb" (1995, p. 31).

Costs

The assessment of costs for any health problem is a complex undertaking that requires making various assumptions about what should be included and excluded from cost estimates. In the case of low birthweight, there are direct and indirect costs. The direct costs are those associated with both the immediate medical care for low-birthweight babies and the longer-term implications that low birthweight has for enduring health problems in childhood. In addition, the health complications of low birthweight place additional burdens on later child care and educational needs. Lewitt et al. (1995) estimated that in 1988, for children aged 0–15 who had been born at low birthweights, the health care, child care, and educational costs directly attributable to their birthweight were between $5.5 billion and $6 billion more than if those children had been normal weight at birth.

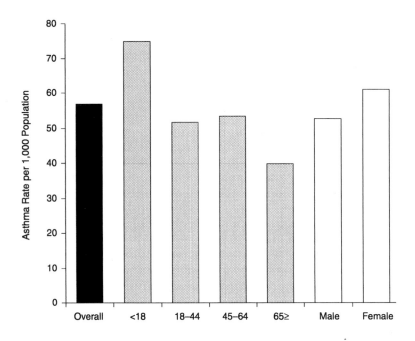

FIGURE 10 Asthma prevalence rate by age, and sex, United States, 1995.

Childhood Asthma

Overall

Asthma is one of the most common chronic health problems in the United States (See Figure 10). In 1995 it was estimated to affect almost 15 million people—almost one-third of them under age 18 (Mannino et al., 1998). Asthma prevalence has increased dramatically over the last 20 years, and what limited comparisons can be made to suggest that the increases observed in the United States may parallel increases in some other industrialized nations such as France, Britain, and Australia (Grant et al., 1999). However, the prevalence of asthma is generally lower in less industrialized countries (Cookson, 1987). The symptoms of asthma—wheezing, breathlessness, and coughing—are brought on by inflammatory processes in the airways and immunoglobulins in response to a wide variety of environmental toxins and allergens such as dust mites, cockroaches, pollens, and particular agents that reduce the overall air quality (Clark et al., 1999). The potentially greater biological vulnerability of children due to their developing immune systems may place them at heightened risk of asthmatic reactions to environmental irritants. Thus, there is a need for much more basic and applied research on asthma. As Grant et al. (1999) state, "Changes in environmental risk factors and exposures may contribute to recent trends, but little information is available relating specific risk factors to either longitudinal asthma trends, geographic variability, or high-risk populations" (p. S1).

Distribution by Race and Socioeconomic Position

Asthma morbidity and mortality are disproportionately higher among disadvantaged children (Weiss et al., 1994). Evans (1992) estimated that asthma is 26% more prevalent among black than white children. Data on socioeconomic and race/ethnicity differences in asthma prevalence among children are limited. However, Figure 11 reveals a growing gap in asthma prevalence between blacks and whites from 1980 to 1994 when averaged across all age groups (Mannino et al., 1998).

Black children also are significantly more likely to be hospitalized for asthma (Figure 12). This is true at every level of zip code income. In fact, even black children living in zip codes where the median income was greater than $40,000 per year are much more likely to be hospitalized for asthma than white children living in the poorest income areas. Understanding what these race/ethnic and socioeconomic differences reflect is a complex task, but it is possible that residential environments for black children are poorer quality, at

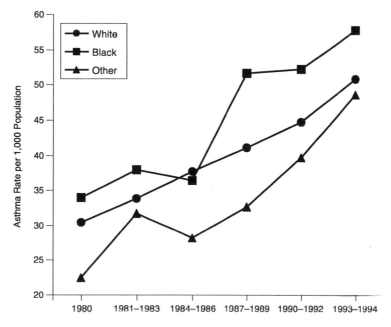

FIGURE 11 Asthma prevalence trends by year and race/ethnicity, United States, 1980–1994.

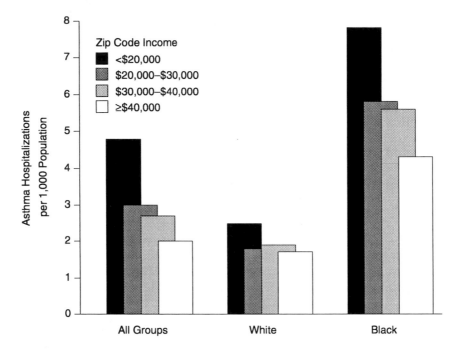

FIGURE 12 Asthma hospitalization for children, aged 1–14, by median household income according to zip code of residence, United States, 1989–1991. SOURCE: NCHS, 1998.

every level of zip code income. U.S. cities are highly segregated residentially (Massey and Denton, 1993), and important environmental differences may exist in levels of inflammatory bioallergens between the residential areas occupied by blacks and whites.

Trends

Prevalence, emergency department treatment, and mortality rates for asthma have all increased in the last 20 years (NHLBI, 1999). Disturbingly, these increases appear faster among children than adults and may reflect the greater biological vulnerability of children to the effects of bioallergens. Figure 13 shows the significantly higher prevalence of asthma among 5- to 14-year-olds in the last 10 years. The sharpest increase has been among the very young (Mannino et al., 1998). Among preschool children, asthma prevalence has increased 160% from 1980 to 1994.

Geographic Distribution

There are no large-scale United States studies assessing geographic varia-tion in emergency department visits or hospitalizations, although self-reported prevalence estimates suggest rates are highest in the western states and lowest in the South (Collins, 1997). Smaller-scale studies also have demonstrated urban-rural differences (Malveaux et al., 1995). In a sample of children in the Bronx in New York, Crain et al. (1994) estimated that there was a cumulative prevalence of asthma of 14.3% and period prevalence of 8.6%. These estimates for inner city children were twice the national average.

Costs

In 1993 there were more than 150,000 hospitalizations for children under age 15 (CDC, 1995). The American Lung Association estimates that the direct health care costs for asthma in the United States are almost $10 billion, with inpatient hospital care being the largest single expenditure. Indirect costs related to both loss of work and missed school days may add up to more than $1 billion annually. It is estimated there are more than 10 million school days missed an-

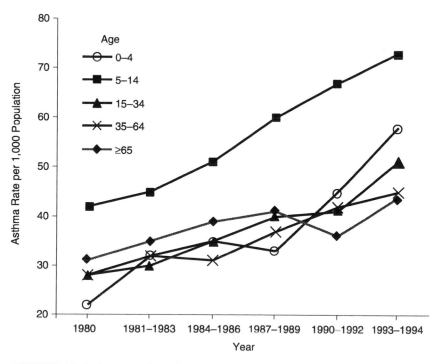

FIGURE 13 Asthma prevalence by year and age, United States, 1980–1994.

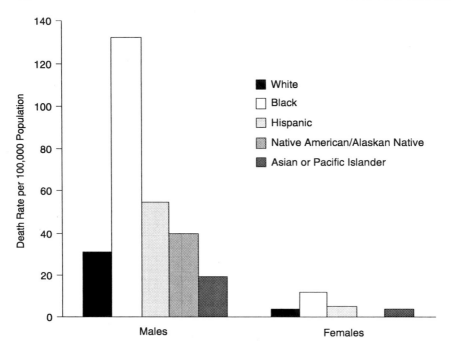

FIGURE 14 Death rates per 100,000 for firearm-related injuries among persons age 15–24 by sex and race/ethnicity, United States, 1996.

nually due to asthma. These productivity losses through work and school are estimated to cost almost $2 billion annually (American Lung Association, 1998).

Firearm-Related Deaths Among Youth and Young Adults

Overall

Nowhere is the important contribution of injuries to the population pattern of death and disability more evident than when considering the health status of youth and young adults. Rates of death from injuries rise from 14.2 per 100,000 population for children age 10–14 to 66.1 per 100,000 population for those age 15–19, and reach a level in the age 20- to 24-year-old group (79.9 per 100,000 population) that is not exceeded until age 75–84. Injuries, including unintentional injuries, homicide, suicide, and legal intervention, are the leading cause of death for 15- to 24-year-olds, accounting for approximately 75% of the 32,443 deaths in this age group in 1996.

Even more striking is the role of firearms in these deaths. Firearm-related injuries accounted for 25.9% of the deaths among 15- to 24-year-olds in 1997 (NCHS, 1997). In 1996, deaths from firearm-related injuries among 15- to 24-year-olds almost reached the level of those due to motor vehicle accidents (24.2

per 100,000 population versus 29.2 per 100,000 population, respectively NCHS, 1998).

Distribution by Race and Sex

The burden of these deaths is not shared equally (Figure 14). While non-Hispanic whites have the highest numbers of deaths from firearm-related injuries, males—and particularly non-Hispanic African American males—have substantially elevated rates of death from firearm-related injuries compared to females and males from other groups. Overall, the age-adjusted 1997 death rate for males from firearm-related injuries was 6.2 times higher than that for females (22.4 per 100,000 population versus 3.6 per 100,000 population) (NCHS, 1998). Among males, in 1996 the lowest rates were among Asian Pacific Islanders (19.6 per 100,000 population) and the highest rates, 6.7 times higher, were among African Americans (131.6 per 100,000 population).

Distribution by Socioeconomic Position

Given that the familiar inverse gradient between measures of socioeconomic position and health outcomes is found for homicide and suicide (Baker et al., 1992), it would not be surprising to find that it also is seen for firearm-related deaths among 15- to 24-year-olds. However, national statistics on this outcome do not generally stratify by socioeconomic position, a general deficiency that has been noted elsewhere (Krieger et al., 1997). Baker et al. (1992) provided some evidence for the association with firearm-related deaths, although not specifically for 15- to 24-year-olds, who account for 25% of all firearm-related deaths. A strong and generally consistent inverse association between per capita income of the area of residence of the decedent and rate of firearm-related deaths (1980–1986) was seen for unintentional injuries, homicide, and suicide related to firearms. For example, areas with a per capita income less than $6,000 compared to areas where it is equal to or greater than $14,000 had rates of unintentional death from firearms, homicide, and suicide that were elevated seven-, three-, and two-fold, respectively.

Trends

There have been substantial trends in firearm-related deaths among 15- to 24-year-olds over the past few decades. From 1970 to 1980 there was a 33% increase, followed by a 16% decrease in 1985, followed by steady increases totaling 158% up to 1993 and gradual declines since then through 1997. From 1993 to 1996, there was a 22% decrease in firearm-related mortality in this group. Although the general direction of these trends has been consistent, there have been variations in magnitude by race/ethnicity. For example, Figure 15

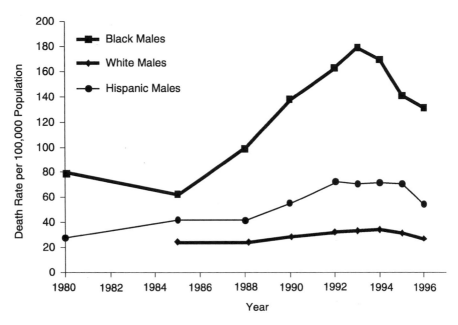

FIGURE 15 Death rates per 100,000 for firearms-related injuries among males, age 15–24, by race/ethnicity, United States, 1980–1996.

illustrates the faster acceleration from 1985 to 1993 of firearm-related deaths among African American and Hispanic men compared to white men.

Geographic Variation

There is substantial geographic variation in the occurrence of firearm-related deaths. The general picture, across all age groups, reflects higher rates of firearm-related homicide in core metropolitan areas compared to rural areas, while there are higher rates of firearm-related unintentional injuries in rural areas (Baker et al., 1992). Fingerhut et al. (1998) analyzed 1979–1995 trends in firearm-related homicide and found similar secular trends for core metropolitan areas, fringe metropolitan areas, different size metropolitan counties, and non-metropolitan counties. Within the overall pattern of geographic differences, there is considerable unexplained heterogeneity. For example, using data available from the Centers for Disease Control and Prevention (CDC) WONDER (on-line), we examined state differences in 1996 firearm-related deaths for 15- to 24-year-old blacks and whites and found substantial variation. On average, death rates from firearm-related injuries were 7.1 (median, 5.8) times higher among blacks than for whites, but the rates of relative disadvantage ranged from 2.4-fold in Texas and 2.7-fold in North Carolina to 12.1-fold in Illinois and 14.6-fold in Massachusetts.

Costs

The calculation of costs of firearm-related injuries and deaths is complex and is hampered by a significant lack of data. Work in this area has generally not reported separate estimates for specific age groups. Nationwide, for all ages, the medical costs of gunshot injuries were recently estimated at $2.3 billion per year (Cook et al., 1999). Total annual medical care expenses, indirect costs for long-term disability, and lost productivity associated with premature death have been estimated at $20.4 billion (Max and Rice, 1993). Because long-term disability and lost productivity costs would be high for firearm-related deaths and injuries to 15- to 24-year-olds, it is likely that a substantial portion of the $20.4 billion reflects costs to children and young adults.

Cardiovascular Disease in Adults

Overall

Heart disease is the leading cause of death in the United States. In 1996, this was true for white males and females, African-American males and females, Asian-American males and females, Hispanic males and females, and American Indian males and females. Overall, deaths from heart disease accounted for 31.7% of all deaths in 1996 (NCHS, 1998) and were responsible for 15.8% of the years of potential life lost before age 75 (NCHS, 1998). Diseases of the heart account for 11.2% of the deaths among those 25–44 years of age, 27.1% among those age 45–64, and 35.7% among those 65 years or older. Coronary heart disease, which accounts for two-thirds of all heart disease deaths, alone accounted for more than 2 million hospital stays in 1995, with an average length of stay of 5.3 days, and almost 10 million physician visits (NHLBI, 1998).

Distribution by Race and Sex

There is considerable variation in rates of death from cardiovascular disease (CVD) by race, ethnicity, and sex (Figure 16). Age-adjusted rates of death for males are 82.1% higher than they are for females (NCHS, 1998). Substantial variation is seen when comparing across race and ethnicity, with the rates for Asian Pacific Islander women, for example, being one-third the rates for African American women, and the rates of death for African American men being more than 2.5-fold greater than for Asian Pacific Islander men. Generally the highest rates are for African American men and women, with the next highest rates being for non-Hispanic white men and women. Problems related to incorrect information on death certificates and census undercounts may lead to systematic biases in rates for some groups, for example, those of Hispanic ethnicity (Goff et al., 1997).

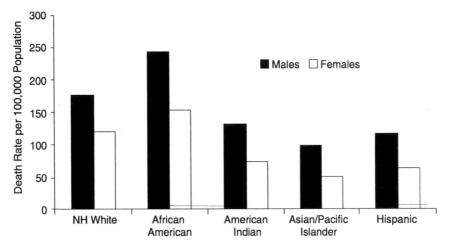

FIGURE 16 Age-adjusted death rates for diseases of the heart by race/ethnicity and sex, United States, 1996. NOTE: NH = non-Hispanic.

Distribution by Socioeconomic Position

There is substantial evidence that various measures of socioeconomic position (SEP) are importantly associated with mortality and morbidity from CVD (Kaplan and Keil, 1993; NHLBI, 1998). Figure 17 shows the inverse association between family income level and heart disease death rates for 25- to 64-year-old non-Hispanic whites and African-Americans. Those in families with incomes less than $10,000 had death rates that are 2.4- to 2.8-fold higher than those with family income greater than $15,000 in 1979–1989. A similar inverse patterning is seen when other measures of SEP, such as education and income of individuals, families, or county of residence are considered (NHLBI, 1995). Other studies have indicated that the impact of SEP on cardiovascular disease (CVD) extends to measures of CVD morbidity as well as subclinical disease (Lynch et al., 1997).

Geographic Variation

There is substantial variation in the geographic distribution of CVD. Generally speaking, death rates from CVD are highest in the southeastern portion of the United States and lowest in the western Mountain states, Alaska, and Hawaii (NHLBI, 1998). Figure 18 shows the similar variation in age-adjusted rates of death from ischemic heart disease among 25- to 74-year-olds in 1996. There also is substantial geographic variation in CVD differentials by race and ethnicity. For example, overall age-adjusted deaths rates from ischemic heart disease among those 25–74 years of age were approximately 3% higher in African-Americans in 1996 than in whites. However, the differential varied widely, from a 20 to 51% excess in California and Nebraska, respectively, to 32–54% lower rates for African-Americans in Washington and Minnesota.

Trends

One of the most remarkable achievements of the latter part of this century has been the substantial decline in death rates from CVD. For example, from 1900 to 1950, rates of death from CVD among those 45–54 years of age increased by 28%, but from 1950 to 1995 these rates declined by 68% (NHLBI, 1998). Given the tremendous burden from CVD in the population, these changes had major consequences. Analyses by the National Heart, Lung, and Blood Institute (NHLBI) indicate that this decline in CVD mortality rates since 1994 translates into more than one million fewer deaths from CVD during that period (NHLBI, 1998). Other analyses indicate that the decline in CVD mortality from 1965 to 1995 accounted for 70% of the 5.6-year gain in life-expectancy seen during that period (Vital Statistics of the United States, 1900–1967; Arriaga, 1984; 1989).

There is substantial demographic and geographic variation in who has benefited from the decline in CVD (Sempos et al., 1988). For example, the average annual percentage decline in age-adjusted coronary heart disease death rates for white males and females was greater than for black males and females from 1980 to 1996. In some periods the differences were substantial—the *annual* percentage decline for males was 50% greater (-3.6% versus -2.4%) for whites than for blacks during 1980–1989. Analyses of these trends also indicate that areas that are better off socioeconomically have benefited more from the declines in CVD mortality (Wing et al., 1988). Barnett et al. (1999), in their analyses of 1984–1993 trends in CHD mortality in North Carolina, found that social class inequalities in coronary heart disease mortality actually widened during this period for both black and white men. Moreover, whereas declines in mortality

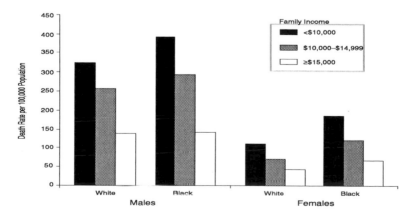

FIGURE 17 Heart disease death rate per 100,000 among persons age 25–64, by sex, race, and family income, United States, 1979–1989.

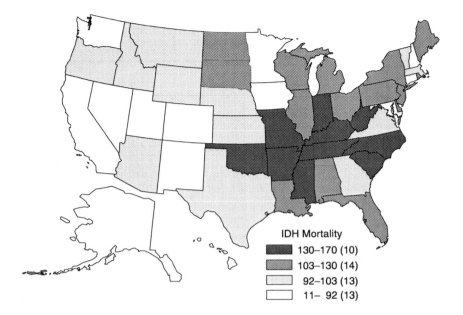

FIGURE 18 Geographic distribution of age-adjusted mortality rates from ischemic heart disease among persons age 24–75, by state, United States, 1996.

were experienced by white men of *all* social classes, with the greatest benefit among those in the highest social class, *only* the highest social class of black men showed any decline at all.

Costs

Given the high population burden of CVD, it is to be expected that CVD is associated with substantial costs. According to recent NHLBI calculations, the direct costs associated with CVD were $171 billion in 1998, and the indirect costs related to morbidity and lost productivity were $103 billion. Thus, while there have been substantial advances in reducing the health burden from CVD, it still is associated with considerable economic costs to society.

Overall Breast Cancer

Overall

Breast cancer is the most commonly diagnosed cancer in women, not counting skin cancers, accounting for one in three cancer diagnoses. Breast cancer is the leading cause of death among women aged 40 to 55 (Henderson,

TABLE 1. Age-Specific Risk of
Developing Breast Cancer

Age	Estimate
25	1 in 19,608
30	1 in 2,525
35	1 in 622
40	1 in 217
45	1 in 93
50	1 in 50
55	1 in 33
60	1 in 24
65	1 in 17
70	1 in 14
75	1 in 10
85	1 in 9
Ever	1 in 8

1995). However, lung cancer mortality rates are higher than breast cancer mortality rates in women overall (American Cancer Society, 1995), and three times as many women will experience heart disease as breast cancer in their lifetime.

Incidence of breast cancer increases greatly with age; more than three-quarters of all cases occur in women over age 50. Current estimates are that one in eight American women will develop breast cancer in her lifetime (Feuer et al., 1993). However, as noted by Feuer et al. (1993), it is important to look at age-specific probabilities because they provide a more accurate estimate of an individual's risk of breast cancer at a specific point in time, compared to lifetime probabilities (see Table 1). In other words, a 50-year-old woman who is currently cancer free has little more than a 2% risk of developing breast cancer over the next 10 years.

Breast cancer also occurs in men but is extremely rare, accounting for less than 1% of the overall incidence of and mortality due to breast cancer.

Distribution by Race and Socioeconomic Position

Breast cancer incident rates vary widely by race/ethnicity within the United States. After age 45, the incidence of breast cancer is higher in white women than in black women; however, age-specific incidence in women less than age 45 is higher in blacks (Kelsey and Bernstein, 1996; Trock, 1996).

Women of other racial or ethnic groups also experience lower incidence of breast cancer than white women. For example, compared to United States-born white women, the incidence of breast cancer is 50% lower in Asian-American women born in China or Japan and 25% lower in United States-born Asian women (Stanford et al., 1995). Figure 19 shows breast cancer incidence rates for

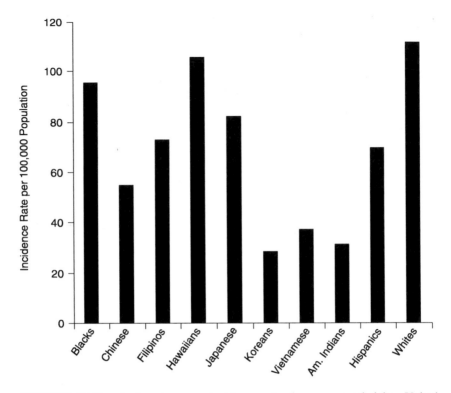

FIGURE 19 Female breast cancer incidence rates by race or ethnicity, United States, 1998–1992. SOURCE: American Cancer Society (1997).

United States women by race/ethnicity, age-adjusted to the 1970 United States population (American Cancer Society, 1995).

Mortality from breast cancer does not follow the same race/ethnicity pattern as that seen for breast cancer incidence. Breast cancer mortality rates among blacks are worse than among whites at all ages in the United States. The National Cancer Institute's (NCI's) Black/White Cancer Survival Study found that the risk of dying in the first 5 years after diagnosis was two times higher among black breast cancer patients than among white patients (Eley et al., 1994). The mortality rate among African American women over all ages is 31.2 per 100,000 population, compared to 26 per 100,000 population for white women (American Cancer Society, 1995). Mortality rates among other racial or ethnic groups, such as those shown in Figure 19, are less than 20 per 100,000 population (Perkins et al., 1995).

Unlike most chronic diseases, incidence rates of breast cancer are positively related to socioeconomic position. Reproductive factors known to increase risk for breast cancer include late age at first full-term pregnancy and low parity, both of which vary by socioeconomic position and likely contribute to the excess risk of breast cancer observed in better-educated, higher-income women (Kelsey and Bernstein, 1996). In contrast to breast cancer incidence, mortality from breast cancer is higher among more socioeconomically disadvantaged women. Growing evidence suggests that this is partly due to a more advanced stage at diagnosis and/or tumor characteristics. For example, Gordon (1995) reported that education and income were inversely related to estrogen receptor-negative tumors, after controlling for age, race or ethnicity, and known breast cancer risk factors. Estrogen receptor-negative breast tumors are strongly associated with poorer survival and, interestingly, are more likely to be diagnosed in African American women than white women.

Trends

Breast cancer incidence increased steadily between 1940 and 1982 and then more markedly between 1982 and 1987, prompting the suggestion, especially in the popular press, that an "epidemic" of breast cancer was occurring (Lantz and Booth, 1998). However, it is clear that a higher prevalence of mammography screenings, earlier diagnoses, and related factors account for a large proportion of this increase (Forbes, 1997; Wun et al., 1995). Moreover, incidence rates in younger women increased only slightly during the same time, and since 1987, incidence rates appear to have stabilized somewhat (Kosary et al., 1995), although this trend varies slightly by race/ethnicity. It has been suggested that the observed increase in breast cancer incidence was partially due to the increased prevalence of risk factors for breast cancer, particularly reproductive factors, such as later age at first birth and smaller family sizes than in previous generations (American Cancer Society, 1995). Until relatively recently, trends in incidence of breast cancer were similar for white women and African American women. Since 1992, however, it appears that the incidence has increased somewhat among African American women while decreasing or remaining stable among whites (American Cancer Society, 1995).

For white women in the United States, the mortality rate from breast cancer was relatively stable between 1940 and 1990 but has improved markedly during the 1990s, with the greatest improvements seen in younger age groups (National Cancer Institute, 1996). In contrast, the mortality rate among African American women increased by more than 19% between 1973 and 1988 and has continued to increase during the 1990s, although this increase has slowed to less than 3% (National Cancer Institute, 1996).

Taken together, the observed trends in breast cancer incidence and mortality suggest that with improved breast cancer management more women are surviving with breast cancer than ever before. However, there is clear evidence that racial disparities in both breast cancer incidence and mortality still exist.

Geographic Variation

Breast cancer incidence varies widely by geographic location. In the United States, evidence suggests that women living in the northern states tend to have higher rates of breast cancer than women living in the southern states (Kelsey and Horn-Ross, 1996). Breast cancer incidence also varies greatly internationally, as seen in Figure 20. The San Francisco Bay area has been identified as having one of the highest rates of breast cancer among white women in the world, with rates that are more than four times greater than in Asian countries and more than 40% higher than in most European countries (Parkin et al., 1997). Recently, it was determined that regional differences in reproductive risk factors (e.g., low parity, late age at first birth), many of which are associated with a more advantaged socioeconomic position, accounted for the high incidence rates of breast cancer in the Bay area (Robbins et al., 1997). Figure 20 also shows how breast cancer incidence varies by race/ethnicity throughout the world. For example, rates among non-Jewish Israeli women are dramatically lower than the rates among Jewish Israeli women. Also, rates in Hawaii vary greatly by ethnicity. Asian women generally have some of the lowest rates of incident breast cancer among developed nations; however, rates in Asia, as well as in central European nations, have risen markedly in recent years (Kelsey and Horn-Ross, 1993). For example, breast cancer incidence in Japanese women more than doubled in the 15-year period from 1970 to 1985, although rates of breast cancer in Japanese women are still dramatically lower than rates in most American women (Kelsey and Bernstein, 1996).

Costs

Breast cancer has enormous direct and indirect costs, as well as psychosocial costs in terms of reduced quality of life, stress, and the psychological demands on the individual, family member, and friends coping with the illness. An estimated $6.6 billion is spent each year in direct medical care costs for breast cancer in the United States alone (Brown and Fintor, 1995). Median survival time for breast cancer patients is nearly a decade; consequently, the greatest proportion (approximately 45%) of medical expenditures for breast cancer is for continuing care (Brown and Fintor, 1995). Nevertheless, with more than 43,000 female breast cancer deaths per year in the United States, it has been calculated that there are more than 800,000 person-years of life lost each year or 19 person-years lost per death (Brown et al., 1993). The nonmedical, indirect, and psychosocial costs of breast cancer have not been quantified but undoubtedly increase several fold the social and economic costs of this disease.

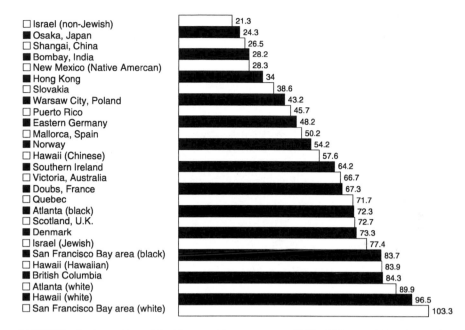

FIGURE 20 Age-adjusted incidence of breast cancer, 1988–1992, per 100,000 population. SOURCE: Adapted from Parkin et al., 1997.

Osteoporosis

Overall

It is estimated that approximately 6 million American men and women have osteoporosis and another 20 million have osteopenia (Looker et al., 1997). Prevalence is dramatically higher in women than in men (see Figure 21). Although peak bone mass is achieved in the second or third decade of life, osteoporosis is rare in individuals less than 50 years of age. In contrast, only 3% of women age 80 or older have normal bone density and 70% have evidence of osteoporosis at one or more skeletal sites (Cooper and Melton, 1996). Thus, osteoporosis can be characterized as a disorder of middle-aged and elderly adults. The greatest public health impact of osteoporosis derives from its accompanying increased risk of fractures. Osteoporotic fractures occur most frequently in the distal forearm, vertebrae, and hip (Cooper and Melton, 1996); indeed, vertebral fractures historically have been considered a defining clinical feature of osteoporosis (Albright et al., 1941). Recent estimates indicate that the age-adjusted incidence of vertebral fracture is more than twice as high as the incidence of hip fracture in women (18 per 1,000 person-years versus 6.2 per 1,000 person-years, respectively) (Melton et al., 1993); both are associated with increased morbidity and mortality in the elderly (Cooper et al. 1993; Melton, 1988).

National data on the epidemiology of osteoporosis and related fractures are somewhat limited, in part, because prior to the advent and widespread use of noninvasive bone densitometry methods such as dual energy x-ray absorptiometry (DEXA), osteoporosis was diagnosed only in the presence of a fracture. However, not all fractures, particularly vertebral fractures, are symptomatic or reach clinical attention. Presently, osteoporosis is defined by the World Health Organization (WHO) as bone mineral density more than 2.5 s.d. (standard deviation) below the young normal mean at one or more skeletal sites (WHO, 1994). Research indicates that a 1 s.d. decrease in femoral bone density is equivalent to a 14-year age increase in risk of hip fracture (Melton et al., 1993). Bone density decreases greatly with age, especially among women, making age one of the strongest risk factors for osteoporosis. However, other factors also influence bone density. For example, among women, bone loss is accelerated after natural or surgical menopause when levels of estrogen drop dramatically.

Other known or suspected risk factors for decreased bone density include tobacco use, physical inactivity, and alcohol abuse (Seeman, 1996; Snow et al., 1996). Each of these is associated with increased risk of fractures. Age-related declines in bone strength also contribute to the increased risk of fractures in elderly populations.

Distribution by Race and Sex

Rates of occurrence of osteoporosis and osteoporotic fractures vary greatly by race and ethnicity, with higher rates consistently observed in whites compared to nonwhites, particularly in North America and northern Europe (Villa and Nelson, 1996). The Third National Health and Nutrition Examination Survey (NHANES III) found a higher prevalence of osteoporosis in whites than blacks or Hispanics for both women and men (Looker et al., 1997). (See Figure 22.) One recent United States study found that age- and sex-adjusted rates of hip fracture for persons over age 50 were nearly three and a half times greater in whites than in blacks (Baron et al., 1994). Hispanics and Asians also have much lower rates of hip fracture than whites (Silverman and Madison, 1988). In addition, the age-related increase in hip fracture is observed in all populations but tends to occur at an earlier age among non-Hispanic whites than Asian, Hispanic, or black populations (Maggi et al., 1991).

Osteoporosis and related fractures occur more frequently in women than in men. NHANES III was the first nationally representative survey to assess bone mineral density using DEXA to determine the prevalence of osteoporosis in the United States adult population (Looker et al., 1995). Femoral bone density was assessed in 14,646 participants age 20 or older (63% of those eligible). Data were age adjusted to the 1980 United States census population, and prevalence of osteoporosis and low bone density or osteopenia (more than 1 but less than 2.5 s.d. below the young normal mean) were determined for women and men age 50 or older (see Figure 21). These data indicate that 15% of American

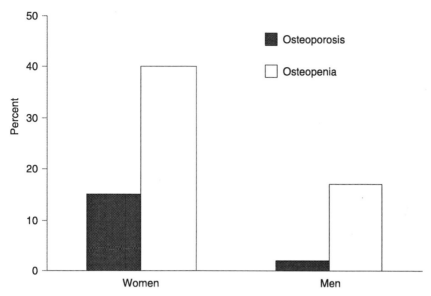

FIGURE 21 Age–adjusted prevalence of osteoporosis and osteopenia of the femur in noninstitutionalized U.S. adults, age 50 and older: NHANES III.

women age 50 or older have osteoporosis and that an additional 40% have osteopenia (Looker et al., 1997). Using the same absolute bone density cutpoint for men as for women (0.56 g/cm^2 for femoral neck bone density), it was estimated that 2% of American men age 50 or over have osteoporosis and another 17% have osteopenia (Looker et al., 1997). However, extrapolating the WHO diagnostic criteria, which did not address osteoporosis or low bone density in nonwhite or male populations, so that the referent was mean bone density in non-Hispanic white men ages 20–29, produced higher estimates. With the male referent, estimates are that 4% of men age 50 or older have osteoporosis and another 33% meet criteria for osteopenia. These estimates thus show that the prevalence of osteoporosis is four to seven times greater in women than men (depending on the referent group used). Other research indicates that the estimated lifetime risk of a hip fracture, distal forearm fracture, or vertebral fracture is three times greater for women than men (39.7% for women and 13.1% for men, respectively) age 50 and older (Melton et al., 1992).

Distribution by Socioeconomic Position

Few data are available that examine osteoporosis or fracture incidence by socioeconomic position. Several of the risk factors for fracture (e.g., alcohol abuse, cigarette smoking, physical inactivity) are known to vary by socioeconomic position, with greater prevalence of these behavioral or life-style factors

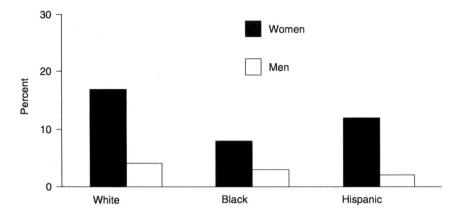

FIGURE 22 Unadjusted prevalence of osteoporosis of femoral bone by race/ ethnicity among noninstitutionalized U.S. adults, age 50 years and older: NHANES III.

among poorer persons. One study reported that hip fracture incidence rates in elderly white women in the United States are higher in regions with greater poverty (Jacobsen et al., 1990). In addition, the use of postmenopausal hormone replacement therapy, which protects against bone loss, is more prevalent among socioeconomically advantaged women (Matthews et al., 1996). However, other factors that appear to protect against age-related bone loss, such as obesity, are more prevalent in lower socioeconomic strata (Sobal and Stunkard, 1989). Moreover, blacks and Hispanics, who disproportionately occupy these lower strata (especially in the United States), are known to have greater bone density and lower rates of osteoporosis and osteopenia (Looker et al., 1997). Clearly, the association between osteoporosis and associated fractures and socioeconomic position is complex, and research is needed to determine what the patterns of association are for men and women of different racial/ethnic groups.

Trends

A lack of data prevents us from knowing if there have been marked trends in the prevalence or incidence of osteoporosis in the past. However, there is evidence that the incidence of hip fractures increased fourfold between 1930 and 1980 in white men and even more dramatically in women (Melton et al., 1987), even after taking into consideration the increase in the elderly population. It has been suggested that the increasing prevalence of sedentary life-styles and greater frailty among the elderly may be contributing to this phenomenon (Cooper and Melton, 1996). Future expectations are that the prevalence of osteoporosis and related fractures will increase substantially because these are problems of the elderly. The number of individuals age 65 or older is expected to increase fivefold in the next 50 years (Cooper et al., 1992). Consequently, it is anticipated that the public health impact of osteoporosis will increase enormously in the coming decades. For example, in 1990, there were more than 1.1 million hip fractures in women and 463,000 hip fractures in men worldwide, and it is predicted that these numbers will increase fourfold by 2050 (Cooper et al., 1992). Interestingly, because of rapidly aging populations, a greater increase in the incidence of hip fractures is expected in Latin American and Asian countries than in North American and European countries in the coming decades, making osteoporosis and related fractures a global public health challenge (Cooper and Melton, 1996).

Geographic Variation

Specific data assessing geographic variations in osteoporosis are sparse. However, there is clear evidence that the incidence of hip fracture varies by geographic region. The highest rates are in Scandinavia, followed by the United States, western Europe, Asia, and Africa (Melton et al., 1987). Rates vary markedly within regions, also. For example, there is a sevenfold difference in incidence of hip fractures within the countries of western Europe (Johnell et al., 1992). A study by Jacobsen and colleagues found interesting regional variations in hip fracture incidence in white women age 65 and older within the United States also (Jacobsen et al., 1990). Data from the Health Care Financing Administration, the Department of Veterans Affairs, the Bureau of the Census, and the Bureau of Health Professions' 1988 Area Resource file were used to examine age-adjusted rates of hip fracture by county for the 48 contiguous states. Figure 23 graphically depicts the findings, which show clear geographic variation, with higher rates in the south. Also, hip fracture incidence rates were positively related to the proportion of elderly below the poverty level and the percentage of farmland in the county, but inversely associated with water hardness and hours of January sunlight. Interestingly, however, regional variations in alcohol consumption, cigarette smoking, obesity, physical activity, or Scandinavian heritage did not account for the observed geographic patterns. The findings suggest that unobserved or unmeasured environmental characteristics and/or individual risk factors are contributing to the geographic variation in hip fracture rates. It is unknown if similar patterns are present for nonwhite populations or men.

Cost

It is difficult to determine the economic costs of osteoporosis, per se. However, the overall cost of fractures is estimated to be $20 billion annually in the United States (Praemer et al., 1992). Recent estimates suggest that hip fractures account for 300,000 hospitalizations annually, with an associated tab of $9 billion in direct medical costs (Bason, 1996). Moreover, it is estimated that hip fractures account for more than 9 years of potential life lost per 1,000 women (Eiskjaer et al., 1992). Because osteoporotic fractures disproportionately affect elderly individuals, the reductions in survival and lost wages associated with osteoporosis are generally determined to be less than similar figures for other diseases, such as the others reviewed in this chapter. Nevertheless, it is clear that osteoporosis and related fractures are an important and growing public health problem of our aging population that have enormous economic costs in terms of increased morbidity and mortality and lost productivity.

MAKING SENSE OF THE DISTRIBUTION OF DISEASE AND ITS DETERMINANTS

The six problems described above illustrate the tremendous heterogeneity there is in the occurrence of diseases and in important public health problems. This heterogeneity by place, race/ethnic group, gender, socioeconomic position, and time ought to be the starting place for most analyses. The extent of this heterogeneity highlights the implausibility that a single set of explanatory determinants will be found or that a single set of interventions will suffice to reduce the population burden from these problems. Instead, we think the heterogeneity points to the importance of the multilevel approach presented in Figure 5. In what follows, we illustrate such an approach to the public health issues previously described. Because such an approach is in its infancy, for the most part the discussion is a mixture of empirical findings, evidence-based speculation, and arguments based on plausibility. Because it is the major focus of this report, for the most part we highlight the potential importance of domains that range from the behavioral to the social and economic.

Economic and Social Policies

Because of the clear relationships between socioeconomic position and these six problems of public health importance, it is likely that actions that have an impact on the socioeconomic position of individuals, families, and communities can potentially reduce the public health burden associated with these problems. Note that this is true even for breast cancer, for although incidence increases with SEP, mortality decreases with increasing SEP (Eley et al., 1994; American Cancer Society, 1995). At the governmental level, policies related to taxation, cash and noncash transfers, and employment may be some of the most important instruments. For example, the introduction of the earned income tax credit resulted in a reduction in the prevalence of children living in families below the poverty line (Plotnick, 1997), presumably with related health effects, and we are still awaiting the results of recent changes in welfare and entitlement policies on the financial status and health of poor families (Danziger et al., 1999). The changes in economic status of individuals and the communities they live in could conceivably lead to better health among pregnant women and women of childbearing age, thereby leading to a reduced risk of low birthweight. Increased SEP also

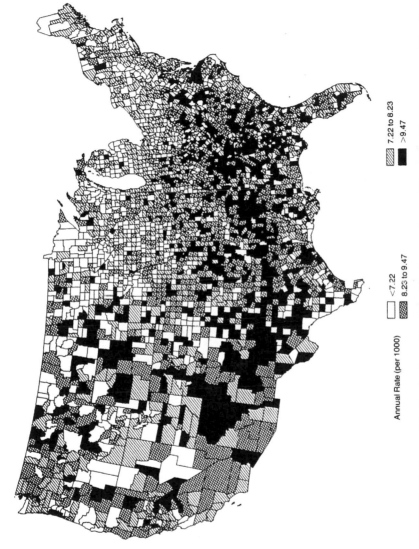

FIGURE 23 Geographic distribution of incident hip fracture in non-Hispanic white women age 65 and older. source: Reprinted, with permission, from Jacobsen et al. (1990). Copyright 1990 by the American Medical Association.

Annual Rate (per 1000)

<7.22
7.22 to 8.23
8.23 to 9.47
>9.47

allows one to mitigate, or move away from, environmental exposures that might be important in the etiology and progression of childhood asthma, to live in environments with lower levels of stress and violence.

Economic policies that alter workforce participation by women may have an effect on reproductive patterns, thereby altering the risk of breast cancer. The same forces may have an impact for both men and women on levels of job strain, which may alter the risk of developing CVD or its risk factors (Schnall et al., 1994) and triggering acute events (Mittleman and Maclure, 1997). Taxation polices also can have a substantial impact on the development and maintenance of unhealthy behaviors such as smoking (Hu et al., 1995). Taxation policies that reduce funding of education also may influence the availability of physical activity at school through reduction in physical education classes (Luepker, 1999). Zoning policies and the design of living, work, and educational environments can conceivably influence the amount and patterns of leisure time and occupational physical activity.

Through mechanisms that are less well understood (Kaplan et al., 1996; Lynch et al., 2000), economic policies that alter the extent of income and wealth inequality in the population may alter disease risks independent of effects on individual incomes or wealth. In addition to being related to risk of death from all causes, increasing income inequality is associated with increased levels of CVD and other diseases (Kennedy et al., 1996; Kaplan and Lynch, 2000). The extent of variations in income inequality, presumably related to government taxation and transfer policies, on infant mortality was shown by Ross et al. (in press) who compared the association between income inequality and infant mortality in metropolitan areas in the United States and Canada. Metropolitan areas in Canada had much lower levels of income inequality than those in the United States and much less geographic variation in income inequality. This combination of decreased income inequality and restriction in the range of income inequality resulting from Canadian economic policies was associated with considerably lower rates of infant mortality in these analyses.

Social policies also can have a substantial impact. The most obvious relates to access to health insurance and state-of-the-art medical care. To the extent that there is no consensus regarding the need for universal access, then we can expect to see substantial variations by SEP and race/ethnicity in low birthweight and the diagnosis and treatment of asthma, as well as screening, treatment, and outcomes of CVD, breast cancer, and osteoporosis. Social policies regarding regulation of gun ownership, types of weapons allowed, safety devices, enforcement of regulations, and policing may all have an impact on firearm-related deaths (Wintemute, 1999). In general, social policies that have an effect on employment, or lack of it, the nature of work, community neighborhood structures, transportation, housing, schools, medical care, and other social institutions may all have an impact on the distribution of public health problems within and between populations and areas. Social policies and norms related to factors such as tobacco and alcohol use also may have a substantial impact because even changes in average consumption levels may influence both the total burden of disease associated with consumption and the prevalence of heavy smoking and drinking (Rose, 1992).

Institutions

In a sense, institutions cannot be separated from the social, cultural, historical, and economic policies that create and sustain them. However, it is important to see the extent to which institutions, such as those related to the worlds of education, work, medical care, the criminal justice system, and housing, may be important determinants of public health problems and solutions. For example, it has been suggested that school and child care environments may increase the risk of childhood asthma and its complications via exposure to secondhand smoke (Bremberg, 1999) and through a lack of support for behavioral self-management strategies (Clark et al., 1999). Similarly, the school environment via promotion of poor nutritional habits through school lunch programs or on-site fast-food outlets, and reduction of school-based physical activity programs may contribute to increased risk of the development of CVD as well as decreased bone mass. The school environment also can support factors related to increased risk of later development of breast cancer, through both dietary and reproductive risk factors. School-related factors also may contribute to patterns of bullying, gang formation, and violence that may lead to firearm-related injuries.

Workplaces, through both working conditions and the physical environment, may increase risk. Stressful working conditions, inflexible working schedules, and afterwork effects of physically and emotionally demanding jobs may all directly contribute to increased risk of CVD (Karasek and Theorell, 1992). Indirectly, they may contribute to patterns of smoking and alcohol use and physical inactivity that increase risks of low-birthweight, breast cancer, CVD, and osteoporosis. Work schedules that make it difficult to utilize preventive or curative services could increase risk of low-birthweight deliveries, CVD, and early detection of breast cancer and osteoporosis.

The physical environment of workplaces and other institutional settings also can increase risk via exposure to tobacco smoke and other toxic substances. In addition, work environments that discourage physical activity in favor of taking elevators or discourage healthy eating via fast-food and vending machine availability also may increase risk of numerous outcomes.

Neighborhoods, Communities, and Living Conditions

A growing literature indicates that characteristics of neighborhoods and communities are associated with variations in health outcomes and individual level risk factors (Macintyre et al., 1993; Kaplan, 1996; Diez-Roux, 1998; Yen and Kaplan 1998, 1999). There are many pathways through which such area differences in health status and risk factors might be generated. Abatement of exposures to lead and other toxins, improvements in ambient air quality, and reduction of diesel exhaust could have an impact on asthma, low birthweight, and possibly osteoporosis. Environmental restrictions on smoking and the sale and consumption of alcoholic beverages, as well as local advertising in support of smoking and drinking, may influence the rates of all six of the public health problems highlighted in this chapter. Neighborhoods differ in the availability of affordable, nutritious food (Troutt, 1993) and in access to preventive and curative services, possibly having an impact on low birthweight, asthma, cardiovascular disease, breast cancer, and osteoporosis. Lack of access to parks and opportunities for safe recreational areas may influence levels of physical activity.

Social and economic characteristics of communities also may have a great influence on public health (Haan et al., 1987; Macintyre et al., 1993; Sampson et al., 1997; Brooks-Gunn et al., 1997; Wing et al., 1988). The extent to which residents of an area feel interconnected, will help each other, and feel responsible for the "commons" is associated with lower rates of violence, much of which is firearm related (Sampson et al., 1997). Levels of social support can be influenced by neighborhood and housing design and may influence birth outcomes (Nuckolls et al., 1972), cardiovascular disease (Kaplan et al., 1988), treatment of childhood asthma (Smyth et al., 1999), and resolution of violence that can lead to firearm-related deaths.

Living conditions, reflected in the quality of housing and residential environments, may be associated with low birthweight, asthma, cardiovascular disease, and osteoporosis and the risk of hip fracture. For example, levels of allergens and exposure to environmental tobacco smoke may be associated with asthma, and conditions that increase the risk of transmission of various infectious agents may thereby lead to exacerbation of asthma (Clark et al., 1999), increased risk of low birthweight (Romero et al. 1988), and possibly, cardiovascular disease (Patel et al., 1995). Environmental hazards in the home may be associated with increased risk of hip fracture (Rubenstein et al., 1988; Grisso et al., 1996), and environmental barriers outside the home could be associated with reduction in physical activity (Kaplan, 1997).

Social Relationships

The quantity, quality, and scope of social relationships can influence the incidence and progression of a variety of health problems (Cohen and Syme, 1985). Social support and social network participation have been shown to be associated with pregnancy complications (Nuckolls et al., 1972), cardiovascular disease (Kaplan et al., 1988), breast cancer prognosis (Spiegel et al., 1989; Reynolds and Kaplan, 1990; Reynolds et al., 1994; Shrock et al., 1999), recovery from hip fracture (Cummings et al., 1988), asthma symptoms (Clark et al., 1999), and pregnancy complications (Nuckolls et al., 1972). Social groups also may influence, in both a positive and a negative direction, the adoption and maintenance of adverse behavioral risk factors such as smoking and excessive alcohol consumption. Clearly, social processes are involved in the promotion or inhibition of violence and its sequelae such as firearm-related mortality. Strain associated with problematic relationships, or overload related to multiple social responsibilities, may increase cardiovascular risk and also may make it more difficult to access preventive or curative services.

Individual Risk Factors

There is ample evidence that the behaviors of individuals, such as tobacco and alcohol consumption, physical inactivity, and diet, are critically associated with important public health problems (McGinnis and Foege, 1993). Because this information is well known and readily available it is not reviewed in this paper. Other individual characteristics related to personality, negative affect, coping, and attitudes also are critically important. For example, considerable evidence now underscores the importance of psychological states related to negative affect and hostility in the pathogenesis and triggering of cardiovascular events and the progression of cardiovascular disease (Mittleman and Maclure, 1995; Everson et al., 1996, 1997), and there is some indication that psychological distress may exacerbate asthma symptoms (Smyth et al., 1999). These states can have indirect impacts on low birthweight, breast cancer, cardiovascular disease, and osteoporosis via their influence on access to and use of preventive and curative services, their impact on social relations, and, possibly, through the influence of psychological states on neuroendocrine and immune pathways.

CONCLUSIONS

We have briefly outlined the heterogeneity in prevalence, distribution, and trends for life expectancy and a number of important public health problems. The usual approach is to adopt either a perspective that privileges individual risk factors, which have been termed by some as the "real" causes of disease (McGinnis and Foege, 1993) or a perspective that similarly privileges an increasingly molecular understanding. Either approach, in our opinion, is likely to be extremely limited in understanding variations in disease incidence or prevalence between groups, places, or across time and consequently will generally be unsuccessful in suggesting effective intervention strategies to reduce the population burden from these problems. Instead, we have tried to argue for an integrated approach that views these problems within a multilevel framework and attempts to build bridges between levels rather than attributing primary importance to one level or another. It is likely that some success will come from efforts at specific levels, but our most complete understanding and most successful intervention attempts may very well come from a multilevel focus. In order to make progress, there is a need for considerably more information on determinants of health that lie "upstream" from individual behaviors.

In an influential book on preventive medicine, the late Geoffrey Rose declared, "The primary determinants of disease are mainly economic and social, and therefore its remedies must be economic and social" (Rose, 1992, p. 129), and a recent report on the "future of medicine" (Hastings Center Report, 1996) called for an effort on the scope of the Human Genome Project directed at understanding the social determinants of health. As work proceeds at a fast pace on both the behavioral and the molecular bases of disease, we need to proceed apace at accumulating knowledge of the upstream determinants of health that include social relations, neighborhoods and communities, institutions, and social and economic policies. Such an effort bridged with expanding knowledge from more "downstream" pursuits could add to the twenty-first century's armamentarium for improving the public's health.

REFERENCES

Albright F, Smith PH, Richardson AM. Postmenopausal osteoporosis: Its clinical features. *Journal of the American Medical Association* 1941; 116:2465–2474.

American Cancer Society. *Breast Cancer Facts and Figures, 1996.* Atlanta: American Cancer Society, 1995.

American Lung Association. *Trends in Asthma Morbidity and Mortality.* Washington, DC: Epidemiology and Statistics Unit, 1998.

Arriaga EE. Measuring and explaining the change in life expectancies. *Demography* 1984; 21(1):83–96.

Arriaga EE. Changing trends in mortality decline during the last decades. In: Ruzicka L, Wunsch G, Kane P, eds., *Differential Mortality: Methodological Issues and Biosocial Factors.* Oxford: Clarendon Press, 1989; 105–129.

Baker SP, O'Neill B, Karpf RS. *The Injury Fact Book,* 2nd ed. New York: Oxford University Press, 1992.

Barnett E, Armstrong DL, Casper ML. Evidence of increasing coronary heart disease mortality among black men of lower social class. *Annals of Epidemiology* 1999; 464–471.

Baron JA, Barrett J, Malenka D, Fisher E, Kniffin W, Bubolz T, Tosteson T. Racial differences in fracture risk. *Epidemiology* 1994; 5:42–47.

Bason WE. Secular trends in hip fracture occurrence and survival: Age and sex differences. *Journal of Aging and Health* 1996; 8:538–553.

Bremberg S. *Evidence-Based Health Promotion for Children and Adolescents in Stockholm County.* Stockholm: Stockholm County Council, 1999.

Brooks-Gunn J, Duncan GJ, Aber JL. *Neighborhood Poverty: Context and Consequences for Children,* Vols. 1 and 2. New York: Russell Sage, 1997.

Brown ML, Fintor L. The economic burden of cancer. In: Greenwald P, Kramer BS, Weed DL, eds., *Cancer Prevention and Control.* New York: Marcel Dekker, Inc., 1995; 69–81.

Brown ML, Hodgson TA, Rice DP. Economic impact of cancer in the United States. In: Schottenfeld D, Fraumeni J, eds., *Cancer Epidemiology and Prevention,* 2nd ed. New York: Oxford University Press, 1993; 255–266.

Annie E. Casey Foundation. *Kids Count Data Book.* Baltimore: The Annie E. Casey Foundation, 1999.

Centers for Disease Control and Prevention. On-line. http://wonder.cdc.gov/

Centers for Disease Control and Prevention. *Vital and Health Statistics. National Hospital Discharge Survey: Annual Summary, 1993.* DHHS Publication No. PHS 95–1782, 1995.

Clark NM, Brown RW, Parker E, et al. Childhood asthma. *Environmental Health Perspectives* 1999; (suppl 3): 421–429.

Cohen S, Syme SL, eds., *Social Support and Health*. Orlando, FL: Academic Press, Inc., 1985.

Collins JG. Prevalence of selected chronic conditions: United States 1990–1992. National Center for Health Statistics. *Vital Health Statistics* 1997; 10:194.

Cook PJ, Lawrence BA, Ludwig J, Miller TR. The medical costs of gunshot injuries in the United States. *Journal of the American Medical Association* 1999; 282(5):447–454.

Cookson JB. Prevalence rates of asthma in developing countries and their comparison with those in Europe and North America. *Chest* 1987; 91(Suppl. 6):97S–103S.

Cooper C, Atkinson EJ, Jacobsen SJ, O'Fallon WM, Melton LJ III. Population-based study of survival after osteoporotic fractures. *American Journal of Epidemiology* 1993; 137:1001–1005.

Cooper C, Campion G, Melton LJ III. Hip fractures in the elderly: A worldwide projection. *Osteoporosis International*. 1992; 2:285–289.

Cooper C, Melton LJ III. Magnitude and impact of osteoporosis and fractures. In: Marcus R, Feldman D, Kelsey J, eds., *Osteoporosis*. San Diego: Academic Press, 1996; 419 434.

Crain EF, Weiss KB, Bijur PE, Hersh M, Westbrook L, Stein RE. An estimate of the prevalence of asthma and wheezing among inner-city children. *Pediatrics* 1994; 94:356–362.

Cummings SR, Phillips SL, Wheat ME, Black D, Goosby E, Wlodarczyk D, Trafton P, Jergesen H, Winograd CH, Hulley SB. Recovery of function after hip fracture. The role of social supports. *Journal of the American Geriatrics Society* 1988; 36(9): 801–806.

Danziger S, Corcoran M, Danziger S, Heflin CM. Work, income and material hardship after welfare reform. Joint Center for Poverty Research Working Paper 114.0, 199–08-01, October 1999. On-line. http://www.jcpr.org/wp/Wpprofile.cfm?ID=114.0.

David RJ, Collins JW. Differing birth weight among infants of U.S.-born blacks, African-born blacks and U.S.-born whites. *New England Journal of Medicine* 1997; 337: 1209–1214.

Diez-Roux AV. Bringing context back into epidemiology: Variables and fallacies in multilevel analysis. *American Journal of Public Health* 1998; 88(2): 216–222.

Eiskjaer S, Østgård SE, Jakobsen BW, Jensen J, Lucht U. Years of potential life lost after hip fracture among postmenopausal women. *Acta Orthopaedica Scandinavica*. 1992; 63:293–296.

Eley JW, Hill HA, Chen VW, Austin DF, Wesley MN, Muss HB, Greenberg RS, Coates RJ, Correa P, Redmond CK, Hunter CP, Herman AA, Kurman R, Blacklow R, Shapiro Sam, and Edwards BK. Racial differences in survival from breast cancer. Results of the National Cancer Institute Black/White Cancer Survival Study. *Journal of the American Medical Association* 1994; 272:947–954.

Evans R. Asthma among minority children: A growing problem. *Chest* 1992; 101:368S–371S.

Everson SA, Goldberg DE, Kaplan GA, Cohen RD, Pukkala E, Tuomilehto J, Salonen JT. Hopelessness and risk of mortality and incidence of myocardial infarction and cancer. *Psychosomatic Medicine* 1996; 5:113–21.

Everson SA, Kaplan GA, Goldberg DE, Salonen R, Salonen JT. Hopelessness and 4-year progression of carotid atherosclerosis: The Kuopio Ishemic Heart Disease Risk Factor Study. *Arteriosclerosis, Thrombosis, and Vascular Biology* 1997; 17:1490–1495.

Fang J, Madhavan S, Alderman MH. Low birth weight: Race and maternal nativity—Impact of community income. *Pediatrics* 1999; 103(1):E5.

Feuer EJ, Wun LM, Boring CC, Flander WD, Timmel MJ, Tong T. The lifetime risk of developing breast cancer. *Journal of the National Cancer Institute* 1993; 85:892–897.

Fingerhut LA, Ingram DD, Feldman JJ. Homicide rates among U.S. teenagers and young adults: Differences by mechanism, level of urbanization, race, and sex, 1987 through 1995. *Journal of the American Medical Association* 1998; 280(5):423–427.

Forbes JF. The incidence of breast cancer: The global burden, public health considerations. *Seminars in Oncology* 1997; 24(1 Suppl 1):S1-20–S1-35.

Goff DC, Nichaman MZ, Chan W, Ramsey DJ, Labarthe DR, Ortiz C. Greater incidence of hospitalized myocardial infarction among Mexican Americans than non-Hispanic whites. The Corpus Christi Heart Project, 1988–1992. *Circulation* 1997; 95(6): 1433–1440.

Gordon NH. Association of education and income with estrogen receptor status in primary breast cancer. *American Journal of Epidemiology* 1995; 142:796–803.

Grant EN, Wagner R, Weiss KB. Observations on emerging patterns of asthma in our society. *Journal of Allergy and Clinical Immunology* 1999; 104(2, Part 2): S1–9.

Grisso JA, Capezuti E, and Schwartz A. Falls as risk factors for fractures. In: Marcus R, Feldman D, Kelsey J, eds., *Osteoporosis*. San Diego: Academic Press, 1996, 599–611.

Haan M, Kaplan GA, Camacho T. Poverty and health: Prospective evidence from the Alameda County Study. *American Journal of Epidemiology* 1987; 125(6):989-98.

Haan MN, Kaplan GA, Syme SL. Socioeconomic status and health: Old observations and new thoughts. In: Bunker JP, Gomby DS, Kehrer BH, eds., *Pathways to Health: The Role of Social Factors*, Menlo Park, CA: Henry J. Kaiser Family Foundation, 1985; 76–135.

Hastings Center Report. The goals of medicine: Setting new priorities. An International Project of the Hastings Center. *Hastings Center Report* November–December 1996; Special Supplement:S-19.

Henderson CI. Breast cancer. In: Murphy GP, Lawrence WL, Lenhard R, eds., *Clinical Oncology*. Atlanta: American Cancer Society; 1995; 198–219.

Hoyert, DL, Kochanek, KD, Murphy, SL. 1999. Deaths: Final data for 1997. *National Vital Statistics Reports* 47:19 (http://www.cdc.gov/nchs/data/nvs47_19.pdf).

Hu TW, Sung HY, Keeler TE. Reducing cigarette consumption in California: Tobacco taxes vs an anti-smoking media campaign. *American Journal of Public Health* 1995; 85(9):1218–1222.

Jacobsen SJ, Goldberg J, Miles TP, Brody JA, Stiers W, Rimm AA. Regional variation in the incidence of hip fracture. *Journal of the American Medical Association* 1990; 264:500–502.

Johnell O, Gullberg B, Allander E, Kanis JA. MEDOS Study Group. The apparent incidence of hip fracture in Europe: A study of national register sources. *Osteoporosis International* 1992; 2:298–302.

Kaplan GA. People and places: Contrasting perspectives on the association between social class and health. *International Journal of Health Services* 1996; 26:507–519.

Kaplan GA. Behavioral, social, and socioenvironmental factors adding years to life and life to years. In: Hickey T, Speers MA, Prohaska TR, eds., *Public Health and Aging*. Baltimore, Johns Hopkins University Press, 1997; 37–52.

Kaplan, GA, Haan MN, Syme SL, Minkler M, Winkleby M. Socioeconomic status and health. In: Amler RW, Dull HB, eds. *Closing the Gap: The Burden of Unnecessary Illness*. New York: Oxford University Press, 1987; 125–129.

Kaplan GA, Salonen JT, Cohen RD, Brand RJ, Syme SL, Puska P. Social connections and mortality from all causes and from cardiovascular disease: Prospective evidence from eastern Finland. *American Journal of Epidemiology* 1988; 128(2):370–380.

Kaplan GA, Keil JE. Socioeconomic factors and cardiovascular disease: A review of the literature. *Circulation* 1993; 88(4):1973–1978.

Kaplan, GA, Pamuk, E, Lynch, JW, Cohen, RD, Balfour, J. Inequality in income and mortality in the United States: Analysis of mortality and potential pathways. *BMJ* 1996; 312:999–1003.

Kaplan GA, Lynch JW. Socioeconomic considerations in the primordial prevention of cardiovascular disease. *Preventive Medicine* in press.

Karasek RA, Theorell T (contributor). *Work: Stress, Productivity, and the Reconstruction of Working Life*. Basic Books: New York 1992.

Kaufman, JS, Cooper, RS, McGee, DL. Socioeconomic status and health in blacks and whites: The problem of residual confounding and the resiliency of race. *Epidemiology* 1997; 8:621–628.

Kelsey JL, Horn-Ross PL. Breast cancer: Magnitude of the problem and descriptive epidemiology. *Epidemiologic Reviews* 1993; 15:7–16.

Kelsey JL, Bernstein L. Epidemiology and prevention of breast cancer. *Annual Review of Public Health* 1996; 17:47–67.

Kennedy BP, Kawachi I, Prothrow-Stith D. Income distribution and mortality: Cross-sectional ecological study of the Robin Hood index in the United States. *British Medical Journal* 1996; 312(7037):1004–1007.

Kosary CL, Ries LAG, Miller BA, Hankey BF, Harras A, Edwards BK. *SEER Cancer Statistics Review, 1973–1992: Tables and Graphs*. National Cancer Institute. NIH Publication No. 95-2789. Bethesda, MD: 1995.

Krieger N, Rowley D, Hermann AA, Avery B, Phillips MT. Racism, sexism, and social class: Implications for studies of health, disease, and well-being. *American Journal of Preventive Medicine* 1993; 9(Suppl 6):82–122.

Krieger N, Williams DR, Moss N. Measuring social class in U.S. public health research: Concepts, methodologies, and guidelines. *Annual Review of Public Health* 1997; 13:341–378.

Lantz PM, Booth KM. The social construction of the breast cancer epidemic. *Social Science and Medicine*. 1998;46:907–918.

Lewitt EM, Schuurman Baker L, Corman H, Shiono PH. The direct cost of low birth weight. In: *The Future of Children*, Vol. 5. Palo Alto, CA: The David and Lucille Packard Foundation, 1995, 35–56.

Looker AC, Johnston CC, Jr, Wahner HW, Dunn WL, Calvo MS, Harris TB, Heyse SP, and Lindsay RL. Prevalence of low femoral bone density in older U.S. women from NHANES III. *Journal of Bone and Mineral Research* 1995; 10:796–802.

Looker AC, Orwoll ES, Johnston CC, Jr., Lindsay RL, Wahner HW, Dunn WL, Calvo MS, Harris TB, and Heyse SP. Prevalence of low femoral bone density in older U.S. adults from NHANES III. *Journal of Bone and Mineral Research* 1997; 12:1761–1771.

Luepker RV. How physically active are American children and what can we do about it? *International Journal of Obesity and Related Metabolic Disorders* 1999; 23(Suppl 2):S12-17.

Lynch JW. Socioeconomic factors in the behavioral and psychosocial epidemiology of cardiovascular disease. In: Schneiderman N, Gentry J, da Silva JM, Speers M, Tomes H., eds., *Integrating Behavioral and Social Sciences with Public Health*. Washington, DC.: APA Press, (in press).

Lynch JW, Davey Smith G, Kaplan GA, House JS. Income inequality and health: A neomaterial interpretation. *British Medical Journal*, in press.

Lynch JW, Kaplan GA, Salonen JT. Why do poor people behave poorly? Variation in adult health behaviors and psycho-social characteristics by stages of the socioeconomic lifecourse. *Social Science and Medicine* 1997; 44:809–819.

MacIntyre S, Maciver S, Sooman A. Area, class, and health: Should we be studying people or places? *Journal of Social Policy* 1993; 22:213–234.

Maggi S, Kelsey JL, Litvak J, Heyse SP. Incidence of hip fracture in the elderly: A cross-national analysis. *Osteoporosis International* 1991; 1:232–241.

Malveaux FJ, Fletcher-Vincent SA. Environmental risk factors of childhood asthma in urban centers. *Environmental Health Perspectives* 1995: 103 (Suppl. 6):59–62.

Mannino DM, Homa DM, Pertowski CA et al. Surveillance for asthma—United States, 1960–1995.Atlants Centers for Disease Control and Prevention 1998; 47:S-1.

Massey D, Denton NA. *American Apartheid: Segregation and the Making of the Underclass.* Cambridge, MA: Harvard University Press, 1993.

Matthews KA, Kuller LH, Wing RR, Meilahn EN, Plantinga P. Prior to use of estrogen replacement therapy, are users healthier than nonusers? *American Journal of Epidemiology* 1996; 143:971–978.

Max W, Rice DP. Shooting in the dark: Estimating the cost of firearm injuries. *Health Affairs* 1993; 12(4):171–185.

McGinnis, JM, Foege WH. Actual causes of death in the United States. *Journal of the American Medical Association* 1993; 270(18):2207–2212.

Melton LJ III. Epidemiology of fractures. In: Riggs BL, Melton LJ III, eds., *Osteoporosis: Etiology, Diagnosis, and Management.* New York: Raven Press, 1988:133–154.

Melton LJ III, Chrischilles EA, Cooper C, Lane AW, Riggs BL. How many women have osteoporosis? *Journal of Bone and Mineral Research* 1992; 7:1005–1010.

Melton LJ III, Lane AW, Cooper C, Eastell R, O'Fallon WM, Riggs BL. Prevalence and incidence of vertebral deformities. *Osteoporosis International* 1993; 3:113–119.

Melton LJ III, O'Fallon WM, Riggs BL. Secular trends in the incidence of hip fractures. *Calcified Tissue International* 1987; 41:57–64.

Mittleman MA, Maclure M. Mental stress during daily life triggers myocardial ischemia (editorial; comment). *Journal of the American Medical Association* 1997; 277(19): 1558–1559.

Murray, CJL, Michaud, CM, McKenna, MT, Marks, JS. *U.S. Patterns of Mortality by County and Race: 1965–1994, U.S. Burden of Disease and Injury Monograph Series.* Cambridge, MA: Harvard Center for Population and Development Studies, 1998.

National Cancer Institute. NCI reports improvements in breast cancer death rate, 1996. On-line. http://cis.nci.nih.gov/fact/625.html.

National Center for Health Statistics. *Health, United States, 1996–1997 Injury Chartbook.* Hyattsville, MD: NCHS, 1997.

National Center for Health Statistics. *Health, United States, 1998 with Socioeconomic Status and Health Chartbook.* Hyattsville, MD: NCHS, 1998.

National Center for Health Statistics. *Health, United States, 1999 with Socioeconomic Status and Health Chartbook.* Hyattsville, MD: NCHS, 1999.

National Heart, Lung, and Blood Institute. *Chartbook of U.S. National Data on Socioeconomic Status and Cardiovascular Health and Disease.* Washington, DC: NIH, June 1995.

National Heart, Lung, and Blood Institute. *Morbidity and Mortality: 1998 Chartbook on Cardiovascular, Lung, and Blood Diseases.* NIH: October 1998. On-line. http://www.nhlbi.nih.gov/resources/docs/cht-book.htm

National Heart, Lung, and Blood Institute. *Asthma Statistics, Data Fact Sheet.* Washington, DC: NIH, 1999.

Nuckolls KB, Cassel J, Kaplan BH. Psychosocial assets, life crisis and the prognosis of pregnancy. *American Journal of Epidemiology* 1972; 5:431–441.

Paneth N. The problem of low birth weight, Vol. 5. In: *The Future of Children.* Palo Alto, CA: The David and Lucille Packard Foundation, 1995, 19–34.

Parkin DM, Whelan SL, Ferlay J, Raymond L, Young J, eds., *Cancer Incidence in Five Continents,* Vol. VII. Lyon, France: International Agency for Research on Cancer; IARC Scientific Publications No. 143; 1997.

Patel P, Mendall MA, Carrington D, et al. Association of *Helicobacter pylori* and *Chlamydia pneumoniae* infections with coronary heart disease and cardiovascular risk factors. *British Medical Journal* 1995; 311:711–714.

Perkins CL, Morris CR, Wright WE, Young JL. *Cancer Incidence and Mortality in California by Detailed Race or Ethnicity, 1988–1992.* Sacramento, CA: California Department of Health Services, Cancer Surveillance Section, 1995.

Plotnick RD. Child poverty can be reduced. *Future of Children* 1997; 7(2):72–87.

Praemer A, Furner S, and Rice DP. *Musculoskeletal Conditions in the United States.* Park Ridge, IL: American Academy of Orthopaedic Surgeons, 1992.

Reynolds P, Kaplan GA. Social connections and risk for cancer: Prospective evidence from the Alameda County Study. *Behavioral Medicine* 1990; 16:101–110.

Reynolds P, Boyd PT, Blacklow RS, Jackson JS, Greenberg RS, Austin DF, Chen VW, and Edwards BK. The relationship between social ties and survival among black and white breast cancer patients. National Cancer Institute Black/White Cancer Survival Study Group. *Cancer Epidemiology, Biomarkers and Prevention* 1994; 3:253–259.

Robbins AS, Brescianini S, Kelsey JL. Regional differences in known risk factors and the higher incidence of breast cancer in San Francisco. *Journal of the National Cancer Institute* 1997; 89:960–965.

Romero R, Mazor M, Wu YK, et al. Infection in the pathogenesis of preterm labor. *Seminars in Perinatology* 1988; 12:262–279.

Rose, G. *The Strategy of Preventive Medicine.* Oxford, UK: Oxford University Press, 1992.

Ross NA, Wolfson MC, Dunn JR, Berthelot J-M, Kaplan GA, Lynch JW. Income inequality and mortality in Canada and the United States: A cross-sectional assessment using census data and vital statistics, *British Medical Journal* 2000; 320:898–902.

Rubenstein LZ, Robbins AS, Schulman BL, Rosado J, Osterweil D, and Josephson KR. Falls and instability in the elderly. *Journal of the American Geriatric Society* 1988; 36:266–278.

Sampson RJ, Raudenbush SW, Earls F. Neighborhoods and violent crime: A multilevel study of collective efficacy. *Science* 1997; 277(5328):918–924.

Schnall PL, Landsbergis PA, Baker D. Job strain and cardiovascular disease (review). *Annual Review of Public Health* 1994; 15:381–411.

Schoendorf KC, Hogue CJ, Kleinman JC, Rowley D. Mortality among infants of black as compared to white college educated parents. *New England Journal of Medicine* 1992; 326:1522–1526.

Seeman E. The effects of tobacco and alcohol use on bone. In: Marcus R, Feldman D, Kelsey J, eds., *Osteoporosis.* San Diego: Academic Press, 1996, 577–597.

Sempos C, Cooper R, Kovar MG, McMillen M. Divergence of the recent trends in coronary mortality for the four major race-sex groups in the United States. *American Journal of Public Health* 1988; 78:1422–1427.

Shrock D, Palmer RF, Taylor B. Effects of a psychosocial intervention on survival among patients with stage I breast and prostate cancer: A matched case-control study. *Alternative Therapies in Health and Medicine* 1999; 5:49–55.

Silverman SL, Madison RE. Decreased incidence of hip fracture in Hispanics, Asians, and blacks: California hospital discharge data. *American Journal of Public Health* 1988; 78:1482–1483.

Smyth JM, Soefer MH, Hurewitz A, Kliment A, Stone AA. Daily psychosocial factors predict levels and diurnal cycles of asthma symptomatology and peak flow. *Journal of Behavioral Medicine* 1999; 22(2):179–193.

Snow CM, Shaw JM, Matkin CC. Physical activity and risk for osteoporosis. In: Marcus R, Feldman D, Kelsey J, eds., *Osteoporosis*. San Diego: Academic Press, 1996; 511–528.

Sobal J, Stunkard AJ. Socioeconomic status and obesity: A review of the literature. *Psychological Bulletin* 1989; 105:260–275.

Spiegel D, Bloom JR, Kraemer HC, Gottheil E. Effect of psychosocial treatment on survival of patients with metastatic breast cancer. *Lancet* 1989; 2:888–891.

Stanford JL, Herrinton LJ, Schwartz SM, Weiss NS. Breast cancer incidence in Asian migrants to the United States and their descendants. *Epidemiology* 1995; 6:181–183.

Trock BJ. Breast cancer in African American women: Epidemiology and tumor biology. *Breast Cancer Research and Treatment* 1996; 40:11–24.

Troutt, DD. *The Thin Red Line: How the Poor Still Pay More*. San Francisco: West Coast Regional Office, Consumers Union of the United States, 1993.

UNICEF. *The State of the World's Children 1998*. Oxford: Oxford University Press, 1998.

Villa ML, Nelson L. Race, ethnicity, and osteoporosis. In: Marcus R, Feldman D, Kelsey J, eds., *Osteoporosis*. San Diego, CA: Academic Press, 1996; 435–447.

Vital Statistics of the United States. Annual publications from the National Center for Health Statistics (and forerunner organization names) for data years 1900 to 1967.

Weiss KB, Sullivan SD. Socio-economic burden of asthma, allergy and other atopic illnesses. *Pediatric Allergy and Immunology* 1994; 5(6 suppl):7–12.

Wing S, Casper M, Riggan W, Hayes C, Tyroler HA. Socioenvironmental characteristics associated with the onset of decline of ischemic heart disease mortality in the United States. *American Journal of Public Health* 1988; (8):923–926.

Wintemute GJ. The future of firearm violence prevention: Building on success. *Journal of the American Medical Association* 1999; 282(5):475–478.

World Health Organization. Assessment of Fracture Risk and Its Application to Screening for Postmenopausal Osteoporosis. WHO Technical Report Series. Geneva: WHO, 1994.

Wun LM, Feuer EJ, Miller BA. Are increases in mammographic screening still a valid explanation for trends in breast cancer incidence in the United States? *Cancer Causes and Control* 1995; 6:135–144.

Yen IH, Kaplan GA. Poverty area residence and changes in physical activity level: Evidence from the Alameda County Study. *American Journal of Public Health* 1998; 88:1709–1712.

Yen IH, Kaplan GA. Poverty area residence and changes in depression and perceived health status: Evidence from the Alameda County Study. *International Journal of Epidemiology* 1999; 28:90–94.

PAPER CONTRIBUTION B
Understanding and Reducing Socioeconomic and Racial/Ethnic Disparities in Health

James S. House and David R. Williams

The initial paper by Kaplan and colleagues and the burgeoning literatures on socioeconomic and racial/ethnic disparities in health establish that such disparities are *large, persistent,* and even *increasing* in the United States and other developed countries, most notably the United Kingdom (Marmot et al., 1987; Preston and Haines, 1991; Adler et al., 1993; Pappas et al., 1993; Evans et al., 1994; Williams and Collins, 1995). Differences across socioeconomic and racial/ethnic groups or combinations thereof range up to 10 or more years in life expectancy and 20 or more years in the age at which significant limitations in functional health are first experienced (see Table 1; House et al., 1990, 1994). Both within and across countries, individuals with the most advantaged socioeconomic and racial/ethnic status are experiencing levels of health and longevity

Dr. House is director of the Survey Research Center in the Institute for Social Research, and professor of sociology, University of Michigan, and Dr. Williams is professor of sociology and research scientist at the Institute for Social Research, University of Michigan. This paper was prepared for the symposium "Capitalizing on Social Science and Behavioral Research to Improve the Public's Health," the Institute of Medicine and the Commission on Behavioral and Social Sciences and Education of the National Research Council, Atlanta, Georgia, February 2–3, 2000. This work has been supported by a Robert Wood Johnson Foundation Investigators in Health Policy Research Award (Dr. House) and by grant MH-57425 from the National Institute of Mental Health and the John D. and Catherine T. MacArthur Foundation Research Network on Socioeconomic Status and Health (Dr. Williams). We are indebted to Debbie Fitch for her work in preparing the manuscript, references, figures, and table.

TABLE 1. United States Life Expectancy, at Age 45 by Family Income (1980 dollars)[a]

Family Income	Females			Males		
	White	Black	Diff.	White	Black	Diff.
All[b]	**36.3**	**32.6**	**3.7**	**31.1**	**26.2**	**4.9**
<$10,000	35.8	32.7	3.1	27.3	25.2	2.1
$10,000–$14,999	37.4	33.5	3.9	30.3	28.1	2.2
$15,000–$24,999	37.8	36.3	1.5	32.4	31.3	1.1
≥$25,000	38.5	36.5	2.0	33.9	32.6	1.3

NOTE: Diff. = difference.

[a]1979–1989; Taken from the National Center for Health Statistics.
[b]1989–1991; Taken from the National Center for Health Statistics.

that increasingly approach the current biologically attainable maxima. Thus, the major opportunity for improving the health of human populations in the United States and most other societies lies in improving the longevity and health of those of below-average socioeconomic or racial/ethnic status.

Accordingly, the reduction of socioeconomic and racial/ethnic disparities in health has been identified by the U.S. Public Health Service and the National Institutes of Health as a major priority for public health practice and research in the first decade of the twenty-first century (USDHHS, 1999; Varmus, 1999). This will involve some combination of either reducing the degree to which disparities in socioeconomic and racial/ethnic status are converted into health disparities or reducing the extent of socioeconomic or racial/ethnic disparities themselves. This will further entail understanding both (1) the psychosocial and biomedical pathways that translate socioeconomic and racial/ethnic disparities into disparities in health, and (2) the broader social, cultural economic, and political processes that determine the nature and extent of socioeconomic and racial/ethnic disparities in our society, and the ways in which individuals become distributed across socioeconomic levels and defined into racial/ethnic groups.

This paper seeks to elucidate what we already know and need yet to learn about reducing socioeconomic and racial/ethnic disparities in health. We first provide a brief overview of the nature of both socioeconomic and racial/ethnic disparities in health and how they are related to each other. Second, we assess current understanding of the pathways or mechanisms by which the socioeconomic or racial/ethnic status of individuals affects their health and the implications of this understanding for reducing socioeconomic and racial/ethnic disparities in health. Third, we explore what is known about how and why communities and societies come to be stratified both socioeconomically and in terms of race/ethnicity, and how these communal and societal patterns of socioeconomic and racial/ethnic stratification affect the socioeconomic and racial/ethnic status of individuals and their health. Finally, we conclude with an assessment of what we know and need to know about how to reduce socioeconomic and racial/ethnic disparities in health and, hence, to improve population health.

Several themes pervade our discussion. First, there are multiple indicators of socioeconomic position and hence multiple indices of socioeconomic disparities in health, and these are best comprehended in a multivariate, causal, and life course framework. Second, socioeconomic and racial/ethnic disparities in health, and the reasons for and means of reducing them, are inextricably related but also distinctive. This also can best be comprehended in a multivariate causal framework. Third, it is important to understand the pathways or mechanisms linking socioeconomic and racial/ethnic status to health. What is most striking and important here is to recognize that socioeconomic and racial/ethnic status shape and operate through a very broad range of pathways or mechanisms, including almost all known major psychosocial and behavioral risk factors for health. Thus, socioeconomic and racial/ethnic status are in the terms of Link and Phelan (1995) the "fundamental causes" of corresponding socioeconomic and racial/ethnic disparities in risk factors and hence health and, consequently, also the fundamental levers for reducing these health disparities. Finally, existing evidence strongly suggests that the nature of the socioeconomic and racial/ethnic stratification of individuals can be changed in ways beneficial to health and, coincidentally, to a broad range of other indicators of individual and societal well-being.

THE NATURE OF SOCIOECONOMIC AND RACIAL/ETHNIC DISPARITIES AND THEIR RELATION TO HEALTH

We take the size, persistence, and even increase of socioeconomic and racial/ethnic disparities as given in Paper Contribution A. Here we seek to clarify the nature of socioeconomic and racial/ethnic status and their relations to each other and to health.

A Multivariate, Causal, and Life Course Framework

Socioeconomic status (SES) refers to individuals' position in a system of social stratification that differentially allocates the major resources enabling people to achieve health or other desired goals. These resources centrally include education, occupation, income, and assets or wealth, which are related to each other and to health in a causal framework first elucidated by Blau and Duncan (1967) and shown in its simplest form in Figure 1A. This model suggests that over the life course, individuals first acquire varying levels and types of education, which in turn help them to enter various types of occupations, which then yield income, which finally enables them to accumulate assets or wealth. Each subsequent variable in this causal chain is generally most affected by the immediately prior variable, with potential residual effects of earlier variables. This model is simple because it omits potential feedback loops other than from assets or wealth to income (e.g., a person's occupation may facilitate further educational attainment) and fails

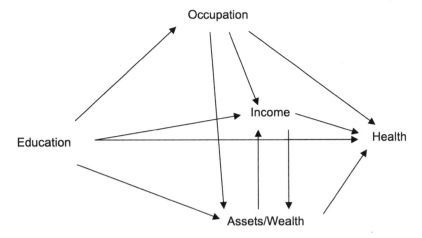

FIGURE 1A. Simple intragenerational causal model relating major indicators of socioeconomic position to each other and to health.

to incorporate variations in each of these indicators that will occur over the life course (e.g., progressions or regressions in terms of occupation or income).

Although this causal framework has been used routinely in the study of socioeconomic attainment, it has seldom been explicitly applied to the study of socioeconomic disparities. It is important, however, that it be utilized more explicitly in future research on the relation of socioeconomic status to health, and especially in thinking about how socioeconomic disparities in health have been or could be reduced. The framework helps, for example, to understand why income is perhaps the strongest and most robust predictor of health (McDonough et al., 1997; Lantz et al., 1998), because to some degree the impacts of all other variables are mediated through it. Also, some health outcomes are more strongly affected by certain socioeconomic indicators than others (education, for example, more strongly affects health behaviors, patterns of which form early in life, and the diseases or health indicators affected most by them). Overall, in the United States, education and income have proved most predictive of health, with occupation often adding little additional explanatory power and assets or wealth somewhat more. More research is needed, however, to estimate explicitly the relative effects on health of these different indicators of socioeconomic position, and how much the total effect of any given variable is spuriously produced by temporally antecedent confounding variables, mediated via temporally subsequent intervening variables, or acts more directly on health (see Sorlie et al., 1995; Lantz et al., 1998 and in press; and Robert and House, 2000 a,b).

From the point of view of reducing health disparities, we need to have such an analysis of the variance in health explained by different socioeconomic factors in order to understand or predict the health effects of planned or unplanned change in each indicator. Further, by adding other variables to Figure 1A,

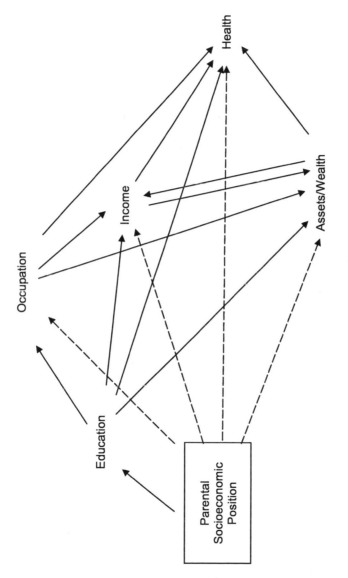

FIGURE 1B Simple intergenerational extension of model in Figure 1A.

86

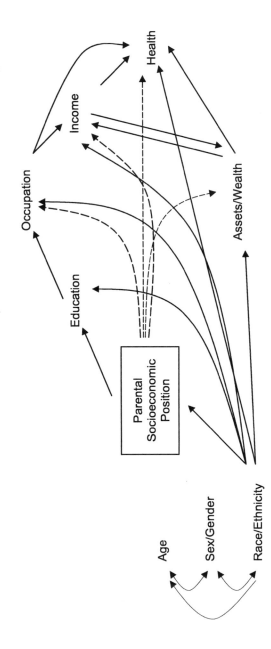

FIGURE 1C Extension of model in Figure 1B incorporating race/ethnicity, sex/gender, and age. NOTE: for clarity of presentation, no arrows are drawn from age and sex/gender to subsequent variables, but these would and should be exactly parallel to those for race/ethnicity.

we can extend our understanding of how disparities in health across these indicators of socioeconomic position may be generated by antecedent factors or mediated via subsequent factors. Several such elaborations are important in thinking about reducing other socioeconomic and racial disparities in health.

First, socioeconomic position (SEP) has to be thought of as an intergenerational as well as intragenerational phenomenon. Thus, parental socioeconomic position may importantly shape childhood well-being and hence educational and later adult socioeconomic attainment and health, as shown in Figure 1B. The work of Barker (e.g., Barker and Osmond, 1986) and others (Kaplan and Salonen, 1990; Elo and Preston, 1992; Blane et al., 1996; Kuh and Ben-Shlomo, 1997) has indicated that childhood socioeconomic position and experiences can have long-term effects on adult health (see also Paper Contribution C). This is sometimes interpreted to mean that childhood socioeconomic position is a more important determinant of health than adult socioeconomic position. However, Figure 1B suggests that most such effects are likely to be channeled through and reinforced by later socioeconomic attainment, and the unique impact of childhood SEP or its sequelae must be evaluated net of later socioeconomic or other experiences. When this is done, the unique effects of childhood SEP on adult health are often found to be small or even nonexistent relative to the effects of later adult socioeconomic attainment and experiences (e.g., Lynch et al., 1994).[*] Thus, although the impact of socioeconomic position on childhood health and well-being is a very important problem in its own right, it cannot and should not be viewed as a major explanation of adult socioeconomic or racial/ethnic disparities in health or hence as the major, preferred, or necessary route for reducing such adult disparities.

However, Figure 1B is also highly simplified, neglecting the changing socioeconomic position of the families of many children. Thus, the socioeconomic position of a child often changes from preschool to elementary school to secondary school and onward through adulthood. Socioeconomic advantage and disadvantage may be viewed as ebbing and flowing or cascading over a person's life course. Although recent socioeconomic position is usually the best predictor of future outcomes, sustained socioeconomic deprivation over time is likely to be even more damaging (Wolfson et al., 1993, Lynch et al., 1997), and uncertainty or variability in socioeconomic position may be deleterious even to those of generally solid middle- or higher-level SEP (McDonough et al., 1997). Thus, knowledge of the full life course of socioeconomic position is ideally desirable for understanding socioeconomic disparities in health and a target for efforts to alleviate such disparities.

Finally, Figures 1A and 1B must be further elaborated, as in Figure 1C, to take account of the impact of more ascribed and relatively fixed social

---

[*]Link and Phelan (in progress) have similarly showed that although cognitive ability contributes to socioeconomic attainment, its effects on health are mediated entirely through such attainments, and it in no way can explain away or make spurious the considerable impact of adult SEP on health.

statuses—most notably for our purposes, race/ethnicity, but also age and gender. Figure 1C reveals two simple but very important truths about racial/ethnic disparities in health. First, racial/ethnic status is a major determinant of every indicator of socioeconomic position, even net of all prior variables in the model. For example, not only are African Americans disadvantaged in terms of level of education, but even given the same education, they are disadvantaged occupationally and in terms of income, and still disadvantaged in income even within the same educational and occupational levels (Featherman and Hauser, 1978). Most egregiously, their assets/wealth lag far behind other Americans of equivalent income, occupation, and education (Oliver and Shapiro, 1995; Conley, 1999). Not surprisingly, then, a great deal of racial/ethnic disparity in health is explainable in terms of the socioeconomic disadvantages associated with membership in the most historically disadvantaged racial/ethnic groups (Williams and Collins, 1995).

However, the second important truth of Figure 1C is that race/ethnicity has effects on health that are independent of socioeconomic differences between racial/ethnic groups (Williams and Collins, 1995; Williams et al., 1997). For example, African Americans generally exhibit poorer health outcomes even when compared to whites with statistically equivalent levels of socioeconomic position (see below and Table 1). Thus, race carries its own burdens for health beyond those associated with socioeconomic disadvantage. We can properly estimate and understand how race/ethnicity and socioeconomic position combine to affect health only within a multivariate framework such as Figure 1C. Further, such a framework can also reveal that race/ethnicity sometimes has salutary effects on health that may compensate in part for the deleterious effects of socioeconomic disadvantages. For example, African Americans exhibit better levels of mental health, and Latinos better levels of infant and child health, than would be expected based on their socioeconomic position. The next major section of this paper focuses on elucidating the pathways or mechanisms through which both socioeconomic position and race/ethnicity affect health, for better as well as for worse.

Due to constraints of space and desire for clarity, Figure 1C fails to represent other important issues for understanding and reducing socioeconomic disparities in health. First is the issue of reciprocal or reverse causality, especially between socioeconomic position and health. Ours and others' discussions of reducing socioeconomic and racial/ethnic disparities in health are predicated on the assumption that, by far, the predominant causal flow is from socioeconomic position and race/ethnicity to health rather than vice versa. This assumption is self-evident for a fixed attribute such as race/ethnicity and is generally borne out in empirical research on socioeconomic position, for example, by introducing baseline controls on health into the framework of Figure 1 (see House and Roberts, 2000:116–117), though clearly health events or shocks can and do affect subsequent labor force participation and income (often more in the short term than in the long term). Second, time and space prevent us from fully and systematically attending to variations by age, sex, race/ethnicity, and other factors in the presence of size of the causal paths/effects in Figure 1, though we will on occasion note such variations (see Robert and House, 2000b:118–120 for more discussion of such issues).

Shape of the Relationship Between SES and Health

Before turning more explicitly to how we may explain and reduce socio-economic and racial/ethnic disparities in health, it is important to clarify our understanding of the shape of the relationship between socioeconomic position and health. An intriguing finding of some research on socioeconomic inequalities in health is that it is not simply that those who are in the lowest socioeconomic groups have worse health than those in higher socioeconomic groups. Rather, a relationship between socioeconomic position and health has been observed across the socioeconomic hierarchy, with even those in relatively high-socioeconomic groups having better health than those just below them in the socioeconomic hierarchy (Adler et al., 1994; Marmot et al., 1991). Perhaps the most important implication of this finding is that it is not just the material, psychological, and social conditions associated with severe deprivation or poverty (such as lack of access to safe housing, healthy food, and adequate medical care) that explain socioeconomic inequalities in health among those already at relatively high levels of socioeconomic position.

Despite some evidence for gradient effects of socioeconomic position on health, it is also important to note the many studies indicating that the relationship of socioeconomic position, especially as indexed by income, to health is monotonic, but not a linear gradient. Although increasingly higher levels of socioeconomic position may be associated with increasingly better levels of health, there are also substantially diminishing returns of higher socioeconomic position to health. For example, studies have found diminishing and even non-existent relationships between income and mortality (Wolfson et al., 1993; Backlund ct al., 1996; Chapman and Hariharan, 1996; McDonough et al., 1997;) or morbidity (House et al., 1990, 1994; Mirowsky and Hu, 1996) at higher levels of income (e.g., above the median). This trend partially reflects a health "ceiling effect" caused by the fact that people in the upper socioeconomic strata maintain overall good health until quite late in life, leaving little opportunity for improvement in health among these groups throughout much of adulthood (House et al., 1994). Thus, it is most important to understand what accounts for socioeconomic inequalities in health across the broad lower range (e.g., lower 40–60%) of socioeconomic position, rather than focusing mainly or only on factors that might explain this relationship across the gradient or at higher levels.

PATHWAYS LINKING INDIVIDUAL SOCIOECONOMIC AND RACIAL/ETHNIC STATUS TO HEALTH

Pathways from SES to Health

We have increased understanding of how and why socioeconomic status has such strong pervasive and even increasing impacts on health. Several aspects of this deserve emphasis. First, access to and utilization of medical care play only a limited role in explaining the impact of socioeconomic factors on health, although research is needed to reassess the size of the role played by medical care. Second, there is no single or small set of factors, psychosocial or physiological, that provides the pathways linking socioeconomic position to health. Rather, what makes socioeconomic position such a powerful determinant of health is that it shapes people's experience of, and exposure to, virtually all psychosocial and environmental risk factors for health—past, present, and future—and these in turn operate through a very broad range of physiological mechanisms to influence the incidence and course of virtually all major causes of disease and health. Thus, in the end, socioeconomic position itself is a fundamental cause (Link and Phelan, 1995) of levels of individual and population health and a fundamental lever for improving health in American society.

The Limited but Insufficiently Understood Role of Medical Care

Several types of evidence point to the limited role of medical care in understanding how and why socioeconomic position affects health. First, there is evidence that modern preventive and therapeutic medical care can account for only a minor fraction of the dramatic improvements in individual and population health over the last 250 years (McKeown, 1976, 1979, 1988; McKinlay and McKinlay, 1977). Even analysts admiring of the impact of medical science on health, for example, estimate that only about 5 years of the 30-year increase in life expectancy in the United States in the twentieth century has been due to preventive or therapeutic medical care (Bunker et al., 1994). The remainder is attributable primarily to increasing socioeconomic development and associated gains in nutrition, public health and sanitation, and living conditions. Second, improvements in access to medical care occasioned by the introduction of national health insurance or service plans have, quite unexpectedly, done little or nothing to reduce socioeconomic differences in health. The rediscovery of the importance of socioeconomic disparities in health as a major public health problem was probably stimulated most by the publication in England in 1980 of the Report of the Working Group on Inequalities in Health, better known as the Black Report after the chair of the working group, Sir Douglas Black, then chief scientist of the U.K. Department of Health and subsequently president of the Royal College of Physicians. The report showed that occupational class differences in health were greater than differences by gender, race, or regional background and, most distressingly, had actually increased between 1949–1953 and

1970–1972 over the first quarter-century of existence of the British National Health Service. Nor did things improve between the early 1970s and 1980s (Marmot et al., 1987). During the 1980s and early 1990s, the British experience was replicated in other developed countries including Canada, where the introduction of national health insurance in the early 1970s had little effect on socioeconomic differences in health (Wilkins et al., 1989). Finally, adjustments for gross access to and utilization of medical care have contributed little or nothing to explaining socioeconomic and racial/ethnic differences in health in our and other data.

However, we believe that the role of medical care in socioeconomic and racial/ethnic health differences deserves renewed examination and research. First, compared to whites, racial/ethnic minorities have lower levels of access to medical care in the United States (Blendon et al. 1989; Trevino et al. 1991). Second, higher incidence rates for racial/ethnic minorities do not fully account for the higher death rates (Schwartz et al. 1990). Later initial diagnosis of disease, comorbidity, delays in medical treatment, and disparities in the quality of care also play a role. There is growing evidence of large racial/ethnic differences in the quality of medical care. Many studies have found racial/ethnic differences in the receipt of therapeutic procedures for a broad range of conditions even after adjustment for insurance status and severity of disease (e.g., Wenneker and Epstein, 1989; Harris et al. 1997). These disparities exist even in contexts where differences in economic status and insurance coverage are minimized, for example, the Veterans Administration Health System (e.g., Whittle et al., 1993) and the Medicare program (e.g., McBean and Gornick, 1994). Recent studies document that these differences in medical treatment adversely affect the health of minority group members (Peterson et al., 1997; Hannan et al., 1999). Moreover, medical care appears to play a modest role in accounting for racial differences in mortality (Woolhandler et al., 1985; Schwartz et al., 1990), and other evidence suggests that medical care has a greater impact on the health status of vulnerable racial and low-SES groups than on their more advantaged counterparts (Williams, 1990). More generally, behind declining socioeconomic and racial/ethnic disparities in gross levels of access to and utilization of medical care may lie in persisting differences in access to more continuous care from a concerned and responsive provider, associated differences in access to and utilization of important standards of preventive care (e.g., blood pressure, prostate and colorectal screening, Pap smears, mammograms, and professional advice on health behaviors), and differences in the timeliness and appropriateness of access to state-of-the-art standards of therapeutic care. Thus, socioeconomic and racial/ethnic disparities in standards and appropriateness of medical care merit increased attention in research and policy.

Psychosocial and Environmental Risk Factors

As evidence grew of the more limited impact of medical care in explaining socioeconomic and racial/ethnic disparities in health, research increasingly established a growing and even predominant role of behavioral and psychosocial risk factors in the etiology and course of human health and disease. First, and still most compelling, was the evidence of the adverse effects of cigarette smoking on mortality and morbidity, especially adult lung cancer and heart disease (e.g., USPHS, 1964). This was followed by increasing evidence of the health risks of other behaviors, including immoderate levels of eating (and hence weight) and of alcohol consumption, lack of exercise, and dietary composition, e.g., fat and fiber (Lalonde, 1975; Berkman and Breslow, 1983, USDHHS, 1990). Evidence has also accumulated on the deleterious health effects of chronic and acute stress in work and life (Theorell, 1982), hostility and depression (Scheier and Bridges, 1995), lack of social relationships and supports (House et al., 1988), and lack of control, efficacy, or mastery (Rodin, 1986), with the impact of lack of social relationships, for example, on all-cause mortality being not incomparable to that of cigarette smoking (House et al., 1988). Notably, these psychosocial factors all tend to affect a broad range of health outcomes, rather than being focused on a single outcome.

Socioeconomic Status and Psychosocial and
Environmental Risk Factors

One factor (e.g., smoking) or a small set of factors (e.g., health behaviors) is sometimes seen as crucial in explaining and alleviating problems of premature morbidity and mortality more generally (e.g., USDHHS, 1990; McGinnis and Forge, 1993) and socioeconomic and racial/ethnic disparities in health in particular (Mechanic, 1989; Satel, 1996). However, increasing evidence suggests that there are few or no analogues in our current problems of public health to the necessary and sufficient microbial causes of many infectious diseases, nor are there any comparable "magic bullets" for treating, preventing, or eradicating them. Rather, the current causes of morbidity and mortality, especially from major chronic diseases, are broadly multifactorial, with no one or few decisive, but the accumulation of many being as debilitating or deadly as a virulent infectious agent (Kunitz, 1987). For example, all major health behaviors combined (i.e., cigarette smoking, immoderate weight and drinking, and lack of physical activity) appear able to explain only 10–20%, at most, of socioeconomic differences in mortality (Lantz et al., 1998). Rather, what is most striking and important about socioeconomic (and, to a lesser degree, racial/ethnic) status is the degree to which it shapes exposure to, and perhaps also the impact of, a wide range of psychosocial and environmental risk factors for health. Our data (House et al., 1992, 1994) and those of others (e.g., Marmot et al., 1991; Lynch et al., 1996) show that lower-SES individuals have a higher prevalence of almost *all* major psychosocial risk factors for health. That is, they manifest higher levels of risky health behaviors such as smoking, lack of exercise, immoderate eating and drinking, and high-fat–low-fiber diets. They also experience more chronic and acute stress due to, for example, their more vulnerable economic status and the higher rates of ill health and death among friends and relatives. They generally report lower levels of social relationships and supports and of personal efficacy or control, along with *higher* levels of hostility and depression.

Figures 2A and 2B show, for national samples of the U.S. population, the distribution and range of these psychosocial risk factors by education and income. The prevalence of each psychosocial risk factor is always highest among those with the lowest level of education and income, with rate ratios (of the lowest- to the highest-SES groups) ranging from 1.1 to 3.8 and averaging 2.0 (see Lantz et al., 1998, for parallel data on health behaviors).

Persons of lower socioeconomic status in adulthood are also more likely to live and work in physical–chemical–biological environments that are hazardous to health. Further, they are more likely to have grown up in lower-socioeconomic environments, which may have residual adverse effects on health in adulthood that research is just beginning to examine (e.g., Power et al., 1990).

At this point we are only beginning to explore the causal pathways and complexities that link socioeconomic position to exposure to behavioral, psychosocial, and environmental risk factors and, in turn, link these risk factors to health outcomes. Our own analyses and those of others find that although any single behavioral, psychosocial, or environmental risk factor, or small set thereof, can account for only a small fraction of the association between SES and health, a set of 10–20 such risk factors can account for 50–100% of the association between a given SES indicator and health outcome. Marmot et al. (1991) and Lynch et al. (1996) have reported that adjusting for 10–20 such risk factors reduces the predictive association of SES with mortality by 50–100%. We get similar results for the cross-sectional relationship between education or income and functional status (House et al., 1994).

Potentials and Limits of Understanding and Intervening in Pathways

Better understanding of the pathways and mechanisms linking socioeconomic and racial/ethnic status to health is often and appropriately seen as crucial to reducing socioeconomic and racial/ethnic disparities in health. Once an intervening variable or mechanism is understood, efforts can be made to reduce this variable or mechanism or to weaken its impact on health, hence reducing the socioeconomic or racial/ethnic disparities in health. To the extent that we are able to decrease smoking and improve other health behaviors, lessen stress, enhance social relationships and supports, modify risky psychological dispositions or reduce exposure to environmental exposures, especially in disadvantaged socioeconomic or racial/ethnic groups, or to moderate their effects on health (e.g., develop a safe cigarette or nicotine delivery system, see Paper Contribution K), we should consequently reduce socioeconomic and racial/ethnic disparities in health. Such intervention strategies have had some beneficial effects in these regards.

94

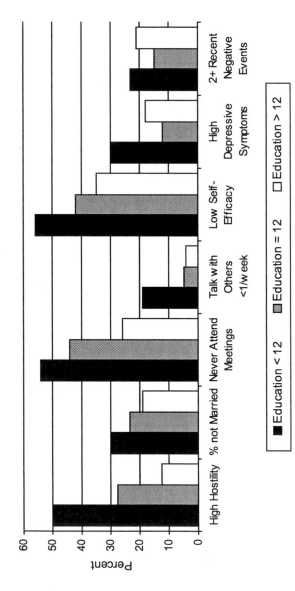

FIGURE 2A Psychosocial risk factors by education for persons 45–64 in the United States. SOURCE: University of Michigan Americans' Changing Lives Survey (1986) and MMPI-II restandardization (1984–1986).

95

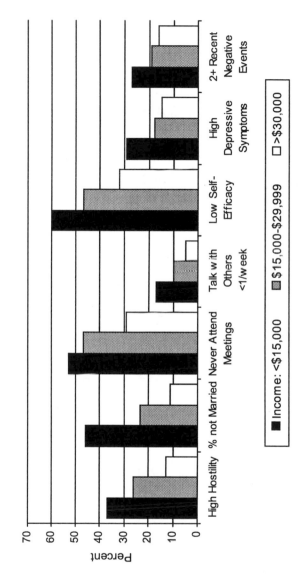

FIGURE 2B Psychosocial risk factors by income for persons 45–64 in the United States. SOURCE: University of Michigan Americans' Changing Lives Survey (1986) and MMPI-II restandardization (1984–1986).

However, we wish to call attention to the often insufficiently recognized limitations of such an approach and to highlight the potential, and indeed necessity, of another and complementary approach. The potential of the pathways strategy is limited in two crucial ways. First, modifying any psychosocial risk factor is a difficult process, and the impact of modifying one or a single risk factor is necessarily limited for the reasons discussed above. Second, where we have had substantial success in reducing a behavioral or psychosocial risk factor (e.g., smoking), this success is often greatest among the more advantaged due to the persistence or even accentuation (e.g., targeting of disadvantaged groups for cigarette advertising) of the causal forces giving rise to the risk factor in less advantaged groups. Thus, as overall levels of smoking have decreased in the United States, socioeconomic differences in smoking have increased (see Paper Contribution K). Finally, it is important to recognize that the mechanisms that currently link socioeconomic status to health are not the same ones that did so in the past or will in the future. Prior socioeconomic differences undoubtedly had more to do with differences in exposure to infectious agents and access to medical care than is currently the case. Indeed, many of the currently most important diseases and risk factors—such as coronary heart disease and its risk factors of smoking, lack of exercise, and high-fat diet—were at one time more characteristic of upper socioeconomic strata, but have become more incident and prevalent in lower socioeconomic strata as these diseases and risk factors have become more deleterious to health. A similar trend has characterized AIDS, which emerged first as a disease among higher socioeconomic strata but has rapidly become more prevalent in disadvantaged socioeconomic and racial/ethnic groups. Thus, whatever the major diseases (or risk factors for them) are in future years, they too are likely to be importantly determined by socioeconomic status (Link and Phelan, 1995).

In sum, as Link and Phelan (1995) have cogently argued, we need to think increasingly of disparities in socioeconomic position as the "fundamental cause" of socioeconomic disparities in health. Hence, ameliorating these socioeconomic disparities themselves may be the best strategy for reducing disparities in health. A parallel, but not identical, argument can be made regarding racial/ethnic disparities, to which we now turn, before returning to evidence that socioeconomic improvement and policy are a major form of health improvement and policy in our and other societies, arguably the most important and essential one for reducing socioeconomic disparities in health.

Understanding Racial/Ethnic Differences in Health

Race/Ethnicity and Health

National mortality data reveal that African Americans (or blacks) have an overall death rate that is more than 1.5 times higher than that of whites (NCHS, 1998). The magnitude of the racial difference in death rates varies by the specific cause of death, but a pattern of elevated death rates for blacks compared to whites exists for almost all the leading causes of death in the United States. In contrast, all other racial/ethnic groups have an overall death rate that is lower than that of whites. However, there is considerable variability for subgroups of these populations and for specific health conditions. All nonblack minorities have considerably lower rates than whites for the two leading causes of death (heart disease and cancer) but higher rates for some conditions. Hispanics have higher mortality rates than non-Hispanic whites for tuberculosis, septicemia, HIV/AIDS, chronic liver disease and cirrhosis, diabetes, and homicide (Sorlie et al., 1993; Vega and Amaro, 1994). Subgroups of the Asian and Pacific Islander population also have elevated mortality rates for some health conditions (Lin-Fu, 1993). For example, the Native Hawaiian population has the highest death rate due to heart disease of any racial group in the United States (Chen, 1993). Similarly, American Indians who receive care from the Indian Health Service (60% of that population) have age-adjusted mortality rates higher than the national average for tuberculosis, alcoholism, diabetes, accidents, homicides, suicides, and pneumonia and influenza (NCHS, 1993).

What Is Race?

Early studies of racial variations in health viewed race as primarily reflecting biological homogeneity and racial differences in health as largely genetically determined. This view predated modern scientific theories of genetics and carefully executed genetic studies. In contrast, scientific evidence suggests that our current racial categories are more alike than different in terms of biological characteristics and genetics (Lewontin, 1972; Gould, 1977; Latter, 1980). All human beings are identical for about 75% of known genetic factors, with about 95% of human genetic variation existing *within* racial groups (Lewontin, 1982). Thus, there is more genetic variation within races than between them, and racial categories do not capture biological distinctiveness. Race is thus more of a social than a biological category, and racial classification schemes have been influenced by larger social and political considerations (Cooper and David, 1986; Williams, in press).

Race and SES

Although not useful as biological markers, current racial/ethnic categories capture an important part of the inequality and injustice in American society (See and Wilson, 1988). There are important power and status differences between groups. For example, in 1995 the poverty rate for Asians was almost twice that of whites, while the rate for blacks and Hispanics was more than three times that of non-Hispanic whites (NCHS, 1998). Data on poverty tell only a part of the story of economic vulnerability. In addition to persons who actually fall below the government's poverty threshold, a large number of persons are only slightly above this level. Many of these persons are at a high risk of becoming poor. The combination of the poor and near-poor (annual income above the poverty threshold but less than twice the poverty level) categories reveals that one in every three persons in the United States falls into this economically vulnerable category —26% of whites, 33% of Asians, 54% of blacks, and 62% of Hispanics (NCHS, 1998). Although there is a strong relationship between race and SES, they are not equivalent. For example, the rate of poverty is three times higher for blacks than for whites, but two-thirds of blacks are not poor, and two-thirds of all poor Americans are white.

Race, SES, and Health

Research reveals that SES differences between races account for much of the racial differences in health. Adjusting racial (black–white) disparities in health for SES sometimes eliminates, but always substantially reduces, these differences (Krieger et al., 1993; Williams and Collins, 1995; Lillie-Blanton et al., 1996). However, race often has an effect on health independent of SES: within levels of SES, blacks still have worse health status than whites.

Table 1 illustrates these issues with life expectancy data. At age 45, white males have a life expectancy that is almost 5 years more than black males (NCHS, 1990). Similarly, the life expectancy at age 45 for white females is 3.7 years longer than that of similarly aged black women. However, there is considerable socioeconomic variation in life expectancy within both racial groups (NCHS, 1998). When we consider the distribution of life expectancy by race and income, two important trends emerge. First, for both racial groups, income is strongly linked to health status. Consistently, persons of lower levels of income report lower life expectancy than their more economically favored peers. Black men in the highest-income group live 7.4 years longer than those in the lowest-income group. The comparable numbers for whites was 6.6 years. Thus, the SES difference within each racial group is larger than the racial difference across groups. A similar pattern is evident for women, although the SES differences are smaller. At age 45, black women in the highest-income group have a life expectancy that is 3.8 years longer than those in the lowest-income group. Among whites, the SES difference is 2.7 years. Moreover, for men and women of both racial groups, increasing levels of income are associated with longer life expectancy. The power of SES in shaping racial differences in health is clearly evident by comparing the highest-SES blacks with the lowest-SES whites, especially among males. High-income black males have a life expectancy that is 5.3 years longer than low-income white males. Thus, the disproportionate concentration of African Americans at lower SES levels is a major factor behind the overall racial differences in health.

The second pattern that clearly emerges in these data is that race is more than socioeconomic status. Consistently, there is an independent effect of race even when SES is controlled. At every level of income, for both men and women, African Americans have lower levels of life expectancy than whites. In these data, the differences are greater at the two lower levels of income than at the two higher-economic- status categories. However, for some indicators of health status such as infant mortality, the racial gap becomes larger as SES increases (NCHS, 1998).

Role of Racism or Discrimination

The construct of racism can structure and inform our understanding of racial inequalities in health (Cooper et al., 1981; Krieger et al., 1993; Hummer, 1996; LaVeist, 1996; Williams, 1997; in press). The term racism refers to an ideology of inferiority that is used to justify the differential treatment of members of racial outgroups by both individuals and societal institutions, usually accompanied by negative attitudes and beliefs toward these groups. Racism has been a central organizing principle within American society and has played a key role in shaping major social institutions and policies (Omi and Winant, 1986; Quadagno, 1994). Historically, ideologies about racial groups were translated into policies and societal arrangements that have limited the opportunities and social mobility of stigmatized groups. The strong association between race/ethnicity and SES in the United States reflects the successful implementation of social policies that were designed to limit societal resources and rewards to socially marginalized groups.

There have been important positive changes in the racial attitudes of whites toward blacks in recent decades and broad current support for the *principle* of equality in most societal institutions (Schuman et al., 1997). At the same time, there is considerably less support for policies that would actually implement equal access to education, housing, jobs, and so forth (Schuman et al., 1997). Moreover, national data on stereotypes reveal that whites view blacks, Hispanics, and Asians more negatively than themselves, with blacks viewed more negatively than all other groups and Hispanics twice as negatively as Asians (Davis and Smith, 1990). Such a high level of acceptance of negative stereotypes of minority groups is an ominous harbinger of widespread societal discrimination. Psychological research indicates that the endorsement of negative racial stereotypes leads to discrimination against minority groups (Devine, 1995; Hilton and von Hippel, 1996). Moreover, well-learned stereotypes are resistant to disconfirmation (Stangnor and McMillan, 1992), and their activation is an automatic process, with individuals spontaneously becoming aware of relevant stereotypes after encountering someone to whom the stereotypes are applicable (Devine, 1989; Hilton and von Hippel, 1996).

Research reveals that considerable racial/ethnic discrimination persists in the United States in domains that affect socioeconomic mobility, such as housing and employment (Kirschenman and Neckerman, 1991; Neckerman and Kirschenman, 1991; Fix and Struyk, 1993). Thus, the advent of civil rights legislation and changes in the racial attitudes of whites have not been sufficient to eradicate discrimination, and there has been remarkable stability over time on multiple dimensions of racial inequality (Economic Report of the President,

1998). For example, the median income of African Americans was 59 cents for every dollar earned by whites in 1996—identical to what it was in 1978.

Racism affects disparities in health in multiple ways. First, racism restricts and truncates socioeconomic attainment. The consequent racial differences in SES and poorer health reflect, in part, the impact of economic discrimination produced by large-scale societal structures. Residential segregation has been a primary mechanism by which racial inequality has been created and reinforced. Racial segregation has determined access to educational and employment opportunities that has importantly led to truncated socioeconomic mobility for blacks and American Indians (Jaynes and Williams, 1987; Massey and Denton, 1993). Residence in segregated neighborhoods can lead to exposure to environmental toxins, poor-quality housing, and other pathogenic living conditions, including inadequate access to a broad range of services provided by municipal authorities (Collins and Williams, 1999). These conditions importantly account for the large racial difference in homicide. The combination of concentrated poverty, male joblessness, and residential instability leads to high rates of single-parent households, and these factors together account for variation in the levels of violent crime (Sampson and Wilson, 1995). Importantly, the association between these factors and violent crime for whites was virtually identical in magnitude with the association for African Americans. Several studies have found a positive association between both adult and infant mortality and residence in segregated areas. One recent study has documented elevated mortality rates for both blacks and whites in cities high on two indices of segregation compared to cities with lower levels of segregation (Collins and Williams, 1999). This pattern suggests that beyond some threshold of segregation, the adverse conditions linked to highly segregated cities may negatively affect the health of all persons who reside there.

Moreover, because of racism, SES indicators are not commensurate across racial groups, which makes it difficult to truly adjust racial differences in health for SES (Kaufman et al., 1997). There are racial differences in the quality of education, income returns for a given level of education or occupational status, wealth or assets associated with a given level of income, the purchasing power of income, the stability of employment, and the health risks associated with occupational status (Williams and Collins, 1995; Kaufman et al., 1997).

Racial differences are especially marked for wealth. Eller (1994) shows that while white households have a median net worth of $44,408, the median net worth is $4,604 for black households and $5,345 for Hispanic ones. Moreover, racial/ethnic differences in wealth are evident at all levels of income and are greatest at the lowest income level. For persons in the lowest quintile of income in the United States, the net worth of whites is 10,000 times higher than that of blacks ($10,257 versus $1).

As noted earlier, systematic discrimination can also affect the quantity and quality of services received, including medical care. Recent research has focused on the potential health consequences of subjective experiences of discrimination. Racism in the larger society can also lead to systematic differences in exposure to personal experiences of discrimination. These experiences of discrimination may be an important part of subjectively experienced stress that can adversely affect health. A growing body of evidence indicates that self-reported measures of discrimination are adversely related to physical and mental health in a broad range of racial/ethnic minority populations (Amaro et al., 1987; Salgado de Snyder, 1987; Krieger, 1990; Dion et al., 1992; Jackson et al., 1996; Krieger and Sidney, 1996; Kessler, et al., 1999; Noh et al., 1999). Two recent studies suggest that exposure to discrimination plays a role in explaining observed racial differences in self-reported measures of health (Williams et al., 1997; Ren, et al., 1999).

A small body of research suggests that the prevalence of negative stereotypes and cultural images of stigmatized groups can adversely affect health status. First, the widespread societal stigma of inferiority can create specific anxieties, expectations, and reactions that can affect health indirectly by having an adverse impact on socioeconomic performance and mobility (Fischer et al., 1996; Steele, 1997). There may also be more direct health effects. Researchers have long identified that one response of minority populations would be to accept the dominant society's ideology of their inferiority as accurate. A few studies have operationalized the extent to which African Americans internalize or endorse these negative cultural images. These studies have found that internalized racism is positively related to psychological distress, depressive symptoms, substance use, and chronic physical health problems (Taylor and Jackson, 1990; Taylor et al., 1991; Williams and Chung, in press).

SOCIOECONOMIC AND RACIAL/ETHNIC CHARACTERISTICS OF SOCIAL SYSTEMS AS DETERMINANTS OF INDIVIDUAL AND POPULATION HEALTH

Individuals occupy particular socioeconomic positions and racial/ethnic status within broader systems of socioeconomic and racial/ethnic stratification at the level of communities, metropolitan areas, regions, nations, and even the world. Research and theory increasingly suggest the importance in at least two ways of these broader stratification systems for individual and population health. First, the nature of socioeconomic and racial/ethnic stratification at these more macrosocial levels is a major determinant of the nature and meaning of the socioeconomic and racial/ethnic status occupied by individuals. For example, the level of economic growth and development in communities, metropolitan areas, regions, nations, and the world and the relative equality or inequality in the distribution of the fruits of economic growth and development shape the absolute and relative levels of income of individuals. In particular, living in an area with lower levels of average income or higher levels of income inequality will increase the likelihood of individuals having low income levels. Similarly, as discussed in the preceding section, higher levels of racial/ethnic segregation are likely to adversely affect the socioeconomic position and other life chances of members of disadvantaged racial/ethnic groups. Second, the socioeconomic and racial/ethnic composition of areas may have effects on individual health that are not mediated through individual socioeconomic and racial/ethnic status. Such effects may be additive or interactive, as shown in Figure 3. The socioeconomic and racial/ethnic characteristics of areas may affect individuals' (and hence population) health independently of individuals' personal socioeconomic and racial/ethnic characteristics, presumably by shaping the nature of the social and physical environment in the area in terms of variables specified in Figure 3 or other unspecified features of the environment that can affect individual health. The area-level socioeconomic, racial/ethnic, and environmental characteristics may also interact with and potentiate or buffer the impact of individual socioeconomic and racial/ethnic status on health. For example, living in a poor area may increase the impact of individual income on health because personal resources become even more consequential in the relative absence of benign environmental influences, and, conversely, living in a better-off area may soften the impact of personal economic deprivation.

Contextual Effects: Real but Limited

Effects of area characteristics on individuals are usually referred to as context effects (e.g., Hauser, 1970, 1974). Evidence of aggregate or ecological correlation between the socioeconomic and racial/ethnic characteristics of areas and the population health parameters of the areas (e.g., mortality rates) are suggestive of context effects, but do not demonstrate them because they fail to control for the characteristics of individuals, which, as shown in Figure 3, may either select people into areas or be shaped by the characteristics of the area. A small number of studies exist that test the effects of area socioeconomic and racial/ethnic characteristics net of individual-level characteristics. As in other areas of research (e.g., Jencks and Mayer, 1990), the general finding is that there are significant effects of context, but that a far greater portion of the variance in individual health outcomes is explained by the socioeconomic and racial/ethnic characteristics of individuals (see Robert, 1999 and Robert and House, 2000a, for reviews of the socioeconomic literature, and Collins and Williams, 1999, for a review of the racial/ethnic literature). However, because social contexts also exert effects on individual characteristics, they remain a potential target for interventions to preomote health.

In recent years, a particular socioeconomic characteristic of areas, income inequality, has received a great deal of attention. Interest in this topic derives from the observation at the population level (as well as at the individual level, e.g., Sorlie et al., 1995) that the relation of income to health is curvilinear, reflecting a pattern of diminishing returns, as shown in Figure 4. Across nations (and within nations over time), growth in average income per capita has had a very powerful effect on population health, presumably reflecting the associated growth both in individual incomes and in public and private social infrastruc-

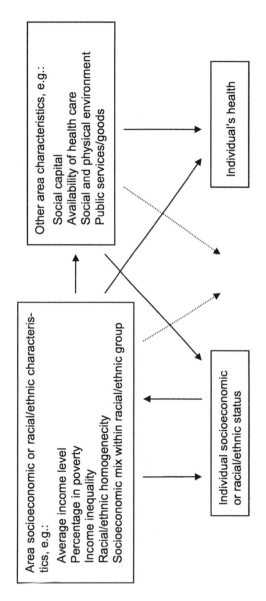

FIGURE 3 Pathways for effects of area socioeconomic and racial/ethnic characteristics on health. NOTE: Dashed lines indicate moderating (or interactive) effects of area characteristics on the relationship of individual racial ethnic status to health.

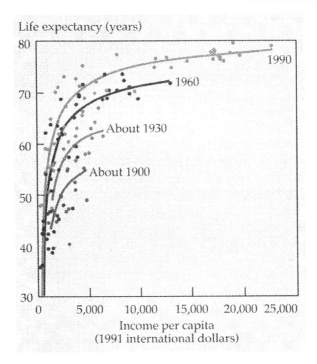

FIGURE 4 Life expectancy and income per capita for selected countries and periods. SOURCE: The World Bank, *World Development Report,* 1993. Reprinted in Wilkinson, 1996:34.

tures productive of health. However, at higher levels of per capita income (e.g., about $5,000 per person, 1991 international dollars), the relationship becomes much weaker. Across countries at this level, however, a number of analyses have found much stronger correlations between income inequality and health (Rodgers, 1979; Wilkinson, 1992, 1996; van Doorslaer et al., 1997). Wilkinson and others have argued that these data, and similar data comparing areas within developed countries (e.g., Ben-Shlomo et al., 1996; Kaplan et al., 1996; Kennedy et al., 1996; Kawachi et al., 1997), reflect strong effects of income inequality per se, operating through variables such as social capital, cohesion, and trust in the population. A large body of conceptual and empirical analyses suggests, on the contrary, that income inequality has its effects primarily via the underlying high level of individuals with relatively low income that necessarily characterizes areas with more unequal incomes, at least given the average levels of income in these populations (Gravelle, 1998; Deaton, 1999; Mellor and Milyo, 1999). Some evidence exists in methodologically sound studies for contextual effects of income inequality, but these are equally or more plausibly interpretable as reflecting a lower investment in public goods, especially for the disadvantaged, in areas or political units characterized by greater income inequality (Robert and House, 2000a; Lynch et al., 2000). Again, these data still suggest that interventions that affect income inequality (or correlates of it) can be a potential means of improving individual or population health, if only or mainly by improving the incomes of more disadvantaged individuals.

In sum, the socioeconomic and, especially, racial/ethnic (due to the powerful deleterious effects of segregation on African Americans discussed at the end of the previous section) characteristics of areas are important components of understanding socioeconomic and racial/ethnic disparities. Hence, they must also be important in policies aimed at alleviating such disparities.

IMPROVING POPULATION HEALTH AND REDUCING SOCIOECONOMIC AND RACIAL/ETHNIC DISPARITIES THROUGH PLANNED SOCIAL POLICY AND UNPLANNED SOCIAL CHANGE

What has been said thus far provides powerful evidence of how social and behavioral science knowledge can contribute to societal and governmental objectives of improving population health and reducing socioeconomic and racial-ethnic disparities in health. It is these socioeconomic and racial/ethnic disparities in health that we believe largely explain why the United States has levels of population health significantly below those of peer nations such as Canada, Japan, or Sweden, and no better than those of many less developed countries (see Figure 5), despite national expenditures on health care and health research that far exceed those of any other nation. Indeed, disadvantaged portions of the U.S. population have levels of health no better than those of some of the least developed nations in the world (McCord and Freeman, 1990).

The main message we want to deliver is that socioeconomic policy and practice and racial/ethnic policy and practice are the most significant levers for reducing socioeconomic and racial/ethnic disparities and hence improving overall population health in our society, more important even than health care policy.

Interventions in Pathways or Mechanisms: Promise and Problems

One of the major reasons for understanding the pathways or mechanisms linking a health outcome to its more distal causes such as socioeconomic and racial/ethnic status is the promise that we may be able to intervene in the pathways or mechanisms, even if we cannot alter the more distal causes, and thus eliminate or mitigate the deleterious effects of the distal cause. Preventive and therapeutic pharmacological interventions via "magic bullets" epitomize this strategy for preventing disease and promoting health. Even if we cannot cradicate the bacteria, viruses, or toxins that cause infectious diseases, we can reduce or eliminate their deleterious effects via vaccination or prophylaxis. Even where

106

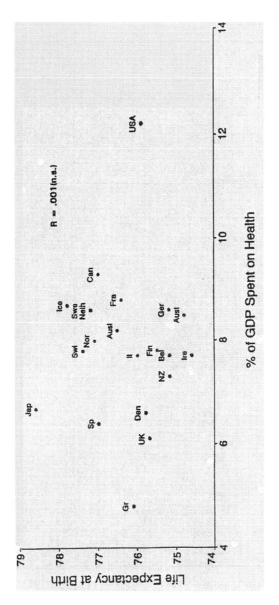

FIGURE 5 Life expectancy at birth by percent of gross domestic product (GDP) spent on health, 1990 (for se-lected OECD countries).

we may only partially understand, much less be able to intervene in, the ultimate causes of disease, as in hypertension, we can mitigate or eliminate its deleterious effects by acting on better-understood intervening mechanisms.

This paradigm of disease prevention and health promotion has great appeal, based on the dramatic instances of its success just alluded to. However, it remains generally more effective and efficient to approach disease promotion from a broader population or public health standpoint where feasible. This has been and may continue to be particularly true for socioeconomic and racial/ethnic disparities in health, for reasons discussed earlier. Returning to the case of cigarette smoking discussed more fully in Paper Contribution K, efforts to understand or intervene in the physiological pathway through which it operates have not yet been successful, and extensive efforts at behavioral and pharmacological interventions to stop smoking behavior at the level of individuals have been only modestly successful. Nevertheless, in the United States at least, we have made major progress in reducing levels of cigarette consumption, due in large part to broader population-wide interventions via pricing, labeling, regulation of pro- and anti-smoking advertising, and increasingly severe restrictions on where and when persons may smoke, all contributing to an increasingly strong set of social norms against smoking. Further, and paradoxically, the success of efforts to reduce smoking may have contributed, as noted above, to the perplexing pattern from which we began—overall improvements in population health but widening socioeconomic and racial/ethnic disparities in health. This is because persons of higher socioeconomic position, especially education, have been much more likely to stop or not start smoking, thus creating a growing inverse association between socioeconomic position and smoking (Moore et al., 1996).

We believe that efforts to intervene on many other psychosocial pathways linking socioeconomic and racial/ethnic status to health are likely to confront similar problems and potentially exacerbate rather than alleviate socioeconomic and racial/ethnic differences in health, unless they very carefully take account of the ways in which these pathways and mechanisms may operate differentially across socioeconomic or racial/ethnic groups. This would be true for plausibly promising interventions such as modifying other health behaviors (eating, drinking, exercise); stress management and reduction; enhancing social relationships and supports, and social capital; or modifying psychological dispositions such as anger or hostility and control or efficacy. This is primarily because such interventions generally presume that the intervening risk factor can be modified largely by individual choice and effort and hence do not alter the strong forces in our systems of socioeconomic and racial/ethnic stratification that produce differences in the first place. These forces include (1) differential access or exposure to opportunities for desirable health behaviors (e.g., areas populated by disadvantaged socioeconomic and racial/ethnic minorities tend to be long on convenience and liquor stores selling cigarettes and junk food and short on supermarkets or groceries selling fresh fruits and vegetables or on safe and supportive venues and facilities for physical activity); (2) the increased risks in disadvantaged socioeconomic groups and areas of stressful events at work or home or of disruptions of social relationships, networks, and support by illness and death; (3) greater exposure to experiences generative of discrimination, hostility, or inefficacy; and (4) heightened exposure to social, and to physical, chemical, and biological environmental hazards. In addition, as noted above, the tendency is for new health problems (e.g., AIDS) and risk factors to arise, which may operate via quite different mechanisms and pathways and yet to become rapidly stratified by socioeconomic and racial/ethnic status.

Nevertheless, there are opportunities for intervening in pathways and mechanisms that offer promise of reducing socioeconomic and racial/ethnic disparities and hence improving overall population health. These must involve, however, sensitivity to the specific sources of risk and also of resilience in disadvantaged socioeconomic and racial/ethnic groups and areas. Let us consider two examples—medical care and sources of resilience and health promotion in disadvantaged racial/ethnic groups.

Medical Care

What we know and do not know about the role of medical care in producing and alleviating socioeconomic and racial/ethnic disparities in health is illustrative. As already noted, there can be no question that wider availability of effective therapeutic and preventive medical care has improved population health, though to a more limited degree than is often presumed. However, Preston and Haines (1991) argued that improvements in medical care may also have exacerbated socioeconomic and racial/ethnic disparities in health to the extent that differential access to care has become more consequential for health. As we have seen, the implementation of national health services or insurance has failed to reduce socioeconomic and racial/ethnic disparities in health to the degree we had hoped or expected, if at all. Growing evidence suggests, however, that gross equalization of access or utilization fails to equalize access to maximally appropriate and effective care.

Addressing three kinds of issues offers promise of reducing socioeconomic and racial/ethnic disparities in the quality and appropriateness of care and hence in health. The first is to recognize that differentials in the ways the medical care system deals with different groups can lead to problems in the delivery of care. If disadvantaged socioeconomic and racial/ethnic groups do not have access to the same type and quality of providers and the same kind of relationships and communication with them as more advantaged persons, the result is likely to be their receiving less regular, preventive, and appropriate care. Second, the focus of the medical care system on different types of care differentially affects the health of different groups. Disadvantaged groups may benefit more from improvements in basic primary and preventive care; advantaged groups, from secondary and tertiary care. Thus, relatively poor societies (e.g., China, Costa Rica, Sri Lanka, Kerala State of India) have achieved "good health at low cost" by focusing their limited resources on ensuring equal access to basic primary and preventive care (Halsted et al., 1985). Finally, as discussed above, even secondary and tertiary care appears to be distributed inequitably by racial/ethnic groups and probably also by socioeconomic status. This may explain why the United States generally lags behind other developed nations in population life expectancy, but surpasses all in life expectancy at age 80, where a high technology system supports a relatively elite set of survivors in the population.

Finally, we must also give more attention in medical care to identifying the ways in which the lives of individuals are constrained by broader social, economic, and political forces. Some evidence suggests that the effectiveness of behavioral interventions varies by the degree that they attend to social situations in which individuals are embedded. Syme's (1978) study of 244 hypertensive patients clearly illustrates how addressing underlying social and economic conditions appears to enhance the management of hypertension and improve the effectiveness of antihypertensive therapy. The patients in this study were matched on age, race, gender, and blood pressure history and randomly assigned to one of three groups. The first group received routine hypertensive care from a physician. In addition to routine hypertensive care, the second group also attended 12 weekly clinic meetings providing health education with regard to hypertension by a health educator and nurse practitioner. In addition to routine hypertensive care, the third group was visited by community health workers who had been recruited from the immediate community and provided with one month of training to address the diverse social and medical needs of persons with hypertension. These outreach lay workers provided information on hypertension but also discussed family difficulties, financial strain, and employment opportunities and, as appropriate, provided support, advice, referral, and direct assistance.

After seven months of follow-up, patients in the third group were more likely to have their blood pressure controlled than patients in the other two groups. In addition, those in the third group knew twice as much about blood pressure and were more compliant with taking their hypertensive medication than patients in the other two groups, and the good compliers in the third group were twice as successful at controlling their blood pressure as good compliers in the health education intervention group. Thus, even the effectiveness of the pharmacological treatment appeared to be enhanced in the group that also addressed the underlying stressful conditions of these hypertensive persons.

A study by Buescher and colleagues (1987) further illustrates how addressing underlying economic and social issues can improve the impact of medical care. This study compared the effectiveness of two approaches to delivering prenatal care in a population of predominantly black low-SES women in Guilford County, North Carolina. One group received prenatal care at the county health department. The other group received prenatal care from private practice physicians. Women who received care from the community-based physicians were twice as likely to have a low-birthweight baby, compared to those visiting the health department. The health department's prenatal care program attempted to comprehensively address the medical and social needs of the pregnant mothers. Prenatal care was provided by nurse practitioners, instead of physicians. Time was devoted during prenatal care visits to counseling the women about nutrition and other aspects of personal care. As appropriate, referrals were made to the Women, Infants and Children Program, which provides nutritional supplements to poor women. These referrals, as well as missed clinic appointments, were followed up aggressively. James (1993) argues that the positive cultural features of this program may have been very important. It appears that the county health department's program offered low-income women an extended network of social support, capable of meeting their needs in much the same way that older, more knowledgeable women have traditionally guided and supported young inexperienced mothers (James, 1993).

Adaptive Attributes of Disadvantaged Groups

One of the major paradoxes in U.S. population health is that African Americans and Latinos are not as disadvantaged on some aspects of health as their socioeconomic positions would lead us to expect. Thus, although African Americans tend to have higher levels of ill health than whites for most indicators of physical health and are also disadvantaged compared to whites on indicators of subjective well-being such as life satisfaction and happiness (Hughes and Thomas, 1998), they have comparable or better health status than whites for other indicators of mental health. Community-based studies using measures of psychological distress show an inconsistent pattern of black–white differences. Some studies show that blacks have higher rates of distress compared to whites, while other studies show higher rates of psychological distress for whites compared to blacks (Dohrenwend and Dohrenwend, 1969; Neighbors, 1984; Vega and Rumbaut, 1991; Williams and Harris-Reid, 1999). However, when rates of psychiatric illness are considered, African Americans have comparable or lower rates of mental illness than whites. In the Epidemiologic Catchment Area Study (ECA), the largest study of psychiatric disorders ever conducted in the United States, there were very few differences between blacks and whites in the rates of both current and lifetime psychiatric disorders. Anxiety disorders, especially phobias, stand out as one area in which blacks had considerably higher rates than Caucasians. In the National Comorbidity Study blacks do not have higher rates of disorder than whites for any of the major classes of disorders (Kessler et al., 1994). Instead, lower rates of disorders for blacks than whites are especially pronounced for the affective disorders (depression) and the substance abuse disorders (alcohol and drug abuse).

These findings emphasize the need for renewed attention to identify the cultural strengths and health-enhancing resources within the black community. Two social institutions—the family and the church—stand out as crucial for the black population. Strong family ties and an extended family system are important resources that may reduce some of the negative effects of stress on the health of black Americans. At the same time, a recognition of the strengths of black families should not be used to romanticize them as if they were a panacea for a broad range of adverse living conditions. While these networks of mutual aid and support do facilitate survival, they are also likely to provide both stress and support. Moreover, it is likely that cutbacks in government-provided social services in recent years have increased the burdens and demands on the support services provided by the black family. The black American church has been the most important social institution in the black community. These churches have historically been centers of spiritual, social, and political life. Black churches may promote mental health by providing a broad range of social and human services to the African-American community, serving as a conduit to the formal mental health system, providing a base for friendship networks, and facilitating collective catharsis and stress reduction through religious rituals and participation (Williams, 1998).

A second paradox is evident for Mexican Americans. In spite of high rates of poverty and comparatively low levels of access to medical care, Mexican Americans tend to have similar or better levels of health than the white population. Moreover, across a broad range of health status indicators foreign-born Hispanics have a better health profile than their counterparts born in the United States. This pattern may reflect the impact of migration. Rates of infant mortality, low birthweight, cancer, high blood pressure, adolescent pregnancy, and psychiatric disorders increase with length of stay in the United States for Hispanics (Vega and Amaro, 1994). It is likely that increasing length of stay and greater acculturation of the Hispanic and Asian population will lead to worsening health. Early studies of acculturation found that rates of heart disease among Japanese increased progressively as they moved from Japan to Hawaii to the U.S. mainland (Marmot and Syme, 1976). As groups migrate from one culture to another, immigrants often adopt the diet and behavior patterns of the new culture. Several behaviors that adversely affect health status appear to increase with acculturation. These include decreased fiber consumption, decreased breast feeding, increased use of cigarettes and alcohol—especially in young women, driving under the influence of alcohol, and use of illicit drugs (Vega and Amaro, 1994). However, the association between acculturation, length of stay in the United States, and the prevalence of disease may be complex. Migration studies of the Chinese and Japanese show that the rates of some cancers, such as prostate and colon, increase when these populations migrate to the United States, while the rates of other cancers, such as liver and cervical, decline (Jenkins and Kagawa-Singer, 1994). Research is needed to identify the extent to which there are specific aspects of culture that promote health and the strategies that may be utilized to facilitate their maintenance over time.

Social and Economic Change and Policy as Major Determinants of Health

For all the reasons discussed to this point, we believe the reduction of socioeconomic and racial/ethnic disparities in health depends most on social changes and public policies that reduce disparities in socioeconomic and racial/ethnic status, or more exactly, ensure that all citizens live under conditions that protect against disease and promote health. We would emphasize that we do not believe that there is evidence that inequality or hierarchy per se produces large social disparities in health, though it may always be a residual difference in any situation of inequality. This is because socioeconomic and other forces of advantage have diminishing returns to health. Thus, the issue is not reducing or eliminating inequality, but reducing or eliminating the relatively severe social and economic deprivations that still characterize the broad lower range (e.g., lower 25–50%) of the U.S. population in terms of socioeconomic and/or racial/ethnic status. The history of our own and other countries suggests that the poor (and truly disadvantaged) need not always be with us, and that as their conditions of life improve so does their health and hence also overall population health.

Improvements in the status of the socioeconomically or racially/ethnically disadvantaged can be made through the provision of either private or public goods or a combination thereof. That is, we can ensure their access to education, income, and other resources that allow them to obtain in the private market housing, health care, and good living and working conditions productive of health. Alternatively we can provide many of these as public goods. Different societies at different times have chosen different mixes, but all have converged on a mix of these strategies. How good is the evidence that they work to reduce health disparities and promote population health? It is both better and worse than we might expect or like.

Macrosocial Change and Health

Not to be ignored is the evidence of history that improvements in the educational, occupational, and income levels of populations have produced massive improvements in population health that in turn improve the human capital necessary for further socioeconomic advancement (see Figure 4). This has included the reduction of health disparities by socioeconomic position, gender, and/or race/ethnicity. Not surprisingly, educational and economic development are major priorities of less developed societies, and also of the developed countries.

Social Welfare and Health

Similarly, evidence from the more developed countries strongly suggests that ensuring that the fruits of development are broadly distributed, especially to the broad lower range of the population, assists in promotion of health. The rise of Sweden and then Japan to the highest levels of population health in the world, and the clearly reduced socioeconomic disparities in the case of Sweden, must be significantly attributed to their emphasis on ensuring good conditions of life for all, albeit via different mixes of social policy and provision of private and public goods.

More Focused Social Policies

One would like to have clearer evidence, however, that specific policies that improve the social and economic status of disadvantaged groups also improve their health. Unfortunately, we have not always evaluated the effects of such policies, and rarely their health impacts, and this remains an agenda for future research. However, limited and developing evidence is at least consistent with our thesis.

At least one study from the evaluation of the negative income tax experiments of the early 1970s shows positive effects on maternal and child health. In a study of expanded income support, Kehrer and Wolin (1979) found that the birthweight of infants born to mothers in the experimental income group was higher than that of those born to mothers in the control group although neither group experienced any experimental manipulation of health services. Improved nutrition, probably a result of the income manipulation, appeared to have been the key intervening factor. Evaluation of the long-term effects of early childhood interventions, such as the Perry preschool study, also suggests long-term effects on socioeconomic factors (median income and rates of home ownership) as well as on other behavior and beliefs (e.g., staying in school, avoiding delinquency and crime, achieving better jobs) that should promote health.

Major Exogenous Income Policies

An ideal test of our thesis would be the examination of social policies that have markedly improved the economic status of all or some of the disadvantaged population. In the United States, two stand out. One is Social Security which has provided an income support program for the elder portion of the population that has, over time, lifted or kept most of them out of poverty. We (Arno and House, in progress) have undertaken to see if one can find evidence that Social Security has also improved the health of the elderly. We have sought to do so by examining the mortality experience of different adult age groups in the population over the course of the century. We hypothesized that the two largest exogenous income improvements from Social Security occurred first at its inception in the late 1930s and second when it was indexed to inflation in the late 1960s and early 1970s. Hence, we expected that one should see discontinuous improvements in the health of the elderly, but not in other age groups, after these two periods. Our initial results, shown in Figure 6, seem to us consistent with this. We recognize that there may be other compelling explanations of these two discontinuities, but we do not believe that others have or would have predicted both of them ex ante or that other explanations can explain both as well or as parsimoniously ex post. Further, these trends are consistent with the evidence that socioeconomic differences in health are markedly reduced among the elderly as compared to working-age adults (House et al., 1990, 1994). The

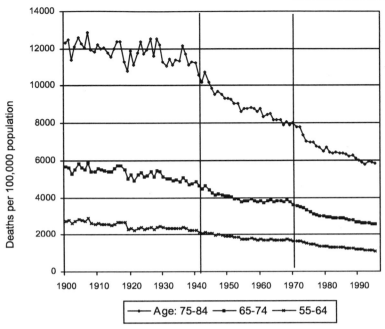

FIGURE 6 Total mortality, United States, 1900–1995.

other major income support program in our country has been the earned income tax credit, but we know of no research on its effects and would certainly see such research as a high priority for the future.

Investment in Public Goods and Infrastructure

Limited data also indicate that efforts to improve the public goods and infrastructures of communities improve the health of their residents. Some research suggests that policy changes to improve neighborhoods can importantly enhance health. Dalgard and Tambs (1997) provide findings from a 10–year follow–up study of residents in five neighborhood types in Norway. This study found that residents in a poorly functioning neighborhood that had experienced dramatic change in its social environment over time reported improved mental health 10 years later. The improvements in the neighborhoods included a new public school, playground extension, establishment of a sports arena and park, organization of activities for adolescents by the sports association of the municipality, establishment of a shopping center with restaurants and a cinema, and a subway line extension into the neighborhood. This effect was not explained by selective migration. Similarly, an intervention in England for a poorly functioning neighborhood also had dramatic effects (Halpern, 1995). Over a 2-year period this intervention refurbished housing, with a special emphasis on making it safe and sheltered from strangers. Changes included improved traffic regulations, improved lighting and strengthening of windows, enclosure of gardens for apartments, closure of alleyways, and landscaping. In this project, residents were involved in the planning process. A 1-year follow-up study, conducted after the intervention had been in place, documented that the changes in the physical environment were associated with changes in the social environment and mental health as well. That is, the contact between neighbors had increased and neighbors reported more trust in each other. Levels of optimism and belief in the future had increased, and residents felt a stronger identification with their neighborhood. In addition, levels of anxiety and depression were significantly reduced among residents. This study reveals that improvement in the quality of life in a neighborhood can increase both the quality of social interaction or cohesion and health (see Paper Contribution I).

The Case of Racial/Ethnic Disparities

Racial/ethnic disparities in health should clearly be reduced by policies that reduce absolute and relative socioeconomic deprivation. However, they also need special approaches, obviously not aimed at changing race/ethnicity per se, but, rather, at changing the way race/ethnicity and associated racial/ethnic status are socially defined and constructed. Again, available evidence suggests there are reduced racial/ethnic disparities in health. Mullings (1989) has suggested that the civil rights movement, for example, had important positive effects on black health. By reducing occupational and educational segregation, it improved the SES of at least a segment of the black population and also influenced public policy to make health care accessible to larger numbers of people. Consistent with this hypothesis, one study found that between 1968 and 1978, blacks experienced a larger decline in mortality rates (on both a percentage and absolute basis) than whites (Cooper et al., 1981).

CONCLUSION

We hope this paper has produced an appreciation that socioeconomic and racial/ethnic disparities in health are the product of a broad and complex system of social stratification that will continue to structure the experience of and exposure to virtually all behavioral and psychosocial risk factors to health, hence producing large, persistent, and even increasing socioeconomic and racial/ethnic disparities in health. These health disparities largely explain why the United States increasingly lags behind other developed and even less developed nations in levels of population health, with the most disadvantaged portions of our population characterized by levels of population health comparable to some of the least developed nations in the world.

Socioeconomic and racial/ethnic disadvantages affect almost all forms of disease; almost all behavioral, psychosocial, and environmental risk factors producing these diseases; and also access to the most appropriate and effective forms of medical care. These effects are persistent over time. Thus, as the major public health problems of society and the risk factors producing them change, they still will be more incident and prevalent among lower socioeconomic classes. Thus, intervening in or changing one or a few major risk factors for health (including inadequate medical care) can have only a limited effect on socioeconomic and racial/ethnic disparities in health, though this effect is clearly enhanced if interventions or changes are attentive to the broader social forces that produce these disparities.

The greatest past accomplishments and future potential for reducing socio-economic and racial/ethnic disparities in health and improving overall population health involve improving socioeconomic status and reducing invidious racial/ethnic distinctions themselves, especially among the more disadvantaged portions of the population. Thus, economic growth and development and progress toward greater racial/ethnic equality have had and can have dramatic effects on individual and population health, especially if these changes impact the more disadvantaged socioeconomic and racial/ethnic groups in our society.

REFERENCES

Adler, N.E., Boyce, T., Chesney, M.A., Cohen, S., Folkman, S., Kahn, R.L., and Syme, S.L. (1994). Socioeconomic status and health: The challenge of the gradient. *American Psychologist,* 49(1), 15–24.

Adler, N.E., Boyce, T., Chesney, M.A., Folkman, S., and Syme, S.L. (1993). Socioeconomic inequalities in health: No easy solution. *Journal of the American Medical Association,* 269, 3140–3145.

Amaro, H., Russo, N.F., and Johnson, J. (1987). Family and work predictors of psychological well-being among Hispanic women professionals. *Psychology of Women Quarterly,* 11, 505–521.

Arno, P., and House, J.S. (in progress). Can socioeconomic policy improve population health and reduce social disparities in health: The case of Social Security.

Backlund, E., Sorlie, P.D., and Johnson, N.J. (1996). The shape of the relationship between income and mortality in the United States. *AEP,* 6, 12–20.

Barker, D.J.P., and Osmond, C. (1986). Infant mortality, childhood nutrition and ischaemic heart disease in England and Wales. *Lancet,* 1, 1077–1081.

Ben-Shlomo, Y., White, I.R., and Marmot, M. (1996). Does the variation in the socioeconomic characteristics of an area affect mortality? *British Medical Journal,* 312, 1013–1014.

Berkman, L.F., and Breslow, L. (1983). *Health and Ways of Living.* New York: Oxford University Press.

Blane, D., Hart, C.L., Smith, G.D., Gillis, C.R., Hole, D.J., and Hawthorne, V.M. (1996). Association of cardiovascular disease risk factors with socioeconomic position during childhood and during adulthood. *British Medical Journal,* 313(7070), 1434–1438.

Blau, P., and Duncan, O.D. (1967). *The American Occupational Structure.* New York: Wiley.

ser, R.M. (1   *Opportunity and Change.* New York: Aca-

nkowski, M Lucas, S.R., Swidler, A., and Voss, K. (1996).
  Cracking t ell Curve Myth. Princeton, NJ: Princeton Uni-

(1993). *Cle nd Convincing Evidence: Measurement of Dis-
ca.* Washing , DC: Urban Institute Press.
.W., Reilly.W., Mentnech, R.M., Fitterman, L.K., Kucken,
3.C. (1996), ffects of race and income on mortality and use of
dicare ben ciaries. *New England Journal of Medicine,* 335

we should ot name human races: A biological view. Pp. 231–
d.), *Ever Si ce Darwin.* New York, W. W. Norton .
v much of c relation between population mortality and unequal
me is a s atistical artifact? *British Medical Journal,* 316, 382–

tal Health and Built Environment.* London: Taylor and Francis.
.A. and Warren, K.S.   (1985). *Good Health at Low Cost: Pro-
ference at the Bellagio   Conference Center,* Bellagio, Italy, April
ork: Rockefeller Foundation.
, M., Burke, J., Stone, D., Kumar, D., Arani, D., Pierce, W., Rafii,
., Sharma, S., Slater, J., and DeBuono, B.A. (1999). Access to
ypass surgery by race/ethnicity and gender among patients who are
rgery. *Medical Care,* 37(1), 68–77.
s, R., and Elixhauser, A. (1997). Racial and gender differences in
s for black and white hospitalized adults. *Ethnicity and Disease,* 7,

Context and convex: A cautionary tale. *American Journal of Soci-
664.
Contextual analysis revisited. *Sociological Methods and Research,* 2

n Hippel, W. (1996). Stereotypes. *Annual Review of Psychology,* 47,

r, R.C., Herzog, A.R., Mero, R. P., Kinney, A.M., and Breslow, M.J.
ocioeconomic status, and health. *Milbank Quarterly* 68(3), 383–411.
er, R.C., Herzog, A.R., Mero, R.P., Kinney, A.M., and Breslow, M.J.
l stratification, age, and health. Pp. 1–32 in K.W. Schaie, D. Blazer,
se (eds.), *Aging, Health Behaviors, and Health Outcomes.* Hillsdale,

is, K., and Umberson, D. (1988). Social relationships and health. *Sci-
40–545.
kowski, J.M., Kinney, A.M., Mero, R.P., Kessler, R.C., and Herzog,
. The social stratification of aging and health. *Journal of Health and So-
or,* 35, 213–234.
Thomas, M.E. (1998). The continuing significance of race revisited: A
ce, class, and quality of life in America, 1972 to 1996. *American Socio-
iew,* 63, 785–795.
(1996). Black–white differences in health and mortality: A review and
l model. *Sociological Quarterly,* 37(1), 105–125.

Blendon, R., Aike
 black and wh
 278–281.
Buescher, P.A., Sm
 care and infant l
 of Obstetrics and
Bunker, J.P., Frazier,
 of medical care. *l*
Chapman, K.S., and H
 between income an
 health analysis. *Jou*
Chen, M.S. (1993). A 1!
 Americans: Compari
 Pacific Islander J. He
Collins, C.A., and William
 of racism? *Sociologica*
Conley, D. (1999). *Being b*
 America. Berkeley, CA:
Cooper, R.S., and David, R.
 public health and epidem
 97–116.
Cooper, R.S., Steinhauer, M.,
 society, and disease: An e:
 ferential mortality. *Internal*
Dalgard, O.S., and Tambs, K. (1
 dinal study. *British Journal*
Davis, J.A., and Smith, T.W. (19
 tional Opinion Research Cent
Deaton, A. (1999). Inequalities in
 per 7141.
Devine, P.G. (1989). Stereotypes an
 nents. *Journal of Personality an*
Devine, P.G. (1995). Prejudice and (
 Advanced Social Psychology.
Dion, K.L., Dion, K.K., and Pak, A.W
 for discrimination-related stress i:
 nadian Journal of Behavioral Scie
Dohrenwend, B.P., and Dohrenwend, E
 order: A Casual Inquiry. New York
Economic Report of the President (1998
 Office.
Eller, T.J. (1994). *Household Wealth an*
 Census, Current Population Reports,
 Printing Office.
Elo, I.T., and Preston, S.H. (1992). Effects
 review. *Population Index,* 58 (2), 186–2
Evans, R.G., Barer, M.L., and Marmor, T.R.
 Others Are Not?: The Determinants of
 deGruyter.

Featherman, D.L, and Ha
 demic Press.
Fischer, C.S., Hout, M., J
 Inequality by Design
 versity Press.
Fix, M., and Struyk, R.J.
 crimination in Amer
Gornick, M.E., Eggers,
 L.E., and Vladeck,
 services among Me
 (11): 791–799.
Gould, S.J. (1977). Why
 236 in S. J. Gould (
Gravelle, H. (1998). Ho
 distribution of inc
 385.
Halpern, D. (1995). Me
Halsted, S.B., Walsh,
 ceedings of a Co
 29–May 3. New Y
Hannan, E.L., van Ryr
 S., Sanborn, T.A
 coronary artery b
 appropriate for s
Harris, D.R., Andrew
 use of procedure
 91–105.
Hauser, R.M. (1970)
 ology, 75, 645–
Hauser, R. (1974).
 (3), 365–375.
Hilton, J.L., and v
 237–271.
House, J.S., Kessl
 (1990). Age,
House, J.S., Kessl
 (1992). Soci
 and J.S. Ho
 NJ: Erlbaum
House, J.S., Lan
 ence, 241, 5
House, J.S., Le
 A.R. (1994
 cial Behav
Hughes, M., an
 study of r
 logical Re
Hummer, R.A
 conceptua

Featherman, D.L, and Hauser, R.M. (1978). *Opportunity and Change.* New York: Academic Press.

Fischer, C.S., Hout, M., Jankowski, M.S., Lucas, S.R., Swidler, A., and Voss, K. (1996). *Inequality by Design: Cracking the Bell Curve Myth.* Princeton, NJ: Princeton University Press.

Fix, M., and Struyk, R.J. (1993). *Clear and Convincing Evidence: Measurement of Discrimination in America.* Washington, DC: Urban Institute Press.

Gornick, M.E., Eggers, P.W., Reilly, T.W., Mentnech, R.M., Fitterman, L.K., Kucken, L.E., and Vladeck, B.C. (1996). Effects of race and income on mortality and use of services among Medicare beneficiaries. *New England Journal of Medicine,* 335 (11): 791–799.

Gould, S.J. (1977). Why we should not name human races: A biological view. Pp. 231–236 in S. J. Gould (ed.), *Ever Since Darwin.* New York, W. W. Norton .

Gravelle, H. (1998). How much of the relation between population mortality and unequal distribution of income is a statistical artifact? *British Medical Journal,* 316, 382–385.

Halpern, D. (1995). *Mental Health and Built Environment.* London: Taylor and Francis.

Halsted, S.B., Walsh, J.A. and Warren, K.S. (1985*). Good Health at Low Cost: Proceedings of a Conference at the Bellagio Conference Center,* Bellagio, Italy, April 29–May 3. New York: Rockefeller Foundation.

Hannan, E.L., van Ryn, M., Burke, J., Stone, D., Kumar, D., Arani, D., Pierce, W., Rafii, S., Sanborn, T.A., Sharma, S., Slater, J., and DeBuono, B.A. (1999). Access to coronary artery bypass surgery by race/ethnicity and gender among patients who are appropriate for surgery. *Medical Care,* 37(1), 68–77.

Harris, D.R., Andrews, R., and Elixhauser, A. (1997). Racial and gender differences in use of procedures for black and white hospitalized adults. *Ethnicity and Disease,* 7, 91–105.

Hauser, R.M. (1970). Context and convex: A cautionary tale. *American Journal of Sociology,* 75, 645–664.

Hauser, R. (1974). Contextual analysis revisited. *Sociological Methods and Research,* 2 (3), 365–375.

Hilton, J.L., and von Hippel, W. (1996). Stereotypes. *Annual Review of Psychology, 47,* 237–271.

House, J.S., Kessler, R.C., Herzog, A.R., Mero, R. P., Kinney, A.M., and Breslow, M.J. (1990). Age, socioeconomic status, and health. *Milbank Quarterly* 68(3), 383–411.

House, J.S., Kessler, R.C., Herzog, A.R., Mero, R.P., Kinney, A.M., and Breslow, M.J. (1992). Social stratification, age, and health. Pp. 1–32 in K.W. Schaie, D. Blazer, and J.S. House (eds.), *Aging, Health Behaviors, and Health Outcomes.* Hillsdale, NJ: Erlbaum.

House, J.S., Landis, K., and Umberson, D. (1988). Social relationships and health. *Science,* 241, 540–545.

House, J.S., Lepkowski, J.M., Kinney, A.M., Mero, R.P., Kessler, R.C., and Herzog, A.R. (1994). The social stratification of aging and health. *Journal of Health and Social Behavior,* 35, 213–234.

Hughes, M., and Thomas, M.E. (1998). The continuing significance of race revisited: A study of race, class, and quality of life in America, 1972 to 1996. *American Sociological Review,* 63, 785–795.

Hummer, R.A. (1996). Black–white differences in health and mortality: A review and conceptual model. *Sociological Quarterly,* 37(1), 105–125.

Blendon, R., Aiken, L., Freeman, H., and Corey, C. (1989). Access to medical care for black and white Americans. *Journal of the American Medical Association, 261,* 278–281.

Buescher, P.A., Smith, C., Holliday, J.L., and Levine, R.H. (1987). Source of prenatal care and infant birth weight: The case of a North Carolina county. *American Journal of Obstetrics and Gynecology, 53,* 204–210.

Bunker, J.P., Frazier, H.S., and Mosteller, F. (1994). Improving health: Measuring effects of medical care. *Milbank Quarterly, 72*(2), 225–258.

Chapman, K.S., and Hariharan, G. (1996). Do poor people have a stronger relationship between income and mortality than the rich? Implications of panel data for health–health analysis. *Journal of Risk and Uncertainty, 12,* 51–63.

Chen, M.S. (1993). A 1993 status report on the health status of Asian Pacific Islander Americans: Comparisons with Healthy People 2000 objectives. *Asian American and Pacific Islander J. Health,* 1, 37–55.

Collins, C.A., and Williams, D.R. (1999). Segregation and mortality: The deadly effects of racism? *Sociological Forum,* 14(3), 495–523.

Conley, D. (1999). *Being Black, Living in the Red: Race, Wealth, and Social Policy in America.* Berkeley, CA: University of California Press.

Cooper, R.S., and David, R. (1986). The biological concept of race and its application to public health and epidemiology. *Journal of Health and Politics, Policy and Law,* 11, 97–116.

Cooper, R.S., Steinhauer, M., Miller, W., David, R., and Schatzkin, A. (1981). Racism, society, and disease: An exploration of the social and biological mechanisms of differential mortality. *International Journal of Health Services,* 11(3), 389–414.

Dalgard, O.S., and Tambs, K. (1997). Urban environment and mental health: A longitudinal study. *British Journal of Psychiatry,* 171, 530–536.

Davis, J.A., and Smith, T.W. (1990). *General Social Surveys, 1972–1990.* Chicago: National Opinion Research Center.

Deaton, A. (1999). Inequalities in income and inequalities in health. *NBER Working Paper 7141.*

Devine, P.G. (1989). Stereotypes and prejudice: Their automatic and controlled components. *Journal of Personality and Social Psychology,* 56, 5–18.

Devine, P.G. (1995). Prejudice and out-group perception. Pp. 467–524 in A. Tesser ed., *Advanced Social Psychology.*

Dion, K.L., Dion, K.K., and Pak, A.W.P. (1992). Personality-based hardiness as a buffer for discrimination-related stress in members of Toronto's Chinese community. *Canadian Journal of Behavioral Science,* 24(4), 517–536.

Dohrenwend, B.P., and Dohrenwend, B.S. (1969). *Social Status and Psychological Disorder: A Casual Inquiry.* New York: Wiley.

Economic Report of the President (1998). Washington, DC: U.S. Government Printing Office.

Eller, T.J. (1994). *Household Wealth and Asset Ownership: 1991. U.S. Bureau of the Census, Current Population Reports, P70-34.* Washington, DC: U.S. Government Printing Office.

Elo, I.T., and Preston, S.H. (1992). Effects of early-life conditions on adult mortality: A review. *Population Index,* 58 (2), 186–212.

Evans, R.G., Barer, M.L., and Marmor, T.R. (1994). Why Are Some People Healthy and Others Are Not?: *The Determinants of Health of Populations.* New York: Aldine deGruyter.

Jackson, J.S., Brown, T.N., Williams, D.R., Torres, M., Sellers, S.L., and Brown, K. (1996). Racism and the physical and mental health status of African Americans: A thirteen year national panel study. *Ethnicity and Disease,* 6(1,2), 132–147.

James, S.A. (1993). Racial and ethnic differences in infant mortality and low birth weight: A psychosocial critique. *Annals of Epidemiology,* 3(2), 131–136.

Jaynes, G.D., and Williams, R. M. (1987). *A Common Destiny: Blacks and American Society.* Washington, DC: National Academy Press.

Jencks, C., and Mayer, S.E. (1990). The social consequences of growing up in a poor neighborhood. Pp. 111–186 in L.E. Lynn, Jr., and M.G.H. McGeary (eds.), *Inner-City Poverty in the United States.* Washington, DC: National Academy Press.

Jenkins, C.N.H., and Kagawa-Singer, M. (1994). Cancer. Pp. 105–147 in N.W.S. Zane, D.T. Takeuchi, and K. N.J. Young (eds.), *Confronting Critical Health Issues of Asian and Pacific Islander Americans.* Thousand Oaks, CA: Sage.

Kaplan, G.A., Pamuk, E.R., Lynch, J.W., Cohen, R.D. and Balfour, J.L. (1996). Inequality in income and mortality in the United States: Analysis of mortality and potential pathways. *British Medical Journal,* 312, 999–1003.

Kaplan, G.A., and Salonen, J.T. (1990). Socioeconomic conditions in childhood and ischaemic heart disease during middle age. *British Medical Journal,* 301, 1121–1123.

Kaufman, J.S., Cooper, R.S., and McGee, D.L. (1997). Socioeconomic status and health in blacks and whites: The problem of residual confounding and the resiliency of race. *Epidemiology,* 8, 621–628.

Kawachi, I., Kennedy, B.P., Lochner, K., and Prothrow-Stith, D. (1997). Social capital, income inequality, and mortality. *American Journal of Public Health, 87, (9),* 1491–1498.

Kehrer, B.H., and Wolin, C.M. (1979). Impact of income maintenance on low birth weight: Evidence from the Gary experiment. *Journal of Human Resources,* 14, 434–462.

Kennedy, B.P., Kawachi, I., and Prothrow-Stith, D. (1996). Income distribution and mortality: Cross sectional ecological study of the Robin Hood index in the United States. *British Medical Journal,* 312, 1004–1007.

Kessler, R.C., McGonagle, K.A., Zhao, S., Nelson, C.B., Hughes, M., Eshleman, S., Wittchen, H.-U., and Kendler, K.S. (1994). Lifetime and 12-month prevalence of DSM-III-R psychiatric disorders in the United States. *Archives of General Psychiatry,* 51, 8–19.

Kessler, R.C., Mickelson, K.D., and Williams, D. R. (1999). The prevalence, distribution, and mental health correlates of perceived discrimination in the United States. *Journal of Health and Social Behavior,* 40, 208–230.

Kirschenman, J., and Neckerman, K.M. (1991). "We'd love to hire them, but . . .": The meaning of race for employers. Pp. 203–232 in C. Jencks, and P. E. Peterson (eds.), *The Urban Underclass.* Washington, DC: The Brookings Institution.

Krieger, N. (1990). Racial and gender discrimination: Risk factors for high blood pressure? *Social Science and Medicine,* 30(12), 1273–1281.

Krieger, N., Rowley, D.L., Herman, A. A., Avery, B., and Phillips, M. T. (1993). Racism, sexism, and social class: Implications for studies of health, disease, and well-being. *American Journal of Preventive Medicine,* 9(6 suppl), 82–122.

Krieger, N., and Sidney, S. (1996). Racial discrimination and blood pressure: The CARDIA study of young black and white adults. *American Journal of Public Health,* 86, 1370–1378.

Kuh, D., and Ben-Shlomo, Y. (1997). *A Lifecourse Approach to Chronic Disease Epidemiology.* Oxford: Oxford University Press.

Kunitz, S.J. (1987). Explanations and ideologies of mortality patterns. *Population and Development Review,* 13(3):379–408.

Lalonde, M. (1975). *A New Perspective in the Health of Canadians.* Ottawa: Information Canada.

Lantz, P.M, House, J.S., Lepkowski, J.M., Williams, D.R., Mero, R.P., and Chen, J. (1998). Socioeconomic factors, health behaviors, and mortality. *Journal of the American Medical Association,* 279, 1703–1708.

Lantz, P.M., Lynch, J.W., House, J.S. Lepkowski, J.M. Mero, R.P., Musick, M.A., and Williams, D.R. (in press). Socioeconomic disparities in health change in a longitudinal study of U.S. adults: The role of health risk behaviors. *Social Science and Medicine.*

Latter, B.D.H. (1980). Genetic differences within and between populations of the major human subgroups. *American Naturalist,* 116, 220–237.

LaVeist, T.A. (1996). Why we should continue to study race but do a better job: An essay on race, racism and health. *Ethnicity and Disease,* 6(1,2), 21–29.

Lewontin, R.C. (1972). The apportionment of human diversity. Pp. 381–386 in T. Dobzhansky, M.K. Hecht, and W.C. Steere (eds.), *EvolutionaryBiology,* Vol 6. New York: Appleton-Century-Crofts.

Lewontin, R. (1982). *Human Diversity.* New York: Scientific American Books.

Lillie-Blanton, M., Parsons, P.E., Gayle, H., and Dievler, A. (1996). Racial differences in health: Not just black and white, but shades of gray. *Annual Review of Public Health,* 17, 411–448.

Lin-Fu, J.S. (1993). Asian and Pacific Islander Americans: An overview of demographic characteristics and health care issues. *Asian and Pacific Islander Journal of Health,* 1, 20–36.

Link, B.G. and Phelan, J. (1995). Social conditions as fundamental causes of disease. *Journal of Health and Social Behavior, (Extra Issue):* 80–94.

Lynch, J.W., Davey-Smith, G., Kaplan, G.A., and House, J.S. (2000). Income inequality and health: Importance to health of individual income, psychosocial environment, or material conditions. *British Medical Journal,* 320, 1200–1204.

Lynch, J.W., Kaplan, G.A., Cohen, R.D., Kauhanen, J., Wilson, T.W., Smith, N.L., and Salonen, J.T. (1994). Childhood and adult socioeconomic status as predictors of mortality in Finland. *Lancet,* 343, 524–527.

Lynch, J.W., Kaplan, G.A., Cohen, R.D., Tuomilehto, J., and Salonen, J.T. (1996). Do cardiovascular risk factors explain the relation between socioeconomic status, risk of all-cause mortality, cardiovascular mortality, and acute myocardial infarction? *American Journal of Epidemiology,* 144, 934–942.

Lynch, J.W., Kaplan, G.A., and Salonen, J.T. (1997). Why do poor people behave poorly? Variation in adult health behaviors and psychosocial characteristics by stages of the socioeconomic lifecourse. *Social Science and Medicine,* 44 *(6),* 809–819.

Marmot, M.G., Davey-Smith, G., Stansfeld, S., Patel, C., North, F., Head, J., White, L. Brunner, E.G., and Feeney, A. (1991). Health inequalities among British civil servants: The Whitehall H Study. *Lancet* 337.

Marmot, M.G., Kogevinas, M., and Elston, M.A. (1987). Social/economic status and disease. *Annual Review of Public Health,* 8, 111–135.

Marmot, M.G., and Syme, S.L. (1976). Acculturation and coronary heart disease in Japanese-Americans. *American Journal of Epidemiology,* 104, 225–247.

Massey, D.S., and Denton, N.A. (1993). *American Apartheid: Segregation and the Making of the Underclass.* Cambridge, MA: Harvard University Press.

McBean, A.M., and Gornick, M. (1994). Differences by race in the rates of procedures performed in hospitals for Medicare beneficiaries. *Health Care Financing Review,* 15(4), 77–90.

McCord C. and Freeman H.P. (1990). Excess mortality in Harlem. *New England Journal of Medicine,* 322, 173–177.

McDonough, P., Duncan, G.J., Williams, D., and House, J. (1997). Income dynamics and adult mortality in the United States, 1972 through 1989. *American Journal of Public Health,* 87 (9), 1476–1483.

McGinnis, M.J., and Forge, W.H. (1993). Actual causes of death in the United States. *Journal of the American Medical Association,* 270, 207–221.

McKeown, T.J. (1976). *The Role of Medicine: Dream, Mirage, or Nemesis.* London: Nuffield Provincial Hospitals Trust.

McKeown, T.J. (1979). *The Role of Medicine: Dream, Mirage, or Nemesis.* Princeton, NJ: Princeton University Press.

McKeown, T.J. (1988). *The Origins of Human Disease.* London: Blackwell.

McKinlay, J.B., and McKinlay, S.J. (1977). The questionable contribution of medical measures to the decline of mortality in the United States in the twentieth century. *Milbank Memorial Fund Quarterly,* 55, 405–428.

Mechanic, D. (1989). Socioeconomic status and health: an explanation of underlying processes. In: Bunker, J.P., Gomby, D.S., Kehrer, B.H. (eds.), *Pathways to Health: The Role of Social Factors.* Menlow Park, CA: Henry J. Kaiser Family Foundation.

Mellor, J., and Milyo, J. (1999). Income Inequality and Individual Health: Evidence from the Current Population Survey. *Robert Wood Johnson Health Policy Scholars Working Paper #8.* Boston University School of Management, Boston.

Mirowsky, J. and Hu, P.N. (1996). Physical impairment and the diminishing effects of income. *Social Forces,* 74(3), 1073–1096.

Moore, D.J., Williams, J.D., and Qualls, W.J. (1996). Target marketing of tobacco and alcohol-related products to ethnic minority groups in the United States. *Ethnicity and Disease,* 6, 83–98.

Mullings, L. (1989). Inequality and African-American health status: Policies and prospects. Pp. 154–182 in W.A. VanHome, and T.V. Tonnesen (eds.), *Twentieth Century Dilemmas—Twenty-First Century Prognoses.* Madison, WI: University of Wisconsin Institute on Race and Ethnicity.

National Center for Health Statistics. (1990). *Mortality Detail Files, 1990, Vol. VII. ICPSR Study #07632.* Ann Arbor, MI: Inter-University Consortium for Political and Social Research.

National Center for Health Statistics. (1993). *Trends in Indian Health—1993.* Rockville, MD: U.S. Department of Health and Human Services.

National Center for Health Statistics. (1998). *Health, United States, Socioeconomic Status and Health Chartbook.* Hyattsville, MD: U.S. Department of Health and Human Services.

Neckerman, K.M., and Kirschenman, J. (1991). Hiring strategies, racial bias, and inner-city workers. *Social Problems,* 38, 433–447.

Neighbors, H.W. (1984). The distribution of psychiatric morbidity in black Americans. *Community Mental Health Journal,* 20, 169–181.

Noh, S., Beiser, M., Kaspar, V., Hou, F., and Rummens, J. (1999). Discrimination and emotional well-being: Perceived racial discrimination, depression, and coping: A study of Southeast Asian refugees in Canada. *Journal of Health and Social Behavior, 40(3),* 193–207.

Oliver, M.L., and Shapiro, T.M. (1995). *Black Wealth/White Wealth: A New Perspective on Racial Inequality*. New York: Routledge.

Omi, M., and Winant, H. (1986). *Racial Formation in the United States: From the 1960s to the 1980s*. New York: Routledge.

Pappas, G., Queen, S., Hadden, W., and Fisher, G. (1993). The increasing disparity in mortality between socioeconomic groups in the United States, 1960 and 1986. *New England Journal of Medicine* 329, 103–109.

Patel, C., and Marmot, M.G. (1988). Efficacy versus effectiveness of relaxation therapy in hypertension. *Stress Medicine*, 4, 283–289.

Peterson, E.D., Shaw, L.K., DeLong, E.R., Pryor, D.B., Califf, R.M., and Mark, D.B. (1997). Racial variation in the use of coronary-revascularization procedures—Are the differences real? Do they matter? *New England Journal of Medicine*, 336(7), 480–486.

Power, C., Manor, O., Fox, A.J., and Fogelman, K. (1990). Health in childhood and social inequalities in young adults. *Journal of the Royal Statistical Society (series A)*, 153, 17–28.

Preston, S.H., and Haines, M.R. (1991). *Fatal Years*. Princeton, NJ: Princeton University Press.

Quadagno, J. (1994). *The Color of Welfare: How Racism Undermined the War on Poverty*. New York: Oxford University Press.

Ren, X.S., Amick, B., and Williams, D.R. (1999). Racial/ethnic disparities in health: The interplay between discrimination and socioeconomic status. *Ethnicity and Disease*, 9(2), 151–165.

Robert, S.A. (1999). Socioeconomic position and health: The independent contribution of community context. *Annual Review of Sociology*, 25, 489–516.

Robert, S.A., and House, J.S. (2000a). Socioeconomic inequalities in health: Integrating individual-, community-, and societal-level theory and research. Pp. 115–135 in G. Albrecht, R. Fitzpatrick, and S. Scrimshaw (Eds.), *Handbook of Social Studies in Health and Medicine*. London: Sage Publishing Company.

Robert, S.A., and House, J.S. (2000b). Socioeconomic inequalities in health: An enduring sociological problem. Pp. 79-97 in C. Bird, P. Conrad, and A. Fremont (Eds.), *Handbook of Medical Sociology*. Upper Saddle River, New Jersey: Prentice Hall.

Rodgers, G.B. (1979). Income and inequality as determinants of mortality: An international cross-section analysis. *Population Studies*, 33, 343–351.

Rodin, J. (1986). Aging and health: Effects of the sense of control. *Science 237*, 143–149.

Salgado de Snyder, V.N. (1987). Factors associated with acculturative stress and depressive symptomatology among married Mexican immigrant women. *Psychology of Women Quarterly*, 11, 475–488.

Sampson, R. J., and Wilson, W. J. (1995). Toward a theory of race, crime, and urban inequality. Pp. 37–54 in J. Hagan, and R. D. Peterson (eds.), *Crime and Inequality*. Stanford, CA: Stanford University Press.

Satel, S. (1996). The politicization of public health. *Wall Street Journal*, Dec. 12, 1996; editorial section: 12.

Scheier, M.F., and Bridges, M.W. (1995). Person variables and health: Personality predispositions and acute psychological states as shared determinants for disease. *Psychosomatic Medicine*, 57, 255–268.

Schuman, H., Steeh, C., Bobo, L., and Krysan, M. (1997). *Racial Attitudes in America: Trends and Interpretations*. Cambridge, MA: Harvard University Press.

Schwartz, E., Kofie, V.Y., Rivo, M., and Tuckson, R.V. (1990). Black/white comparisons of deaths preventable by medical intervention: United States and the District of Columbia 1980–1986. *International Journal of Epidemiology,* 19, 591–598.

See, K.O., and Wilson, W.J. (1988). Race and ethnicity. Pp. 233–242 in N.J. Smelser (Ed*.), Handbook of Sociology.* Beverly Hills: Sage Publications.

Sorlie, P.D., Backlund, E., Johnson, N.J., and Rogot, E. (1993). Mortality by Hispanic status in the United States. *Journal of the American Medical Association,* 270, 2464–2468.

Sorlie, P.D., Backlund, E., and Keller, J.B. (1995). U.S. mortality by economic, demographic, and social characteristics: The National Longitudinal Mortality Study. *American Journal of Public Health,* 85 (7), 949–956.

Stangnor, C., and McMillan, D. (1992). Memory for expectancy-congruent and expectancy-incongruent information: A review of the social and social development literatures. *Psychological Bulletin,* 111, 42–61.

Steele, C.M. (1997). A threat in the air: How stereotypes shape intellectual identity and performance. *American Psychologist,* 52(6), 613–629.

Syme, S.L. (1978). Drug treatment of mild hypertension: Social and psychological considerations. *Annals New York Academy of Science,* 304, 99–106.

Taylor, J., and Jackson, B. (1990). Factors affecting alcohol consumption in black women, Part II. *International Journal of Addictions,* 25(12), 1415–1427.

Taylor, J., Henderson, D., and Jackson, B.B. (1991). A holistic model for understanding and predicting depression in African American women. *Journal of Community Psychology,* 19, 306–320.

Theorell, Töres G.T. (1982). Review of research on life events and cardiovascular illness. *Advance Cardiology,* 29, 140–147.

Trevino, F.M., Moyer, M.E., Valdez, R.B., and Stroup-Benham, C.A. (1991). Health insurance coverage and utilization of health services by Mexican Americans, mainland Puerto Ricans, and Cuban Americans. *Journal of the American Medical Association,* 265, 2233–2237.

U.S. Department of Health and Human Services (1990*). Healthy People 2000: National Health Promotion and Disease Prevention Objectives.* DHHS publication 91-50212 Washington, DC: U.S. Department of Health and Human Services.

U.S. Department of Health and Human Services. (1999). *Healthy People 2010 Objectives: Draft for Public Comment.*http://web.health.gov/healthypeople/2010Draft/object.htm

U.S. Public Health Service (1964). U.S. Surgeon General's Advisory Committee on Smoking and Health. *Smoking and Health.* U.S. Public Health Service, Washington, DC.

van Doorslaer, E., Wagstaff, A., Bleichrodt, H., Calonge, S., Gerdtham, U.-G., Gerfin, M., Geurts, J., Gross, L., Hakkinen, U., Leu, R.E., O'Donnell, O., Propper, C., Puffer, F., Rodriguez, M., Sundberg, G., and Winkelhake, O. (1997). Income-related inequalities in health: Some international comparisons. *Journal of Health Economics,* 16, 93–112.

Varmus H.E. (1999). Statement before the House and Senate Appropriations Subcommittees on Labor, Health and Human Services, and Education, February 23–24. http://www.nih.gov/welcome/director/022299.htm

Vega, W.A., and Amaro, H. (1994). Latino outlook: Good health, uncertain prognosis. *Annual Review of Public Health,* 15, 39–67.

Vega, W.A., and Rumbaut, R.G. (1991). Ethnic minorities and mental health. *Annual Review of Sociology,* 17, 351–383.

Wenneker, M.B., and Epstein A.M. (1989). Racial inequalities in the use of procedures for patients with ischemic heart disease in Massachusetts. *Journal of the American Medical Association*, 261, 253–257.

Whittle, J., Conigliaro, J., Good, C.B., and Lofgren, R.P. (1993). Racial differences in the use of invasive cardiovasular procedures in the Department of Veterans Affairs. *New England Journal of Medicine*, 329, 621–626.

Wilkins, R., Adams, O. and Brancker, A. (1989). Changes in mortality by income in urban Canada from 1971 to 1986. *Health Reports (Statistics Canada catalogue 82-003*, 1(2), 137–174.

Wilkinson, R.G. (1992). Income distribution and life expectancy. *British Medical Journal*, 301, 165–168.

Wilkinson, R.G. (1996). *Unhealthy Societies: The Afflictions of Inequality*. New York: Routledge.

Williams, D.R. (1990). Socioeconomic differentials in health: A review and redirection. *Social Psychology Quarterly,* 53(2), 81–99.

Williams, D.R. (1992). Black–white differences in blood pressure: The role of social factors. *Ethnicity and Disease,* 2, 126–141.

Williams, D.R. (1997). Race and health: Basic questions, emerging directions. *Annals of Epidemiology,* 7(5), 322–333.

Williams, D.R. (1998). African-American health: The role of the social environment. *Journal of Urban Health: Bulletin of the New York Academy of Medicine*, 75, 300–321.

Williams, D.R. (1999). Race, SES and Health: The added effects of racism and discrimination. *Annals of the New York Academy of Sciences*, 896: 173–188.

Williams, D.R. (in press). Racial variations in adult health status: Patterns, paradoxes and prospects. In N. Smelser, W.J. Wilson, and F. Mitchell (eds.), *America Becoming: Racial Trends and Their Consequences*. Washington, DC: National Academy Press.

Williams, D.R., and Chung, A.-M. (in press). Racism and health. In R. Gibson, and J. S. Jackson (eds.), *Health in Black America* . Thousand Oaks, CA: Sage Publications.

Williams, D.R., and Collins, C. (1995). U.S. socioeconomic and racial differences in health. *Annual Review of Sociology,* 21, 349–386.

Williams, D.R., and Harris-Reid, M. (1999). Race and mental health: Emerging patterns and promising approaches. Pp. 295–314 in A. V. Horwitz, and T. L. Scheid (eds.), *A Handbook for the Study of Mental Health: Social Contexts, Theories, and Systems*. New York: Cambridge University Press.

Williams, D.R., Yu, Y., Jackson, J.S., and Anderson, N.B. (1997). Racial differences in physical and mental health: Socio-economic status, stress and discrimination. *Journal of Health Psychology,* 2, 335–351.

Wolfson, M., Rowe, G., Gentleman, J.F., and Tomiak, M. (1993). Career earnings and death: A longitudinal analysis of older Canadian men. *Journal of Gerontology,* 48(4), S167–179.

Woolhandler, S., Himmelstein, D.U., Silber, R., Bader, M., Harnly, M., and Jones, A.A. (1985). Medical care and mortality: Racial differences in preventable deaths. *International Journal of Health Services,* 15, 1–11.

PAPER CONTRIBUTION C
Preconception, Prenatal, Perinatal, and Postnatal Influences on Health

Carol C. Korenbrot and Nancy E. Moss

After more than a decade of impressive public health efforts to improve the health of infants at birth in the United States, health status indicators indicate that little progress has been made. The United States still ranks 25th in infant mortality among nations reporting to the World Health Organization (Petrini et al., 1997). While there have been reductions in infant mortality, the ranking remains as low as in 1985 when major policy and program reforms of prenatal care were initiated in the United States to reduce infant mortality and the ethnic disparities in the health outcome by focusing on reductions in low-birthweight (Institute of Medicine, 1985; U.S. Department of Health and Human Services, 1985). There have not been increases in low-birthweight rates, nor has there been any significant reduction in the ethnic disparities in infant mortality or low-birthweight rates (Figure 1) (Centers for Disease Control and Prevention, 1999). This remains true in spite of improvements in the early and continuous use of prenatal care (Figure 2) and a reduction in contributing health behaviors including smoking in pregnancy and teenage childbearing (Petrini et al., 1997; Ventura et al., 1999). The lack of measurable gains is not explained by increases in mul-

Carol C. Korenbrot, Ph.D., is adjunct professor, Institute for Health Policy Studies and the Department of Obstetrics, Gynecology and Reproductive Sciences, University of California, San Francisco, and Nancy E. Moss, Ph.D., is a consultant. This paper was prepared for the symposium, "Capitalizing on Social Science and Behavioral Research to Improve the Public's Health," the Institute of Medicine, and the Commission on Behavioral and Social Sciences and Education of the National Research Council, Atlanta, Georgia, February 2–3, 2000.

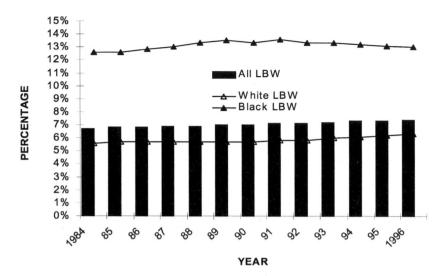

FIGURE 1. Percentage of low birthweight: United States, 1984–1996. SOURCE: National Center for Health Statistics, prepared by March of Dimes, Perinatal Data Center. 1997.

tiple births, births to older women, or changes in medical practice such as induction of labor or cesarean sections before full gestation (Kramer, 1998; Ventura et al., 1999). Birth outcomes in the United States have behaved less like indicators of poor health care and health behaviors, and more like indicators of deeper disparities among women of different social classes and ethnicities (Collins et al., 1997; O'Campo et al., 1997; Roberts, 1997; Johnson et al., 1999). The lack of improvement in indicators of the health of babies at birth is discouraging to public health professionals, but comes as no surprise to social and behavioral scientists.

Public health practice has not fully embraced the contributions that social science and behavioral research have to offer in the design of programs and policies for maternal and infant health (Mechanic, 1995; Grason et al., 1999; Hogue, 1999). The public health model for a healthy start in life is broader than the medical model and addresses disparities in health education, nutrition, and psychosocial conditions of families (Bennett and Kotelchuck, 1997). Public health professionals have long recognized the need to ameliorate effects of social policies that discriminate against economically and ethnically vulnerable populations (Aday, 1993). Public health programs for pregnant women have not had measurable effects on the country's poor pregnancy outcomes in recent years and have had limited effects on infant mortality (Willinger et al., 1998; U.S. Department of Health and Human Services, 1999). To have larger effects on maternal and infant health, innovative programs and policies need to address social, economic, cultural, political, and psychological antecedents of disparities.

Social structure, the positions people hold within it, and the nature of the social relations that result from these positions are important antecedent factors in determining resources that affect health (Link and Phelan, 1995; Kennedy et al., 1996; Kiwachi and Kennedy, 1997). Gender, socioeconomic position, and racial segregation contribute to the ideological and cultural context in which social relationships occur (Williams, 1990; Benderly, 1997). These, in turn, affect people's everyday lives. Thus, it is not difficult to see health as "the product of social relationships between . . . groups, with these relationships expressed through people's everyday living and working conditions, including daily interactions with others" (Krieger, 1994). Social and economic relations are causal, explicitly shaping the production and distribution of individual and population health and disease at different points across the life span (Evans, 1995; Moss, 2000a).

The resources that are differentially associated with social and economic status include knowledge, income, wealth and assets, power, prestige, social networks, and psychological well-being. Availability and deprivation of these resources over time structure and differentiate the life course of individual men and women (Table 1) (Link and Phelan, 1995; Moss, 2000a). The cumulative effect of deprivation of social and material support over the life course is associated with stressful living and working conditions. Trajectories of stress and deprivation across a number of dimensions, including social class and ethnicity, may explain a higher prevalence of poor birth outcomes in groups such as African Americans (Geronimus, 1992). By contrast, resources are hypothesized to influence the ability of people to avoid health risks such as stress and to minimize their consequences if they occur (Rowley, 1998). In this framework, stress and health behaviors are mediating factors that occur in the context of an individual's social and economic position, the socioeconomic characteristics of a

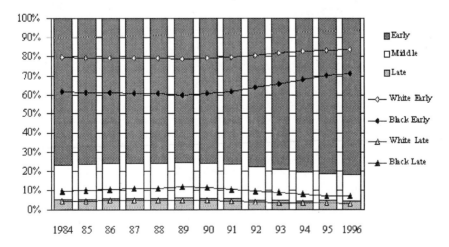

FIGURE 2. Onset of prenatal care use: United States, 1984–1996. SOURCE: National Center for Health Statistics, prepared by March of Dimes, Perinatal Data Center, 1997.

community, and the psychosocial environment that they create (Krieger, 1994). Addressing behaviors alone, without attention to the structural and psychosocial context in which they occur, will not reduce socioeconomic and racial or ethnic disparities in outcomes. While alternative frameworks such as social selection have been proposed as explanations for health disparities (Rutter and Quine, 1990; Syme, 1998), longitudinal research continues to provide stronger support for social position as a determinant rather than consequence of health. The latter approach offers rich new opportunities to develop and test social and health policies and programs that may ultimately promote health and reduce disparities among mothers and infants.

This chapter explores the opportunities offered by social and behavioral research to develop public health policies and programs that reduce or eliminate social class and ethnic disparities shaping health at birth. We use low-birthweight as the primary indicator of morbidity and mortality risk in infancy because of its links with maternal morbidity and infant morbidity, development, and mortality, as well as health conditions that can endure through childhood or appear later in life (Institute of Medicine, 1985; Hack et al., 1995; Paneth, 1995). The chapter begins with an overview of how social class, race or ethnicity, and gender roles and relations are hypothesized to affect maternal health before and during pregnancy and infant health at birth. We then examine how psychosocial factors could be a critical route for mediating the effects of social class and race or ethnicity on behaviors known to affect maternal and infant health. Following the overview of sociodemographic and psychosocial factors, we examine recent public health policy and program interventions designed to address social class and ethnic disparities in health at birth. The paper concludes with opportunities for social and behavioral research that can contribute to the design and evaluation of innovative policies and programs directed at reducing socioeconomic and racial or ethnic disparities to improve maternal and infant health. Our purpose is not to provide an exhaustive summary of the vast literature relating to these issues, but rather to provide a framework in which to take a fresh look at a persistent public health challenge.

SOCIODEMOGRAPHIC ANTECEDENTS AND OUTCOMES

The sociodemographic factors that best predict health at birth are social class and race or ethnicity. In the United States, poverty and wealth are closely related to ethnicity and "race" which have independent and interdependent effects on birth outcomes (Krieger, 1991; Lillie-Blanton and LaVeist, 1996). These social and demographic antecedents together shape gender, social, and economic roles and hierarchies that women experience throughout their lives (Table 1). In this section of the paper we first explore contextual effects of social class or "socioeconomic status" (SES in the public health literature) (Krieger et al., 1997), with an emphasis on gender-based, role-related, and life span issues-for reproductive-age women that could help to explain disparities in health out-

TABLE 1. Examples of Social, Economic, Psychological, and Behavioral Concepts That Could Help Explain Socioeconomic Status and Ethnic Disparities in Health at Birth

Sociodemographic Factors		Psychosocial Factors		Biological System	Health Outcomes
Antecedents	Potential Mediators	Environmental Resources and Stressors	Psychological and Behavioral Resources and Stressors		
Socioeconomic Status (SES)	Gender-based roles or hierarchies	*Stressors or life events:*	*Vulnerabilities:*	Endocrine	*Preconception:* Maternal weight at birth
Education	Social and economic roles or hierarchies (and marital status) (and age)	Mediator	Distress	Cardiovascular	Hypertension
Income		Modifier of mediator effect	Anxiety	Fetal growth	Diabetes
Occupation		Confounder of mediator effect	Depression	Immune	
		Social supports or deprivation	*Adaptation:*	Neural	*Prenatal:* Complications of pregnancy
		Socioeconomic discrimination	Coping		
		Access to health care	Self-esteem		*Perinatal:* Preterm birth
			Mastery or control		Small for gestational age
Race or Ethnicity	Acculturation	Racial discrimination	*Behaviors:*		Low birthweight
Ethnic Origins	Residential segregation	Community characteristics	Health behaviors		Congenital anomalies
Nativity			Use of health care		
					Postnatal: Neonatal or infant mortality

comes at birth (Grason et al., 1999; Minkovitz and Baldwin, 1999). We address race and ethnicity with an emphasis on the national origins and acculturation of different groups, highlighting similarities and differences across groups. Sociocultural factors associated with SES and ethnicity influence health and health choices (Link and Phelan, 1995). While we recognize the crucial influence of women's psychosocial characteristics and behaviors on infant health at birth, our emphasis in this section is on "upstream" sociodemographic antecedents.

Socioeconomic Disparities

Socioeconomic indicators such as education, income, and occupation have been consistently associated with low-birthweight, preterm birth, and infant mortality (Rutter and Quine, 1990; Savitz et al., 1996). SES captures "living conditions and life chances, skill levels and material resources, relative power and privilege" (Williams and Collins, 1995). This very capturing of so many aspects of life history and everyday experience makes SES a powerful and persistent antecedent of many pregnancy outcomes, though it has rarely been measured by more than education in most epidemiological studies (Williams, 1990; Feinstein, 1993; Moss, 2000a). Effects of SES on health at birth are not confined to the lowest-SES groups; as with many other health indicators, there is a gradient of effects across SES strata (Adler et al., 1994). The incidence of low-birthweight, for example, decreases as levels of maternal education increase, with progressively better outcomes for women who have completed high school, had some college, or graduated from college (Figure 3). The gradient implies

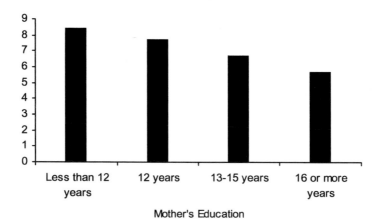

FIGURE 3. Percentage of low-birthweight live births among mothers 20 years of age and over by mother's education, United States, 1996. Less than 12 years includes persons with 12 years of schooling but no high school diploma. Twelve years includes persons with a high school diploma or GED. Thirteen to 15 years includes persons without a degree and persons with associate's degrees. Sixteen years or more includes all persons with a baccalaurate degree or higher.

that it is *not only* poverty, the severe deprivation of social and material resources, socioeconomic discrimination, and exposure to health risks that contribute to SES disparities. Rather, the relative deprivation and adverse exposures are mediating factors that affect women over a range of SES levels (Carstairs, 1995; Robert and House, 2000).

Gender, social, and economic roles and hierarchies may also contribute to gradients in pregnancy outcomes by determining the relative risks and resources to which women are differentially exposed prior to and during the reproductive period (Table 1) (Wilkinson, 1997; Weisman, 1998; Minkovitz and Baldwin, 1999). A clear understanding of the relative effects of these mediators is important in designing effective policies and programs. For example, if status in a social hierarchy is detrimental to health, then merely increasing cash assistance and food vouchers for those in poverty, without simultaneously reducing inequality, may afford little health benefit (Adler et al., 1994). On the other hand, deprivation of material assets such as car and home ownership that affect the everyday conditions of life may be as important a dimension of social class as education or income in predicting health outcomes, particularly for women (Arber, 1991). We will need to better understand why socioeconomic gradients in health at birth develop in order to reduce disparities.

The health of reproductive-age women is shaped beginning with their own health at birth and continuing through childhood and adolescence with conditions that develop prior to becoming pregnant (Power et al., 1997; 1998). Lower-SES women are at greater risk for the illnesses and conditions that complicate pregnancy (Pamuk et al., 1998). For example, hypertension exhibits a steep socioeconomic effect. Poor women are 1.6 times as likely as high-income women to be hypertensive (Pamuk et al., 1998). Diabetes is also more prevalent among women of low SES, and the death rate for diabetes among low-income women is three times that for high-income women (Pamuk et al., 1998). Even behavior change is socioeconomically structured. Cigarette smoking among adults 25 and over declined between 1974 and 1995, but rates were down 49% for college-educated women, compared with a drop of 13% among those who did not finish high school (Pamuk et al., 1998). In 1995 the least educated women were twice as likely to smoke as the most educated. Risks of nutritional deficiencies are higher in lower-SES groups and nutrition prior to and during pregnancy, including folic acid intake, is linked to higher rates of congenital anomalies (Centers for Disease Control and Prevention, 1998). Often, these socioeconomically-structured behaviors have their roots in women's everyday experiences (Moss, 2000a).

The life span perspective suggests how social factors in maternal health over generations contribute to the SES gradient in health and disease of subsequent generations during infancy, childhood, and beyond (Elo and Preston, 1992; Barker, 1998). The dependence of offspring health on the health of the prior generation is clearly shown in birthweights. Women who were themselves low-birthweight, are more likely to give birth to low-birthweight babies (Sanderson et al., 1995).

Gender-Based Roles and Hierarchies

As women make the transition to pregnancy, many of the gender-based issues that they find problematic are magnified by SES and could contribute to
SES gradients in outcomes (Benderly, 1997). Social constructs of masculinity
and femininity are arguably nowhere more pronounced than around issues of
sexuality and reproduction (Lane and Cibula, 2000). Assumptions about what is
natural, biologically determined, or even divinely ordained, for men and women
shape the views and experiences women have of sex, contraception, and pregnancy, as well as their health behaviors and interactions with the health care
system (Ruzek et al., 1997; Weisman, 1997). They also affect the power and
effectiveness women have in implementing their views, whether in bedrooms or
the workplace. Unintended pregnancies, for example, occur at higher rates in
low-SES women (Institute of Medicine, 1995) and lead to a complex array of
situations that women must deal with before they decide whether or not to accept the pregnancy (U.S. Department of Health and Human Services, 1991; Institute of Medicine, 1995). An unintended pregnancy does not necessarily mean
that the child is unwanted, but it does mean that many of the transitions required
of women are not anticipated or planned. As a result, the pregnancy may be
more stressful, particularly if there are limited resources to overcome competing
demands.

Low SES may be associated with more traditional and conservative views of
women's roles: that sex is man's business and child rearing is woman's work, as
well as the socially and culturally sanctioned hierarchical dominance by men over
women. Some men use traditional views of masculinity and femininity to exert
power over women that may be harmful to the health and well-being of women in
pregnancy. This can result in forced sex, lack of condom use, domestic violence,
and little sharing in care giving for children (Amaro, 1995; Weisman, 1997).
When women become pregnant, hierarchical views and behaviors may be responsible for the increase in exposure to domestic violence and emotional abuse
(O'Campo et al., 1995; Crowell and Burgess, 1996). While domestic violence is
found in all socioeconomic strata, the traditional view that it is a man's job to
support his spouse and children economically can backfire on lower-SES women
if their partners face more frustrations than men in upper-SES strata in succeeding in the role. Abuse of women has serious ramifications because of the greater
risk for homicide, effects on children in the household, and the long-term emotional and physical consequences for women and their families.

Social and Economic Roles and Hierarchies

Failure to consider role demands in women's lives unnecessarily limits our
understanding of maternal health in pregnancy and childbirth and the impact on
pregnancy outcomes (Benderly, 1997; Zapata and Bennett, 1997). Becoming a
mother increases the role demands for women, which in turn may strain material
and social resources in ways that vary across socioeconomic strata. Each role,

including that of mother-to-be, is associated with normative expectations in women, partners, families, and communities, although there are cultural as well as socioeconomic variations. When expectations of a particular role are not fulfilled or demands are particularly heavy, stress or "strain" arises (Pritchard and Teo, 1994). Strain increases proportionally to the number of roles a woman must play as well as to the role transitions she makes during her childbearing years (Young, 1996; Weisman, 1997).

For women, the roles of education, work, and motherhood interact in complex ways. In the United States and other western industrialized nations, the actual period of childbearing in a woman's life is much shorter than the duration of her potential childbearing, although countries vary in the expectation that women will work outside the home and participate actively in community affairs. The trend in the United States in recent decades has been for women to obtain high school and post-high school college degrees, enter the workforce, delay or forgo marriage, and delay or forgo child rearing (Minkovitz and Baldwin, 1999). The proportion of women with high school and college degrees now exceeds that of men (Grason et al., 1999). There has been a substantial increase in the proportion of women 20 to 30 years of age in the labor market, the prime years for healthy childbearing (Grason et al., 1999). The decline in labor force participation that used to occur between ages 20 and 24 when women left the labor force for motherhood, has progressively disappeared with women born since 1945. Yet, despite concerns that rising participation in the labor force would expose pregnant women to more stress, employed women generally report better health status and birth outcomes than do women who are not employed (Moss and Carver, 1993; Pugliesi, 1995). This can be a reflection of selection of healthier women into the labor force (the "healthy worker effect") or of the psychosocial and material benefits that accrue from employment. Still, long work weeks of physically demanding work have been found to lead to fetal growth reductions (Hatch et al., 1997). Women working in higher-status occupations during pregnancy may obtain psychosocial and material benefits that protect against any strain of work or multiple roles (Landsbergis and Hatch, 1996). The ability to control work pace, physical demands, generosity of sick and maternity leave, and other factors may all affect how healthy a woman is when she becomes pregnant and how much care a working woman can give her pregnancy (Brett et al., 1997; Wergeland and Strand, 1998). Effects on gestational hypertension have been associated with low-decision latitude and job complexity among women in lower-status jobs (Landsbergis and Hatch, 1996). In contrast to the United States, in some European countries (e.g., France) substantial research programs have led to equitable social policies that protect the mother and fetus from work that is detrimental to their health (DiRenzo et al., 1998).

In addition to role demands of school, work, and motherhood, women are likely to be primarily responsible for housework and caregivers for a child, partner, or family member. Because there has been little progress in gender equity in household responsibilities, women, especially low-SES women, continue to be responsible for most "second shift" household work and caregiving for children

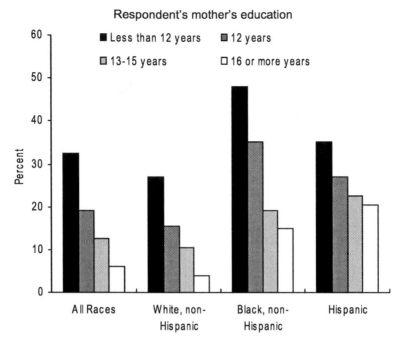

FIGURE 4 Percentage of women 20–29 years of age who had a teenage birth, by respondent's mother's education and respondent's race and Hispanic origin: United States, 1995. NOTE: Education level is for the infant's maternal grandmother. SOURCE: 1995 National Survey of Family Growth (Pamuk et al., 1998).

and adults in the household. Women's traditional role in caring for the home must be juggled along with other roles. Studies have shown that household work for women who have had a child can have its own measurable strains on subsequent birth outcomes (Pritchard and Teo, 1994). The issue of caregiving for children is of particular importance for low-SES women because they have fewer material resources to pay for child care, available child care is usually of poor quality (Fuller and Kagan, 2000), and they are more likely to depend on family and friends. The recent change in social policy that is moving mothers on welfare into paid employment while there is limited access to affordable, quality child care in many communities will be an important change for low-SES women and may potentially affect pregnancy outcomes (O'Campo and Rojas-Smith, 1998; Wise et al., 1999).

In every major ethnic group, there is an SES gradient in the percentage of women who have had teen births (Figure 4) (Pamuk et al., 1998). Birth rates to teens are particularly high in the United States, relative to other industrialized nations, and the extent to which poorer women give birth at younger ages because of lack of options in social and economic roles is of particular concern. At the same time, the demands of balancing schooling, work, and motherhood are likely to place greater strain on teenagers than on older women.

Socioeconomic variations in communities and neighborhoods, independent of individual socioeconomic characteristics, are associated with differences in pregnancy outcomes. For example, living in wealthier communities than expected after adjustment for parental education and marital status has been associated with lower odds of very low-birthweight babies for both black and white women in Chicago (Collins et al., 1997). Similarly, living in neighborhoods in Chicago with large proportions of unemployment and poverty has shown greater association with individual low-birthweight outcomes than individual education, even after adjustment for other community and individual factors (Roberts, 1997). Others have shown interactions of neighborhood-level per capita crime rates, unemployment, average wealth, and income with individual low-birthweight outcomes in Baltimore (O'Campo et al., 1997). A household class measure (based on working class and non-working class characteristics of employment) at the level of census block group in California served as a better predictor of individual birth outcomes than did the mother's own social class (Krieger, 1991). The woman's socioeconomic context may provide additional information about SES gradients not captured by individual-level factors.

We have suggested that socioeconomically structured roles and material conditions, along with gender hierarchies, partially explain differential demands and resources of childbearing women. The fewer the resources—social and material—the more likely they are to be overwhelmed by demands, contributing to a socioeconomic gradient in health for mothers and their infants. Most public health policies and programs are predicated upon deficit models of the high-risk conditions and behaviors of women and families in poverty, without attention to antecedent socioeconomic structural factors and without strategies for building on the strengths and resilience of those low-SES women (Hogue and Hargraves, 1993; Edin and Lein, 1997; Stack, 1997). We turn now to ethnic disparities, which provides a further opportunity to examine the strengths of adaptation and maximization of resources as well as the negative effects of stress and deprivation.

"Racial" and Ethnic Disparities

Public health research has focused on the concept of race, largely believing that physical differences between groups of people are important in determining health and disease (Polednak, 1989; Osborne and Feit, 1992; Centers for Disease Control and Prevention with the National Institute of Child Health and Human Development, 1993; Bennett and Kotelchuck, 1997). The terms race and ethnicity are frequently used in public health without regard to social and cultural biases of researchers that obscure the social origins of disease and support the status quo, rather than stimulate change (Williams, 1994). In fact, race is an ill-defined, socially agreed-upon mixed measure of ethnicity, skin color, and nationality, without regard to genetics and lacking in scientific rigor. There is

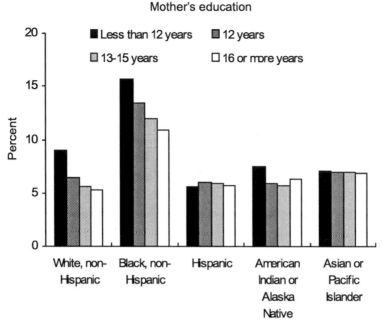

FIGURE 5. Low-birthweight live births among mothers 20 years of age and over by mother's education, race, and Hispanic origin: United States, 1996. SOURCE: Pamuk et al., 1998.

growing agreement that groups defined by race are social, not biological, in nature (LaVeist, 1994). There is no clearer example of this than the pregnancy outcome, low-birthweight. Low-birthweight, while a poor indicator of the impact of prenatal care, is still a robust indicator of sociodemographic characteristics of different populations. There is a marked socioeconomic gradient in low-birthweight for white and black ethnic groups, but there is no gradient for Latino and Asian American or Pacific Islanders (Figure 5). Subsumed under "race" in the United States are key sociodemographic characteristics that help to explain differences in pregnancy outcomes among ethnic groups: ethnic origins and history (their country and class of origin, whether they are indigenous or came as slaves, refugees, or voluntary immigrants), the length of time and social conditions since arriving in the United States (generations, years, or months), and their acculturation to dominant ethnic norms in the United States (food, language, behaviors, and other ethnic traditions).

African Americans

In the United States, African Americans occupy a unique position socially, culturally, and politically such that the most powerful sociodemographic factor in determining birth outcomes is being black. There is a strong socioeconomic gradient for low-birthweight (as for other pregnancy outcomes) among black women, and the low-birthweight rate is twice as high as the rate for white women at every education level (Figure 5) (Kleinman and Kessel, 1987; McGrady et al., 1992; Schoendorf et al., 1992). While African Americans are disproportionately represented in lower socioeconomic groups, not all of the differential in birth outcomes for African Americans is explained by SES (Starfield et al., 1991; Williams and Collins, 1995; Roberts, 1997). One potential explanation for the disparity is that education does not have the same social or economic returns (salary, benefits, or occupational status) for blacks as it does for whites (Figure 6) (Krieger et al., 1993). But even this is not a sufficient explanation for observed black/white differences. For one, black/white differences persist even in the military with universal employment and health coverage,

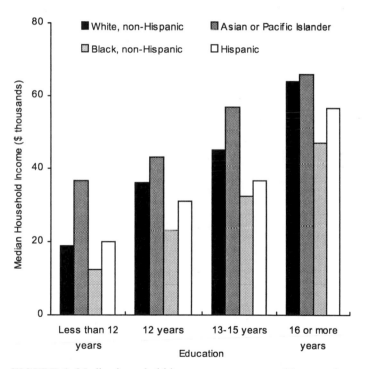

FIGURE 6. Median household income among women 25 years of age and over by education, sex, race, and Hispanic origin: United States, 1996. NOTES: Median income is based on total household income (earnings and other income) and is not adjusted for work status or number of hours worked by household members. Median is calculated using actual reported household income, not grouped data. Educational attainment is as of March 1997. SOURCE: U.S. Bureau of the Census (Pamuk et al., 1998).

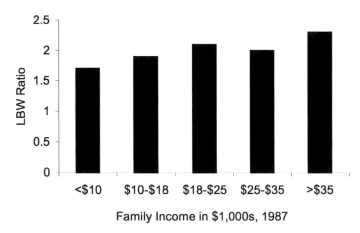

FIGURE 7. Ratios of low birthweight (black/white) by income (Schoendorf et al., 1992).

though disparities are reduced (Adams et al., 1993; Alexander et al., 1993; Barfield et al., 1996). Furthermore, differences persist across the socioeconomic spectrum; in fact, the black/white ratio of poor outcomes actually *increases* with income (Figure 7) (Schoendorf et al., 1992). Nor are these striking differences fully explained by health behaviors. For example, the smoking rates during pregnancy are almost twice as high for *whites* as blacks at every level of education (except college graduates) (Pamuk et al., 1998). The prevalence of chronic and intergenerational health disparities in women of reproductive age may explain part of the difference. For example, 30% percent of middle- and high-income black women 20 years and older are hypertensive, a rate comparable to that for poor white women, and hypertension is a major risk factor for adverse outcomes (Flack et al., 1995).

The weathering hypothesis has been advanced to explain life course differences in birth outcomes between black and white women (Geronimus, 1992). Using evidence from black/white neonatal mortality ratios that increase with age of the mother, the theory helps to explain ethnic disparities in health at birth by showing that black and white women "weather" at different rates (Geronimus, 1986, 1987). This occurs because different life circumstances undermine or promote health through a cascade of advantages and disadvantages throughout the life course. Changes over time occur in part because of age-dependent trajectories of risky behaviors such as smoking and using drugs, as well as community-level environmental exposures (e.g., to lead-based paint) and access to health services (Geronimus, 1992). The weathering framework also suggests how intergenerational effects on health occur, by connecting physical manifestations of weathering such as maternal hypertension, cigarette smoking, and blood-lead levels to infant health.

Another approach to explaining racial differences in birth outcomes looks at the effect of racial segregation and discrimination as expressed both in interpersonal behaviors and in community-level characteristics. Investigators have developed conceptual frameworks that include racial segregation and racism, as well as SES as contributing factors to disparities in health (Williams, 1996; Polednak, 1997). Data from the most segregated metropolitan areas show that a high black infant mortality rate persisted from 1980 to 1990, contributing substantially to the black/white disparity in overall mortality (Polednak, 1996). Besides residential segregation, other community features are associated with health disparities. In a hospital-based case-control study, African American mothers who rated their neighborhoods unfavorably in terms of police protection, protection of property, personal safety, friendliness, delivery of municipal services, cleanliness, quietness, and schools were 1.7 to 3.2 times as likely to deliver a very low-birthweight infant as those who rated the neighborhoods favorably (Collins et al., 1998). Geronimus and her collaborators examined the effects on excess mortality of residence in geographic areas that vary in population-level patterns of disadvantage and segregation, showing that environmental and psychosocial factors in different communities create sharp disparities in death rates among black and white men and women (Geronimus et al., 1996). They argue for looking beyond individual-level chronic burdens of everyday deprivation to population-level indicators of hardship.

Differences in health status of women of African descent born in the United States compared to those born outside the United States (a nativity effect) provide evidence consistent with the hypothesis that historically and socially constructed racism and segregation may have deleterious effects on health. Birth outcomes among Africans and other blacks who migrate to the United States are better than those of U.S.-born blacks (Table 2) (Cabral et al., 1990; Kleinman et al., 1991; Friedman et al., 1993; Morton-Mitchell et al., 1999). Caribbean- and African-born black women have better low-birthweight rates than U.S.-born black women (9, 10, and 14%, respectively) although they are not as low as those of whites (Morton-Mitchell et al., 1999). In a hospital-based study that controlled for income, the foreign-born group had higher prevalence of protective factors such as education and marriage and lower prevalence of risk factors such as teenage births, low pre-pregnancy weight for height, and number (but not early onset) of prenatal care visits (Cabral et al., 1990). Ethnic differences persisted even after adjustment for multiple sociodemographic, obstetric risk, and health behavior variables, with adjusted outcomes best for Haitians and worst for American blacks. The explanation in part may be a "healthy migrant effect." People who put energy and resources into migrating at any SES level may have better health than those who stay behind. This effect may be more prominent at lower-SES levels and less prominent at higher SES levels. Universal birth information on low-birthweight and infant mortality from the countries of origin for the immigrant black women would help to shed light on this issue (Kleinman et al., 1991; Howell and Blondel, 1994; Guendelman et al., 1995; Abraido-Lanza et al., 1999). It also remains to be demonstrated whether black women born outside the United States have stress and adaptation patterns before, during, and after pregnancy similar to those of U.S.-born blacks (Table 1) and whether, as they reside longer in this country, they develop stress patterns and birth outcomes that resemble those of U.S.-born blacks (see discussion of acculturation in the next section).

Racism is hypothesized to influence health disparities by increasing psychological stress and reducing adaptive resources of the individual (such as self-esteem, self-efficacy) and of the community and culture (such as social support) (Williams, 1996). Stress increases due to negative attitudes and beliefs about groups distinguishable from the predominant ethnic group (prejudice) and differential treatment of members of those groups (discrimination) (Williams, 1996). Fundamental to racism are assumptions that groups of people can be ranked by the superiority or inferiority of particular characteristics that "explain" their hierarchical position. The internalization of cultural stereotypes is hypothesized to lead to negative self-evaluations that adversely affect psychological well-being and healthy behaviors. The stress of life events that can be linked to ethnic minority status is one form of socially induced stress long recognized in mental health literature that is now being investigated for its contributions to physical health (Thoits, 1983; Lipton et al., 1993).

Latinos and Asian Americans or Pacific Islanders

As with African American women born outside the United States, foreign-born Latina and Asian American or Pacific Islander women have better birth outcomes than those of their U.S.-born peers (Table 2). One potential reason is because of the healthy migrant or nativity effect described above. An alternative—or complementary—explanation is that immigrants have sociocultural strengths that favor better birth outcomes. One test of the healthy migrant hypothesis is to compare birth outcomes in the countries of origin with those of foreign-born women in the United States. Evidence consistent with the hypothesized effect, for example, is that low-birthweight rates in Japan (7.5% in 1994 and 1995) are higher than those of Japanese American women giving birth in the United States (6.9% in 1994) (Alexander et al., 1996; Hirayama and Wallace, 1998). Unfortunately, many other key countries of origin for the non-native-born U.S. population do not have universal reporting of pregnancy outcomes comparable to that of the United States, so such comparisons are difficult (Howell and Blondel, 1994). Better cross-national, preferably longitudinal data on women's sociodemographic characteristics, migration trajectories, and birth outcomes are needed to help sort out these effects.

The lack of a socioeconomic gradient in birth outcomes for Latina and Asian American or Pacific Islander women is consistent with the healthy migrant hypothesis. Latina and Asian American women of low SES have better birth outcomes than low-SES white women, the so-called birth paradox (Figure 5) (Singh and Yu, 1996a). The advantage over white women, however, does not hold for women at higher SES levels. For women with college degrees, low-birthweight rates are better for white women than either Hispanic or Asian American women. Among Asian Americans, the low-birthweight advantage is observed only for non-high school graduates. One of the problems with socio-economic analyses that are not stratified by country of birth and ethnic sub-group, however, is that there is striking heterogeneity in outcomes among ethnic subgroups of Latina and Asian women (Table 2) (Singh and Yu, 1994, 1996b; Zane et al., 1994). For Latinas, lowest rates of low-weight births are generally observed in Mexican Americans and Cuban Americans and higher rates in Puerto Ricans, regardless of whether they are born in the United States (Table 2). Among Asians, the lowest rates of low-weight births are generally observed in Chinese and Japanese Americans and higher rates in Filipino women, regard-less of their nativity (Singh and Yu, 1996b). The heterogeneity in outcomes between ethnic subgroups persists for both U.S.-born and foreign-born women in each group (Table 2). Nor are the differences explained by SES, as measured by education. For example, nearly 34% of the foreign-born Chinese Americans had 16 or more years of education (mean of 13.2 years) and a low-birthweight rate of 4.7%, while more than 40% of foreign-born Filipinos had high levels of education (mean 13.8 years) and a low-birthweight rate of 7.1%. Similarly, Mexican Americans had fewer years of education than Puerto Ricans or Cubans, but better birthweight outcomes. When adjusted for sociodemographic factors including education, there remain systematic ethnic differences in odds of low-birthweight and preterm birth, increasing from Chinese to Japanese and Filipino groups, and with the odds highest among the U.S.-born (Singh and Yu, 1996b).

Cultural explanations for both nativity and ethnic subgroup effects and in pregnancy outcomes need further exploration. Understanding acculturation, the process of adapting to the host country, is one promising direction. Accultura-tion includes the extent to which the beliefs and practices of immigrants adhere to their traditional culture, adhere to their host country culture, or combine both (Nagata, 1994; Landrine and Klonoff, 1996). As a general rule, acculturation increases with length of time in the host country. Among Hispanic ethnic sub-groups, outcomes have been found to vary with acculturation to the United States; for example, the longer non-native-born women reside in the United States, the poorer their perinatal outcomes tend to be (Williams et al., 1986; Guendelman et al., 1990). Acculturation is associated with a direct effects on birth outcomes and indirect effects through effects on health behaviors, like smoking (Scribner and Dwyer, 1989; Cobas et al., 1996). Second-generation Hispanic women report a higher prevalence of health risk behaviors such as smoking and drinking than first-generation women (Guendelman et al., 1990). In a study with multiple measures of acculturation, acculturation was not associ-ated with birthweight, gestational age, or smoking, though it was associated with alcohol and drug use (Zambrana et al., 1997). Instead, language and time in the United States affected gestational age and birthweight through a mediating vari-able, prenatal stress (see below).

TABLE 2. Low-Birthweight Outcomes and Selected Sociodemographic Characteristics by Maternal Nativity Status and Race or Ethnicity, 1985 Through 1987

Characteristics	Non-Hispanic Whites	Blacks	Chinese	Japanese	Filipinos	Other Asians	Mexicans	Puerto Ricans	Cubans	Central and South Americans
U.S.-Born Mothers										
Low-birthweight, % per 1,000 births	5.5	13.1	6.5	6.5	8.0	6.3	6.6	9.4	7.0	6.8
Maternal age <20 years, %	9.6	24.4	2.3	3.8	15.9	9.8	22.7	26.4	19.1	25.3
Maternal education <12 years, %	14.9	32.3	3.2	2.9	13.8	12.3	42.3	43.8	22.4	29.9
Maternal education >16 years, %	19.2	6.5	54.3	41.4	8.5	37.1	3.8	4.5	14.3	13.6
Mean Education, years	13.0	11.9	14.8	14.4	12.6	13.7	11.4	11.4	12.6	12.3
Unmarried, %	14.0	64.0	8.9	10.2	29.0	18.9	29.6	54.2	23.2	65.1
Nonmetropolitan county, %	40.0	33.3	10.4	19.3	21.7	20.4	29.8	6.0	9.1	9.5
Live birth order >4%	8.1	13.9	3.9	3.7	9.4	7.2	15.0	8.0	3.5	5.1
Prenatal care in first trimester, %	81.1	61.2	89.8	88.0	74.2	76.1	62.7	57.1	66.6	65.8
No prenatal care, %	1.1	3.8	0.4	0.5	1.0	1.5	3.7	9.4	4.4	2.8
Number of live births	2,013,179	1,657,672	6,281	13,011	8,849	9,805	333,073	58,066	3,968	3,454

Foreign- or Puerto Rican-Born Mothers

Low-birthweight, % per 1,000 births	5.2	8.8	4.7	5.9	7.1	6.4	5.0	8.7	5.6	5.7
Maternal age < 20 years, %	4.1	6.7	0.6	1.4	3.4	5.3	13.1	14.5	4.8	7.7
Maternal education <12 years, %	11.2	28.1	15.2	5.5	12.7	23.7	74.6	46.7	19.5	35.8
Maternal education >16 years, %	26.6	13.9	33.8	39.0	42.2	30.9	2.6	5.5	16.2	8.3
Mean education, years	13.3	11.8	13.2	14.0	13.8	12.3	8.2	11.1	12.6	11.3
Unmarried, %	9.2	40.4	2.8	5.2	9.2	8.6	25.9	50.0	14.9	36.8
Nonmetropolitan county, %	21.4	6.6	9.1	16.7	14.8	20.1	15.7	6.5	3.5	3.0
Live birth order >4%	8.7	13.7	4.3	4.3	7.1	16.5	20.9	16.1	5.9	11.5
Prenatal care in first trimester, %	82.5	60.8	80.8	82.8	78.2	70.2	57.1	58.3	83.5	59.2
No prenatal care, %	1.1	5.6	1.0	0.9	0.9	1.8	5.7	9.2	1.4	5.8
Number of live births	94,428	124,335	44,291	10,908	54,211	164,674	407,309	51,808	25,967	132,913

SOURCE: Data were derived from the Linked Birth and Infant Death data sets, 1985, 1986, and 1987 cohorts (Singh and Yu, 1996a).

Changes in pregnancy outcomes with acculturation can happen quickly in the host country. Controlling for sociodemographic factors, Mexican immigrants who had lived in the United States 5 years or more were found to have more pregnancy complications resulting in higher rates of preterm birth than more recent immigrants (Guendelman et al., 1995). Longer residents also had fewer planned pregnancies. The length of U.S. residence appears to be associated with an increase in low-birthweight through a decrease in length of gestation, rather than through slowing fetal growth (Guendelman et al., 1995; Zambrana et al., 1997).

Psychological stress is believed to be one of the key mechanisms through which acculturation contributes to health disparities among immigrant ethnic groups. Social, economic, and cultural stressors are thought to accumulate over time with experiences in the host country. Stressors include the adjustment of moving from a rural to an urban area, separation from family, language barriers, unrealized expectations, and changes in gender roles (Perez, 1983; Menville, 1987). If not moderated sufficiently by social, economic, or cultural resources, then some women cope with the stress by adopting host country behaviors such as smoking, or alcohol and drug use (Marin et al., 1989). Acculturation is a complex process, however, with complicated effects. Acculturation among Latinas is associated with increased self-esteem, independent of social support, marital status, religion, or education (Flaskerud and Uman, 1996). Young Vietnamese adults were more acculturated and bicultural, and reported themselves as healthier than older, foreign-born Vietnamese, but they experienced more family conflict and dissatisfaction with their current lives in the United States (Leong and Johnson, 1994). Nevertheless, they had lower than expected levels of distress compared to their elders because of their perceived positive well-being. Because stress and adaptation are hypothesized to play a role in mediating effects of racial or ethnic disparities on birth outcomes, we turn next to a detailed presentation of what is currently known about stress and adaptation in pregnancy.

PSYCHOSOCIAL ANTECEDENTS AND OUTCOMES

Psychosocial characteristics such as stress and adaptation, and associated behaviors, affect women's health before, during, and after pregnancy (Lederman, 1995a; Weisman, 1997). They are shaped in turn by social factors such as material and social resources or deprivation, residential segregation, and racism (Table 1) (Cohen et al., 1997). While studies have not yet documented SES gradients in stress and adaptation, and are only beginning to investigate ethnic differences in stress and adaptation, there is growing evidence that these factors are associated with reproductive health and pregnancy outcomes, and need to be better understood (Hogue, 1999). Better understanding of stress and adaptation may help to explain socioeconomic and ethnic disparities in health, and why some women do well in spite of their SES and ethnic health risks. Since the majority of pregnancies and births in every group are healthy, studying stress and adaptation within as well as across groups is important. To explore further how stress and adaptation affect childbearing women, we summarize evidence from studies of ethnic disparities in outcomes as a function of measures of stress and adaptation, and describe trials of social support designed to prevent or reduce stress among pregnant women.

Stress and Adaptation

Psychological stress and how women adapt to stress have long been suspected of playing a role in adverse birth outcomes (Lazarus and Folkman, 1984; Lobel and Dunkel-Schetter, 1990; Lobel, 1994). Stress is a process in which social or physical environmental demands are placed on the adaptive capacity of an individual, resulting in psychological changes, which in turn can lead to biological changes (Cohen et al., 1997). The social or physical environment can, however, also supply resources (such as social supports) to help individuals adapt and improve their individual abilities to cope with stress. To complicate matters further, the pregnancy is itself an internal stress with its own biological stress response that develops to protect the unborn baby (Wadhwa et al., 1996; 1997). What appears to happen in pregnant women who have high levels of acute, chronic, or intergenerational stress in their environments is that either their prenatal stress effects are heightened or their protective stress response is inhibited from its full development, and fetal growth or the length of gestation becomes vulnerable to external stresses (Wadhwa et al., 1993). The result would be a low-birthweight or preterm birth.

Research on stress and adaptation effects on birth outcomes has focused largely on constructs of psychological stress that depend on measuring stressful life events (Cohen et al., 1997). In more recent research, it is the woman's perception of potentially stressful events that is measured (Lobel, 1994; Lederman, 1995a). Adaptation is generally captured in measures of coping skills or social support. Potentially confounding factors that are adjusted in thorough studies of such effects include psychological factors (such as trait anxiety) and obstetric risks. Defining and measuring stress and adaptation in diverse SES and ethnic groups is difficult because of differences in the definition, interpretation, and experience of stress and coping skills (Tracy and Mattar, 1999).

Recent studies of birth outcomes in African American women have found associations of stress and adaptation with birth outcomes. The odds of very low-birthweight were three times as high for African American mothers exposed to three or more stressful life events during pregnancy when compared to women with fewer events (Collins et al., 1998). Neighborhoods that could be characterized as stressful were also associated with higher odds of low-birthweight for infants of African American mothers. African American women who had more respect for themselves, believed they did things the same as most people, and had more people in their social networks all had higher-weight babies, and term delivery was associated with positive self-attitude (Edwards et al., 1994). Among African American women, social support, life events the year prior to pregnancy, and mental health were associated with birthweight through their effects on smoking behavior (McCormick et al., 1990).

Acculturation effects on stress and outcomes have been explored in two recent studies comparing Mexican immigrants with Mexican Americans. Greater "integration" in the United States was associated with significantly more prenatal stress, which in turn was associated with preterm birth (Zambrana et al., 1997). Integration was measured by length of time in the country and use of English and was the only acculturation dimension with a significant relationship to stress or outcomes. Stress had direct effects on gestational age and indirect effects on birthweight (Rini et al., 1999). The effects of ethnicity on birthweight were entirely explained by personal resources (mastery, optimism, self-esteem) and interaction effects of ethnicity with income, education, marital status, and age on personal resources. Latina women had weaker personal resources than white non-Hispanics, and women with weaker resources had lower birthweights. There was no difference in prenatal stress between the two groups, however, and women with higher prenatal stress had shorter gestational ages. These studies with multiple measures of psychological SES and ethnicity are particularly promising for beginning to understand how ethnic effects on health at birth are produced.

Clinical depression may also affect pregnancy outcomes. Depression for women occurs at particularly high rates during the reproductive years, as well as in pregnancy and the postpartum period (Ruderman and O'Campo, 1999). In inner-city women with depression measured in the third trimester, higher odds of low-birthweight and preterm birth were found, even after adjustment for demographic, health behavior, and obstetric risks (Steer et al., 1992). Among African Americans, but not whites, women with high depression scores at their first prenatal visit were found to have higher rates of preterm births (Orr and Miller, 1995). A deeper understanding of the contributions of psychological stress and depression to birth outcomes could add considerably to our understanding of how SES gradients and ethnic disparities in outcomes arise (Hogue, 1999).

Social Support

The hypothesis that stress during pregnancy contributes to poor pregnancy outcomes and that social support could "buffer" against stress or enhance adaptation has led to numerous trials of social support services in clinical settings. Nearly all have been with poor women, several with Latinas, and one with African American women. Beneficial effects on birthweight have been documented for social support, but not as a buffer to high levels of stress. Intimate social support from a partner or family member appears to improve fetal growth, even for women with low levels of stress, (Lederman, 1995a; Hoffman and Hatch, 1996). Trials in which social support was provided through the health care systems, however, have produced highly variable results, indicating that there is no reliable model as yet for reducing disparities in low-birthweight.

Randomized trials of social support in pregnancy were conducted with women of varying levels of psychosocial risk (Spencer et al., 1989; Blondel et al., 1990; Oakley et al., 1990; Bryce et al., 1991; Villar et al., 1992; Langer et al., 1996) and women with high levels of measured stress and low social support (Rothberg and Lits, 1991; Norbeck et al., 1996). The amount and type of psychosocial support varied a great deal among the studies. In one study, nurses provided emotional support and health education, and helped women to cope with pregnancy-related problems. In other trials, nurses helped women to mobilize support from their network (Villar et al., 1992; Langer et al., 1996; Norbeck et al., 1996). One study had a lay home visitor provide household help and some advice when necessary (Spencer et al., 1989), while the others had midwives increase their emotional support (Oakley et al., 1990; Bryce et al., 1991). Intervention groups had lower rates of preterm birth in only four of the six trials reporting rates, and none showed significantly lower odds of preterm birth (Blondel, 1998). The pooled odds ratio was 1.4 (95% confidence interval [CI], 0.9–1.9). In two other trials for women at high risk of preterm birth, either women (Collaborative Group on Preterm Birth Prevention, 1993) or public clinic sites (Hobel et al., 1994) were randomized. Nurses provided preterm birth education and general emotional support. In the former study, there was no significant difference between groups. In the second study, although the rate of preterm births was lower in the intervention group (7.3% compared to 9.1%), the odds of preterm birth were not significantly lower. Among women in the trial who were randomized to social work support, there was no advantage to social work intervention. The results are consistent with at least three different interpretations: (1) it is difficult to provide sufficient social support during pregnancy in clinical encounters to overcome psychosocial contributions to poor birth outcomes, (2) it is difficult to demonstrate an effect unless the women with reducible psychosocial risks are identified and evaluated by themselves, or (3) there is no reliable effect of psychosocial support services during pregnancy in clinical encounters.

POLICY AND PROGRAM STRATEGIES

Since reducing infant mortality in the United States became a prime public health policy goal in the mid-1980s, the evidence that any of the policy or program changes have lead to measurable improvements in the health of infants at birth is modest at best. What is humbling is that public health efforts that attempted to deal with SES and ethnic disparities using public health professional expertise, have had little if any significant impact on the disparate birth outcomes. No single type of public health effort has led to reliable, reproducible impact on low-birthweight or preterm birth outcomes (Alexander and Korenbrot, 1995). The efforts have been associated with national improvements in the United States of prenatal care, teenage pregnancy, smoking in pregnancy, and reduction in infant deaths due to sudden infant death syndrome (SIDS) (Pamuk et al., 1998; Willinger et al., 1998; Ventura et al., 1999). Yet there has been no conclusive impact on the birth outcomes. We review here briefly some of the major public health efforts that have been made, and their associated impacts. We do so not to demonstrate what has already worked but to document what has been tried. In looking for reasons why changes in birth outcomes are so difficult to achieve with traditional public health interventions, we present first national-level efforts that have attempted to reduce socioeconomic health disparities of infants, and then ethnic-specific efforts at the community level that have attempted to reduce racial or ethnic health disparities of infants. At the conclusion of this section, we point to lessons learned and ignorance revealed that point to new opportunities for future research and development of public health policy and program strategies.

Reducing Socioeconomic Health Disparities at Birth

The public policy and program strategies that have attempted to reduce the effects of differences in socioeconomic status on infants have emphasized improving access to and content of health care services that low-income pregnant women receive and improving material resources of low-income women (Hughes and Simpson, 1995). Innovations were implemented at the societal, community, family, and individual levels, but all focused almost exclusively on pregnant women. None have revealed models that reliably or reproducibly reduce population rates of low-birthweight or infant mortality, though there is evidence of limited success in some groups of participants.

Expanded Access to Perinatal Health Care for Low-Income Women

Beginning in 1984 a series of policy reforms of the federal Medicaid program in the Health Resources and Services Administration (HRSA) removed the requirement that pregnant women be eligible for welfare in order to obtain health care coverage for pregnancy-related medical care (Coughlin et al., 1994). Changes in Medicaid policies not only expanded income criteria for eligibility so that women with household incomes up to twice the poverty level eventually were eligible, but also provided the states incentives for establishing early and continuous coverage of care before eligibility applications were fully processed (presumptive eligibility) and uninterrupted coverage in pregnancy (continuous eligibility) (Sardell, 1990; Dubay et al., 1995). Access to prenatal care and use of prenatal care improved for low-income pregnant women for Medicaid in many states, but not all (Piper et al., 1990; Braveman et al., 1993; Epstein and Newhouse, 1998). Studies evaluating the impact of Medicaid improvements found variable effects on prenatal care use and little impact on pregnancy outcomes (Piper et al., 1990; 1994a; 1994b; California Department of Health Services, 1996; Haas et al., 1996; Epstein and Newhouse, 1998). Nationwide, vital statistics revealed that the early and continuous use of prenatal care improved, without associated impact on birth outcomes (Figures 1–3). States that increased payments to physicians for obstetric care, thus expanding the capacity of the health system accessible to low-SES women, were among the more successful states in eventually improving early and continuous use of prenatal care (Dubay et al., 1995). California attained "universal coverage" (more than 95% of pregnant women covered by private and public insurance) by 1994, but low-birthweight and preterm births in the state did not improve (California Department of Health Services, 1996). Evidence from a variety of sources indicates that Medicaid coverage of pregnant women is inadequate to compensate for socioeconomic deprivation (Haas et al., 1996; Moss and Carver, 1998). On the other hand, women who use food from the U.S. Department of Agriculture's Supplemental Nutrition Program for Women, Infants and Children (WIC) during pregnancy have better birthweight and infant mortality rates than women who do not, even after adjustment for a number of characteristics to reduce selection bias (Stockbauer, 1987; Moss and Carver, 1998).

Psychosocial Services for Low-Income Women

Enhanced prenatal care services that include nutrition, psychosocial, and health education services along with obstetric care have developed in the public health sector of the nation's health care system largely through the efforts of the Bureau of Maternal and Child Health in HRSA. Most states by 1990 offered enhanced prenatal services to low-income women through public health services and some through Medicaid. Two basic models have been used for the service delivery: public health sites provide the support services for all obstetric providers, or physician offices and public or private clinics provide their own enhanced services (McLaughlin et al., 1992; Simpson et al., 1997). Enhanced prenatal care services in statewide Medicaid programs have demonstrated effects on outcomes, though effects have been variable and largely limited to particular groups who are likely to be at higher psychosocial risk. The one randomized control trial of psychosocial, nutrition, and health education services found that the services were related to higher mean birthweights for women who had not given birth before, but not those who had (McLaughlin et al., 1992). In observational trials, the services have been associated with infant mortality or low-birthweight rates statewide (Buescher et al., 1991), for black women only (Reichman and Florio, 1996), for women with a minimal number of visits (Korenbrot et al., 1995), medically high-risk women (Baldwin et al., 1998), or with no impact on low-birthweight rates (Piper et al., 1996). Part of the variation in impact could be the result of variation in quality of content and delivery of the psychosocial services. In a stratified random sample of 27 ambulatory prenatal care sites of five practice setting types, the quality and extent of psychosocial services varied at the individual and site level and with provider credentials (Wilkinson et al., 1994; 1998). The differences in birth outcomes observed with differences in the measure of quality of care, however, varied at the individual level and did not depend on the credentials of the psychosocial service provider or the site of care (Homan and Korenbrot, 1998; Wilkinson et al., 1998). There is no conclusive evidence that these services improve outcomes for low-income women in general, and they may at best have an impact on birth outcomes only in some women with elevated, but reducible, psychosocial risks.

National Healthy Start Program

As an alternative to Medicaid reform, which was a change in health care coverage for pregnant women across the country, the national Healthy Start program provided funding to a limited number of local areas in the country (Mason, 1991). The program was started in 1990 to assist communities with high infant mortality rates in developing innovative, multidimensional community approaches to reducing infant mortality. Community-level consortia at most sites developed collaborative partnerships of local and state agencies, the private sector, schools, and other community and social organizations, sharing people and resources in the efforts. The projects developed their own interventions, and over the course of the 5-year demonstration there were nine models of intervention that evolved (Healthy Start National Resource Center, 1999). Projects developed different combinations and versions of the models. For example, three projects developed Family Resource Centers with an array of services available at one community site. Services included high school graduate equivalency degree (GED) classes, food vouchers through the food stamps and WIC programs, cash assistance through the welfare program, on-site Medicaid links, health education, and life planning. Not all of the Family Resource Centers provided all these services, however. Other models of intervention used in the same community might include enhanced clinical services, risk prevention and reduction, facilitating services, training and education, or adolescent programs. The primary issues addressed by the projects regardless of intervention models were to include teenage pregnancy and schooling, inadequate prenatal care, poor nutrition, and absence of family and community support, as well as the use of tobacco, alcohol, and drugs.

Results of the national evaluation of the Healthy Start program are to be released in the Spring of 2000. Preliminary results released in 1998 indicated no consistent impacts on birth outcomes (Local Evaluations, 1998). The national evaluation results are anxiously awaited for final lessons to be drawn.

National Fetal–Infant Mortality Review

The National Fetal–Infant Mortality Review (NFIMR) program begun in 1992 established community-level FIMRs to examine health, behavior, and psychosocial factors, as well as health and social service factors, in families that experience fetal and infant deaths. Initiated by the American College of Obstetricians and Gynecologists (ACOG) in partnership with other major professional societies, the federal government, the March of Dimes, the Robert Wood Johnson Foundation, and private organizations, the reviews were devised and carried out at the local community level. The communities selected to participate had high levels of infant mortality, with demonstrated local professional support, community consensus of need, and commitment of local resources for review activities. Major aspects of the FIMR programs included: examining social, economic, cultural, safety, and health systems factors associated with fetal and infant mortality through review of individual cases; planning a series of interventions and policies that addressed these factors to improve the services systems and community resources; participating in community-based interventions and policies; and assessing the progress of the interventions (NFIMR, 1997). The quantitative impact of the FIMRs has not been formally evaluated, but one study where infant mortality rates declined more than statewide rates occurred in Aiken County, South Carolina, which mounted an impressive sociopolitical and public health response to the findings of its FIMR task force.

In Aiken County, the coroner who started reviewing the cases and causes of infant death noticed a growing number of deaths that appeared to have socially linked causes as a growing differential between blacks and whites (Papouchado and Townsend, 1999). The coroner notified the newly elected mayor. The deaths proved to be "a red flag for a host of serious societal problems." Together women began a cascade of community reforms that put rural police on bicycles to get to know their community, its children, and its parents ("MOMS and COPS"), not to jail them for neglect or abuse or put their children in protective services but to find out what people needed to take care of their pregnancies and infants and to help them get it. A growing number of community participants (more than 70 members from institutions, agencies, civic groups, and religious groups) that had been the Infant Mortality Task Force (a medical model) turned into the Growing into Life: Healthy Community Collaborative (a social model). A virtual organization, the collaborative operated on the principle of a "minimum of bureaucracy and territorialism," and an expanded mission to address issues of domestic violence, poverty, lack of education, and other psychosocial issues. No small part of the efforts of the collaborative were to discover and take on a pocket of corruption in the state capital, and win, to get their local needs—and those of other communities in the state like themselves—addressed. During the mayor's first term, the running 3-year averages for infant mortality in Aiken declined steadily from 11.6 to 7.9 per 1,000 live births, while statewide the rates fell from 10.5 to 8.3 live births. The Aiken County experience, like that of some Healthy Start and other FIMR projects, is illustrative of case studies that lead to theories of community interventions that develop multilevel and multidimensional policies and strategies over time, involving community partnerships that potentially could begin to reverse disparities in health at birth.

Reducing Ethnic Health Disparities at Birth

National public health interventions addressing the reduction in ethnic disparities in maternal and infant health have been developed largely as research demonstration projects, rather than government policy or program initiatives.

Although in a few of the original Healthy Start sites described above there were ethnic-specific program strategies for African Americans, by and large the efforts to engage specific ethnic minority communities in culturally adapted programs have been funded by research rather than administrative government funds. The demonstration projects that have attempted to reduce the effects of differences in ethnic disparities on infants have emphasized having members of the ethnic communities themselves participate in the assessment of the communities, assets and needs and plan changes in public health services. Innovations were implemented at the community, family, and individual levels. We present descriptions of two such research demonstration projects, one that involved African American women in four communities across the continental United States and the other that involved three Asian American ethnic groups in one community in Hawaii. These projects focused on the role of stress and adaptation in mediating effects of ethnicity in birth outcomes: (1) starting with qualitative research methods to ascertain the needs of the women in the communities in their own terms, and (2) ending with quantitative epidemiological and psychological research methods to analyze effects of stress and adaptation during pregnancy.

Demonstration Projects with African American Women

In 1993 the Centers for Disease Control and Prevention (CDC), together with the National Institutes of Health (NIH), held a conference to announce research demonstration projects to determine what could be done to reduce the ethnic disparities in preterm birth rates for black and white women (Centers for Disease Control and Prevention with the National Institute of Child Health and Human Development, 1993). The result was the introduction of the concept of community empowerment to maternal and infant health research demonstration projects. The concept grew out of social action ideology of the 1960s and was popularized to describe both traditional and innovative social work practices and interventions to counteract the effects of social, economic, and racial hierarchies (Braithwaite, 1992). Empowerment is the psychological resource needed to reduce the effects of powerlessness, real or imagined, learned helplessness, alienation, and loss of sense of control over life (Rappaport, 1984). It takes on different forms in different people and contexts. The concept of political empowerment of African Americans, and especially African American women, is more complex than merely increasing social capital (LaVeist, 1992). The question of what will engage African American women to become more attuned to "wellness" is the primary question that these programs address. Birth outcomes and stress measurements in African American women participants in the projects will be released in the year 2000, so we present some of the findings of the qualitative research phase of the community-based projects.

Four coordinated demonstration projects in this program use qualitative ethnographic, community-partnered, and participatory research methods (Cornwall and Jewkes, 1995). The guiding principles of the research approach are (1) there is a high degree of community participation; (2) the community identifies issues that it wants to address; (3) the research has as its purposes both collective learning and action to address the issue; (4) methods of research are flexible and appropriate to the community; and (5) the goal of the demonstration project is to benefit the community. The researchers collected data and synthesized their qualitative research findings to define two fundamental efforts to reduce disparities: (1) understanding disparities and defining prevention efforts are dependent on understanding context; and (2) all aspects of methodology from research to action should promote and support prevention. Presenters then documented experiences of black women. The analyses contrast the expectations of public health professionals with the life experiences of African American women with regards to pregnancy and prenatal care. The findings illustrate the gap in mutual understanding to be closed before there can be effective behavior change on the parts of both professionals and women participants. For example, public health professionals ask questions such as, Why do women practice unhealthy behaviors? And, What can we do to promote healthier life-styles? The implicit assumptions were that women have clear lifestyle choices ("good" versus "bad"), women choose unhealthy life-styles, and individual behavior is independent of social forces. African American women revealed that in their view, women are not passive victims, but their options are limited and constrained by social environment (housing, material resources, service availability, violence—both illegal activity and law enforcement, racism), and they are living "between a rock and a hard place." Women with risky behaviors, they found, are often actually choosing the "lesser of the two evils" rather than the bad over the good. This contrast with views of those in the medical professions who provide prenatal care to improve maternal and infant health. For example, Diana, a worker in a fast-food restaurant, had been diligent about her prenatal appointments except for two: her doctor insisted on an amniocentesis, which she did not want to have. She states that she would love a baby with Down's syndrome anyway. Her doctor said she was crazy. In another case, "A non-black obstetrician told the ethnographer that she teaches residents that even if a patient states that she misses her appointments because of child care or work difficulties, she is still irresponsible."

Policy recommendations of an interdisciplinary group of researchers, clergy, media, and community members reviewing the qualitative findings from the projects include (1) address women's health before pregnancy; (2) increase use of alternative providers who can address social issues; (3) improve provider cultural competence; (4) utilize "peer-to-peer" education model in reproductive health; (5) expand communication and collaboration between public health and social sectors (e.g., criminal justice system); (6) integrate the empowerment of women and communities into public health interventions; (7) improve advocacy to make racial and ethnic disparities a national issue; and (8) adjust grant-making strategies for the research and intervention to accommodate nontraditional collaboration (additional partners will improve ability to address social factors).

Demonstration Project with Asian American and
Pacific Islander Women

In 1990 a research demonstration project funded by the National Center for Nursing Research at NIH was unique in its ethnic-specific approach to improving birth outcomes by improving the psychological adaptation of women to pregnancy and parenting (Affonso et al., 1992). The Malama Na Wahine Hapai (Caring for Pregnant Women) community perinatal program in the Hilo-Puna area of the island of Hawaii was developed for three ethnic subgroups of Asian American and Pacific Islanders (Japanese, Filipino, and Hawaiian) that had been found to have significantly higher rates of low-birthweight outcomes than the white majority ethnic group in the area (Korenbrot et al., 1994). Significantly lower rates of risk-adjusted preterm birth and low-birthweight outcomes were observed in program participants compared to a local comparison group (Affonso et al., 1999a). Findings also included significant stress reduction and improvement in cognitive adaptation (meaning mastery and self-esteem) as pregnancy progressed, compared to women in a comparison group (Affonso et al., 1999b).

The Malama project combined conceptually based theory from academic psychology, partnerships with both community leaders and traditional healers of the three ethnic groups, and focus groups with women from each ethnic group, to develop culturally sensitive program strategies (Affonso et al., 1993a; Affonso et al., 1993b, 1994, 1996). The primary Malama administrators and caregivers were public health nurses. A Neighborhood Women's Health Watch (NWHW) of local community women from the three ethnic groups, participated as partners in caregiving activities with the nurses and also provided transportation or child care or helped as "buddies" to those women who needed additional support in maintaining the visit structure. Other family members, particularly spouses, were encouraged to participate in program activities, including couples' group sessions that addressed the emotional and physical aspects of pregnancy. A van was available for transportation of women to both individual appointments and group sessions because the women indicated that in this rural area, transportation was a major barrier to their use of health care. While there are limitations to the generalizations that can be made from such a demonstration project and the birth outcome findings because of the quasi-experimental design limitations, the approach to reducing ethnic disparities in outcomes with multilevel, multidimensional program strategies deserves further investigation and replication (Lederman, 1995b).

NEW RESEARCH OPPORTUNITIES

The preceding overview indicates that while our knowledge base of factors associated with SES and ethnic disparities in health at birth is large, our understanding is very limited. We have much to learn about how stress, depression, and social support, which are shaped by social class, racism, and gender roles and hierarchies, contribute to disparities in outcomes. From this understanding, we can develop better interventions at the community and policy levels. In order to proceed with a sound basis for intervention, research is needed on (1) the concepts that underlie not only SES and race or ethnicity, but the psychosocial factors that mediate the effects of these antecedents; (2) the pathways by which the mediating factors link to health outcomes at birth; and (3) how our understanding of these pathways can be translated into policies and programs that reduce disparities in health at birth. To achieve these goals, public health research will need to integrate theories, methods, and data from the social and behavioral sciences.

Reconceptualizing Antecedents and Mediating Factors

The sociodemographic and psychosocial factors that influence the health of childbearing women and of infants need to be reconceptualized for public health policies and programs in the context of women's lives. The gender, social, economic, and culturally driven roles and hierarchies that evolve from SES and race or ethnicity, and the social context of stress and adaptation, can reinforce long-held prejudices and perpetuate stereotypes, or they can be used to rejuvenate health policy and programs (Williams, 1996). Interdisciplinary public health research that uses the theories and methods of anthropology, sociology, psychology, political science, and economics is needed. The reigning paradigms of different disciplines shape the research questions that are asked and identify research issues that are often neglected outside disciplinary boundaries. The concepts and data relevant to pregnancy outcomes and infant mortality require a scrutiny of values and expansion of meaning systems as they relate to class, gender, ethnicity, and other forms of social differentiation, as well as psychological stress and adaptation in different sociocultural and sociopolitical settings. Applying social science theories and methods to problems of women and pregnancy will encourage clarification of implicit assumptions, so that mutual understanding across disciplines can grow to address the improvement of health at birth (Mechanic, 1995). The lack of conceptual theory behind the casual use of sociodemographic variables has been a drawback to progress in public health research and practice (Krieger et al., 1997). Public health has a fresh opportunity to expand upon and refine social science and behavioral theories in the process of creating innovative interventions.

Incorporating social sciences and behavioral research methods can also bring to the development of policies and programs the integration of qualitative and quantitative techniques. Much has been written on the strengths and limitations of both approaches; it is not repeated here (Baum, 1995; Devers and Rundall, 1998). In the presentation of this paper, we have integrated qualitative evidence with quantitative evidence, particularly where uncertainty is high, as in generalizing about women's experiences in different SES and ethnic groups (see "Sociodemographic Antecedents" section) or describing characteristics of "successful" community demonstration projects (see "Program and Policy Strategies" section). We emphasize the importance of obtaining qualitative information before we further quantify the sociodemographic and environmental stressors and resources that affect health outcomes for individual women and design programs to reduce disparities. We argue against a rush to reductionist approaches to the concepts until multiple dimensions have been devised, operationalized, and validated for a variety of socioeconomic and ethnic groups, accounting for the difficulties in translating and operationalizing concepts without the participation from beginning to end of people who have experienced these factors in their own lives.

Research is needed that conceptualizes the positive resources that women of reproductive age from varied socioeconomic and ethnic groups have in their families and communities. The vast majority of babies are healthy; the challenge to public health research is whether it can move from a focus on risk toward a better understanding of resources and resilience.

Documenting Causal Mechanisms

Additional work is needed on the concepts and measures that are used to track socioeconomic effects on pregnancy outcomes. We know very little about what factors produce socioeconomic gradients in preconception, prenatal, perinatal, and postnatal health. As an example, we need only consider what education captures in the context of maternal health. Education shows effects on health at birth (Figure 4), but we have done little to understand why (Kogan and Alexander, 1998). Is it maternal intelligence? Receptivity to information? Ability to interact with bureaucratic agents? A proxy for social support? A measure of social prestige? A combination of factors or all of the above? In public health research, we have used "education" as a variable of convenience for "socioeconomic status" in order not to ask people about their incomes or classify their occupations, while paying little attention to the dimensions of social class in this country that might better capture the concept of social class (Yen and Moss, 1999).

Once concepts are expanded and validated, there are new opportunities to improve the evidence of causality for antecedents and mediating factors. The time, money, and effort invested in public health efforts to reduce disparities in birth outcomes, to little or no effect, have created pressure to demonstrate causation prior to new social investments. Most of the quantitative relationships between antecedents and outcomes in this overview were measures of association, with varying degrees of inference dependent on study design characteristics. A systematic review is needed to sort the most and least likely mediating factors, while limiting the biases of reviewers (Cochrane Collaboration, 1997). Few studies include the multidimensional, multilevel path modeling that distinguishes mediating, modifying, and confounding effects. Improvements in analytic approaches and more sophisticated causal reasoning, are needed to draw conclusions about social causation (Mechanic, 1995; Smith and Torrey, 1996; Holzman et al., 1998). Prospective, longitudinal studies would isolate preconception and life span effects of SES and ethnicity. Multilevel hierarchical models (to separate environmental from personal sources of effect) are needed to control for individual-level effects when social causation hypotheses are being tested.

Causal research calls for larger samples. Many of the studies reviewed did not have sufficient sample size to test birth outcome hypotheses for different socioeconomic or ethnic groups, nor could they distinguish the birthweight or gestational age outcomes that may be infrequent but contribute to ethnic health disparities. Larger studies would also reduce bias in variation of unmeasured modifying and confounding variables. There were unexpectedly low rates of low-birthweight, for example, in some samples of African American and Mexican American women that raise issues about participation bias among cautious respondents. To have more women participate will take greater efforts to build trust in research. Participatory research is one promising approach (Cornwall and Jewkes, 1995).

Translating Research into Policies and Programs

There are new opportunities to apply the findings of conceptually based, causally tested research to policy and program intervention. Although public health projects are sometimes built on social science knowledge, they have rarely been informed by social science theory (Mechanic, 1995). We have learned that there are no impressive or reliable "quick fixes" that reduce disparities. Policies and programs have generally addressed a narrow range of factors; they often operate for only a few years. The tide of generations of complex and multiple influences that have created disparities in this country will not be reversed in a 9-month period for individuals or a decade for populations. Project directors frequently look to see where they can concentrate their efforts and funds for the greatest impact, when what may be needed to make an impact is a broad array of changes addressing many of the consequences of social, economic, political, historical, and cultural realities. Public health professional expertise is necessary but not sufficient; we have already emphasized the importance of a multidisciplinary approach. New approaches should take into account experiences prior to and during the reproductive years, not just the 9 months of pregnancy. Many interventions focus exclusively on the prenatal period for an impact on outcomes. But the women at highest risk of having low infant weights at birth had low birthweights themselves (Sanderson et al., 1995). They are likely to have continued health complications (Haas and McCormick, 1997). It may take long periods of time to achieve and maintain enough change in the socioeconomic environment, families, and individuals to overcome deprivation or disadvantage.

Interventions should address community change. Promising program strategies indicate that communities may well be the proper units to address disparities in health at birth, but making social changes for health impacts is a relatively new endeavor for many community members who are involved. Each community is unique, and a variety of models for community change that address socioeconomic status and ethnic disparities are needed for communities to draw on. Communities need better ways to define needs, measure activities, and monitor progress toward goals while maintaining community involvement. Intervention strategies involve identifying institutions that can serve as leverage points for stimulating change. Success depends upon motivating the involvement and resources of community members as the basis of planning and implementing change.

REFERENCES

Abraido-Lanza, A. F., Dohrenwend, B. P., Ng-Mak, D. S., and Turner, J. B. (1999). Latino mortality paradox: A test of the "Salmon bias" and healthy migrant hypotheses. *American Journal of Public Health*, 1543–1548.

Adams, M. M., Read, J. A., Rawlings, J. S., Harlass, F. B., Sarno, A. P., and Rhodes, P. H. (1993). Preterm delivery among black and white enlisted women in the United States Army. *Obstetrics and Gynecology, 81*, 65–71.

Aday, L. A. (1993). *At Risk in America: Health Care Needs of Vulnerable Populations in the United States.* San Francisco: Jossey-Bass.

Adler, N. E., Boyce, W. T., Chesney, M. A., Folkman, S., Kahn, R. L., and Syme, S. L. (1994). Socioeconomic status and health: The challenge of the gradient. *American Psychologist, 49*, 15–24.

Affonso, D. D., Mayberry, L. J., Graham, K., Shibuya, J., and Kunimoto, J. (1993a). Prenatal and postpartum care in Hawaii: A community-based approach. *Journal of Obstetric and Gynecological Neonatal Nursing, 22*, 320–325.

Affonso, D. D., Mayberry, L. J., Shibuya, J., Kunimoto, J., Graham, K., and Sheptak, S. (1993b). Themes of stressors for childbearing women in the island of Hawaii. *Journal of Family and Community Health Care, 16*, 9–19.

Affonso, D. D., DeLeon, P. H., Raymond, J. S., and Mayberry, L. J. (1994). Promoting community partnerships: Public policy initiatives related to prenatal care. *Clinical Psychology Science and Practice, 1*, 13–24.

Affonso, D. D., Korenbrot, C. C., De, A., and Mayberry, L. J. (1999a). Birth outcomes and costs of a culturally-based perinatal program in Hawaii. *Asian Pacific Islander Journal Health, 7*, 10–24.

Affonso, D. D., De, A., Korenbrot, C. C., and Mayberry, L. J. (1999b). Cognitive adaptation: Women's health perspective for reducing stress during child bearing. *Journal of Women's Health and Gender-Based Medicine, 8*, 1–10.

Alexander, G. R., Baruffi, G., Mor, J. M., Kieffer, E. C., and Hulsey, T. C. (1993). Multiethnic variations in the pregnancy outcomes of military dependents. *American Journal of Public Health, 83*, 1721–1725.

Alexander, G. R., and Korenbrot, C. C. (1995). The role of prenatal care in preventing low birth weight. *Future of Children, 5*, 103–120.

Alexander, G. R., Mor, J. M., Kogan, M. D., Leland, N. L., and Kieffer, E. (1996). Pregnancy outcomes of U.S.-born and foreign-born Japanese Americans. *American Journal of Public Health, 86*, 820–824.

Amaro, H. (1995). Love, sex, and power: Considering women's realities in HIV prevention. *American Psychologist, 50*, 437–447.

Arber, S. (1991). Class, paid employment and family roles: Making sense of structural disadvantage, gender, and health status. *Social Science and Medicine, 32*, 425–436.

Baldwin, L. M., Larson, E. H., Connell, F. A., Nordlund, D., Cain, K. C., Cawthon, M. L., Byrns, P., and Rosenblatt, R. A. (1998). Effect of expanding Medicaid prenatal services on birth outcomes. *American Journal of Public Health, 88*, 1623–1629.

Barfield, W. D., Wise, P. H., Rust, F. P., Rust, K. J., Gould, J. B., and Gortmaker, S. L. (1996). Racial disparities in outcomes of military and civilian births in California. *Archives of Pediatric and Adolescent Medicine, 150*, 1062–1067.

Barker, D. J. P. (1998). *Mothers, Babies, and Health in Later Life*. Edinborough: Churchill Livingstone.

Baum, F. (1995). Researching public health: Behind the qualitative-quantitative methodological debate. *Social Science and Medicine, 40*, 459–468.

Benderly, B. L. (1997). *In Her Own Right: Institute of Medicine's Guide to Women's Health Issues*. Washington, DC: National Academy Press.

Bennett, T. (1997). "Racial" and ethnic classification: Two steps forward and one step back? *Public Health Reports, 112*, 477–480.

Bennett, T., and Kotelchuck, M. (1997). Mothers and infants. In J. Kotch (Ed.), *Maternal and Child Health: Programs, Problems and Policy in Public Health* (pp. 85–114). Gaithersburg, MD: Aspen.

Blondel, B., Breart, G., Llado, J., and Chartier, M. (1990). Evaluation of the home visiting system for women with threatened preterm labor: Results of a randomized controlled trial. *European Journal of Obstetrics, Gynecology and Reproductive Biology, 34*, 47–58.

Blondel, B. (1998). Social and medical support during pregnancy: An overview of the randomized controlled trials. *Prenatal and Neonatal Medicine, 3*, 141–144.

Braithwaite, R. L. (1992). Coalition partnerships for health promotion and empowerment. In R. L. Braithwaite (Ed.), *Health Issues in the Black Community* (pp. 321–338). San Francisco: Jossey-Bass.

Braveman, P., Bennett, T., Lewis, C., Egerter, S., and Showstack, J. (1993). Access to prenatal care following major Medicaid eligibility expansions. *Journal of the American Medical Association, 269*, 1285–1289.

Brett, K. M., Strogatz, D. S., and Savitz, D. A. (1997). Employment, job strain, and preterm delivery among women in North Carolina. *American Journal of Public Health, 87*, 199–204.

Bryce, R. L., Stanley, F. J., and Garner, J. B. (1991). Randomized controlled trial of antenatal social support to prevent preterm birth. *British Journal of Obstetrics and Gynecology, 98*, 1001–1008.

Buescher, P. A., Roth, M. S., Williams, D., and Goforth, C. M. (1991). An evaluation of the impact of maternity care coordination on Medicaid birth outcomes in North Carolina. *American Journal of Public Health, 81*, 1625–1629.

Cabral, H., Fried, L. E., Levenson, S., Amaro, H., and Zuckerman, B. (1990). Foreign-born and U.S.-born black women: Differences in health behaviors and outcomes. *American Journal of Public Health, 80*, 70–71.

California Department of Health Services (1996). Adequacy of prenatal care utilization—California 1989-1994. *Morbidity and Mortality Weekly Report, 45(30)*, 653–656.

Carstairs, V. (1995). Deprivation indices: Their interpretation and use in relation to health. *Journal of Epidemiology and Community Health, 49*, S39–S44.

Centers for Disease Control and Prevention. (1998). Use of folic acid-containing supplements among women of child bearing age—United States, 1997. *Journal of the American Medical Association, 279*, 1430.

Centers for Disease Control and Prevention. (1999). Achievements in public health, 1900-1999: Healthier mothers and babies. *Morbidity and Mortality Weekly Report,* 48(38), 849–858.

Centers for Disease Control and Prevention and the National Institutes of Health. (1993). Conference on Preterm Delivery and Other Pregnancy Outcomes Among Black Women. Atlanta: Reproductive Health Branch.

Cobas, J. A., Balcazar, H., Benin, M. B., Keith, V. M., and Chong, Y. (1996). Acculturation and low-birthweight infants among Latino women: A reanalysis of HHANES data with structural equation models. *American Journal of Public Health, 86,* 394–396.

The Cochrane Collaboration. (1997). *The Cochrane Collaboration Handbook Version 3.0.2.* London: British Medical Journal Publishing Group

Cohen, S., Kessler, R. C., and Gordon, L. U. (1997). Strategies for measuring stress in studies of psychiatric and physical disorders. In S. Cohen, R. C. Kessler, and L. U. Gordon (Eds.), *Measuring Stress: A Guide for Health and Social Scientists* (pp. 3–26). New York: Oxford University Press.

Collaborative Group on Preterm Birth Prevention (1993). Multicenter randomized controlled trial of preterm birth prevention. *American Journal of Obstetrics and Gynecology, 169,* 352–366.

Collins, J. W., Herman, A. A., and David, R. J. (1997). Very-low-birthweight infants and income incongruity among African American and white parents in Chicago. *American Journal of Public Health, 87,* 414–417.

Collins, J. W., David, R. J., Symons, R., Handler, A., Wall, S., and Andes, S. (1998). African American mothers' perception of their residential environment, stressful life events, and very low-birthweight. *Epidemiology, 9,* 286–289.

Cornwall, A., and Jewkes, R. (1995). What is participatory research? *Social Science and Medicine, 41,* 1667–1676.

Coughlin, T. A., Ku, L., Holahan, J., Heslam, D., and Winterbottom, C. (1994). State responses to the Medicaid spending crisis: 1988 to 1992. *Journal of Health Policy, Politics, and Law, 19,* 837–864.

Crowell, N.A., and Burgess, A. (Eds). (1996). *Understanding Violence Against Women.* Washington, DC: National Academy of Sciences.

Devers, K. J., and Rundall, T. G. (1998). Qualitative methods in health services research. *Health Services Research, 34,* Part II.

DiRenzo, G. C., Moscioni, P., Perazzi, A., Papiernik, E., Breart, G., and Saurel-Cubizolles, M. J. (1998). Social policies in relation to employment and pregnancy in European countries. *Prenatal and Neonatal Medicine, 3,* 147–156.

Dubay, L. C., Kenney, G. M., Norton, S. A., and Cohen, B. C. (1995). Local responses to expanded Medicaid coverage for pregnant women. *Milbank Quarterly, 73,* 535-563.

Edin, K., and Lein, L. (1997). *Making Ends Meet: How Single Mothers Survive Welfare and Low-Wage Work.* New York: Russell Sage Foundation.

Edwards, C. H., Cole, O. J., Oyemade, U. J., Knight, E. M., Johnson, A. A., Westney, O. E., Laryea, H., West, W., Jones, S., and Westney, L. S. (1994). Maternal stress and pregnancy outcomes in a prenatal clinic population. *Journal of Nutrition, 124,* 1006S–1021S.

Elo, I. T., and Preston, S. H. (1992). Effects of early-life conditions on adult mortality: A review. *Population Index, 58,* 186–212.

Epstein, A., and Newhouse, J. P. (1998). Impact of Medicaid expansion on early prenatal care and health outcomes. *Health Care Finance Review, 19,* 85–98.

Evans, R. G. (1995). Introduction. In R.G. Evans, M.L. Barer, and T.R. Marmor (Eds.), *Why Are Some People Healthy and Others Not? The Determinants of Health of Populations*. New York: Aldine de Gruyter.

Feinstein, J. S. (1993). The relationship between socioeconomic status and health. *Milbank Quarterly, 71*, 279–322.

Flack, J. M., Amaro, H., Jenkins, W., Kunitz, S., Levy, J., Mixon, M., and Yu, E. (1995). Panel I: Epidemiology of minority health. *Health Psychology, 14*, 592–600.

Flaskerud, J. H., and Uman, G. (1996). Acculturation and its effects on self-esteem among immigrant Latina women. *Behavioral Medicine, 22*, 123–133.

Friedman, D. J., Cohen, B. B., Mahan, C. M., Lederman, R. I., Vezina, R. J., and Dunn, V. H. (1993). Maternal ethnicity and birthweight among blacks. *Ethnicity and Disease, 3*, 255–269.

Fuller, B., and Kagan, S. (2000). *Remember the Children: Mothers Balance Work and Child Care Under Welfare Reform*. Berkeley, CA: University of California.

Geronimus, A. T. (1986). Effects of race, residence and prenatal care on the relationship of maternal age to neonatal mortality. *American Journal of Public Health, 76*, 1416–1421.

Geronimus, A. T. (1987). On teenage child bearing and neonatal mortality in the United States. *Population Development Review, 13*, 245–279.

Geronimus, A. T. (1992). Weathering hypothesis and the health of African American women and infants: Evidence and speculations. *Ethnicity and Disease, 2*, 207–221.

Geronimus, A. T., Waidman, T. A., Hillemeier, M. M., and Burns, P. B. (1996). Excess mortality among blacks and whites in the United States. *New England Journal of Medicine, 335*, 1552–1558.

Grason, H., Hutchins, J., and Silver, G. (Eds.) (1999). *Charting a Course for the Future Of Women's and Perinatal Health*. Rockville, MD: Maternal and Child Health Bureau, U.S. Department of Health and Human Services.

Guendelman, S., and English, P. B. (1995). Effect of United States residence on birth outcomes among Mexican immigrants: An exploratory study. *American Journal of Epidemiology, 142*, S30–S38.

Guendelman, S., English, P., and Chavez, G. (1995). Infants of Mexican immigrants. Health status of an emerging population. *Medical Care, 33*, 41–52.

Guendelman, S., Gould, J. B., and Hudes, M. (1990). Generational differences in perinatal health among Mexican American population: Findings from HHANES 1982–1984. *American Journal of Public Health, 80*, 61–65.

Haas, J. S., Berman, S., Goldberg, A. B., Lee, L. W., and Cook, E. F. (1996). Prenatal hospitalization and compliance with guidelines for prenatal care. *American Journal of Public Health, 86*, 815–819.

Haas, J. S., and McCormick, M. C. (1997). Hospital use and health status of women during the 5 years following the birth of a premature, low-birthweight infant. *American Journal of Public Health, 87*, 1151–1155.

Hack, M., Klein, N. K., and Taylor, H. G. (1995). Long-term developmental outcomes of low-birthweight infants. *Future of Children, 5*, 176–196.

Hatch, M., Ji, B. T., Shu, X. O., and Susser, M. (1997). Do standing, lifting, climbing, or long hours of work during pregnancy have an effect on fetal growth? *Epidemiology, 8*, 530–536.

Healthy Start National Resource Center (1999). http://www. healthystart.net/.

Hirayama, M., and Wallace, H. M. (1998). *Infant Mortality in Japan and the United States*. Tokyo: Mother and Children's Health Organization.

Hobel, C. J., Ross, M. G., Bemis, R. L., Bragonier, J. R., Nessim, S., Sandhu, M., Bear, M. B., and Mori, B. (1994). The West Los Angeles Preterm Birth Prevention Project. I. Program impact on high-risk women. *American Journal of Obstetrics and Gynecology, 170,* 54–62.

Hoffman, S., and Hatch, M. C. (1996). Stress, social support and pregnancy outcome: A reassessment based on recent research. *Paediatric and Perinatal Epidemiology, 10,* 380–405.

Hogue, C. J. R., and Hargraves, M. A. (1993). Class, race and infant mortality in the United States. *American Journal of Public Health, 83,* 9–12.

Hogue, C. J. R. (1999). Gender, race and class: From epidemiologic association to etiologic hypotheses. In M. Goldman and M. Hatch (Eds.), *Women and Health* (pp. 15-23). San Diego: Academic Press.

Holzman, C., Paneth, N., and Fisher, R. (1998). Rethinking the concept of risk factors for preterm delivery: Antecedents, markers and mediators. *Prenatal and Neonatal Medicine, 3,* 47–52.

Homan, R., and Korenbrot, C. C. (1998). Explaining variation in birth outcomes of Medicaid-eligible women with variation in the adequacy of prenatal support services. *Medical Care, 36,* 190–201.

Howell, E. M., and Blondel, B. (1994). International infant mortality rates: Bias from reporting differences. *American Journal of Public Health, 84,* 850–852.

Hughes, D., and Simpson, L. (1995). Role of social change in preventing low-birthweight. *Future of Children, 5,* 187–102.

Institute of Medicine (1985). *Preventing Low Birthweight.* Washington, DC: National Academy Press.

Institute of Medicine (1995). *The Best Intentions: Unintended Pregnancy and the Well-Being of Children and Families.* Washington, DC: National Academy of Sciences.

Johnson, T., Drisko, K., Gallagher, J., and Barela, C. (1999). Low birth weight: A women's health issue. *Women's Health Issues, 9,* 223–230.

Kennedy, B. P., Kiwachi, I., and Prothrow-Stith, D. (1996). Income distribution and mortality: Cross sectional ecological study of the Robin Hood index in the United States. *British Medical Journal, 312,* 1004–1008.

Kiwachi, I., and Kennedy, B. P. (1997). Health and social cohesion: Why care about income inequality? *British Medical Journal, 314,* 1037-1041.

Kleinman, J. C., and Kessel, S. S. (1987). Racial differences in low-birthweight. *New England Journal of Medicine, 317,* 749–753.

Kleinman, J. C., Fingerhut, L. A., and Prager, K. (1991). Differences in infant mortality by race, nativity status and other maternal characteristics. *American Journal of the Diseases of Children, 145,* 194–199.

Kogan, M. D., and Alexander, G. R. (1998). Social and behavioral factors in preterm birth. *Prenatal and Neonatal Medicine, 3,* 29–31.

Korenbrot, C., Affonso, D., Mayberry, L., and Paul, S. M. (1994). Associations of the use of prenatal care with low-birthweight in Asian Pacific women in Hawaii. *Asian American Pacific Islander Journal of Health, 2,* 181–194.

Korenbrot, C. C., Gill, A., Clayson, Z., and Patterson, E. (1995). Evaluation of California's statewide implementation of enhanced perinatal services as Medicaid benefits. *Public Health Reports, 110,* 125–133.

Kramer, M. S. (1998). Preventing preterm birth: Are we making any progress? *Prenatal and Neonatal Medicine, 3,* 10–12.

Krieger, N. (1991). Women and social class: A methodological study comparing individual, household and census measures as predictors of black/white differences in reproductive history. *Journal of Epidemiology and Community Health, 45*, 35–42.

Krieger, N., Rowley, D. L., Herman, A. A., Avery, B., and Phillips, M. T. (1993). Racism, sexism and social class. *American Journal of Preventive Medicine, 9*, 82–122.

Krieger, N. (1994). Epidemiology and the web of causation: Has anyone seen the spider? *Social Science and Medicine, 39*, 887–903.

Krieger, N., Williams, D. R., and Moss, N. E. (1997). Measuring social class in U.S. public health research: Concepts, methodologies, and guidelines. *Annual Review of Public Health, 18*, 341–378.

Landrine, H., and Klonoff, E. A. (1996). *African American Acculturation: Deconstructing Race and Reviving Culture.* Thousand Oaks, CA: Sage.

Landsbergis, P. A., and Hatch, M. C. (1996). Psychosocial work stress and pregnancy-induced hypertension [see comments]. *Epidemiology, 7*, 346–351.

Lane, S. D., and Cibula, D. A. (2000). *Gender and Health.* In G. L. Albrecht, R. Fitzpatrick, and S. C. Scrimshaw (Eds.). *Handbook of Social Studies in Health and Medicine* (pp. 136–153). Thousand Oaks CA: Sage.

Langer, A., Farnot, U., Garcia, C., Barros, F., Victora, C., Belizan, J. M., and Villar, J. (1996). The Latin American trial of psychosocial support during pregnancy: Effects on mother's wellbeing and satisfaction. Latin American Network for Perinatal and Reproductive Research (LANPER). *Social Science and Medicine, 42*, 1589–1597.

LaVeist, T. A. (1992). Political empowerment and health status of African Americans: Mapping a new territory. *American Journal of Sociology, 97*, 1080–1095.

LaVeist, T. A. (1994). Beyond dummy variables and sample selection: What health services researchers ought to know about race as a variable. *Health Services Research, 29*, 1–16.

Lazarus, R. S., and Folkman, S. (1984). *Stress, Appraisal and Coping.* New York: Springer.

Lederman, R. P. (1995a). Relationship of anxiety, stress, and psychosocial development to reproductive health. *Behavioral Medicine, 21*, 101–112.

Lederman, R. P. (1995b). Treatment strategies for anxiety, stress, and developmental conflict during reproduction. *Behavioral Medicine, 21*, 113–122.

Leong, F.T.L. and Johnson, M.C. (1994). Motheres of Vietnamese Americans: Psychological distress and high–risk factors. *Asian American and Pacific Islander Journal of Health, 2*, 31–48.

Lillie-Blanton, M., and LaVeist, T. (1996). Race or ethnicity, the social environment and health. *Social Science and Medicine, 43*, 83–91.

Link, B. G. and Phelan, J.. (1995). Social conditions as fundamental causes of disease. *Journal of Health Society and Behavior, Supplementary Issue*, 80–94.

Lipton, R. B., Liao, Y., Cao, G., Cooper, R. S., and McGee, D. (1993). Determinants of incident non-insulin-dependent diabetes mellitus among blacks and whites in a national sample. The NHANES I Epidemiologic Follow-Up Study. *American Journal of Epidemiology, 138*, 826–839.

Lobel, M., and Dunkel-Schetter, C. (1990). Conceptualizing stress to study effects on health: Environmental, perceptual and emotional components. *Anxiety Research, 3*, 213–230.

Lobel, M. (1994). Conceptualizations, measurement, and effects of prenatal maternal stress on birth outcomes. *Journal of Behavioral Medicine, 17*, 225–272.

Local Evaluations of the Healthy Start Projects (1998). American Public Health Association Annual Meeting, Washington, DC.

Marin, G., Perez-Stables, E. J., and Marin, B. (1989). Cigarette smoking among San Francisco Hispanics: The role of acculturation and gender. *American Journal of Public Health, 79*, 196–199.

Marmot, M., Ryff, C. D., Bumpass, L. L., Shipley, M., and Marks, N. F. (1997). Social inequalities in health: Next questions and converging evidence. *Social Science and Medicine, 44*, 901–910.

Mason, J. O. (1991). Reducing infant mortality in the United States through "Healthy Start." *Public Health Reports, 106*, 479–483.

McCormick, M. C., Brooks-Gunn, J., Shorter, T., Holmes, J. H., Wallace, C. Y., and Heagarty, M. C. (1990). Factors associated with smoking in low-income pregnant women: Relationship to birth weight, stressful life events, social support, health behaviors and mental distress. *Journal of Clinical Epidemiology, 43*, 441–448.

McGrady, G. A., Sung, J. F., Rowley, D. L., and Hogue, C. J. (1992). Preterm delivery and low birth weight among first-born infants of black and white college graduates. *American Journal of Epidemiology, 136*, 266–276.

McLaughlin, F. J., Altemeier, W. A., Christensen, M. J., Sherrod, K. B., Dietrich, M. S., and Stern, D. T. (1992). Randomized trial of comprehensive prenatal care for low-income women: Effect on infant birth weight. *Pediatrics, 89*, 128–132.

Mechanic, D. (1995). Emerging trends in the application of the social sciences to health and medicine. *Social Science and Medicine, 40*, 1491–1496.

Menville, M. (1987). Mexican women adapt to migration. *International Migration Review, 12*, 235–255.

Minkovitz, C., and Baldwin, K. (1999). Social context of women's health. In H. Grason, J. Hutchins, and G. Silver (Eds.), *Course for the Future of Women's and Perinatal Health* (pp. 5–24). Rockville, MD: Maternal and Child Health Bureau, U.S. Department of Health and Human Services.

Morton-Mitchell, I. M., Ibrahim, A. R., and Bekele, Y. (1999). In search of protective factors: Examining the differences in factors related to preterm birth among U.S.-born, Caribbean-born and Africa-born black mothers. Presented at the Maternal, Infant and Child Health Epidemiology Program Workshop, Atlanta GA.

Moss, N.E. (2000a). Socioeconomic inequalities and women's health. In M. Goldman, and M. Hatch (Eds.), *Women and Health* (pp. 541–552). San Diego: Academic Press.

Moss, N. E. (2000b). Gender equity and socioeconomic inequality: A framework for the patterning of women's health. Presented at CICRED Seminar Social and Economic Patterning of Health Among Women, Tunis, Tunisia.

Moss, N., and Carver, K. (1993). Pregnant women at work: Sociodemographic perspectives. *American Journal of Industrial Medicine, 23*, 541–557.

Moss, N., and Carver, K. (1998). The effect of WIC and Medicaid on infant mortality in the United States. *American Journal of Public Health, 88*, 1354–1361.

Nagata, D. K. (1994). Assessing Asian American acculturation and ethnic identity: Need for a multidimensional framework. *Asian American Pacific Islander Journal of Health, 2*, 108–124.

National Fetal and Infant Mortality Review. (1997). Report on projects funded by the Robert Wood Johnson Foundation and ACOG District IV. Washington, DC: American College of Obstetricians and Gynecologists.

Norbeck, J. S., DeJoseph, J. F., and Smith, R. T. (1996). A randomized trial of an empirically derived social support intervention to prevent low-birthweight among African American women. *Social Science and Medicine, 43*, 947–954.

Oakley, A., Rajan, L., and Grant, A. (1990). Social support and pregnancy outcome. *British Journal of Obstetrics and Gynecology, 97*, 155–162.

O'Campo, P., Gielen, A. C., Faden, R. R., Xue, X., Kass, N., and Wang, M. (1995). Violence by male partners against women during the child bearing year: A contextual analysis. *American Journal of Public Health, 85*, 1092–1097.

O'Campo, P., Xue, X., Wang, M., and Caughy, M. O. (1997). Neighborhood risk factors for low-birthweight in Baltimore: A multilevel analysis. *American Journal of Public Health, 87*, 1113–1118.

O'Campo, P., and Rojas-Smith, L. (1998). Welfare reform and women's health: Review of the literature and implications for state policy. *Journal of Public Health Policy, 19*, 420–446.

Orr, S. T., and Miller, C. A. (1995). Maternal depressive symptoms and the risk of poor pregnancy outcome. Review of the literature and preliminary findings. *Epidemiological Review, 17*, 165–171.

Osborne, N. G., and Feit, M. D. (1992). Use of race in medical research. *Journal of the American Medical Association, 267*, 275–279.

Pamuk, E., Makuc, D., Heck, K., Reuben, C., and Lochner, K. (1998). *Socioeconomic Status and Health Chartbook: Health, United States, 1998*. Hyattsville, MD: National Center for Health Statistics, U.S. Department of Health and Human Services.

Paneth, N. (1995). Problem of low-birthweight. *Future of Children, 5*, 19–34.

Papouchado, K., and Townsend, S. R. (1999, May). When spider webs unite they can tie up a lion. Presented at Maternal and Child Health Branch Annual Conference. *"Capitalizing" on Our Resources*, Sacramento, CA.

Perez, R. (1983). Effects of stress, social support and coping style on adjustment to pregnancy. *Hispanic Journal of Behavioral Science, 5*, 141–161.

Petrini, J., Foti, H., and Damus, K. (1997). *March of Dimes StatBook: Statistics for Monitoring Maternal and Infant Health, 1997*. Wilkes-Barre, PA: March of Dimes Birth Defects Foundation.

Piper, J. M., Ray, W. A., and Griffin, M. R. (1990). Effects of Medicaid eligibility expansion on prenatal care and pregnancy outcome in Tennessee. *Journal of the American Medical Association, 264*, 2219–2223.

Piper, J. M., Mitchel, E. F., and Ray, W. A. (1994a). Expanded Medicaid coverage for pregnant women to 100 percent of the federal poverty level. *American Journal of Preventive Medicine, 10*, 97–102.

Piper, J. M., Mitchel, E. F., and Ray, W. A. (1994b). Presumptive eligibility for pregnant Medicaid enrollees: Its effects on prenatal care and perinatal outcome. *American Journal of Public Health, 84*, 1626–1630.

Piper, J. M., Mitchel, E. F., and Ray, W. A. (1996). Obstetric care provider density and delayed onset of prenatal care. *Medical Care, 34*, 1066–1070.

Polednak, A. P. (1989). *Racial and Ethnic Differences in Disease*. New York: Oxford.

Polednak, A. P. (1996). Trends in U.S. urban black infant mortality, by degree of residential segregation. *American Journal of Public Health, 86*, 723–726.

Polednak, A. P. (1997). *Segregation, Poverty and Mortality in Urban African Americans*. New York: Oxford.

Power, C., Hertzmann, C., Matthews, S., and Manor, O. (1997). Social differences in health: Life-cycle effects between ages 23 and 33 in the 1958 British birth cohort. *American Journal of Public Health, 87*, 1499–1503.

Power, C., Matthews, S., and Manor, O. (1998). Inequalities in self-rated health: Explanations from different stages of life. *Lancet, 351*, 1009–1014.

Pritchard, C. W., and Teo, P. Y. (1994). Preterm birth, low-birthweight and the stressfulness of the household role for pregnant women. *Social Science and Medicine, 38,* 89–96.

Pugliesi, K. (1995). Work and well-being: Gender differences in the psychological consequences of employment. *Journal of Health, Society and Behavior, 36,* 57–71.

Rappaport, J. (1984). Studies in empowerment: Introduction to the issue. *Prevention Human Services, 3,* 1–7.

Reichman, N. E., and Florio, M. J. (1996). The effects of enriched prenatal care services on Medicaid birth outcomes in New Jersey. *Journal of Health Economics, 15,* 455–476.

Rini, C. K., Dunkel-Schetter, C., Wadhwa, P. D., and Sandman, C. A. (1999). Psychological adaptation and birth outcomes: The role of personal resources, stress, and sociocultural context in pregnancy. *Health Psychology, 18,* 333–345.

Robert, S. A., and House, J. S. (2000). Socioeconomic inequalities in health: Integrating individual-, community-, and societal-level theory and research. In G. L. Albrecht, R. Fitzpatrick, and S. C. Scrimshaw (Eds.), *Handbook of Social Studies in Health and Medicine* (pp. 115–135). Thousand Oaks, CA: Sage.

Roberts, E. M. (1997). Neighborhood social environments and the distribution of low-birthweight in Chicago. *American Journal of Public Health, 87,* 597–603.

Rothberg, A. D., and Lits, B. (1991). Psychosocial support for maternal stress during pregnancy: Effect on birth weight. *American Journal of Obstetrics and Gynecology, 165,* 403–407.

Rowley, D. L. (1998). Beyond the medical model: Research on social factors and preterm delivery. *Prenatal and Neonatal Medicine, 3,* 170–172.

Ruderman, M., and O'Campo. P. (May 1999). Depression in women. In H. Grason, J. Hutchins, and G.Silver (Eds.), *Charting a Course for the Future of Women's and Perinatal Health,* pp. 147–166. Rockville MD: Maternal and Child Health Bureau, U.S. Department of Health and Human Services.

Rutter, D. R., and Quine, L. (1990). Inequalities in pregnancy outcome: A review of psychosocial and behavioural mediators. *Social Science and Medicine, 30,* 553–568.

Ruzek, S. B., Clarke, A. E., and Olesen, V. L. (Eds.). (1997). *Social, behavioral and feminist models of women's health.* Columbus OH: Ohio State University Press.

Sanderson, M., Emmanuel, I., and Holt, V. (1995). Intergenerational relationship between mother's birthweight, infant birthweight and infant mortality in black and white mothers. *Paediatric and Perinatal Epidemiology, 9,* 391–405.

Sardell, A. (1990). Child health policy in the U.S.: The paradox of consensus. *Journal of Health Politics, Policy and Law, 15,* 271–304.

Savitz, D. A., Olshan, A. F., and Gallagher, K. (1996). Maternal occupation and pregnancy outcome. *Epidemiology, 7,* 269–274.

Schoendorf, K. C., Hogue, C. J., Kleinman, J. C., and Rowley, D. (1992). Mortality among infants of black as compared with white college-educated parents. *New England Journal of Medicine, 326,* 1522–1526.

Scribner, R., and Dwyer, J. H. (1989). Acculturation and low-birthweight among Latinos in the Hispanic HANES. *American Journal of Public Health, 79,* 1263–1267.

Simpson, L., Korenbrot, C. C., and Greene, J. D. (1997). Enhanced prenatal services: Birth outcomes in public and private practice settings for low-income women. *Public Health Reports, 112,* 122–132.

Singh, G. K., and Yu, S. M. (1994). Pregnancy outcomes among Asian Americans. *Asian American Pacific Islander Journal of Health, 2,* 63–78.

Singh, G. K., and Yu, S. M. (1996a). Adverse pregnancy outcomes: Differences between US- and foreign-born women in major U.S. racial and ethnic groups. *American Journal of Public Health, 86,* 837–843.

Singh, G. K., and Yu, S. M. (1996b). Birthweight differentials among Asian Americans. *American Journal of Public Health, 84,* 1444–1449.

Smith, P. M., and Torrey, B. B. (1996). Future of the behavioral and social sciences. *Science, 271,* 611–612.

Spencer, B., Thomas, H., and Morris, J. (1989). A randomized controlled trial of the provision of a social support service during pregnancy: The South Manchester Family Worker Project. *British Journal of Obstetrics and Gynecology, 96,* 281–288.

Stack, C. B. (1974/1997). All our kin: Strategies for survival in a black community. New York: Basic Books.

Starfield, B., Shapiro, S., Weiss, J., Kung-Yee, L., Ra, K., Paige, D., and Wang, X. (1991). Race, family income and low birth weight. *American Journal of Epidemiology, 134,* 1167–1174.

Steer, R. A., Scholl, T. O., Hediger, M. L., and Fischer, R. L. (1992). Self-reported depression and negative pregnancy outcomes. *Journal of Clinical Epidemiology, 45,* 1093–1099.

Stockbauer, J. W. (1987). WIC prenatal participation and its relation to pregnancy outcomes in Missouri: A second look. *American Journal of Public Health, 77,* 813–818.

Syme, S. L. (1998). Social and economic disparities in health: Thoughts about intervention. *Milbank Quarterly, 76,* 493–503.

Thoits, P. A. (1983). Dimensions of life events that influence psychological distress: An evaluation and synthesis of the literature. In H. B. Kaplan (Ed.), *Psychosocial Research: Trends in Theory and Research* (pp. 1–16). New York: Academic Press.

Tracy, L. C., and Mattar, S. (1999). Depression and anxiety disorders. In E. J. Kramer, S. L. Ivey, and Y. Ying. (Eds.), *Immigrant Women's Health: Problems and Solutions* San Francisco, CA: Jossey-Bass.

U.S. Department of Health and Human Services. (1985). *Report of the Secretary's Task Force on Black and Minority Health.* Washington, DC: U.S. Government Printing Office.

U.S. Department of Health and Human Services. (1991). *Healthy People 2000: National Health Promotion and Disease Prevention Objectives.* Washington, DC: U.S. Government Printing Office.

U.S. Department of Health and Human Services. (1999). *Goal 1—Eliminate Disparities in Infant Mortality Rates.* http://www.raceandhealth.hhs.gov/ 3rdpgBlue/3pgGoalsInfant.htm.

Ventura, S. J., Martin, J. A., Curtin, S. C., and Mathews, T. J. (1999). *Births: Final data for 1997. National Vital Statistics Reports, 47* (18). Hyattsville MD: National Center for Health Statistics.

Villar, J., Farnot, U., Barros, F., Victora, C., Langer, A., and Belizan, J. M. (1992). A randomized trial of psychosocial support during high-risk pregnancies. *New England Journal of Medicine, 327,* 1266–1271.

Wadhwa, P. D., Sandman, C. A., Porto, M., Dunkel-Schetter, C., and Garite, T. J. (1993). The association between prenatal stress and infant birth weight and gestational age at birth: A prospective investigation. *American Journal of Obstetrics and Gynecology, 169,* 858–865.

168 PROMOTING HEALTH

Wadhwa, P. D., Dunkel-Schetter, C., Chicz-DeMet, A., Porto, M., and Sandman, C. A. (1996). Prenatal psychosocial factors and the neuroendocrine axis in human pregnancy. *Psychosomatic Medicine, 58*, 432–446.

Wadhwa, P. D., Sandman, C. A., Chicz-DeMet, A., and Porto, M. (1997). Placental CRH modulates maternal pituitary adrenal function in human pregnancy. *Annals of the New York Academy of Sciences, 814*, 276–281.

Weisman, C. S. (1997). Changing definitions of women's health: Implications for health care and policy. *Maternal and Child Health Journal, 1*, 179–189.

Weisman, C. S. (1998). *Women's Health Care: Activist Traditions and Institutional Change.* Baltimore: Johns Hopkins University Press.

Wergeland, E., and Strand, K. (1998). Work pace control and pregnancy health in a population-based sample of employed women in Norway. *Scandinavian Journal of Work, Environment and Health, 24*, 206–212.

Wilkinson, D. S., Korenbrot, C. C., and Fuentes-Afflick, E. (1994). Nonclient factors in the reporting of prenatal psychosocial risk assessments. *American Journal of Public Health, 84*, 1511–1514.

Wilkinson, D. S., Korenbrot, C. C., and Greene, J. D. (1998). A performance indicator of psychosocial services in enhanced prenatal care of Medicaid-eligible women. *Maternal Child Health Journal, 2*, 131–143.

Wilkinson, R. G. (1997). Health inequalities: Relative or absolute material standards. *British Medical Journal, 314*, 591–595.

Williams, D. R. (1990). Socioeconomic and racial differences in health: A review and redirection. *Social Psychology Quarterly, 53*, 81–99.

Williams, D. R. (1994). The concept of race in health services research: 1966 to 1990. *Health Services Research, 29*, 261–274.

Williams, D. R. (1996). Racism and health: a research agenda. *Ethnicity and Disease, 6*, 1–6.

Williams, D. R., and Collins, C. (1995). U.S. socioeconomic and racial differences in health: Patterns and explanations. *Annual Review of Sociology, 21*, 349–386.

Williams, R. L., Binkin, N. H., and Clingman, E. J. (1986). Pregnancy outcomes among Spanish-surname women in California. *American Journal of Public Health, 76*, 387-391.

Willinger, M., Hoffman, H. J., Wu, K., Hou, J., Kessler, R. C., Ward, S. L., Keens, T. G., and Corwin, M. J. (1998). Factors associated with the transition to non-prone sleep positions of infants in the United States: National infant sleep position study. *Journal of the American Medical Association, 280*, 329–335.

Wise, P., Chavkin, W., and Romero, D. (1999). Assessing the effects of welfare reform policies on reproductive and infant health. *American Journal of Public Health, 89*, 1514–1521.

Yen, I. and Moss, N. (1999, May 11-12). Unbundling education: A critical discussion of what education confers and how it lowers risk for disease and death. Presented at the meeting of the New York Academy of Sciences, Socioeconomic Status and Health in Industrial Nations: Social Psychological and Biological Pathways. Bethesda, MD.

Young, R. (1996). The household context for women's health care decisions: Impacts of U.K. policy changes. *Social Science and Medicine, 42*, 949–963.

Zambrana, R. E., Scrimshaw, S., Collins, N., and Dunkel-Schetter, C. (1997). Prenatal health behaviors and psychosocial risk factors in pregnant women of Mexican origin: Role of acculturation. *American Journal of Public Health, 87*, 1022–1026.

Zane, N. W. S., Takeuchi, D. T., and Young, K. N. (1994). Overview of Asian and Pacific Islander Americans. In N.W.S. Zane, D.T. Takeuchi, and K.N. Young (Eds.),

Confronting Critical Health Issues of Asian and Pacific Islander Americans (pp. 1–32). Thousand Oaks, CA: Sage.

Zapata, B. C., and Bennett, T. (1997). Women's health: A life cycle. In J. Kotch (Ed.), *Maternal and Child Health: Programs, Problems and Policy and Public Health* (pp. 253–277). Gaithersburg, MD: Aspen.

The Healthy Development of Young Children: SES Disparities, Prevention Strategies, and Policy Opportunities

Allison Sidle Fuligni, Ph.D., and Jeanne Brooks-Gunn, Ph.D.[1,2]

In 1994, the federal government passed the Goals 2000: Educate America Act, which adopted into law six national goals for improving the education system. Foremost on this list was Goal 1: *"By the year 2000, all children in America will start school ready to learn"* (National Education Goals Panel, 1998). Now that the new millennium has arrived, examination of the status of young children entering school shows that we have fallen short of meeting this goal. In this paper, we explore some reasons that the nation is not appreciably nearer to

[1]Allison Sidle Fuligni, Ph.D., is a research scientist at the Center for Children and Families, Teachers College at Columbia University. Jeanne Brooks-Gunn, Ph.D., is a Virginia and Leonard Marx Professor of Child Development and Education and director at the Center for Children and Families at Teachers College, Columbia University.

[2]We wish to thank Brian Smedley, Marie McCormick, Hortensia Amaro, and the Institute of Medicine Committee on Capitalizing on Social Science and Behavioral Research to Improve the Public's Health for their support in the writing of this paper. We are grateful for the support of the MacArthur Network on the Family and the Economy, the National Institute of Child Health and Human Development Research Network on Child and Family Well-Being, and the Administration of Children, Youth and Families and National Institute for Mental Health Research Consortium on Mental Health in Head Start. We are also grateful to Penny Hauser-Cram, Amado Padilla, and Deborah L. Coates for their insightful comments on an earlier draft of this paper. Rebecca Fauth provided valuable editorial assistance in the production of the manuscript. Correspondence regarding this paper should be addressed to Allison Sidle Fuligni, Center for Children and Families, Teachers College, Columbia University, Box 39, 525 West 120th Street, New York, NY 10027; asf27@columbia.edu.

achieving this laudatory outcome and offer research and policy strategies that may help move the nation in this direction.

The Goal 1 Technical Planning Group (1993, p. 1) also highlighted three objectives for families and communities necessary to support school readiness:

Objective 1. All children will have access to high quality and developmentally appropriate preschool programs that help prepare children for school;

Objective 2. Every parent in America will be a child's first teacher and devote time each day helping his or her preschool child learn; parents will have access to the training and support they need; and

Objective 3. Children will receive the nutrition and health care needed to arrive at school with healthy minds and bodies, and the number of low-birthweight babies will be significantly reduced through enhanced prenatal health systems.

Clearly, the interplay of all of these objectives is necessary to ensure that young children are in the optimal state of physical, emotional, and intellectual well-being when they enter school.

DEFINING HEALTHY DEVELOPMENT FOR YOUNG CHILDREN

The dimensions of school readiness outlined by the Goal 1 Technical Planning Group (1993) include aspects of physical health, as well as social, emotional, and cognitive development. These five dimensions are listed below (from Love et al., 1994, pp. 4–5):

Physical well-being and motor development
• *Physical development* (rate of growth and physical fitness)
• *Physical abilities* (gross motor skills, fine motor skills, oral motor skills, and functional performance)
• *Background and contextual conditions of [physical] development* (vulnerabilities, such as prenatal alcohol exposure; environmental risks, such as harmful aspects of the community environment; health care utilization; and adverse conditions, such as disease and disability)

Social and emotional development
• *Emotional development* (feeling states regarding self and others, including self-concept; emotions, such as joy, fear, anger, grief, disgust, delight, horror, shame, pride, and guilt; and the ability to express feelings appropriately, including empathy and sensitivity to the feelings of others)
• *Social development* (ability to form and sustain social relationships with adults and friends, and social skills necessary to cooperate with peers; ability to

form and sustain reciprocal relationships; understanding the rights of others; ability to treat others equitably and to avoid being overly submissive or directive; ability to distinguish between incidental and intentional actions; willingness to give and receive support; ability to balance one's own needs against those of others; creating opportunities for affection and companionship; ability to solicit and listen to others' points of view; being emotionally secure with parents and teachers; being open to approaching others with expectations of positive and prosocial interactions, or trust)

Approaches toward learning
• *Predisposition* (gender, temperament, and cultural patterns and values)
• *Learning styles* (openness to and curiosity about new tasks and challenges, task persistence and attentiveness, tendency toward reflection and interpretation, and imagination and invention)

Language usage
• *Verbal language* (listening, speaking, social uses of language, vocabulary and meaning, questioning, and creative uses of language)
• *Emerging literacy* (literature awareness, print awareness, story sense, and writing process)

Cognition and general knowledge
• *Knowledge* (physical knowledge, logicomathematical knowledge, and social-conventional knowledge)
• *Cognitive competencies* (representational thought, problem solving, mathematical knowledge, and social knowledge).

Domains of child well-being could be conceived somewhat differently. For instance, health is sometimes divided into four broad categories: (1) physical health, (2) emotional well-being and behavioral competence, (3) cognitive and linguistic development, and (4) social competencies (McCormick and Brooks-Gunn, 1989). Starfield (1992a) describes a "profile of health" encompassing five domains: (1) physical activity and physical fitness, (2) physical and emotional symptoms, (3) self-perceptions of health and satisfaction with health, (4) achievement of developmental and social relationship milestones, and (5) "resilience" (presence of characteristics influencing future good health). Brooks-Gunn and Duncan (1997) list four domains of well-being that are applicable to young children: (1) physical health (including birthweight, growth, and conditions such as blood-lead levels); (2) cognitive ability (measured by intelligence, verbal ability, and achievement test scores); (3) school achievement; and (4) emotional and behavioral outcomes. Each of these conceptualizations emphasizes the importance of considering multiple domains of functioning when assessing health and well-being. It is noteworthy that scholars and policy makers from a variety of disciplines have converged on broadening their definitions of child well-being: educators have recently added physical and emotional health; health scholars now include emotional health, communication, and relationships; economists also focus on these factors in addition to human capital indicators; and psychologists include more than cognitive, social, and emotional aspects of development. However, these broad constructs are subsumed under a variety of rubrics—health, development, healthy development, well-being, and of most significance here, school readiness.

In using such domains to define school readiness for young children, we wish to emphasize several points. First, broad conceptualizations include domains that are usually considered under the rubric of health, defined by the World Health Organization (WHO, 1978) as: "a state of complete physical, mental, and social well-being and not merely the absence of disease or infirmity." In addition to physical health, other competencies are required under this definition. Second, under such definitions, competencies as well as liabilities or dysfunction are emphasized. Hence, healthy development can be considered to include more than simply the absence of disease. Third, competencies with social cognitive components are included, such as engagement, motivation, and curiosity. On the other hand, we must not limit ourselves to observing only competencies, because many conditions—such as asthma, limitations on daily activities, or low literacy—have important effects on children's abilities to engage in family, school, and peer activities. Thus, there is clearly a need for a balanced view of health and development that encompasses the absence of conditions that limit children's lives as well as the presence of factors and features that enhance their lives.

Fourth, many definitions of health do not consider the comorbidity or co-occurrence of various conditions or features. We know that limitations often co-occur. For instance, a child with poor self-regulation will often also exhibit aggressive behavior; low levels of literacy often co-occur with attentional difficulties; and a fussy or irritable temperament may be associated with less responsive relationships between the child and the mother. Physical health problems also tend to co-occur: during a span of several years, children who experience one type of medical condition are significantly more likely to also experience other types of illnesses or psychosocial conditions (Starfield, 1992a). In addition, physical conditions have associations with emotional and behavioral outcomes and abilities. For instance, high blood-lead levels are associated with hyperactivity, impulsivity, being easily frustrated, and having difficulty following directions (Loeber, 1990). Children who are in poor health are more likely to experience limitations in their abilities to engage in age-appropriate activities, which may have consequences for their development of peer relationships (Starfield, 1992a; Klebanov et al., 1994).

Although a detailed examination of comorbidity of health and developmental conditions is beyond the scope of this chapter, we wish to underscore the importance of considering patterns of limitations and abilities within individual children. In addition to the burdens of co-occurrence of multiple limiting factors for some children, patterns in which children experience limitations in combination with positive competencies will result in quite different outcomes. For example, a child with a chronic health condition such as asthma, but with very high literacy and language abilities, will be in a very different position in terms of establishing relationships with peers and succeeding in school than a child with similar health conditions but poor communication skills or poor emotional self-regulation.

Based on these considerations, we believe that in order for children to be considered ready to learn they must be healthy in all of the domains discussed above. They should be free from physically limiting conditions and be on a normal trajectory of development in physical, social, emotional, and cognitive domains. (It is important to note, however, that there remains a longstanding debate regarding what constitutes "normal development" and what the relevant cutoff points would be).

With this vision of the health and development of the whole child in place, we return to assessment of the nation's progress on the first education goal—that of school readiness. Although definite strides have been made toward improving the health and well-being of young children, the basic objectives of Goal 1 have not been met for all children, leaving many unprepared physically, mentally, and/or socially for learning in school. The National Education Goals Panel has measured progress on Goal 1, in part by assessing indicators including health risks at birth, full immunization rates at various ages, regularity of reading to children by parents, and preschool participation. (1) From 1994 to 1996, the rate of infants being born with one or more health risks decreased, but only to 34%. (2) Rates of full immunization of 2-year-olds increased from 1994 to 1997, but only to 78%. (3) Rates of regular parental reading to preschoolers increased from 1993 to 1996, but only to 72%. (4) Rates of preschool participation increased, but no change in the disparity of preschool participation rates between children from high- and low-income families occurred from 1991 to 1996 (National Education Goals Panel, 1998).

In an innovative exploration of teacher and parent perceptions of school readiness, Lewit and Baker (1995) compared the responses from three different studies of kindergarten teachers and families to estimate rates of school readiness. In the first, teachers rated the most important characteristics of school readiness; these were physical health, communication skills, enthusiasm, taking turns, and the ability to sit and pay attention. In a second study, a sample of 7,000 kindergarten teachers estimated that only 65% of their students in the fall of 1990 were ready for school. The third study used the most important characteristics of school readiness identified by teachers above and found that in a sample of 2,126 parents of kindergartners, only 63% reported that their children had been rated highly by their teacher in all five of the characteristics listed above. Although the estimation techniques used here are not the most straightforward, they suggest that as many as one-third of kindergartners may not be considered by their teachers to be ready for school. It is also interesting to note that teachers often emphasize the importance of the physical health of children as well as the children's social-emotional skills (including sitting still and taking turns). Contrary to expectations, teachers are less concerned about traditional academics as evidenced by their lack of concentration on the cognitive abilities of children. Rather, teachers focus on the children's communication skills, which include verbal, cognitive, and social-emotional aspects.

In a recent study using a nationally representative sample of 3,595 kindergarten teachers, rates of readiness are reported somewhat differently (Rimm-Kaufman et al., in press). Teachers reported that 16% of children experienced serious difficulties upon entering kindergarten, and more than one-third of teachers reported that specific problems were experienced by about half the class or more. This study highlighted the specific arenas in which children are perceived as having difficulty upon school entry. For instance, 46% of teachers reported that a majority of their class had difficulty following directions, 34% had a majority with difficulty working independently, 20% said a majority of the class had problems with social skills, and 14% reported that half or more of the class had communication or language problems.

In the remainder of this chapter, we explore the health and development of young children in the context of optimizing healthy development and school readiness. We first discuss socioeconomic disparities in health and development. Next, we describe possible mechanisms or pathways through which socioeconomic status may operate to affect child health and development. Third, we present links between this conceptual work on processes and existing strategies for prevention of poor developmental outcomes in young children. We conclude with discussion of future directions for policy-oriented research and intervention.

SOCIOECONOMIC DISPARITIES IN HEALTH AND DEVELOPMENTAL OUTCOMES

Socioeconomic status (SES) accounts for large differences in physical and emotional health outcomes for adult populations. These differences appear across the income distribution and cannot be explained by the differential access to health care (Marmot et al., 1984, 1991; Marmot and Shipley, 1996), or educational attainment (Adler et al., 1994) of different SES groups (Brooks-Gunn et al., 1999). Among children, SES is also a strong predictor of health and development (e.g., Brooks-Gunn and Duncan, 1997; Duncan and Brooks-Gunn, 1997). In this section, we present SES disparities in young children's outcomes, including cognitive and language development, emotional health, and physical health, and discuss the relative importance of separate factors of SES (e.g., parental education and family income) for each.

Questions to Be Addressed

Several questions are addressed in terms of SES disparities in the health and development of young children. First, we must ask whether young children are more or less ready for school as a function of SES. If the answer is yes, then the problem of SES disparities goes beyond a simple equity issue because it affects children's ability to do well in school academically, emotionally, and socially.

Second, if we do find associations between SES and school readiness, we want to know which aspects of SES are responsible for the associations, in order to make policy decisions for raising the competencies of low-SES children. For instance, different programs might be designed depending on whether parental education or family income is more important for child outcomes. If maternal education seems to be more highly related, we might want to emphasize programs that increase mothers' human capital, such as GED completion programs, dropout prevention, or literacy programs. On the other hand, if family income is more predictive, then economic policies may be more beneficial, such as increasing the Earned Income Tax Credit, the minimum wage, or housing subsidies. If both aspects of SES are important, then programs should combine these approaches, and of course, if neither is particularly relevant, we should be looking elsewhere for ways to reduce SES disparities in child outcomes.

Strategies may focus on the parent, the family, or the child, or some combination. For instance, to affect some outcomes, we might want to alter parental behavior toward the child by teaching parenting skills and reducing the emotional distress of the parent, or we might want to enhance the human capital or wages of the parents themselves through training and education programs. For other outcomes, family living conditions may be the target, through reducing environmental toxins in the household or neighborhood. Or services may be targeted directly to the child, as in high-quality child care programs. All of these approaches require the support and involvement of the parent, through either direct participation or enabling the child to participate by bringing the child to the intervention program site.

Third, if we do find SES differences, what are the outcomes that are most affected? Again, this bears on the types of remedies that should be proposed. If language and literacy are strongly related to SES, then prevention might focus on literacy programs in the home and/or academically oriented child care. If emotional problems are more prevalent among low-SES children, intervention might focus on impulse control and self-regulation through parenting skills training, a child care program, or reduction of lead exposure in the living quarters. If health problems such as asthma are disproportionally present in lower-SES groups, yet another set of programs should be designed to reduce the disparities, such as improving parent knowledge for identifying and treating health problems; removing roaches, dust, and other allergens from the living environment; and/or improving access to medical treatment.

Fourth, we must address the issue of which children and families should be served by such interventions. If intervention programs are not universal, the feasibility of targeting services should be considered in order to provide appropriate services to the families that are most likely to benefit. For instance, programs that are most highly associated with gains in literacy skills for mothers with low literacy skills might use maternal education to define eligibility, whereas a program that has been shown to have the strongest consequences for low-birthweight rather than normal-birthweight infants would be targeted to that population.

Fifth, are there any implications of early SES disparities for later health and development, even after the entrance to school? Some work suggests that this is the case. In a sample of more than 11,000 British adults, inequalities in health status at age 33 were linked to several causes early in life, including SES at birth for the whole sample and poor housing during childhood for the women (Power et al., 1998). Such findings indicate the importance of reducing differences in material resources early in life for reducing lifelong health disadvantages.

Research on Education and Income as Indicators of SES

Let us begin this discussion by reviewing what is known from the research about SES and child development. There are three main lines of research addressing this topic. First, effects of parental education have been examined by developmentalists from a human capital standpoint. Second, a focus on family income considers the importance of material resources to health and development (Wachs and Gruen, 1982; Hoff-Ginsberg and Tardiff, 1995). Both of these categories arc often subsumed under the broad domain of SES (with the addition of parent's occupational status, which has not received much attention in the literature on young children). Within the category of family income, the literature has addressed issues of depth of poverty, persistence of poverty, and timing of poverty since all provide a richer exploration of the effect of money (or lack of it) on child development.

The third topic is neighborhood income. Neighborhood characteristics are receiving increased attention in the literature on young children (Brooks-Gunn et al., 1997a,b; Leventhal and Brooks-Gunn, 2000). We focus here on neighborhood income, recognizing, however, that other structural features of neighborhoods might be important. In much of the research, it is nearly impossible to separate the association between neighborhood income and other features, such as the percentage of unemployed adult males, percentage of single mothers, percentage of families receiving welfare, or percentage of adults with a college education. All of these features overlap with income, resulting in multicolinearity when all variables are included together in a regression (Brooks-Gunn et al., 1997b; Sampson et al., 1997).

Associations Between SES and Child Outcomes

In the following sections, we briefly review research showing the relationships between these three components of SES on three domains of child outcomes: (1) cognitive, language, and early schooling; (2) emotional and behavioral development; and (3) physical health. In the findings reported below, other important factors are statistically controlled, including family structure, ethnicity, and maternal age. When reporting effects of family income, maternal education is controlled, and vice versa, so that wherever possible we are reporting the independent effects of the SES indicator in question.

Cognitive, Linguistic, and Early Schooling Outcomes

The number of years of schooling of the mother has been shown to have a consistently significant effect on child outcomes. In two large samples (the Children of the National Longitudinal Survey of Youth [NLSY] and the Infant Health and Development Program [IHDP]), effects of mother's education on child language, achievement, and IQ scores ranged from .10 to .29, for children from 2 to 8 years of age. Even after controlling for family income, effects ranged from .07 to .18 (Duncan et al., 1994; Smith et al., 1997).

Although many studies of SES effects on early cognitive abilities have not examined family income separately from other SES indicators, recent analyses have shown that income does affect cognitive outcomes at a young age. In the National Longitudinal Study of Youth-Child Supplement (NLSY-CS) and the IHDP, effects were found on several different cognitive indicators, using several different measures of income (Smith et al., 1997). Total family income was positively associated with verbal scores and achievement test scores as well as intelligence test scores for children ranging in age from 3 to 8 years (Duncan et al., 1994; Smith et al., 1997; Klebanov et al., 1998). Effect sizes for family income ranged from .20 to .32, even after controlling for mothers' education. For families that experienced persistent poverty (below the poverty level at four different time points), children's cognitive scores averaged 6 to 9 points lower than those of children who had never lived in poverty. Living in poverty for only some but not all of the early years was associated with smaller differences compared to children who had never lived in poverty (Smith et al., 1997).

The effects of family income are nonlinear. Children whose family incomes were below 50% of the poverty level had scores 7 to 12 points lower than children who were near-poor (just over the poverty level); whereas those who were slightly less poor (50–100% of the poverty level) had scores ranging from 4 to 7 points lower than the near-poor group (Smith et al., 1997). Although the timing of poverty did not show a significant relationship with early measures of IQ, verbal ability, or achievement scores in the NLSY or IHDP data (Duncan et al., 1994; Smith et al., 1997), analysis from the Panel Study of Income Dynamics

(PSID) showed that family income in the early childhood years is more strongly related to the ultimate years of schooling the child completes than is family income at any other period in the child's life (Duncan et al., 1998).

Links between neighborhood income, defined in terms of structural characteristics of neighborhoods at the census-tract level, and child cognitive outcomes have been documented starting at age 3 and continuing through age 6. Residing in an affluent neighborhood (defined as the proportion of residents with incomes over $30,000) was positively associated with intelligence test scores at age 3 for children in the IHDP (Brooks-Gunn et al., 1993; Chase-Lansdale et al., 1997). Similarly, at ages 5 and 6, residing in a high-SES neighborhood was associated with higher IQ, verbal ability, and reading achievement scores, after controlling for family and individual characteristics (Chase-Lansdale and Gordon, 1996; Chase-Lansdale et al., 1997 Duncan et al., 1994). It is the presence of high-income neighbors relative to middle income ($10,000 to $30,000 per year) that makes a difference in these cognitive and achievement outcomes, not the presence or absence of low-income neighbors. We will return to possible reasons for such findings in the next section.

Emotional Health Outcomes

Studies of the prevalence of emotional health or behavior problems tend to find that overall, approximately one-quarter of all preschoolers have reported behavior problems (e.g., Richman et al., 1975); however, higher rates are often associated with low SES. Again using data from IHDP and NLSY, effects of maternal education on emotional health are found. In both samples, maternal education is related to fewer internalizing problems, and maternal education is associated with fewer externalizing problems in the IHDP sample only (Brooks-Gunn et al., 1997; Chase-Lansdale et al., 1997).

Links between family poverty and child behavioral problems have also been noted in the research. Among children ages 3 to 17 years in the 1988 National Health Interview Survey Child Health Supplement, parents of poor children were more likely to report that they had had an emotional or behavioral problem lasting 3 months or more (Brooks-Gunn and Duncan, 1997). Higher family income-to-needs ratio is associated with lower levels of externalizing problems in the IHDP and NLSY samples at ages 3 through 6 (Brooks-Gunn et al., 1993; Chase-Lansdale et al., 1997).

Findings are less strong for neighborhood income effects on emotional and behavioral outcomes in young children. However, there are links between externalizing behaviors and the presence of low-income neighbors as opposed to middle-income neighbors (Duncan et al., 1994; Chase-Lansdale et al., 1997).

Physical Health Outcomes

Patterns of physical health problems and conditions reveal higher rates of illness among poor children (Starfield, 1992a; Brooks-Gunn and Duncan, 1997). For instance, parents of poor children are nearly twice as likely as those of nonpoor children to report that their children are in fair to poor health; blood-lead levels are three times more likely to be dangerously high among poor children; childhood immunization is three times more likely to be delayed for poor children, and the percentage of children with conditions limiting school activity is two to three times higher among poor children (Starfield, 1992a; Brooks-Gunn and Duncan, 1997). Growth stunting and short-stay hospital episodes are also twice as common among poor children (Brooks-Gunn and Duncan, 1997), and duration of poverty is strongly related to growth stunting (Korenman and Miller, 1997).

It is difficult to estimate the effect of neighborhood income on health outcomes for young children. We do know that in addition to the direct effects of poverty on nutrition and access to preventive health care, the higher rates of health problems among poor children are partially due to hazardous and unsafe living conditions of poor housing and dangerous neighborhoods (Starfield, 1992b). However, since most studies do not control for family-level indicators of poverty or human capital, it is impossible to distinguish between neighborhood and family-level indicators of physical health. This research tends to look at the prevalence of child health indicators by health district using aggregate data only, without individual-level data. Some research on disparities in low-birthweight births has combined neighborhood-level and individual-level data, and concluded that residence in low-income neighborhood has an independent association with lower rates of prenatal health care and higher incidence of low-birthweight births (Gould and LeRoy, 1988; Collins and David, 1990; O'Campo et al., 1997).

Summary

We find that maternal education, family income, and neighborhood income each have independent effects on child cognitive, emotional, and physical outcomes. Maternal education tends to be strongly associated with all types of cognitive assessments (cognitive, verbal, and school achievement measures), but more strongly associated with internalizing than externalizing behavior problems. Family income also affects cognitive assessments and is more predictive of externalizing problems. When other aspects of family poverty are assessed, such as persistence and extreme poverty, stronger effects are seen. Finally, a few links between neighborhood poverty and early childhood outcomes have been documented, net of family-level influences. In particular, the presence of affluent neighbors has been associated with cognitive and school achievement outcomes, whereas the presence of low-income neighbors leads to more external-izing behavior problems. Generally, family income produces the strongest ef-fects (twice as large as maternal education for IQ outcomes), and maternal edu-cation effects are somewhat smaller. During these early years, neighborhood income produces only small effects, although the importance of neighborhood characteristics may increase as children grow older and have more direct contact with environments outside the family (Chase-Lansdale et al., 1997).

Although these SES indicators account for a substantial portion of the vari-ance in child outcomes, other factors are important as well. Low levels of family income and maternal education each represent risk factors for children. Research has suggested that an accumulation of multiple risk factors in areas of family structure (e.g., parental unemployment, father's absence, teen parenthood), hu-man capital (e.g., maternal education, maternal verbal ability), and mental health (e.g., maternal depression, stressful life events) is associated with lower IQ scores as early as age 2 to 4 years (Sameroff et al., 1987; Law and Brooks-Gunn, 1994; Klebanov et al., 1998) and more behavior problems by age 3 (Liaw and Brooks-Gunn, 1994). Poverty and cumulative risk interact, so that although poor children tend to experience more risks, nonpoor children in the highest-risk groups, as early as 2 to 4 years of age, have IQ scores resembling those of high-risk poor children (Liaw and Brooks-Gunn, 1994).

Child characteristics have also been left out of this discussion so far. Birth-weight and neonatal status can have lasting effects on cognitive and emotional development in addition to contributing to ongoing physical health conditions. However, debate continues as to whether these child health characteristics influ-ence children similarly across all SES levels or whether the effects are stronger for lower-SES children, a phenomenon that has been termed "double jeopardy" (Werner and Smith, 1982; Parker et al., 1988; McCormick et al., 1992). Al-though some evidence indicates that child gender and SES interact, the bulk of the research to date suggests few interactions between gender and SES for young children; for instance, the presence of high-income neighbors was related to age 5 IQ scores for boys only in the NLSY data (Brooks-Gunn, 1995). Gener-ally, SES effects are quite similar for boys and girls.

SES effects also tend to be similar for blacks and whites, although SES may be more highly associated with some child outcomes for whites than blacks. For instance, poverty is associated with the likelihood of having a low-birthweight baby, after controlling for mother's age, education, marital status, and smoking status, but only for white and not for black mothers (Brooks-Gunn and Duncan, 1997). In the NLSY, long-term poverty was associated with growth stunting for whites, but not for blacks (Korenman and Miller, 1997). One reason that SES may be more highly associated with child outcomes for whites is that the SES distribution is truncated for blacks (and other children of color). We are also likely to see the intergenerational effects of SES upon blacks, probably because blacks who are in the middle class are more likely to have had parents who were poor or who had less education than whites in similar current economic conditions (Brooks-Gunn et al., 1996; Phillips et al., 1998). Such intergenerational links may also be seen for low-birthweight disparities between black and white children (see Paper Contribution C). Further explanation of SES disparities for blacks and whites may come from patterns of racial and ethnic segregation among poor urban blacks and Hispanics (Massey and Eggers, 1990). The segregation of poor black and Hispanic families into concentrated areas leads to effects on employment opportunities, access to health care, and the quality of schools. For example, in the NLSY, the black-white test score gap is reduced by controlling not only for maternal education, but also for the quality of the school the mother had attended. In other words, over and above the number of years of schooling mothers completed and the mother's cognitive ability scores, black mothers had attended poorer-quality schools and this affected child IQ scores for black children (Phillips et al., 1998).

In the next section, we move beyond the findings of SES disparities in health and developmental outcomes for young children to consider pathways by which SES may be having these effects. It is important to note that selection bias plagues all of the research cited in this section. It is possible, for example, that unmeasured family characteristics are really accounting for the links between child outcome and parental education or family income. Several attempts have been made to overcome this pervasive bias. First, regressions have been conducted that include family demographic variables believed to be linked to poverty or education, resulting in decreases of effect sizes for education, family income, and neighborhood income. Second, researchers have put in, when available, measures of mothers' verbal or cognitive abilities due to the possibility that mothers with greater cognitive skills may have a higher education or income than those with lower cognitive skills. Without this precaution, these ability effects could be wrongly attributed as SES effects. (Analyses using NLSY and IDHP data do control for cognitive or receptive language ability.) Finally, other possible controls include, for example, sibling analyses wherein sibling outcomes are compared with income at various points during childhood. Using this technique to control for many possible unmeasured characteristics, Duncan and his colleagues (1998) still found income effects.

PROCESSES OPERATING IN SES LINKS TO CHILD HEALTH

Why does SES affect child health and development in the ways described above? How can we explain the processes by which SES factors such as family income, maternal education, and neighborhood income affect children's cognitive, linguistic, social, emotional, and physical well-being? In this section, we consider three levels of influences: the family, child care settings, and the neighborhood. Having a theoretical understanding of these processes is crucial for the development of intervention programs aimed to decrease SES disparities in child well-being.[3] The importance of having a well-developed "theory of change" when developing programs is discussed in more detail in the final section of this paper.

Family Processes

The role of family processes in SES disparities in young children's health and development has been studied much more extensively than the roles of child care settings or neighborhood processes. Much of the focus of this work has been on four family processes: (1) parent's emotional and physical health, (2) the provision of stimulating experiences in the home, (3) parental sensitivity, and (4) parental harshness.

General models have hypothesized that low-SES (as well as the specific experience of job loss) is associated with family financial strain, which in turn influences parental mental health and parenting behavior (Elder, 1974; McLoyd, 1990, 1998; Conger et al., 1997). The proposed pathways differ somewhat from scholar to scholar: some believe that parenting behavior may be directly influenced by financial strain, while others believe that such effects are usually mediated through parental mental health. Social support is often thought to be a moderator of the link between financial strain and parental mental health (McLoyd, 1998; Jackson et al., in press). This general model is presented in Figure 1.

Most of this research has focused on effects on adolescents; however, several research groups are examining young children's achievement and cognitive outcomes (Jackson et al., in press; Klebanov et al., 1998). About one-third to one-half of the effects of SES on achievement and cognition seem to operate through maternal mental health and parenting behavior. For example, a study of low-wage-earning single mothers in New York City found some support for the model in Figure 1. Specifically, maternal education and earnings were directly related to financial strain, which in turn affected maternal depressive symptoms. Depressive affect was associated with single African-American mothers' provision of intellectual stimulation, emotional support, and warmth to their 3- to 5-year-old children. Completing the link, preschoolers' scores on a school readiness measure directly related to these parenting practices; however, the indirect pathway from financial strain to depression to parenting did not significantly predict school readiness (Jackson et al., in press). Linver and colleagues (1999) found that for low-birthweight children from the eight-site Infant Health and Development Program, with heterogeneous SES and ethnic ba-

---

[3]For this discussion, we focus primarily on cognitive, social, and emotional well-being, drawing parallels, when appropriate, to physical health outcomes for children. A discussion of the wide range of physical outcomes is beyond the scope of this paper.

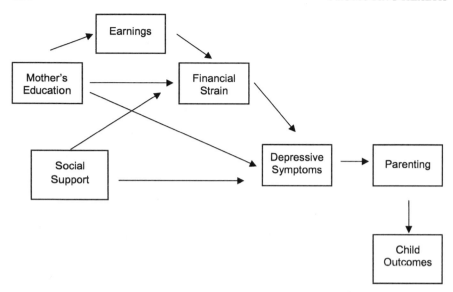

FIGURE 1 Proposed model for SES effects on parental mental health, parenting, and child outcomes.

ckgrounds, a significant indirect relationship between family income and IQ scores at 3 and 5 years was mediated by the home learning environment and authoritative parenting. This model accounted for 84% of the variance in child IQ. Both of these studies focus on maternal emotional distress, given the high proportion of single mothers in IHDP in general and the exclusive focus on mothers in the New York City study. These results parallel those for fathers reported by Elder (1974) in his work on the children of the Great Depression, that paternal emotional distress and parenting mediated the link between job loss and child outcomes (see also Conger et al., 1992, for a similar model for children from rural farm families).

Similar results are found for linking these pathways with children's emotional problems. Jackson et al. (in press) found significant indirect effects of financial strain on preschoolers' behavior problems, mediated by maternal depressive symptoms and parenting behaviors. Likewise, Linver and colleagues (1999) report a significant link between family income and home learning environment, which is associated with fewer child behavior problems (accounting for about one-third of the variance in child behavior problems). However, these researchers did not find evidence for maternal emotional distress as a mediator of the link between family income and either IQ or problem behaviors.

Similar pathways could be operating for parent's physical health, with low SES being associated with parental health problems and these health problems affecting parents' ability to provide warm, consistent, or stimulating environments for their children. Comparable work examining parenting variables as pathways for SES effects has not been conducted for young children's physical health and well-being. However, physical health problems might be as prevalent as emotional distress in low-SES mothers.

Neighborhood Processes

Researchers from many varying fields have attempted to define the potential mechanisms by which characteristics of neighborhoods may affect children. These neighborhood mechanisms fall into the categories of resources (e.g., availability and accessibility of quality schools, child care, recreational activities, services, and opportunities); relationships (e.g., parental characteristics, support networks available to parents, and the quality and structure of the home environment); and norms or collective efficacy (existence of formal and informal institutions to monitor residents' behavior and the presence of physical risk to residents) (Leventhal and Brooks-Gunn, 2000). We have hypothesized that the effects of neighborhood-level SES disparities on outcomes for children may be both direct and indirect. For very young children, most effects are likely to be indirect, as parents control the child's access to neighborhood resources, relationships, and collective norms (Klebanov et al., 1994; Leventhal and Brooks-Gunn, 2000; in press).

Indeed, living in a poor neighborhood has been linked to less cognitively stimulating home environments for 3- to 4-year-olds in the IHDP and the NLSY, and less maternal warmth in the IHDP (Klebanov et al., 1994, 1997), setting the stage for indirect effects on children through these parenting variables. Neighborhood effects on social support are curvilinear: lower levels of social support are found among those living in low-income as well as affluent neighborhoods, relative to middle-income neighborhoods (Klebanov et al., 1997). These studies have also linked parenting characteristics (cognitively stimulating environment and maternal warmth) to preschoolers' cognitive outcomes. Although the complete model, showing neighborhood effects on cognitive outcomes being mediated by home learning environments, was not statistically significant for preschoolers, it was for young school-aged children. In both the IHDP and the NLSY, living in a neighborhood with affluent neighbors was associated with higher verbal and ability scores as well as lower behavior problem scores, and these effects were mediated by the cognitive stimulation parents provided in the home (Klebanov et al., 1997, 1998).

Again, we need to specify the processes through which neighborhood income operates to affect children's outcomes, even when the effect is indirect, through parenting and home environments. Neighborhood income is similar to family income in that it is a structural feature. The question here is how neighborhood residence might influence parental provision of stimulating experiences, sensitivity, and warmth. Three general processes that may be operating are presented above: institutional resources, relationships, and norms or collective efficacy. Institutional resources include the availability of learning, social and recreational activities, child care, schools, and health care services. These resources may be of most interest regarding children's achievement outcomes since the availability of libraries, museums, and learning programs in the community may affect parent's provision of such experiences outside the home and, in turn, children's school readiness and achievement. Social and recreational activities may affect children's physical and social development, and the availability of quality child health care may affect parent's usage of health care services for their children and, in turn, children's physical health.

In terms of relationships, there are several possible ways for parental relationships to be involved in the links between neighborhood characteristics and child outcomes. One extends the theory underlying Figure 1: perhaps neighborhood poverty affects parental mental health, which influences parenting behaviors and, ultimately, child outcomes. Furthermore, access to neighborhood sources of social support may help alleviate the stress of living in poor or dangerous neighborhoods, and this may reduce the negative effects of parent stress on child outcomes (McLoyd, 1990; Conger et al., 1994). Parental warmth, sensitivity, harshness, supervision, and monitoring are all dimensions of parenting that could both be affected by neighborhood characteristics and affect child outcomes. There is evidence that living in poor neighborhoods is associated with harsher parenting, though a link between this association and outcomes for adolescents shows an interaction effect, such that in particularly high-risk neighborhoods, having a highly controlling parent is actually positive for adolescent academic, behavioral, and social outcomes (Gonzales et al., 1996; Lamborn et al., 1996).

The structural features of neighborhoods, such as income, residential stability, family stability, and ethnic heterogeneity, determine the extent to which formal and informal institutions are in place to monitor and socialize the behaviors of the residents. The dimension of norms and collective efficacy has mostly been examined in the context of direct effects on problem behavior of adolescents (e.g., Sampson, 1997; Sampson et al., 1997). However, one line of work suggests that young children (ages 2 to 5 years) experience most exposure to aggressive peers in neighborhood settings and play aggressively in unstructured, unsupervised settings. Furthermore, low-SES children are most likely to be involved in these types of settings that expose them to aggressive peers, possibly putting them at risk for behavior problems (Sinclair et al., 1994). Kupersmidt and her colleagues (Kupersmidt et al., 1995) have found that living in a middle-SES neighborhood can protect poor black children of single parents from developing aggressive behavior, perhaps because of the higher prevalence of successful adult or peer role models outside the family. For all three of these proposed mechanisms between neighborhood income and child outcomes, the links for young children are mostly speculative at this point.

Child Care Settings

A third setting that may mediate between SES and child outcomes is non-parental child care. Child care for infants and young children is extremely expensive, so very low income families spend a much higher proportion of their income on child care (25–33%) than affluent families (6% of their income) (Phillips and Bridgman, 1995). Family income is associated with the quality of nonparental care that young children receive. When children receive care from relatives or in home-based arrangements, lower family income is associated with lower quality of these settings (Galinsky et al., 1994; National Institute of Child Health and Human Development [NICHD] Early Child Care Research Network, 1997). For children in center-based care, the associations are somewhat different: the quality of center-based care is higher for the lowest-income families (with income-to-needs ratios of less than 1.0, indicating that families are below the poverty line), who receive subsidies for purchasing child care and who may qualify for high-quality intervention programs, such as Head Start, than for less poor families (families with incomes above the poverty line). In fact, a curvilinear association is found—middle-income families receive lower-quality center-based care than high- or low-income families (Phillips et al., 1994; NICHD Early Child Care Research Network, 1997).

The curvilinear findings relating child care quality and family income illustrate two different processes that may be operating in families' use of out-of-home child care. First, highly educated and employed families purchase high-quality child care in order to continue their high rates of employment. The high usage of child care among this group is exemplified by the fact that children from high-income families are more likely to enter care as early as ages 3–5 months and those whose mothers' income is high (as a proportion of total family income) are most likely to enter care even before 3 months; whereas children from families who are continuously poor or continuously receiving assistance are more likely to enter care later or not at all (NICHD Early Child Care Research Network, 1997). On the other hand, families who are in the lowest-income groups may qualify for high-quality government-subsidized child care as they continue schooling, job training, or working in low-wage jobs.

An important aspect of quality in center-based child care is the number and stability of caregivers, which requires generating enough income to pay and retain a larger staff. Thus, centers that generate more income, either through charging high rates to parents or through government subsidies (e.g., Head Start or universal pre-kindergarten programs) are more likely to provide optimal levels of staffing. The government-funded Head Start programs have indeed been found to be of relatively high quality in comparison with many other center-based programs, including school-based, nonprofit, for-profit, and preschool centers (Zill et al., 1998).

These findings suggest that it is the families in the middle whose children may experience the poorest center-based care, while children from poor families experience poor-quality home-based child care. Researchers are only now beginning to explore child care quality at a neighborhood level. We look forward to future data that will see whether neighborhood residence is associated with quality of child care available to families.

We do have extensive evidence of the impact of child care quality on child outcomes (e.g., Whitebook et al., 1990; Cost, Quality, and Child Outcomes Study Team, 1995, 1999). For instance, children who experienced poor-quality early child care settings exhibit lower math and language scores, worse peer relations, and more behavior problems in second grade (Cost, Quality and Child Outcomes Study Team, 1999). Within Head Start classrooms, classroom quality is associated with early literacy and math skills (Zill et al., 1998). These two strands of research taken together, one demonstrating links between low family income and the quality of child care settings, and the other linking the quality of early child care to young children's cognitive, social, and emotional outcomes, illustrate the potential usefulness of considering the child care setting as another mechanism by which SES operates to affect young children.

It is important to note that the majority of the child care quality literature does not control for possible selection bias—the unmeasured family characteristics, such as parental education and family income, that may be accounting for the links between child care and children's developmental outcomes. Such controls are needed to ensure that higher-income families and/or better-educated mothers are not selecting higher-quality settings. It is unclear, otherwise, whether it is the quality of the child care setting or the characteristics of the home environment independent of the quality of child care accounting for the links. In many analyses of the NICHD child care study, the relatively large effects of maternal education and income level are controlled. Additionally, when examining children younger than 3 years of age, the influences of home environment and maternal parenting are stronger than the quality of child care. While the effects of quality of the child care setting are still present, they are not as prominent when compared with models lacking such controls. Another complication arises due to the curvilinear association between income and quality of child care, due to some low-income families receiving child care subsidies for the use of Head Start facilities that are higher in quality than other child care centers (Zill et al., 1998). The quality of Head Start programs varies, although none of these programs are of the poorest quality, which unfortunately is found in other for-profit, locally run child care centers.

LINKS BETWEEN THE CONCEPTUAL WORK AND
PREVENTION STRATEGIES

In recognition of the poorer cognitive, linguistic, social, emotional, and health outcomes of young children from low-SES families, intervention efforts have been designed and conducted in attempts to minimize or prevent these disparities early in life. Prevention strategies have been undertaken in each of the areas discussed above: family-level interventions, child care services, and neighborhood-level interventions. Below, we review the relative successes of such efforts to support and improve the health and development of young children.

Family-Level Interventions

Prevention efforts that focus on the family as the mechanism by which low SES affects young children include home-visiting programs, intergenerational or family literacy programs, and family support programs. Many of these programs focus on the mother or family, without offering direct services to the child, while others include a direct child component. Given this variation, findings are mixed with respect to effects on child outcomes. Some programs show beneficial effects on mothers and weaker effects on children.

Home-Visiting Programs

Home-visiting programs tend to focus on the parent, often beginning service delivery in the prenatal period and continuing through the first months or years of the child's life. A professional (often a nurse) or paraprofessional may visit the home on a weekly, biweekly, or monthly basis, offering a curriculum focused on improving parental functioning and promoting preventive health care usage. A well-known example is the Nurse Home Visitation Program (NHVP) (Olds et al., 1999), aimed at promoting children's health and development, as well as the economic self-sufficiency of low-income families. Some home-visiting programs also include an educational component, to show parents intellectually stimulating ways of interacting with their young children. Two large-scale examples of these are Parents as Teachers (PAT), serving parents of diverse socioeconomic backgrounds with children ages 0 to 3 (Wagner and Clayton, 1999), and the Home Instruction Program for Preschool Youngsters (HIPPY), which is designed to train low-income parents of preschoolers to engage in specific educational activities with their preschool-aged children (Baker et al., 1998).

Home-visiting programs that do not provide other services (e.g., center-based early education for the children) tend to report few effects on child cognitive and linguistic outcomes. In a review of 19 home-visiting programs, 15 of which placed specific emphasis on promoting children's cognitive and linguistic development, only 6 found significant benefits for these outcomes (Olds and Kitzman, 1993). Similarly, a review of 16 home-based programs, 14 of which assessed cognitive outcomes, showed only 9 with immediate positive gains (Benasich et al., 1992). The well-known NHVP reported no intervention effects on children at ages 3 and 4 years, except for the children of mothers who were heavy smokers during pregnancy, at the beginning of the program. These children had mental development scores comparable to children of nonsmoking mothers, about 5 points higher than children whose mothers were heavy smokers during pregnancy but did not receive the home-visiting treatment. There was also less incidence of lower birthweight among adolescent mothers who smoked—an effect that may be partly mediated through program effects on smoking (Olds et al., 1999). A recent evaluation of HIPPY, which is designed specifically to enhance the cognitive skills and school readiness of preschool children but provides its treatment only to the parent (through weekly lessons on activities to engage in with children), found few cognitive effects on children, and these were not consistently replicated across different cohorts of this evaluation (Baker et al., 1998). Similarly, the PAT program, which provides monthly home visits to teach mothers about parenting and stimulating their children, found only modest and inconsistent effects on child cognitive outcomes in two recent demonstrations (Wagner and Clayton, 1999).

In the domain of social and emotional well-being, some home-visiting programs have documented important effects. In the short-term some (but not all) home-visiting programs have improved children's self-confidence and social skills at age 3 years, reduced problem behaviors at 6 years, and improved the quality of mother-infant and mother-child interactions (Olds and Kitzman, 1993). The IHDP, which provided both home-visiting services and a center-based child care component, found significantly fewer mother-reported behavior problems at 2 and at 3 years, especially for children whose mothers had lower levels of education (IHDP, 1990). Also, treatment effects tended to be seen in those children whose mothers rated them as having difficult temperaments at age 1 (Brooks-Gunn et al., 1993). However, these effects were only significant for the heavier low-birthweight children when they were 5 years old (Brooks-Gunn et al., 1994).

Since many home-visiting programs begin prenatally and often focus on the importance of preventive health care, we might expect to see more effects in the area of children's health. However, a recent issue of the journal *The Future of Children*, devoted to recent evaluations of home-visiting programs (the Comprehensive Child Development Program [CCDP], Hawaii Healthy Start, Healthy Families America [HFA], HIPPY, NHVP, and PAT), reported no program effects on children's immunization rates or the number of well-child medical visits (Gomby et al., 1999). The Hawaii Healthy Start program, designed to promote positive parenting, enhance child development, ensure that children have a regular physician and "medical home," and prevent child abuse and neglect, did report a treatment effect on the number of children who had regular medical providers familiar with their needs (Duggan et al., 1999). Home visiting may also improve the physical well-being of children by improving parents' care and treatment of children through decreased stress, more understanding of child development and child rearing, and improved safety of home environments (Gomby et al., 1999). Fewer reported cases of abuse and neglect were found in the home-visited families of the Elmira NHVP (Olds et al., 1999) and a teen-parent demonstration of PAT (Wagner and Clayton, 1999), but not in the Hawaii Healthy Start program, nor in HFA (Gomby et al., 1999). Some home-visiting programs have also reported reductions in the number of hospital visits in the first 4 years of life, particularly those resulting from injuries and ingestions (Olds et al., 1999), and differences in maternal attitudes and behaviors related to abuse and neglect (Gomby et al., 1999). A review of 17 home-based interventions found only 2 with positive effects on child immunizations and well-baby visits out of the 5 that assessed this outcome; all 6 of the evaluations assessing signs of child maltreatment found positive intervention effects (Brooks-Gunn et al., 2000a).

Family Literacy Programs

Intergenerational, or family literacy programs, are designed to enhance the skills of both the young child and one or more adult family members in order to improve the well-being and future prospects for the entire family (St. Pierre and Swartz, 1995). These programs tend to offer a combination of early childhood education, adult education, and parenting education, and vary in the extent to which these services are provided exclusively in center-based settings or in a combination of center- and home-based services. Children are expected to benefit both directly from the child-focused component and indirectly from the two parent-focused services. Family resources and well-being are expected to be influenced by improved educational and occupational status of adults participating in adult education, and parenting education is expected to improve both the provision of literacy and cognitively stimulating parent-child activities and the amount of literacy-related materials in the home environment (St. Pierre and Swartz, 1995).

Evaluations of family literacy programs lack the rigor of the home-visiting program evaluations described above (in particular, few studies have been conducted using randomly assigned control groups). One evaluation of the national Even Start Family Literacy Program that randomized treatment at five sites found positive program effects on school readiness and language scores for 3- and 4-year-old program participants (St. Pierre et al., 1995). Pre-test/post-test designs have been used to document improved preschool cognitive outcomes for children in Even Start and other, smaller-scale family literacy programs (Heberle, 1992; Philliber et al., 1996; Richardson and Brown, 1997; St. Pierre et al., 1998; Tao et al., 1998).

Given their focus on literacy, family literacy program evaluation has not focused on child outcomes beyond cognitive and language achievement. The research to date does not provide data on social, emotional, or behavioral outcomes for children, nor does it follow the children longitudinally to assess the stability of the cognitive gains into the school years.

However, the effects of family literacy programs on parents and home environments have been examined. Participation in parenting education as part of a family literacy program is associated with modest improvements in parents' own literacy skills as measured by standardized assessment tests and improved rates of GED attainment (Heberle, 1992; St. Pierre and Swartz, 1995; Richardson and Brown, 1997; Tao et al., 1997). Furthermore, Even Start participants had larger gains than control group families on the number of reading materials for children in the home, but there were no treatment-control differences on measures of parent-child reading interactions or parental educational expectations for their children (St. Pierre et al., 1995). Although most evaluations tend not to measure effects on maternal mental and physical health, even as they postulate effects on these areas, one national evaluation of Even Start reported no program effects on maternal depression or locus of control. Neither were there measurable pretest/post-test program effects on family income, perceived social support, family resources, or parental employment (St. Pierre et al., 1995).

Family Support Programs

Traditionally, family support programs were community-based efforts designed to offer a broad array of support and information that could be accessed on a voluntary basis by all families in the community. According to this "universal access" model, the programs are designed for all families, not targeted to a special population. However, because of the growing crisis among certain groups of families, such as those living in poverty, poor housing, and poor neighborhoods, family support programs have emerged that are specifically designed for families that are considered to be "at risk." The populations that have been the focus of such specialized efforts include families who are environmentally at risk because of low income or low education of the parents, or families with children who are biologically at risk due to conditions such as premature birth, low birthweight, or developmental disability (Barnes et al., 1995).

Because of their definition as grass roots, preventive efforts to serve the individual needs of families, "family support programs" are actually quite variable in the design of their programs and the services they provide. What these programs have in common is the goal to serve the family as a system: to serve multiple members of the family with appropriate educational services, to help empower family members to achieve their personal goals by giving them relevant skills and strategies, to bring families together to share common problems and solutions, and to provide links to other social and health services available in the community as needed. Programs go about these goals in many different ways, some offering home-visiting services, others providing center-based child care, and some simply serving as community centers. All programs seek to improve the lives of children and families by improving parents' education and resources, improving parents' understanding of child development and parenting skills, improving the resources available to children in the home, and improving the health care and education they receive outside the home.

A comprehensive review of 87 different family support programs has been conducted by Abt Associates and Yale University's Bush Center in Child Development and Social Policy (Barnes et al., 1995). Overall, findings suggest that universal access programs show an inconsistent pattern of short-term effects on child development, with the strongest effects occurring for children from higher-risk families and attending center-based interventions. However, many of these studies are weakened by the fact that they did not use control or comparison groups. Among programs that specifically targeted environmentally at-risk families, mixed results were also found: similarly to the results reported above, home-visiting programs show only a few effects on infant cognitive development, with no evidence for long-term effects, whereas center-based interventions serving preschool-aged children document stronger short- and long-term effects on cognitive development, school-based indicators, and some positive effects on parental caregiving and child health and health care service use (Barnes et al., 1995).

Summary of Family-Level Interventions

The three types of family-focused intervention described above (home-visiting programs, two-generation literacy programs, and family support programs) tend to overlap somewhat in their definitions. For instance some would argue that some of the family literacy programs fall under the definition of family support programs, and many family support programs serving families with infants utilize a home-visiting approach. What they have in common is a focus on improving child outcomes by serving the family. Services may focus on the mother or family, seeking to influence child outcomes indirectly.

Findings for effects on parents are relatively few: for universal-access programs, some associations have been found for increased parent knowledge of child development, parenting attitudes and behaviors, and improved parental feelings of social support, coping, and reduced family stress (Pfannenstiel and Seltzer, 1989; Pfannenstiel et al., 1991; Barnes et al., 1995). Physical health, education, and employment effects on mothers in universal-access family support programs have not been reported (Barnes et al., 1995). In programs specifically targeting at-risk families, positive effects have been found on home learning environment, parenting attitudes, and parent child interactions (e.g., Andrews et al., 1982; Travers et al., 1982; Johnson and Walker, 1991; Quint et al., 1994; St. Pierre et al., 1994), but almost no effects on parent mental health are reported (Barnes et al., 1995). Although many programs are successful in getting mothers with low education to continue schooling and complete GEDs, there have not been strong effects of program participation on high school graduation or employment (Barnes et al., 1995).

A recent review has focused specifically on the effects of early intervention programs on parents, and also found variation based on program type (Brooks-Gunn et al., 2000a). Among home-visiting programs for infants and toddlers, program effects on mothers included greater maternal work force participation and reduced use of welfare and food stamps (Olds et al., 1986a,b; 1988; 1994, 1995, 1997; Kitzman et al., 1997), more supportive and less harsh parenting (Field et al., 1980; Gray and Ruttle, 1980; Larson, 1980; Madden et al., 1984; Barrera et al., 1986; Olds et al., 1988, 1994; Lieberman et al., 1991), and some effects on home environment and child-rearing attitudes (e.g., Field et al., 1980; Gray and Ruttle, 1980; Larson, 1980; Ross, 1984; Barrera et al., 1986; Osofsky, Culp and Ware, 1988; Erickson et al., 1992; Olds et al., 1994). Family-focused interventions including a center-based component (particularly the IHDP, Teenage Pregnancy Intervention Program, and the Yale Child Welfare Project) found some positive effects on maternal education and employment (Andrews et al., 1982; Brooks-Gunn et al., 1994; Field et al., 1982; Seitz and Apfel, 1994), and maternal mental health (Klebanov et al., 1993). Six out of seven studies reporting on parenting behaviors found that program participation improved the quality and sensitivity of parent-child interactions, but only two of four studies assessing children's home environment found positive effects of program participation (Brooks-Gunn et al., 2000a).

Although family-focused intervention programs aim to affect children both directly and indirectly through improving outcomes for parents and families, few evaluations have directly tested these pathways. Three exceptions are worth noting (Brooks-Gunn et al., 2000a). First, an analysis of Abecedarian and Project CARE programs tested both the quality of the home environment and parental authoritarian attitudes as possible mediators of program effects on children. The analysis showed a direct effect of the quality of the home environment on children's cognitive test scores, but none of this effect was mediated through the effect of the intervention upon the home environment. Furthermore, there was no direct relationship between parents' authoritarian attitudes and child outcomes, so this pathway was ruled out (Burchinal et al., 1997). Second, IHDP data were used to test the pathway from program effects on parents to child outcomes. The data supported a pathway, similar to that found in Figure 1, by which participation in the intervention program reduced maternal depression, which was associated with improved parenting behaviors and, in turn, affected child test scores. The treatment also had a direct effect on parenting in addition to the indirect one through depression (Linver et al., 1999). A third test of this pathway was conducted in an attempt to link program participation to child outcomes through its effect on parents' ability to cope with stressful life events (Klebanov et al., in press). Although intervention affected depression, it did not affect coping. Instead, the authors found that the intervention affected maternal mental health only for those mothers with a large number of stressful life events and that child test scores and depressive symptoms at age 3 were positively influenced by the intervention through its effects on mothers with high depression and a high number of stressful life events. Evaluation research explicitly testing these types of pathways is important for assessing the effects of interventions that seek to influence children's development through affecting the family. As we discuss below in our conclusion, more research of this type is needed.

Early Childhood Education Interventions

The research findings above have suggested that providing a direct intervention component to the child may have the strongest impact on child outcomes. Indeed, many interventions designed to enhance the healthy development of children from low-SES families have focused on the provision of high-quality, developmentally appropriate center-based child care. Model preschool programs, such as the Perry Preschool, and large-scale public programs such as Head Start, each emerged in the 1960s War on Poverty—a movement to enhance the learning experiences and other support of children from poor families. These programs often also include a focus on services for the family, but the main centerpiece is the provision of services directly to the child outside the home. Examples of programs combining center-based services with other forms of family support include the Perry Preschool, the Houston Parent Child Development Center, and the IHDP.

Several recent reviews have summarized the findings of the many evaluations that have been conducted on center-based interventions (Barnett, 1995; Yoshikawa, 1995; Bryant and Maxwell, 1997; Brooks-Gunn et al., 2000a; Farran, 2000). Center-based programs beginning in infancy, such as the Carolina Abecedarian program and the IHDP, have shown immediate and strong effects on children's IQ scores (IHDP, 1990; Brooks-Gunn et al., 1994; Campbell and Ramey, 1994). Programs for preschool-aged children have smaller but still significant effects on IQ. Across 11 early education programs that served poor children in the 1960s and 1970s, IQ gains for program children averaged 7.42 points higher than those for control group children (Royce et al., 1983). Barnett (1995) reported that 11 of 12 model preschool programs showed significant IQ effects, but only 1 out of 5 large-scale public programs positively affected IQ scores.

The findings by some researchers that early IQ gains from these programs may diminish over time as children from program and control groups progress through school (e.g., Royce et al., 1983; McKey et al., 1985; Lee et al., 1990) have led researchers to consider the importance of the ongoing schooling and support received by children through the transition to schooling and beyond (Lee and Loeb, 1995; Head Start Bureau, 1996). The continuation of supports for these children does appear to be associated with better long-term outcomes, including higher IQ scores, reduced rates of grade retention and special education placement, and fewer delinquent behaviors (Campbell and Ramey, 1994, 1995; Burchinal et al., 1997; Reynolds, 1997).

In addition to IQ and school-related outcomes, early childhood intervention programs have documented long-term effects on children's social and emotional outcomes. For instance, the Perry Preschool has documented lasting effects on reducing delinquent behaviors at age 14 and less involvement with the criminal justice system at ages 19 and 27 (Schweinhart et al., 1993). In a summary across 40 early intervention studies, Yoshikawa (1995) identified four programs with particular success in reducing antisocial and delinquent behavior. In addition to the Perry Preschool, these include the Syracuse University Family Development Research Project (Lally et al., 1988), the Yale Child Welfare Project (Seitz and Apfel, 1994), and the Houston PCDC (Johnson and Walker, 1987). Important associations are noted between early program effects on child verbal and cognitive abilities and on parents' parenting skills and these long-term outcomes (Yoshikawa, 1995).

Participation in early childhood education intervention may improve children's physical well-being in several ways. First, programs require that children be up-to-date on their immunizations in order to participate. Second, referrals may be made to necessary health services, some of which may be provided on-site. Third, vision, hearing, and developmental screenings may be conducted at the center, identifying children with delays or deficits in these areas. Fourth, nutritious meals and snacks provided at centers may substantially improve the diets of economically disadvantaged children (Gomby et al., 1995). However, few studies have focused on children's physical health.

Overall, the research points to strong effects of high-quality center-based child care programs for economically disadvantaged children. Effects are found in cognitive, literacy, emotional, and behavioral domains, and long-term effects are seen in related adult outcomes such as high school graduation, employment, less welfare use, and less delinquent behavior. Many researchers have therefore concluded that in order to achieve effects on the child, direct early childhood education is needed, in addition to the provision of comprehensive services to the family (Barnett, 1995; Yoshikawa, 1995; Bryant and Maxwell, 1997; Berlin et al., 1998).

Neighborhood-Focused Interventions

The research presented earlier suggests growing evidence that neighborhood environments may operate independently of family characteristics to influence child outcomes. Accordingly, an argument could then be made for focusing intervention for low-SES children on improving the characteristics of poor neighborhoods. Interventions focusing on the neighborhood (as opposed to focusing on individuals or families) are emerging and are termed "comprehensive community initiatives." These initiatives target the physical, economic, and social conditions of neighborhoods in order to improve the lives of the low-income individuals and families living there (Connell et al., 1995; Brown and Richman, 1997; Roundtable on Comprehensive Community Initiatives for Children and Families, 1997). Thus, comprehensive community initiatives expect to directly influence individuals, families, and communities, and they also expect to have an indirect effect on individuals and families through their effect on communities (Berlin et al., in press).

Comprehensive community initiatives (CCIs) represent a new approach to increasing the social capital of a community by improving the number and quality of connections among residents of the community (Brooks-Gunn, 1995). Although many have been developed, few have focused directly on young children. Berlin and her colleagues have argued that CCIs typically incorporate many of the qualities that are found to be associated with developmental outcomes for young children, including a focus on neighborhood social capital, comprehensive approaches to service delivery, provision of high-quality services, and the development of trusting relationships between service providers and recipients. Specifically, these authors recommend that "through their support of anti-poverty policies and programs and through system reform and community building strategies, CCIs can directly and indirectly support young children's most pressing developmental needs for supportive home and out-of-home experiences that promote both emotional security and learning" (Berlin et al., in press, p. 26).

At this point, there is no research to support the effectiveness of the CCI approach in improving the developmental outcomes of low-SES children. However, we believe such initiatives can be beneficial for poor children if (1) they do in fact improve the community characteristics that have been found to influence children's healthy development, such as neighborhood income and employment levels, and (2) they include high-quality child care as a form of direct service to young children.

CONCLUSIONS AND OPPORTUNITIES FOR FUTURE RESEARCH

There is great interest currently in positive child development and health, which is being discussed under the rubric of positive child outcomes, well-being, and health (Moore et al., in press). There are parallels to this approach in the literature on adult outcomes, with new work on positive well-being that grows out of more clinically oriented approaches such as those of Erikson,

Maslow, and Allport (e.g., Green et al., 1993). In this context, we need more consideration of what positive health or well-being looks like for children. Discussions should be initiated across disciplines to work toward acceptable definitions of well-being. For example, definitions of well-being might include trust and security in the family context, curiosity and exploration, age-appropriate self-regulatory behavior, and age-appropriate autonomy (Moore et al., in press).

In this paper, we have considered healthy development of the whole child to include outcomes in all of these domains and discussed how SES seems to operate to create disparities in the health and well-being of poor versus more affluent children. In particular, we have focused on the arenas of the family, child care setting, and neighborhood as important contexts in which SES may be operating. Interventions targeting these contexts have been described, and their relative success has been evaluated.

In general, the research suggests that economically disadvantaged children benefit from high-quality, center-based child care programs, augmented by services that support other family members and the family as a whole. However, beyond this general finding, attention must be paid to subgroups of participants who may benefit the most. Aspects of programs (e.g., duration, intensity, and mode of service delivery), participants (e.g., maternal education and the number of risk factors the family has), and the interactions between the program and participants (e.g., the degree of participation of the family and the match between program services and the individual needs of the family) all work to influence the effectiveness of a program (Berlin et al., 1998). Program evaluations should incorporate all of these factors to assess program success more accurately.

We have attempted to illustrate the importance of considering the possible pathways through which SES may affect young children by reporting findings of the few studies that have explicitly tested such models. Exploring the processes linking SES and child health and development is critical in the design of prevention strategies and policies that are conceptually driven. For instance, most program developers to date have not explicated the ways in which they expect their interventions to influence children. The theoretical bases for the programs have not been spelled out. Recently, however, prevention scholars have begun to outline their theories of change in order to articulate program goals and the ways in which specific program components are thought to relate to these goals (Weiss, 1995; see also Barnard, 1998; Berlin et al., 1998). Services should be designed to address the stated goals as directly as possible—when attempting to influence parenting behavior, parenting education should be offered; if attempting to influence child behavior, direct early childhood education should be provided. We believe that the "theory of change" approach is crucial in order to design the most effective programs, as well as to document the successes of such programs—an important component in ensuring their continued funding. We expect that such efforts will continue in the next decade.

In addition to knowing the specific goals and methods of achieving those goals, Barnard (1998) points out that levels of implementation often fall short of optimum program goals. The "implementation gap" represents the difference between the amount, or "dose," of intervention that is prescribed by the program and the actual amount of intervention that participating families receive. This gap should be measured when assessing program effects in order to determine levels of implementation or doses that result in positive outcomes for children and families and those that do not.

Examining the theory of change of a specific program goes beyond determining the theory held by the program's designers. Theories of change may vary even within programs, according to different program staff members. For instance, discussions with staff members at Early Head Start site visits as part of the implementation study of the Early Head Start Research and Evaluation Project (Mathematica Policy Research, 1999), reveal variation in what staff mention as important. Many Early Head Start staff mention that strengthening relationships is an important goal, both relationships between parent and child and relationships between parents and program staff. If strengthening relationships is considered to be an important goal of the staff implementing the intervention, it is important to find effective ways of measuring these when evaluating program effectiveness. Barnard (1998) also asserts that an emphasis on the participant-staff relationship is essential for successful intervention programs. Similarly for child physical health, the relationships between medical care providers and parents are an important component in the successful administration of medical recommendations and treatments.

We believe that the range of what are considered to be "good outcomes" should be broad enough to truly capture young children's healthy development. In part, this means accepting maternal outcomes and parenting outcomes as important in their own right, as well as focusing on children's social, emotional, and physical health. The overwhelming historical focus on IQ and cognitive outcomes has not represented this broad conceptualization of healthy development and arguably has resulted in underestimation of the effects of intervention programs on children.

In fact, the broad conceptualization of child development and well-being presented in our introduction to this paper may not go far enough. To determine what constitutes "success" of an early intervention program, we must attend to the views of the parents and families served. Parents may have their own theories of change and these voices must be heard in order to develop programs that will successfully engage parents and, via parents' participation, children. Parents' goals for their children and reasons for participating in intervention programs may be somewhat different from those espoused by program designers. For instance, parent perceptions of program success may be more deeply rooted in cultural or moral values, or religious beliefs, than in such things as school readiness. In a study of the different views held by parents and service providers, Goldenberg and Gallimore (1995) described how immigrant Latino parents would sacrifice school activities that might further their children's academic skills if they perceived the activities as possible threats to their child's moral development. These parent's viewed the *buen camino* (good path) as being primarily moral. Program designers should "listen" to these parental voices, attempting to take into account the cultural background of the families served, not just as a token to represent cultural sensitivity but to really provide services that are perceived as meaningful and important to the families served.[4]

This argument leads to the issue of "top-down" versus "bottom-up" program design (e.g., Brooks-Gunn, 1995; Leventhal et al., 1997). The philosophy of top-down design assumes that the problems of low-income children and families are similar across different communities, and therefore standard programs may be brought into the community and have a positive effect. Bottom-up design involves the input of community members to identify the problems and needs specific to their community in order to tailor-make a program that addresses those needs. While many of the issues faced in poor communities do seem to be universal, such as few neighborhood resources, poor-quality housing, or unsafe streets, individual communities will differ in their cultural or ethnic makeup, which will have implications both for what family members value in terms of program goals and the steps that must be taken to foster trust and community buy-in of a new program.

One of the big gaps in the literature on the efficacy of early childhood intervention programs is that studies have not looked at the efficacy of such programs for immigrant children. With the growing population of immigrant children who may need special early childhood services (Lewitt and Baker, 1994), this is a critical area of inquiry. Part of the reason for this gap is a cohort effect: many of the interventions that have been evaluated served children in the 1960s, 1970s, and early 1980s, before the recent new waves of immigration to this country. Another reason is that there has been differential access to some programs for immigrant families. For instance, in the IHDP, a decision was made in the early stages of program design that program services could not be provided in all the languages spoken by families that would otherwise qualify for the trial. Families who could not receive services in English were excluded from participating. One-quarter of the IHDP families did indicate that a language other than English was spoken in their home, but they were proficient enough to receive services in English. Thus, there is less information available about the efficacy of family- and child-focused services for children from other countries and children who are not English language proficient. Such exclusion criteria, while arguably necessary for a smaller-scale clinical trial, are not appropriate for larger-scale provision of services to needy families. There are rich data being

---

[4]We are grateful to P. Hauser-Cram for providing this example in her review of an earlier version of this paper.

collected about differential beliefs relating to health practices, educational practices, and socialization practices in different groups, and these should be helpful in informing culturally sensitive program development (see, e.g., Greenfield and Cocking, 1994; Garcia Coll et al., 1995; Harkness and Super, 1995). The gap in the research on efficacy of intervention programs in immigrant populations can hopefully be remedied in the next decade, as several studies currently in the field are attending to the issue by adding oversamples of Latinos and other minority populations, and ensuring that at least some program intervention staff are fluent in the languages spoken by the families they serve (Brooks-Gunn et al., 2000).

Even if programs continue to improve their ability to address the needs of families, there remains the issue of discrimination against certain minority populations. In our discussion of SES disparities in the health and well-being of young children, we have not addressed the probability that racial discrimination may be a root of many disparities seen, especially vis-à-vis access to health services, the continued and increasing segregation of poor neighborhoods, and the experiences of minority children in their communities, schools, and other social institutions. Racial discrimination probably also plays a role both in the access of minority children and families to early intervention services, and in their interactions with program staff members. Coates (1992) argues that the specific experiences of African-American youth, in terms of the racism they experience and the strength of their extended family connections, may make interventions at the level of the social network particularly beneficial for this group. Intervention efforts for younger children and families must also attend to the experiences of discrimination faced by the families they serve. Programs need to identify barriers affecting service participation of certain groups and to develop culturally diverse services and skills (Coates and Vietze, 1996). Attention to eliminating discriminatory attitudes and practices, even at their most subtle levels, continues to be a necessary process for programs and society as a whole if we hope to have a significant effect on reducing SES disparities in children's outcomes.

We have argued for the importance of considering social and emotional development as indicators of healthy development and school readiness, and have highlighted teachers' concerns about children's behavioral functioning in the classroom. Parents of young children also express concern about these areas of functioning. In fact, in families of children with disabilities studied in the Early Intervention Collaborative Study, parents' well-being was more strongly affected by children's behavior problems and difficulty with self-regulation than by the type of disability the child had or the child's cognitive abilities (P. Hauser-Cram, personal communication, February 2, 2000). This finding suggests that parenting may be affected by children's problem behaviors.

The estimates of emotional or behavioral disorders in young children range from 7 to 22%, with approximately 9% having severe emotional disorders, and social-emotional problems are disproportionately found among children in low-income groups (Knitzer, in press). However, rates of referral into mental health services for emotional disturbances among Head Start children are relatively low: only 4% of those with identified disabilities are diagnosed with an emotional or behavioral disability (Knitzer, in press). There may be a stigma associated with identifying young children with emotional or behavioral problems, yet young children from poor families are much more likely to have parents with depressive symptoms, who may have difficulty forming warm, nurturing relationships with their children. Early emotional experiences lay the groundwork for children's developing emotional self-regulation and will be important for later school performance. Thus, it appears that sufficient attention is not being paid to children's emotional and behavioral development in intervention efforts for low-income children (Lara et al., 2000).

Mental health services for young children living in conditions that are associated with emotional disorder (e.g., low-income families with depressed mothers) should be more widely available, with attention to prevention rather than the more stigmatizing classification and diagnosis. Some intervention studies have found stronger effects on children's test scores and attachment security for children with depressed mothers (Lyons-Ruth et al., 1990) and children whose mothers had low cognitive scores or poor social skills (Barnard et al., 1988). The IHDP had stronger effects on maternal distress outcomes among mothers with lower levels of education and less active coping strategies (Klebanov et al., in press). These findings point to the particular efficacy of intervention for children in families at risk for poor mental health outcomes.

Returning to our initial discussion of the goal of ensuring that by 2000 all children will start school ready to learn, we believe that the current progress falls short of the needs of America's young children. To be optimally ready to learn when entering school, today's youngest children need families and neighborhoods that can support them economically, physically, and emotionally. Interventions targeting needy families, with services addressing these broad categories (i.e., economic support, nutritional support, health care, child care, parental education and employment, parenting education, and neighborhood economic and social stability) are clearly needed, but such expenditures must be made with the awareness of where success has and has not been achieved in previous programs. Guarded optimism is warranted, based on findings in several areas: the long-term effects of small-scale, child-focused early education programs, such as the Perry Preschool; the few findings indicating intervention effects on children mediated by effects on parenting; and home-based programs that may influence parent behaviors. Combining comprehensive intervention approaches with careful theory- and research-based goal setting will improve the settings in which young children develop and help ensure that they enter school ready in every way to learn.

Based on the findings and discussion above, we present a number of specific recommendations for early childhood intervention:

1. If programs want to have positive effects on child cognitive, literacy, and school outcomes, they most likely must provide intensive programs directly to the child. Child- and family-focused programs will need to offer high-quality, center-based care to children on a consistent basis, not just by providing care while the parents attend meetings and parenting classes but for a substantial amount of time each week.

2. High-quality center-based child care should also be a component of programs striving to influence social and emotional development. Less evidence supports the effectiveness of center-based programs on these outcomes (as compared to cognitive and school achievement), largely because either social and emotional well-being have not been the primary focus of preschool-type interventions, measurement of such outcomes has been weak, and/or theories of change have not been made explicit. Preschool intervention programs need to be more explicit about their social and emotional goals and to develop specific intervention components, including preventive mental health and physical health services to foster these goals.

3. Although early education research has found benefits from intensive intervention and long-term intervention (e.g., 2 years or more), the focus in many programs is often on the preschool years. Projects should consider expanding infant/toddler services. If these services are expanded, efforts would also have to be made to retain families for longer periods of time and to provide some service continuity over child care and school transitions (just as the health care field has done).

4. Service providers, whether from the education, health, or social service sector, must pay attention to research on quality. Lessons from the well-developed field of assessing child care quality could be a beacon for such efforts. For example, issues of promoting staff development, reducing child-staff ratios, providing developmentally appropriate curriculum and continuity of care for the child, and adhering to safety regulations are all important for child well-being (Whitebook et al., 1990; Cost, Quality and Child Outcomes Study Team, 1995, 1999; Howes et al., 1995). Recent longitudinal data from more than 800 children who had attended 170 different child care centers suggests that early child care quality is associated with math and language skills as well as peer relations and behavior problems in second grade (Cost, Quality and Child Outcomes Study Team, 1999).

The National Association for the Education of Young Children has outlined the characteristics of developmentally appropriate practices in early childhood settings (Bredekamp and Copple, 1997), and these practices form the basis for an extensive observational research measure of early childhood classrooms (Early Childhood Environment Rating Scale [ECERS]; Harms and Clifford, 1990; Harms et al., 1998). Research assessing child care environments using this measure has found that across a diverse sample of child care centers, quality is generally in the medium range (3 to 5 points on a scale from 1 to 7), with more than 11% scoring below the minimal quality rating of 3 points (Cost, Quality and Child Outcomes Study Team, 1999). A recent assessment using the ECERS in Head Start classrooms found somewhat different results: although the average quality score was 4.9 (indicating "good" quality), only 1.5% of classrooms had an overall score of 3 ("minimal"), and no Head Start classrooms had scores below 3 points, indicating an "inadequate" environment (Zill et al., 1998). These findings suggest that technical assistance and monitoring of service quality could use the Head Start experience as a guidepost. The ECERS instrument can also be used as an internal self-assessment, and many programs would benefit from using such a tool to guide quality improvement efforts.

The early childhood education field has done a better job of defining quality than have other types of programs. Intervention scholars targeting health and behavior should similarly delineate factors of program quality in order to create an ECERS-like scale for other types of interventions.

5. More programs should consider how they can facilitate continuity of services for families as children progress through preschool and elementary school. Programs must be realistic about the number of families they can keep in the program through the transition to elementary school. Are pieces of the program, such as literacy activities in the home, more tailored to preschoolers than to school-aged children? Do different techniques need to be used to help parents with children of different ages? What types of links are programs forging with elementary schools and existing preschools (including, but not limited to, Head Start)? Attention to all of these issues will be important for continuing to serve children throughout these early years.

6. Programs should work on defining what full implementation is. This is important for medical interventions as well. Benchmarks should be created regarding the percentage of families served with particular services, the intensity of services, staff training, the percentage of families served for only a brief time, and links to other service agencies in the community. Often, evaluations are conducted on programs that are not being fully implemented, and this reduces the likelihood of getting positive results. Currently, the Early Head Start Research and Evaluation Project is paying more attention to the definitions of full implementation across a variety of dimensions (Mathematica Policy Research, 1999). Measures of levels of intervention received by families (or participation levels) can be included in analyses to determine effects for high-participation versus low-participation families.

7. Program designers and program staff should spend some time explicating their theories of change—their philosophies about how their program helps children and how it may help children differently for different types of outcomes (emotional, cognitive, school success). Programs may need to hire a facilitator to guide this process. Awareness of different theories of change held by staff

members within programs and the theories of change held by parents in the families served by the program will be important in this process.

8. Given a program's theory of change (see recommendation 7, above) and the research literature to date, specific programs should consider what their primary goals are. Given funding constraints, some programs may not be able to be all things to all members of a family. A program may be more likely to influence adult literacy and perhaps parent-child literacy activities in the home, rather than strongly influencing child outcomes. Programs should focus their resources on the areas they are most likely to influence.

9. Programs should realistically consider the intensity of the services they offer to families. There is a trade-off between the amount of intervention that can be provided and the number of families that can be served. If a program can only offer thin services in order to serve all families, there may be no positive child outcomes at all. Instead, programs should determine how many families can be served with a program that is intense enough to make a difference. In particular, with the evidence that high-risk families may be most likely to benefit from program participation, the question then is whether high-risk families are receiving high enough doses of intervention. Often, these families may be the hardest to reach because of barriers to their participation: transportation difficulties, the convergence of multiple family crises making program participation a lower priority, substance abuse, domestic abuse, mental health problems, and many more. So in many cases, these families may actually be receiving the lowest levels of service.

The question then becomes whether or not we should specifically target different bundles of services for different subgroups of families. Even within groups of families with low education or low income, differential treatment effects can be seen. For instance, in the IHDP, the treatment had a stronger effect on children's cognitive test scores when mothers experienced fewer negative life events (Klebanov et al., in press). Some families with high numbers of risk factors may be overwhelmed, making it harder for them to attend to the services they are receiving. It may be necessary to individualize some services for families experiencing high numbers of negative life events, who may not be helped by the standard package of services.

10. A related issue has to do with whether some services should be universal. This is not to be confused with the more extensive services that are needed for poor children. However, when programs become known as "where the poor kids go," this contributes to the labeling and stigmatization of children and families, may reduce participation rates, and contributes to continued stereotyping and segregation in our society (P. Hauser-Cram, personal communication, February 2, 2000). Thus, some may argue that high-quality early childhood programs should be made more universally available, and indeed, we are beginning

to see movement in this direction with the introduction of universal pre-kindergarten programs in many states, and home-visiting programs for all babies born in some counties and states. Universal services, then, are converging, with newborns and 4-year-olds currently being served in many areas. Policymakers should consider whether early childhood and family services should be made available to all families consistently from birth, or at least starting at age 3.

11. Projects will need to tailor both core and support services to be responsive (and relevant) to the needs of working parents by scheduling them on off-hours, providing more home-based services, and providing supports such as transportation, child care, and meals to help remove barriers to participation. Since working parents have less time, coordination of services will be important, so that more services, such as child care and parenting education, are offered at the same site. While these issues are important for all parents, the problems will be even more serious when programs include parents who are moving from welfare to work. Consistent with this recommendation, programs have to consider the changing needs of poor parents, especially in light of welfare reform.

Concluding Remarks

The study of early childhood interventions is not a new topic. In fact, some of the conclusions are strikingly similar to those made by Urie Bronfenbrenner more than 25 years ago in a review of the effects of early intervention (Bronfenbrenner, 1974). We conclude, as did Bronfenbrenner, that high-quality early childhood programs can have significant effects on cognitive outcomes for children, especially when the children are from low-income families and especially when the programs provide both child and family services. What has changed in the more than 30 years since the programs that began in the 1960s and 1970s were first evaluated is a change from deficit models to models focusing on the strengths of families. Families are considered to be at risk due to the inequities of opportunities and differential obstacles faced by low-income families. The field has broadened its focus to consider the multiple contexts in which children develop and consider the interrelationships among parents, program staff, and neighborhood providers, all of whom jointly provide opportunities for growth. With the increased numbers of mothers of young children in the workforce, we have learned more about the difficulties families have managing family and work responsibilities, and the limited choices that families often have in procuring high-quality child care. We have made strides in addressing questions about who ought to be targeted in early intervention efforts, how to successfully integrate services, how programs affect outcomes for mothers and other family members, what effects programs have on outcomes other than child IQ, and how staff and family perceptions influence program processes and outcomes.

At the same time, some of Bronfenbrenner's statements have stood the test of time over a quarter of a century. Parents need supports in multiple arenas of functioning. High-quality programs can make a difference in the health and well-being of children and families. And finally, there are no quick fixes—families need intensive services of substantial duration in order to reap significant benefits.

REFERENCES

Adler, N. E., Boyce, T., Chesney, M. A., Cohen, S., Folkman, S., Kahn, R. L., and Syme, S. L. (1994). Socioeconomic status and health: The challenge of the gradient. *American Psychologist, 49*, 15–24.

Andrews, S. R., Blumenthal, L. B., Johnson, D. L., Kahn, A. J., Ferguson, C. J., Lasater, T. M., Malone, P. E., and Wallace, D. B. (1982). The skills of mothering: A study of parent child development centers. *Monographs of the Society for Research in Child Development, 47*(6), Serial No. 198.

Baker, A., Piotrkowski, C. S., and Brooks-Gunn, J. (1998). The effects of the Home Instruction Program for Preschool Youngsters (HIPPY) on children's school performance at the end of the program and one year later. *Early Childhood Research Quarterly, 13*, 571–588.

Barnard, K. E. (1998). Developing, implementing, documenting interventions with parents and young children. In L.J. Berlin (Ed.), Opening the black box: Understanding how early intervention programs work [Special Issue]. *Zero to Three, 18*, 23–29.

Barnes, H.V., Goodson, B.D., and Layzer, J.I. (1995). *Review of Research on Supportive Interventions for Children and Families: Vol. 1*. Cambridge, MA: Abt Associates, Inc.

Barnett, W. S. (1995). Long-term effects of early childhood programs on cognitive and school outcomes. *The Future of Children, 5*, 25–50.

Barrera, M. E., Rosenbaum, P. L., and Cunningham, C. E. (1986). Early home intervention with low-birthweight infants and their parents. *Child Development, 57,* 20–33.

Benasich, A. A., Brooks-Gunn, J., and Clewell, B. C. (1992). How do mothers benefit from early intervention programs? *Journal of Applied Developmental Psychology, 13*, 311–362.

Berlin, L.J., Brooks-Gunn, J., and Aber, J. L. Promoting early childhood development through comprehensive community initiatives. *Children's Services*.

Berlin, L.J., O'Neal, C. R., and Brooks-Gunn, J. (1998). What makes early intervention programs work? The program, its participants, and their interaction. In L.J. Berlin (Ed.), Opening the black box: What makes early child and family development programs work? [Special Issue]. *Zero to Three, 18*, 4–15.

Bredekamp, S., and Copple, C. (1997). *Developmentally Appropriate Practice in Early Childhood Programs*. Washington, DC: National Association for the Education of Young Children.

Bronfenbrenner, U. (1974). Is early intervention effective? *Teachers College Record, 76*(2), 279–303.

Brooks-Gunn, J. (1995). Strategies for altering the outcomes for poor children and their families. In P. L. Chase-Lansdale and J. Brooks-Gunn (Eds.), *Escape from Poverty: What Makes a Difference for Children?* (pp. 87–117). Cambridge: Cambridge University Press.

Brooks-Gunn, J., Berlin, L.J., and Fuligni, A. S. (2000a). Early childhood intervention programs: What about the family? In J. P. Shonkoff and S. J. Meisels (Eds.), *Hand-*

book of Early Childhood intervention (2nd ed. pp. 549–588). New York: Cambridge University Press.

Brooks-Gunn, J., Berlin, L.J., Leventhal, T., and Fuligni, A. (2000). Depending on the kindness of strangers: Current national data initiatives and developmental research. *Child Development 71*, 257-267.

Brooks-Gunn, J., and Duncan, G. J. (1997). The effects of poverty on children. *The Future of Children, 7*(2), 55–71.

Brooks-Gunn, J., Duncan, G. J., and Aber, J. L. (Eds.). (1997a). *Neighborhood Poverty: Vol. 1. Context and Consequences for Children.* New York: Russell Sage Foundation.

Brooks-Gunn, J., Duncan, G. J., and Aber, J. L. (Eds.). (1997b). *Neighborhood Poverty: Vol. 2. Policy Implications in Studying Neighborhoods.* New York: Russell Sage Foundation.

Brooks-Gunn, J., Duncan, G. J., and Britto, P. R. (1999). Are socioeconomic gradients for children similar to those for adults? In D. P. Keating and C. Hertzman (Eds.), *Developmental Health and the Wealth of Nations* (pp. 94–124). New York: Guilford Press.

Brooks-Gunn, J., Duncan, G. J., Klebanov, P. K., and Sealand, N. (1993). Do neighborhoods influence child and adolescent development? *American Journal of Sociology, 99*(2), 353–395.

Brooks-Gunn, J., Duncan, G. J., Leventhal, T., and Aber, J. L. (1997c). Lessons learned and future directions for research on neighborhoods in which children live. In J. Brooks-Gunn, G. J. Duncan and J. L. Aber (Eds.), *Neighborhood Poverty: Vol. 1. Context and Consequences for Children* (pp. 279–297). New York: Russell Sage Foundation.

Brooks-Gunn, J., Klebanov, P. K., and Duncan, G. J. (1996). Ethnic differences in children's intelligence test scores: Role of economic deprivation, home environment, and maternal characteristics. *Child Development, 67*, 396–408.

Brooks-Gunn, J., McCarton, C., Casey, P., McCormick, M., Bauer, C., Bernbaum, J., Tyson, J., Swanson, M., Bennett, F., Scott, D., Tonascia, J., and Meinert, C. (1994a). Early intervention in low birthweight, premature infants: Results through age 5 years from the Infant Health and Development Program. *Journal of the American Medical Association, 272*, 1257–1262.

Brooks-Gunn, J., McCormick, M. C., Shapiro, S., Benasich, A. A., and Black, G. (1994b). The effects of early education intervention on maternal employment, public assistance, and health insurance: The Infant Health and Development Program. *American Journal of Public Health, 84*, 924–931.

Brown, P., and Richman, H. A. (1997). Neighborhood effects and state and local policy. In J. Brooks-Gunn, G. J. Duncan and J. L. Aber (Eds.), *Neighborhood Poverty: Vol. 1. Context and Consequences for Children* (pp. 161–184). New York: Russell Sage Foundation.

Bryant, D., and Maxwell, K. (1997). The effectiveness of early intervention for disadvantaged children. In M.J. Guralnick (Ed.), *The Effectiveness of Early Iintervention* (pp. 23–46). Baltimore: Brookes.

Burchinal, M. R., Campbell, F. A., Bryant, D. M., Wasik, B. H., and Ramey, C. T. (1997). Early intervention and mediating processes in cognitive performance of children of low-income African-American families. *Child Development, 68*, 935–954.

Campbell, F., and Ramey, C. (1994). Effects of early intervention on intellectual and academic achievement: A follow-up study from low-income families. *Child Development, 65*, 684–698.

Campbell, F., and Ramey, C. (1995). Cognitive and school outcomes for high risk African-American students at middle adolescence: Positive effects of early intervention. *American Educational Research Journal, 32*, 743–772.

Chase-Lansdale, P. L., and Gordon, R. A. (1996). Economic hardship and the development of five- and six-year-olds: Neighborhood and regional perspectives. *Child Development, 67*, 3338–3367.

Chase-Lansdale, P. L., Gordon, R. A., Brooks-Gunn, J., and Klebanov, P. K. (1997). Neighborhood and family influences on the intellectual and behavioral competence of preschool and early school-age children. In J. Brooks-Gunn, G. J. Duncan and J. L. Aber (Eds.), *Neighborhood Poverty: Vol. 1. Context and Consequences for Children* (pp. 79–118). New York: Russell Sage Foundation.

Coates, D. L. (1992). Social network analysis as mental health intervention with African-American adolescents. In F. C. Serafica, A. I. Schwebel, R. K. Russell, P. D. Isaac, and L. B. Myers (Eds.), *Mental Health of Ethnic Minorities* (pp. 5–37). New York: Praeger.

Coates, D. L., and Vietze, P. M. (1996). Cultural considerations in assessment, diagnosis, and intervention. In J. W. Jacobson and J. A. Mulick (Eds.), *Manual of Diagnosis and Professional Practice in Mental Retardation* (pp. 243–256). Washington, DC: American Psychological Association.

Collins, J. W., and David, R. J. (1990). The differential effect of traditional risk factors on infant birthweight among blacks and whites in Chicago. *American Journal of Public Health, 80*(6), 679–681.

Conger, R. D., Conger, K. J., and Elder, G. H., Jr. (1997). Family economic hardship and adolescent adjustment: Mediating and moderating processes. In G. J. Duncan and J. Brooks-Gunn (Eds.), *Consequences of Growing up Poor* (pp. 288–310). New York: Russell Sage Foundation.

Conger, R. D., Conger, K. J., Elder G. H., and Lorenz, F. O. (1992). A family process model of economic hardship and adjustment of early adolescent boys. *Child Development, 63*, 526–541.

Conger, R. D., Ge, X., Elder, G., Lorenz, F., and Simons, R. (1994). Economic stress, coercive family process and developmental problems of adolescents. *Child Development, 65*, 541–561.

Connell, J. P., Walker, G., and Aber, J. L. (1995). How do urban communities affect youth? Using social science research to inform the design and evaluation of comprehensive community initiatives. In J. P. Connell, A. C. Kubisch, L. B. Schorr, and C. H. Weiss (Eds.), *New Approaches to Evaluating Community Initiatives: Vol. 1. Concepts, Methods, and Contexts* (pp. 93–124). Washington, DC: The Aspen Institute.

Cost, Quality and Child Outcomes Study Team (1995). *Cost, Quality, and Child Outcomes in Child Care Centers*. Denver: Economics Department, University of Colorado at Denver.

Cost, Quality and Child Outcomes Study Team (1999). *The Children of the Cost, Quality, and Outcomes Study Go to School: Executive Summary*. Chapel Hill, NC: Frank Porter Graham Child Development Center, University of North Carolina at Chapel Hill.

Duggan, A. K., McFarlane, E. C., Windham, A. M., Rohde, C. A., Salkever, D. S., Fuddy, L., Rosenberg, L. A., Buchbinder, S. B., and Sia, C. C. J. (1999). Evaluation of Hawaii's Healthy Start Program. *Future of Children, 9*(1), 66–90.

Duncan, G. J., and Brooks-Gunn, J. (1997). Income effects across the life span: Integration and interpretation. In G. J. Duncan and J. Brooks-Gunn (Eds.), *Consequences of Growing up Poor* (pp. 596–610). New York: Russell Sage Foundation.

Duncan, G. J., Brooks-Gunn, J., and Klebanov, P. K. (1994). Economic deprivation and early childhood development. *Child Development, 65,* 296–318.

Duncan, G. J., Brooks-Gunn, J., Yeung, W. J., and Smith, J. R. (1998). How much does childhood poverty affect the life chances of children? *American Sociological Review, 63,* 406–423.

Elder, G. H., Jr. (1974). *Children of the Great Depression: Social Change in Life Experience.* Chicago: University of Chicago Press.

Erickson, M. F., Korfmacher, J., and Egeland, B. (1992). Attachments past and present: Implications for therapeutic intervention with mother-infant dyads. *Development and Psychopathology, 4,* 495–507.

Farran, D. C. (2000). Another decade of intervention for children who are low income or disabled: What do we know now? In J. P. Shonkoff and S. J. Meisels (Eds.), *Handbook of Early Childhood Intervention* (2nd ed., pp. 510–548). New York: Cambridge University Press.

Field, T., Widmayer, S., Greenburg, R., and Stoller, S. (1982). Effects of parent training on teenage mothers and their infants. *Pediatrics, 69,* 703–707.

Field, T. M., Widmayer, S. M., Stringer, S., and Ignatoff, E. (1980). Teenage, lower-class, black mothers and their preterm infants: An intervention and developmental follow-up. *Child Development, 51,* 426–436.

Galinsky, E., Howes, C., Kontos, S., and Shinn, M. (1994). *The Study of Children in Family Child Care and Relative Care.* New York: Families and Work Institute.

Garcia Coll, C. T., Meyer, E. C., and Brillon, L. (1995). Ethnic and minority parenting. In M. H. Bornstein (Ed.), *Handbook of Parenting: Vol. 2. Biology and Ecology of Parenting* (pp. 189–209). Mahwah, NJ: Lawrence Erlbaum Associates.

Goal 1 Technical Planning Group. (1993). *Reconsidering children's early development and learning: Toward shared beliefs and vocabulary.* Draft report to the National Education Goals Panel. Washington, DC: National Education Goals Panel.

Goldenberg, C., and Gallimore, R. (1995). Immigrant Latino parents' values and beliefs about their children's education: Continuities and discontinuities across cultures and generations. *Advances in Motivation and Achievement: Vol. 9* (pp. 183–228). Greenwich, CT: JAI Press.

Gomby, D. S., Culross, P. L., and Behrman, R. E. (1999). Home visiting: Recent program evaluations—Analysis and recommendations. *Future of Children, 9*(1), 4–26.

Gomby, D. S., Larner, M. B., Stevenson, C. S., Lewit, E. M., and Behrman, R. E. (1995). Long-term outcomes of early childhood programs: Analysis and recommendations. *Future of Children, 5*(3), 6–24.

Gonzales, N. S., Cauce, A., Friedman, R. J., Mason, C. A. (1996). Family, peer, and neighborhood influences on academic achievement among African-American adolescents: One-year prospective effects. *American Journal of Community Psychology, 24*(3), 365–387.

Gould, J. B., and LeRoy, S. (1988). Socioeconomic status and low birthweight: A racial comparison. *Pediatrics, 82*(6), 896–904.

Gray, S. W., and Ruttle, K. (1980). The Family-Oriented Home Visiting Program: A longitudinal study. *Genetic Psychology Monographs, 102,* 299–316.

Green, D. P., Goldman, S. L., and Salovey, P. (1993). Measurement error masks bipolarity in affect ratings. *Journal of Personality and Social Psychology, 64*(6), 1029–1041.

Greenfield, P. M., and Cocking, R. R. (Eds.). (1994). *Cross-Cultural Roots of Minority Child Development*. Hillsdale, NJ: Lawrence Erlbaum Associates.

Harkness, S., and Super, C. (1995). Culture and parenting. In M. H. Bornstein (Ed.), *Handbook of Parenting: Vol. 2. Biology and Ecology of Parenting* (pp. 211–234). Mahwah, NJ: Lawrence Erlbaum Associates, Publishers.

Harms, T., and Clifford, R. M. (1990). *The Early ChildhoodEnvironment Rating Scale*. New York: Teachers College Press.

Harms, T., Clifford, R. M., and Cryer, D. (1998). *Early Childhood Environment Rating Scale: Rev. ed.* New York: Teachers College Press.

Head Start Bureau (1996). *Head Start Children's Entry into Public School: An Interim Report on the National Head Start-Public School Early Childhood Demonstration Study*. Washington, DC: Department of Health and Human Services.

Heberle, J. (1992). PACE: Parent and child education in Kentucky. In T. G. Sticht, M.J. Beeler, and B.A. McDonald (Eds.), *The Intergenerational Transfer of Cognitive Skills: Vol. I. Programs, Policy, and Research Issues* (pp. 136–148). Norwood, NJ: Ablex.

Hoff-Ginsberg, E., and Tardiff, T. (1995). Socioeconomic status and parenting. In M. H. Bornstein (Ed.), *Handbook of Parenting: Vol. 2. Biology and Ecology of Parenting* (pp. 161–188). Mahwah, NJ: Lawrence Erlbaum Associates.

Howes, C., Smith, E., and Galinsky, E. (1995). *The Florida Child Care Quality Improvement Study: Interim Report*. New York: Families and Work Institute.

Infant Health and Development Program (IHDP) (1990). Enhancing the outcomes of low-birthweight, premature infants. *Journal of the American Medical Association, 263*, 3035–3042.

Jackson, A. P., Brooks-Gunn, J., Huang, C., and Glassman, M. (in press). Single mothers in low-wage jobs: Financial strain, parenting, and preschoolers' outcomes. *Child Development*.

Johnson, D. L., and Walker, T. (1987). Primary prevention of behavior problems in Mexican-American children. *American Journal of Community Psychology, 15*(4), 375–385.

Johnson, D. L., and Walker, T. (1991). A follow-up evaluation of the Houston Parent-Child Development Center: School performance. *Journal of Early Intervention, 15*(3), 226–236.

Kitzman, H., Olds, D. L., Henderson, C. R., Hanks, C., Cole, R., Tatelbaum, R., McConnochie, K. M., Sidora, K., Luckey, D. W., Shaver, D., Engelhardt, K., James, D., and Barnard, K. (1997). Effect of prenatal and infancy home visitation by nurses on pregnancy outcomes, childhood, childhood injuries, and repeated childbearing: A randomized controlled trial. *Journal of the American Medical Association, 278*, 644–652.

Klebanov, P. K., Brooks-Gunn, J., Chase-Lansdale, P. L., and Gordon, R. A. (1997). Are neighborhood effects on young children mediated by features of the home environment? In J. Brooks-Gunn, G. J., Duncan, and J. L. Aber (Eds.), *Neighborhood poverty: Vol. 1. Context and Consequences for Children* (pp. 79–118). New York: Russell Sage Foundation.

Klebanov, P. K., Brooks-Gunn, J., and Duncan, G. J. (1994). Does neighborhood and family poverty affect mothers' parenting, mental health, and social support? *Journal of Marriage and the Family, 56*, 441–455.

Klebanov, P. K., Brooks-Gunn, J., McCarton, C., and McCormick, M. C. (1998). The contribution of neighborhood and family income to developmental test scores over the first three years of life. *Child Development, 69*, 1420–1436.

Klebanov, P. K., Brooks-Gunn, J., and McCormick, M. C. (1994b). Classroom behavior of very low birthweight elementary school children. *Pediatrics, 94*(5), 700–708.

Klebanov, P. K., Brooks-Gunn, J., and McCormick, M. C. (in press). Maternal coping strategies and emotional distress: Results of an early intervention program for low birthweight young children. *Developmental Psychology.*

Knitzer, J. (in press). Early childhood mental health services: A policy systems development perspective. In J. P. Shonkoff and S. J. Meisels (Eds.), *Handbook of Early Childhood Intervention* (2nd ed.). New York: Cambridge University Press.

Korenman, S., and Miller, J. E. (1997). Effects of long-term poverty on physical health of children in the National Longitudinal Survey of Youth. In G. J. Duncan and J. Brooks-Gunn (Eds.), *Consequences of Growing up Poor* (pp. 70–99). New York: Russell Sage Foundation.

Kupersmidt, J. B., Griesler, P. C., DeRosier, M. E., Patterson, C. J., and Davis, P. W. (1995). Childhood aggression and peer relations in the context of family and neighborhood factors. *Child Development, 66*, 350–375.

Lally, R. J., Mangione, P. L., and Honig, A. S. (1988). The Syracuse University Family Development Research Program: Long-range impact of an early intervention with low-income children and their families. In D.R. Powell (Ed.), *Advances in Applied Developmental Psychology: Vol. 3. Parent Education as Early Childhood Intervention: Emerging Directions in Theory, Research, and Practice* (pp.79–104). Norwood, NJ: Ablex.

Lamborn, S. D., Dornbusch, S. M., and Steinberg, L. (1996). Ethnicity and community context as moderators of the relations between family decision making and adolescent adjustment. *Child Development, 67*, 283–301.

Lara, S. L., McCabe, L. M., and Brooks-Gunn, J. (2000). From horizontal to vertical management models: A qualitative look at Head Start staff strategies for addressing behavior problems [Special Issue on "Mental Health and Head Start"]. *Early Education and Development 2* (3), 283–306.

Larson, C. P. (1980). Efficacy of prenatal and postpartum home visits on child health and development. *Pediatrics, 66*, 191–197.

Lee, K., and Brooks-Gunn. (under review). *Maternal conceptions of development and social skills: Its consequences on children's outcomes.*

Lee, V. E., Brooks-Gunn, J., Schnur, E., and Liaw, F. (1990). Are Head Start effects sustained? A longitudinal follow-up comparison of disadvantaged children attending Head Start, no preschool, and other preschool programs. *Child Development, 61*, 495–507.

Lee, V. E., and Loeb, S. (1995). Where do Head Start enrollees end up? One reason why preschool effects fade out. *Educational Evaluation and Policy Analysis, 17*, 62–82.

Leventhal, T., and Brooks-Gunn, J. (2000). The neighborhoods they live in: The effects of neighborhood residence upon child and adolescent outcomes. *Psychological Bulletin, 126*, 309–337.

Leventhal, T., and Brooks-Gunn, J. (in press). Changing neighborhoods and child well-being: Understanding how children may be affected in the coming century. *Advances in Life Course Research.*

Leventhal, T., Brooks-Gunn, J., and Kamerman, S. (1997). Communities as place, face, and space: Provision of services to poor, urban children and their families. In J. Brooks-Gunn, G.J. Duncan, and J. L. Aber (Eds.), *Neighborhood Poverty: Policy Implications in Studying Neighborhoods: Vol. 2. Policy Implications in Studying Neighborhoods* (pp. 182–205). New York: Russell Sage Foundation.

. Children i⌐ Development, public policy, and practice. In
), *Handbool⌐d Psychology: Vol. 4. Child Psychology in*
⌐–210). New⌐hn Wiley and Sons, Inc.

Brooks-Gu⌐ld Roth, J. (in press). What are good child out-
⌐ornton (Ed.⌐*Well-Being of Children and Families: Research*
Ann Arbor.⌐niversity of Michigan Press.

⌐oals Panel.⌐. *The National Education Goals Report: Building*
⌐*ners, 1998.*⌐ington, DC: U.S. Government Printing Office.

Care Resea⌐etwork (1997). Poverty and patterns of child care.
⌐ and J. Bro⌐unn (Eds.), *Consequences of Growing up Poor* (pp.
York: Russ⌐age Foundation.

X., Wang, ⌐., and Caughy, M. (1997). Neighborhood risk factors
⌐eight in Balt⌐re: A multilevel analysis. *American Journal of Public*
⌐1113–1118.

⌐rode, J., He⌐rson, C. R., Kitzman, H., Powers, J., Cole, R., Sidora,
⌐, Pettitt, L.⌐., and Luckey, D. (1997). Long-term effects of home
⌐naternal lif⌐course and child abuse and neglect: Fifteen-year follow-
⌐mized trial⌐*Journal of the American Medical Association, 278,* 637–

⌐erson, C. R., Chamberlin, R., and Tatelbaum, R. (1986a). Preventing
⌐nd neglect. A randomized trial of nurse home visitation. *Pediatrics, 78,*

⌐erson, C. R., Chamberlin, R., and Tatelbaum, R. (1988). Improving the
⌐levelopment of socially disadvantaged mothers: A randomized trial of
⌐visitation. *American Journal of Public Health, 78,* 1436–1445.

⌐rson, C., and Kitzman, H. (1994). Does prenatal and infancy nurse home
⌐ave enduring effects on qualities of parental caregiving and child health
⌐nonths of life? *Pediatrics, 93,* 89–98.

⌐nderson, C. R., Kitzman, H., and Cole, R. (1995). Effects of prenatal and
⌐arse home visitation on surveillance of child maltreatment. *Pediatrics, 95,*

⌐ienderson, C. R., Kitzman, H. J., Eckenrode, J. J., Cole, R. E., and Tatel-
⌐. C. (1999). Prenatal and infancy home visitation by nurses: Recent find-
⌐*ure of Children, 9*(1), 44–65.

⌐Henderson, C. R., Tatelbaum, R., and Chamberlin, R. (1986b). Improving
⌐very of prenatal care and outcomes of pregnancy: A randomized trial of
⌐ome visitation. *Pediatrics, 77,* 16–28.

⌐ and Kitzman, H. (1993). Review of research on home visiting for pregnant
⌐ and parents of young children. *Future of Children, 3,* 53–92.

⌐D., Culp, A. M., and Ware, L. M. (1988). Intervention challenges with ado-
⌐t mothers and their infants. *Psychiatry, 51,* 236–241.

⌐Greer, S., and Zuckerman, B. (1988). Double jeopardy: The impact of poverty
⌐rly child development. *Pediatric Clinics of North America, 35,* 1227–1240.

⌐iel, J. C., and Seltzer, D. A. (1989). New parents as teachers: Evaluation of an
⌐ parent education program. *Early Childhood Research Quarterly, 4,* 1–18.

⌐iel, J. C., Lambson, T., and Yarnell, V. (1991). *Second wave study of the Par-*
⌐*as Teachers Program: Final Report.* Research and Training Associates, Inc.

⌐, W. W., Spillman, R. E., and King, R. (1996). Consequences of family literacy
⌐adults and children: Some preliminary findings. *Journal of Adolescent and Adult*
⌐*eracy, 39*(7), 558–565.

Lewit, E. M., and Bake
    children. *Future of*
Lewit, E. M., and Baker
    139.
Liaw, F., and Brooks-Gu
    children's cognitive a
    chology, 23(4), 360–37
Lieberman, A. F., Weston,
    outcome with anxiously
Linver, M. R., Brooks-Gunn,
    tional Health as Mediators
    Children's Cognitive Abil.
    376–378.
Loeber, R. (1990). Development
    linquency. *Clinical Psycholog*
Love, J. M., Aber, L., and Brooks-
    Progress Toward Achieving t
    Mathematica Policy Research, I
Lyons-Ruth, K., Connell, D. B., Gr
    social risk: Maternal depression
    development and security of attach.
Madden, J., O'Hara, J., Levenstein, P.
    home program on mother and child.
Marmot, M. G., and Shipley, M. J. (199
    persist after retirement? 25 year follc
    study. *BioMedical Journal, 313*(7066)
Marmot, M. G., Shipley, M. J., and Rose, G
    nations of a general pattern. *Lancet, i,* 1
Marmot, M. G., Smith, G., Stansfeld, S., Pat
    ner, E., and Feeney, A. (1991). Health in
    Whitehall II study. *Lancet, 337,* 1387–139
Massey, D. S., and Eggers, M. L. (1990). The
    concentration of poverty, 1970–1980. *Ame*
    1188.
Mathematica Policy Research, Inc. (1999). *Over*
    and Evaluation Project. Princeton, NJ: Mathe
McCormick, M. C., and Brooks-Gunn, J. (1989).
    cents. In H. Freeman and S. Levine (Eds.),
    347–380). Englewood Cliffs, NJ: Prentice Hall.
McCormick, M. C., Brooks-Gunn, J., Workman-Dan
    (1992). The health and developmental status of
    school age. *Journal of the American Medical Asso*
McKey, R. H., Condelli, L., Granson, H., Barrett, B.
    (1985). *The Impact of Head Start on Children, Fe*
    Report of the Head Start Evaluation, Synthesis, and
    DC: CSR.
McLoyd, V. C. (1990). The impact of economic hardship
    Psychological distress, parenting, and socioeconomic
    ment, 61, 311–346.

214

McLoyd, V. C. (1998
    W. Damon (Ed
    Practice (pp. 13
Moore, K., Evans, J.
    comes? In A. T
    and Data Needs
National Education
    a Nation of Lea
NICHD Early Child
    In G. J. Duncar
    100–131). New
O'Campo, P., Xue,
    for low birthw
    Health, 87(7),
Olds, D. L., Ecken
    K., Morris, P
    visitation on
    up of a rando
    643.
Olds, D. L., Hend
    child abuse a
    65–78.
Olds, D. L., Hend
    life-course
    nurse home
Olds, D., Hende
    visitation l
    at 25–50 m
Olds, D. L., He
    infancy n
    365–372.
Olds, D. L., P
    baum, R
    ings. *Fu*
Olds, D. L.,
    the del
    nurse h
Olds, D. L.
    wome
Osofsky, J
    lesce
Parker, S.
    on e
Pfannens
    earl
Pfannens
    ent
Phillibe
    for
    Li

Lewit, E. M., and Baker, L. G. (1994). Child indicators: Race and ethnicity—Changes for children. *Future of Children, 4*(3), 134–144.

Lewit, E. M., and Baker, L. S. (1995). School readiness. *Future of Children, 5*(2), 128–139.

Liaw, F., and Brooks-Gunn, J. (1994). Cumulative familial risks and low-birthweight children's cognitive and behavioral development. *Journal of Clinical Child Psychology, 23*(4), 360–372.

Lieberman, A. F., Weston, D. R., and Pawl, J. H. (1991). Preventive intervention and outcome with anxiously attached dyads. *Child Development, 62,* 199–209.

Linver, M. R., Brooks-Gunn, J., and Kohen, D. (1999). Parenting Behavior and Emotional Health as Mediators of Family Poverty Effects Upon Young Low Birthweight Children's Cognitive Ability. *Annals of the New York Academy of Sciences, 896,* 376–378.

Loeber, R. (1990). Development and risk factors of juvenile antisocial behavior and delinquency. *Clinical Psychology Review, 10,* 1–41.

Love, J. M., Aber, L., and Brooks-Gunn, J. (1994). *Strategies for Assessing Community Progress Toward Achieving the First National Educational Goal.* Princeton, NJ: Mathematica Policy Research, Inc.

Lyons-Ruth, K., Connell, D. B., Grunebaum, H. U., and Botein, S. (1990). Infants at social risk: Maternal depression and family support services as mediators of infant development and security of attachment. *Child Development, 61,* 85–98.

Madden, J., O'Hara, J., Levenstein, P. (1984). Home again: Effects of the mother-child home program on mother and child. *Child Development, 55,* 636–647.

Marmot, M. G., and Shipley, M. J. (1996). Do socioeconomic differences in mortality persist after retirement? 25 year follow-up of civil servants from the first Whitehall study. *BioMedical Journal, 313*(7066), 1177–1180.

Marmot, M. G., Shipley, M. J., and Rose, G. (1984). Inequalities in death-specific explanations of a general pattern. *Lancet, i,* 1003–1006.

Marmot, M. G., Smith, G., Stansfeld, S., Patel, C., North, F., Head, J., White, L., Brunner, E., and Feeney, A. (1991). Health inequalities among British civil servants: The Whitehall II study. *Lancet, 337,* 1387–1393.

Massey, D. S., and Eggers, M. L. (1990). The ecology of inequality: Minorities and the concentration of poverty, 1970–1980. *American Journal of Sociology, 95*(5), 1153–1188.

Mathematica Policy Research, Inc. (1999). *Overview of the Early Head Start Research and Evaluation Project.* Princeton, NJ: Mathematica Policy Research, Inc.

McCormick, M. C., and Brooks-Gunn, J. (1989). Health care for children and adolescents. In H. Freeman and S. Levine (Eds.), *Handbook of Medical Sociology* (pp. 347–380). Englewood Cliffs, NJ: Prentice Hall.

McCormick, M. C., Brooks-Gunn, J., Workman-Daniels, K., Turner, J., and Peckham, G. (1992). The health and developmental status of very low birthweight children at school age. *Journal of the American Medical Association, 267*(16), 2204–2208.

McKey, R. H., Condelli, L., Granson, H., Barrett, B., McConkey, C., and Plantz, M. (1985). *The Impact of Head Start on Children, Families, and Communities: Final Report of the Head Start Evaluation, Synthesis, and Utilization Project.* Washington, DC: CSR.

McLoyd, V. C. (1990). The impact of economic hardship on black families and children: Psychological distress, parenting, and socioeconomic development. *Child Development, 61,* 311–346.

McLoyd, V. C. (1998). Children in poverty: Development, public policy, and practice. In W. Damon (Ed.), *Handbook of Child Psychology: Vol. 4. Child Psychology in Practice* (pp. 135–210). New York: John Wiley and Sons, Inc.

Moore, K., Evans, J., Brooks-Gunn, J., and Roth, J. (in press). What are good child outcomes? In A. Thornton (Ed.), *The Well-Being of Children and Families: Research and Data Needs.* Ann Arbor, MI: University of Michigan Press.

National Education Goals Panel. (1998). *The National Education Goals Report: Building a Nation of Learners, 1998.* Washington, DC: U.S. Government Printing Office.

NICHD Early Child Care Research Network (1997). Poverty and patterns of child care. In G. J. Duncan and J. Brooks-Gunn (Eds.), *Consequences of Growing up Poor* (pp. 100–131). New York: Russell Sage Foundation.

O'Campo, P., Xue, X., Wang, M. C., and Caughy, M. (1997). Neighborhood risk factors for low birthweight in Baltimore: A multilevel analysis. *American Journal of Public Health, 87*(7), 1113–1118.

Olds, D. L., Eckenrode, J., Henderson, C. R., Kitzman, H., Powers, J., Cole, R., Sidora, K., Morris, P., Pettitt, L. M., and Luckey, D. (1997). Long-term effects of home visitation on maternal life course and child abuse and neglect: Fifteen-year follow-up of a randomized trial. *Journal of the American Medical Association, 278,* 637–643.

Olds, D. L., Henderson, C. R., Chamberlin, R., and Tatelbaum, R. (1986a). Preventing child abuse and neglect: A randomized trial of nurse home visitation. *Pediatrics, 78,* 65–78.

Olds, D. L., Henderson, C. R., Chamberlin, R., and Tatelbaum, R. (1988). Improving the life-course development of socially disadvantaged mothers: A randomized trial of nurse home visitation. *American Journal of Public Health, 78,* 1436–1445.

Olds, D., Henderson, C., and Kitzman, H. (1994). Does prenatal and infancy nurse home visitation have enduring effects on qualities of parental caregiving and child health at 25–50 months of life? *Pediatrics, 93,* 89–98.

Olds, D. L., Henderson, C. R., Kitzman, H., and Cole, R. (1995). Effects of prenatal and infancy nurse home visitation on surveillance of child maltreatment. *Pediatrics, 95,* 365–372.

Olds, D. L., Henderson, C. R., Kitzman, H. J., Eckenrode, J. J., Cole, R. E., and Tatelbaum, R. C. (1999). Prenatal and infancy home visitation by nurses: Recent findings. *Future of Children, 9*(1), 44–65.

Olds, D. L., Henderson, C. R., Tatelbaum, R., and Chamberlin, R. (1986b). Improving the delivery of prenatal care and outcomes of pregnancy: A randomized trial of nurse home visitation. *Pediatrics, 77,* 16–28.

Olds, D. L., and Kitzman, H. (1993). Review of research on home visiting for pregnant women and parents of young children. *Future of Children, 3,* 53–92.

Osofsky, J. D., Culp, A. M., and Ware, L. M. (1988). Intervention challenges with adolescent mothers and their infants. *Psychiatry, 51,* 236–241.

Parker, S., Greer, S., and Zuckerman, B. (1988). Double jeopardy: The impact of poverty on early child development. *Pediatric Clinics of North America, 35,* 1227–1240.

Pfannenstiel, J. C., and Seltzer, D. A. (1989). New parents as teachers: Evaluation of an early parent education program. *Early Childhood Research Quarterly, 4,* 1–18.

Pfannenstiel, J. C., Lambson, T., and Yarnell, V. (1991). *Second wave study of the Parents as Teachers Program: Final Report.* Research and Training Associates, Inc.

Philliber, W. W., Spillman, R. E., and King, R. (1996). Consequences of family literacy for adults and children: Some preliminary findings. *Journal of Adolescent and Adult Literacy, 39*(7), 558–565.

Phillips, D., and Bridgman, A. (Eds.). (1995). *New Findings on Children, Families, and Economic Self-Sufficiency.* Washington, DC: National Academy Press.

Phillips, M., Brooks-Gunn, J., Duncan, G. J., Klebanov, P., and Crane, J. (1998). Family background, parenting practices, and the black-white test score gap. In C. Jencks and M. Phillips (Eds.), *The Black-White Test Score Gap* (pp. 103–145). Washington, DC: Brookings Institution Press.

Phillips, D., Voran, M., Kisker, E., Howes, C., and Whitebook, M. (1994). Child care for children in poverty: Opportunity or inequity? *Child Development, 65,* 472–492.

Power, C., Matthews, S., and Manor, O. (1998). Inequalities in self-rated health: Explanations from different stages of life. *Lancet, 351,* 1009–14.

Quint, J. C., Polit, D. F., Bos, H., and Cave, G. (1994). *New Chance: Interim Findings on a Comprehensive Program for Disadvantaged Young Mothers and Their Children.* New York: Manpower Demonstration Research Corporation.

Reynolds, A. J. (1997, April). *Long-Term Effects of the Chicago Child-Parent Center Program Through Age 15.* Paper presented at the biennial meeting of the Society for Research on Child Development, Washington, DC.

Richardson, D. C., and Brown, M. (1997). *Family Intergenerational Literacy Model. Fact Sheet and Impact Statements.* Oklahoma City, OK: National Diffusion Network.

Richman, N., Stevenson, J., and Graham, P. J. (1975). Prevalence of behaviour problems in three year old children: An epidemiological study in a London borough. *Journal of Child Psychology and Psychiatry, 12,* 5–33.

Rimm-Kaufman, S. E., Pianta, R. C., and Cox, M. J. (in press). Teachers judgments of problems in the transition to kindergarten. *Early Childhood Research Quarterly.*

Ross, G. S. (1984). Home intervention for premature infants of low-income families. *American Journal of Orthopsychiatry, 54,* 263–270.

Roundtable on Comprehensive Community Initiatives for Children and Families. (1997). *Voices from theFfield: Learning from the Early Work of Comprehensive Community Initiatives.* Washington, DC: The Aspen Institute.

Royce, J. M., Darlington, R. B., and Murray, H. W. (1983). Pooled analyses: Findings across studies. In *As the Twig is Bent. . . . Lasting Effects of Preschool Programs.* Hillsdale, NJ: Lawrence Erlbaum Associates.

Sameroff, A. J., Seifer, R., Barocas, R., Zax, M., and Greenspan, S. (1987). Intelligence quotient scores of 4-year old children: Social and environmental risk factors. *Pediatrics, 79,* 343–350.

Sampson, R. J. (1997). Collective regulation of adolescent misbehavior: Validation results from eighty Chicago neighborhoods. *Journal of Adolescent Research, 12*(2), 227–244.

Sampson, R. J., Raudenbush, S. W., and Earls, F. (1997). Neighborhoods and violent crime: A multilevel study of collective efficacy. *Science, 277,* 918–924.

Schweinhart, L.J., Barnes, H. V., Weikart, D. P., Barnett, W. S., and Epstein, A. S. (1993). *Significant Benefits: The High/Scope Perry Preschool Study Through Age 27.* Ypsilanti, MI: High/Scope Press.

Seitz, V., and Apfel, N. H. (1994). Parent-focused intervention: Diffusion effects on siblings. *Child Development, 65,* 677–683.

Sinclair, J. J., Pettit, G. S., Harrist, A. W., Dodge, K. A., and Bates, J. E. (1994). Encounters with aggressive peers in early childhood: Frequency, age differences, and correlates of risk behaviour problems. *International Journal of Behavioral Development, 17*(4), 675–696.

Smith, J. R., Brooks-Gunn, J., and Klebanov, P. K. (1997). Consequences of living in poverty for young children's cognitive and verbal ability and early school achievement. In G. J. Duncan and J. Brooks-Gunn (Eds.), *Consequences of Growing up Poor* (pp. 132–189). New York: Russell Sage Foundation.

St. Pierre, R., Goodson, B., Layzer, J., and Bernstein, L. (1994). *National Evaluation of the Comprehensive Child Development Program: Report to Congress.* Cambridge, MA: Abt Associates Inc.

St. Pierre, R. G., Ricciuti, A., and Creps, C. (1998). *Synthesis of State and Local Even Start Evaluations: Draft.* Cambridge, MA: Abt Associates.

St. Pierre, R. G., and Swartz, J. P. (1995). The Even Start Family Literacy Program. In S. Smith (Ed.), *Advances in Applied Developmental Psychology: Vol. 9. Two Generation Programs for Families in Poverty: A New Intervention Strategy* (pp. 37–66). Norwood, NJ: Ablex Publishing Corporation.

St.Pierre, R., Swartz, J., Gamse, B., Murray, S., Deck, D., and Nickel, P. (1995). *National Evaluation of the Even Start Family Literacy Program: Final Report.* Washington, DC: U.S. Department of Education.

Starfield, B. (1992a). Child and adolescent health status measures. *The Future of Children, 2*(2), 25–29.

Starfield, B. (1992b). Effects of poverty on health status. *Bulletin of the New York Academy of Medicine, 68,* 17–24.

Tao, F., Gamse, B., and Tarr, H. (1998). *National Evaluation of the Even Start Family Literacy Program: 1994–1997 Final Report.* Washington, D.C.: U.S. Department of Education, Planning and Evaluation Service.

Tao, F., Swartz, J., St. Pierre, R., and Tarr, H. (1997). *National Evaluations of the Even Start Family Literacy Program.* Washington, DC: U.S. Department of Education.

Travers, J., Nauta, M. J., Irwin, N. (1982). *The Effects of a Social Program: Final Report of the Child and Family Resource Program's Infant-Toddler Component.* Cambridge, MA: Abt Associates Inc.

Wachs, T. D., and Gruen, G. E. (1982). *Early Experience and Human Development.* New York: Plenum Press.

Wagner, M. M., and Clayton, S. L. (1999). The Parents as Teachers program: Results from two demonstrations. *Future of Children, 9*(1), 91–115.

Weiss, C. H. (1995). Nothing as practical as a good theory: Exploring theory-based evaluation for Comprehensive Community Initiatives for children and families. In J. P. Connell, A. C. Kubisch, L. B. Schorr, and C. H. Weiss (Eds.), *New Approaches to Evaluating Community Initiatives: Vol. 1. Concepts, Methods, and Contexts* (pp. 65–92). Washington, DC: The Aspen Institute.

Werner, E. E., and Smith, R. S. (1982). *Vulnerable but Invincible: A Longitudinal Study of Resilient Children and Youth.* New York: Adams.

Whitebook, M., Howes, C., and Phillips, D. A. (1990). *Who Cares? Child Care Teachers and the Quality of Care in America: Final Report, National Child Care Staffing Study.* Oakland, CA: Child Care Employee Project.

World Health Organization (1978). *Primary Health Care.* Report of the International Conference on Primary Health Care, Alma Ata, USSR. Geneva: World Health Organization.

Yoshikawa, H. (1995). Long-term effects of early childhood programs on social outcomes and delinquency. *Future of Children, 5*(3), 51–75.

Zill, N., Resnick, G., McKey, R. H., Clark, C., Connell, D., Swartz, J., O'Brien, R., and D'Elio, M. (1998). *Head Start Program Performance Measures: Second Progress Report.* Washington, DC: U.S. Department of Health and Human Services.

Preadolescent and Adolescent Influences on Health

Cheryl L. Perry, Ph.D.

Adolescence, the stage of development between childhood and adulthood, and approximately the second decade of the life cycle, was first presented as a subject for scientific inquiry only a century ago by G. Stanley Hall (1904) and was characterized as the developmental stage of "storm and stress." Manifestations of storm and stress included adolescents' tendencies to contradict their parents, experience mood changes, and engage in antisocial behaviors (Arnett, 1999). After nearly 100 years of research, this picture of adolescence seems both limited in scope and too broad a generalization (even if the tendencies are still familiar and relevant). In particular, as we enter the twenty-first century, adolescence is viewed as part of life span development, with continuities from childhood, unique developmental challenges and tasks, and implications for adulthood. Adolescence is also examined within context, so that adolescence is seen as a dynamic developmental process that is influenced by proximal and distal social environments. The manifestation of this developmental process can be seen in adolescents' behaviors, behaviors that cause considerable concern in American society. Thus, this paper attempts to provide a snapshot of the dynamics of adolescence and adolescent behavior, what factors influence the adoption or maintenance of behavior, examples of how changes in behavior

Dr. Perry is professor, Division of Epidemiology, School of Public Health, University of Minnesota. This paper was prepared for the symposium, "Capitalizing on Social Science and Behavioral Research to Improve the Public's Health," the Institute of Medicine, and the Commission on Behavioral and Social Sciences and Education of the National Research Council, Atlanta, Georgia, February 2–3, 2000.

have been achieved, and the implications of this research for healthful adolescent development in the twenty-first century.

DEVELOPMENTAL INFLUENCES DURING ADOLESCENCE

The Dynamics of Adolescence

Adolescence is a time of metamorphosis. Some changes are biologically—and others socioculturally—determined. The latter are often referred to as the "developmental tasks" of adolescence and are discussed in the next section. From a biological viewpoint, during adolescence, children become adults. They experience puberty, acquire reproductive capabilities, and secondary sexual characteristics, and grow to reach full adult height (Susman, 1997). Hormones are primarily responsible for the biological changes in adolescence (Hopwood et al., 1990; Buchanan et al., 1992). The primary hormones begin to differ by gender at about age 11 (Susman, 1997), with the most dramatic biological changes occurring during early adolescence, between the ages of 12 and 16 (Tanner, 1978). The timing of biological changes differs by gender and racial or ethnic group (Money, 1980; Susman, 1997). On average, females mature 1–2 years ahead of males, and reach their full adult height by age 14 (Marshall and Tanner, 1970); African American females mature even earlier than white females (Kaplowitz and Oberfield, 1999). Interestingly, the age of pubertal onset, as measured by menarche in females, has become younger throughout the past century, most likely due to improved nutritional intake (Wyshak and Frisch, 1982; Hopwood et al., 1990; Herman-Giddens et al., 1997; Kaplowitz and Oberfield, 1999).

Hormonal changes have been "blamed" for their influence on adolescent mood and behavior. Recent provocative research suggests that hormones do influence behavior; the direct effects are small but stable and may be mediated by the social environment (Buchanan et al., 1992; Brooks-Gunn et al., 1994; Susman, 1997). For example, Olweus et al. (1988) found that boys with relatively higher testosterone levels were more likely to become aggressive if they were provoked. Thus, some boys might never exhibit aggressive behavior in a social environment without provocation. Similarly, Udry (1988) found that testosterone levels were a strong predictor of sexual involvement among young adolescent girls. This relationship was attenuated or eliminated by their involvement in sports or having a father in the home. Again, the hormone-behavior relationship existed, but did not manifest in particular environments.

Substantial research has been done on the timing of puberty relative to peers (Silbereisen et al., 1989). Early maturers are differentiated from on-time and late maturers in terms of the development of secondary sexual characteristics, height velocity, and menarche (Silbereisen and Kracke, 1993). Most studies in the United States have found that early maturation among boys is positive for them, with early maturers reporting more confidence, less dependence, and greater popularity than their peers (Nottelmann et al., 1990; Petersen and Taylor, 1980).

For girls, the picture is more mixed, with studies showing more negative affect, lower self-esteem, and greater contact with deviant peers among early-maturing females (Brooks-Gunn, 1988; Brooks-Gunn and Warren, 1989; Silbereisen and Kracke, 1993). However, these associations with early maturation may be mediated by social, cultural, and socioeconomic factors (Clausen, 1975; Silbereisen and Kracke, 1993). For example, in homes where the father was absent, females matured at significantly younger ages (Surbey, 1990). Also, closeness of mothers to their daughters was associated with slower maturational development among girls (Steinberg, 1989; Silbereisen and Kracke, 1993). Thus, even for biological changes that are examined relative to age-mates or peers, the rate of maturation may be mediated by the social context of the adolescent.

Changes in cognitive processes also occur during preadolescence and adolescence. These changes may be the result of continued brain growth during adolescence and more efficient neural processing (Crockett and Petersen, 1993; Brownlee, 1999). Pre- and young adolescents are concrete thinkers (Blum and Stark, 1985). To experience something, concrete thinkers need to see, feel, touch, smell, or hear it, rather than being able to rely on abstract descriptions. By middle or late adolescence, formal operational or abstract thinking is possible (Blum and Stark, 1985; Crockett and Petersen, 1993). Rather than strictly relying on experience, abstract thinkers can generate hypotheses, possible solutions, rules, and ideals using symbols and abstractions. Adolescents can learn to arrange pieces of information into multiple combinations, understand words that are not reflecting real life, think about thinking, and conceptualize ideals. However, many adolescents may not attain formal operational thinking levels (Flavell, 1985) or may revert to concrete thinking in unfamiliar or emotionally charged situations (Hamburg, 1986).

The level and sophistication of thinking has important implications for adolescents' behavior. As concrete thinkers, young adolescents cannot truly comprehend abstract concepts such as "health" or project the outcomes of their current behavior into the future (Blum and Stark, 1985). Even as adolescents learn to think abstractly, this occurs through trial, error, and experimentation. Messages about health behaviors, therefore, that rely on long-term consequences or fail to provide relevant and concrete examples will have little meaning to many adolescents. Likewise, adolescents may misperceive that others are preoccupied with them, confusing their own thoughts with the thoughts of others (Arnett, 1992). This can lead to a sense of invulnerability and participation in reckless behavior (Elkind, 1967; Arnett, 1992). The lack of rational and abstract thinking abilities leaves adolescents particularly vulnerable to messages from the social environment that portray some behaviors, such as smoking, drinking, and sexual behavior, as potentially functional and rewarding (Perry, 1999a), even though the longer-term consequences may be dire for them.

In terms of biology, then, adolescents are maturing earlier than in previous times; so physically, they become adults at a younger age, yet do not have the cognitive capabilities to cope with a complex social environment as adults. Additionally, the changes within and between adolescents are not synchronous—there are enormous differences in the rate and timing of these changes. This sets the stage for a kind of "prolonged" adolescence, during which young people are expected to become prepared to become adults in our society, mentally and socially, yet with physical bodies that are already mature. This tension may contribute to some of the problems associated with adolescents, such as precocious or unprotected sexual behavior, which have a biological as well as a social etiology (Hine, 1999).

The "Tasks" of Adolescence

Puberty and the associated physical and cognitive changes are perhaps the only parts of adolescence that are culture-free; that is, adolescents worldwide experience these metamorphoses. Yet, as the examples above indicate, even biological changes interact with social environmental factors to influence adolescent behavior. Still, from within specific cultures and subcultures come the answers to the question, What are adolescents supposed to achieve during this developmental stage? These achievements are considered the psychosocial tasks of adolescence (Havighurst, 1972; Hill, 1980; Hill and Holmbeck, 1986; Masten et al., 1995).

For adolescents in the United States, the specific tasks have been described in psychological and social terms, and include accomplishments related to autonomy, sexuality, attachment, intimacy, achievement, and identity (Havighurst, 1972; Hill and Holmbeck, 1986). Adolescents strive to accomplish these tasks (1) to become independent and able to make their own decisions, (2) to understand their changing social-sexual roles and sexual identity, (3) to change their relationships with their parents, (4) to transform acquaintances into deeper friendships, (5) to focus their ambitions on their futures, and (6) to transform their images of themselves to accommodate their physical and psychosocial changes. These tasks have been characterized as the driving forces in adolescent behavior (Havighurst, 1972). Adolescents are more likely to think of themselves as being adults when these psychosocial tasks, rather than particular events, such as high school graduation, are achieved (Scheer et al., 1996). However, these tasks may also be changing in scope and interpretation as greater cultural and ethnic diversity is found throughout the United States.

Recent research has examined the continuity and coherence of developmental tasks in childhood and adulthood, using sophisticated methodologies. Masten et al. (1995) defined developmental tasks as "broad dimensions of effective behavior evaluated in comparison to normative expectations for people of a given age" (p. 1636). They observed three areas of competence in late childhood and adolescence (academic achievement, rule-abiding conduct, and getting along with peers) and two additional areas that emerge in adolescence (holding a job for pay and romantic relationships). Using structural equation modeling techniques, they examined the coherence of these areas of competence and demonstrated the continuity of the three childhood areas into late adolescence. Notably, rule-abiding or rule-breaking conduct in late childhood strongly predicted such conduct in adolescence, thus "demonstrating the stability of anti-social behavior by late childhood" (Masten et al., 1995, p. 1654). Adolescent conduct problems in adolescence were also associated with lower academic achievement and being able to hold a job. This suggests that focusing attention on early conduct problems and competencies in childhood should be beneficial for academic and job achievements, as well as reducing conduct problems, in adolescence (Moffitt, 1993; Masten et al., 1995). Additionally, this study strongly underlines the need to examine early precursors to some adolescent behaviors as an avenue to early prevention and intervention.

The promotion of positive youth development is complementary to the goal of healthfully achieving the developmental tasks of childhood or adolescence (Catalano et al., 1999). As Bronfenbrenner and Morris (1998, p. 996) note:

> Especially in its early phases, but also throughout the life course, human development takes place through progressively more complex reciprocal interactions between an active, evolving, biopsychological human organism and the person, objects, and symbols in its immediate external environment. To be effective, the interaction must occur on a fairly regular basis over extended periods of time.

The authors then describe the developmental process for adolescents as a series of interactions within particular social contexts—families, schools, neighborhoods, and communities—that progressively shape young people and their behavior (Jessor, 1993). These interactions, and resulting behavior, are also determined by the time in history and the culture of the young person (Elder, 1974; Hine, 1999; Vega and Gil, 1998). Thus, the way in which youth develop, and whether they have the resources and environmental supports to achieve developmental tasks, serve as the background against which healthful or unhealthful behavior in the United States should be examined.

Threats to Health Among Preadolescents and Adolescents

Adolescence is the developmental period that has been characterized as the physically healthiest in the life cycle: adolescents have outgrown most of the childhood infectious diseases and are not yet old enough to suffer from the chronic diseases that plague adults (Ozer, Brindis et al., 1998). Yet, even a brief review of adolescent health issues suggests otherwise. Adolescents engage in a range of behaviors that impact their current and future risk of injury or premature death; many of these behaviors have their onset during this developmental stage (Blum, 1998; Perry, 1999b).

The United States continues to lead the developed world in adolescent mortality rates, even though there has been a significant decline in these rates in the past 10 years (Blum, 1998). Unintentional injuries, homicide, and suicide are the primary causes of adolescent mortality, accounting for four out of five deaths (Ozer et al., 1998). Among these deaths, more than half are due to motor vehicle collisions (CDC, 1993), and a third of those are related to alcohol use.

Fortunately, the fatal collision rate has been declining since 1980, primarily due to environmental and policy changes such as improved highway construction, safer cars, and a uniform 21-year-old drinking age (Blum, 1998). Of recent concern is the startling increase in the young adolescent suicide rate, which has risen 35% since 1990 among those 10 to 14 years old (Blum, 1998).

The mortality rates among adolescents show notable differences by ethnic or racial group and gender. Although there has been a 14% decline overall in mortality rates over the past decade, there has been a 17% decline among white males, and an 11% increase among African American males (Blum, 1998). Also among African American males, death from homicide is nine times higher than among white males, reaching epidemic proportions (Ozer et al., 1998). Suicide rates, however, are higher among white adolescents. In general, males are more likely than females to die from any type of injury (although females are more likely to attempt suicide, males are more likely to commit suicide). Among those 15–19 years old, males are about two times more likely to die of any unintentional injury and five times more likely to die of homicide or suicide than females (Ozer et al., 1998).

The major causes of adolescent morbidity are also behavioral, with differences in subgroups of adolescents who engage in particular risk-related behaviors, as shown in Table 1. The behaviors of most concern are tobacco, alcohol, and drug use; precocious and unprotected sexual behavior; unhealthful eating practices; sedentariness; violence; and deviant, risky behaviors. Although these are being reviewed separately, there is significant covariation among these health behaviors, making some adolescents at increased risk for a range of short-term and long-term health problems (Jessor and Jessor, 1977; U.S. DHHS, 1994; Lytle et al., 1995).

Drug Use

The gateway drugs—tobacco, alcohol, and marijuana—require particular attention during adolescence because they are initiated during this period; cause injury, illness, and death during adolescence and in adulthood; and are precursors to "heavier" drugs such as cocaine, hallucinogens, and heroin (U.S. DHHS, 1994). In addition, the majority of adolescents in the United States engages in each of these behaviors before they graduate from high school—74% have tried a cigarette, 84% have had an alcoholic drink, and 52% have used marijuana (CDC, 1998). Clearly, societal and personal decisions concerning tobacco, alcohol, and marijuana use are an integral part of examining adolescence in the United States, as the entire population can be considered "at risk."

There are important differences in tobacco, alcohol, and marijuana use by ethnic or racial group and gender. These differences are particularly important to note as the United States continues to become increasingly multicultural (Vega and Gil, 1998). Overall, African American adolescents smoke, drink, and use illegal drugs at significantly lower rates than white and Hispanic adolescents

TABLE 1 Adolescent Health Risk Behaviors: Prevalence and Risk Status by Racial or Ethnic Group and Gender

Behavior	Prevalence (%) 9th–12th Grades	Greatest Risk by Race or Ethnicity[a]					By Gender[b]	
		Whites	Blacks	Hispanics	Asians	American Indians	Female	Male
Smoking (past month)	36.4%	X				X	X	X
Alcohol use (past month)	50.8%	X				X	X	X
Marijuana use (past month)	25.2%	X				X	X	X
Sexual intercourse (ever)	48.4%		X			X		X
Pregnant or made pregnant (ever)	6.5%			X			X	
High fat intake (past day)	37.7%		X	X				X
Insufficient fruits and vegetables (past day)	70.7%						X	
Dieting (past month)	39.7%	X		X			X	
Insufficient vigorous activity (<3 times in past week)	36.2%		X	X			X	
Fighting (past year)	36.6%		X	X	X			X
Carried weapon (past month)	18.3%			X				X
Carried gun (past month)	5.9%		X	X				X
Riding with a drinking driver (past month)	36.6%			X				
Drove after drinking (past month)	16.9%	X	*	X				X

[a]Does not take into account subcategories of racial or ethnic groups or acculturation. Data are from the 1997 Youth Risk Behavior Surveillance System for white, black, and Hispanic high school students (CDC, 1998). Data for American Indians and Asians come from the Monitoring the Future Study and other non-nationally representative studies (U.S. DHHS, 1998) for drug use, sexual behavior, and fighting only.

[b]Males were significantly more likely than females to report smokeless tobacco use and episodic heavy drinking, and to initiate sexual intercourse at a younger age.

CDC, 1998). White students are more likely to smoke cigarettes than Hispanic students (U.S. DHHS, 1998). National data from American Indian and Asian students have only recently become available from the Monitoring the Future study (Johnston et al., 1998; U.S. DHHS, 1998), and rates of tobacco, alcohol, and marijuana use among American Indians are consistently as high or higher than among white students, while Asian students' use was similar to African Americans and lower than other racial or ethnic groups (Beauvais, 1992; Gruber et al., 1996; Neumark-Sztainer et al., 1996; Epstein et al., 1998; U.S. DHHS, 1998; Chen et al., 1999).

Several authors make note, and this is relevant across all behaviors, that the classification of ethnic or racial groups masks significant differences within groups, such as differences between American Indian tribal groups and whether they live on or off reservation lands, and subcategories of Asians (Chinese, Japanese, Korean, etc.) and Hispanics (Gruber et al., 1996; Epstein et al., 1998; Bell et al., 1999). The classifications also do not account for levels of acculturation among recent immigrant groups and differences in drug use based on level of acculturation (Vega et al., 1993; Chen et al., 1999).

Gender differences in drug use among adolescents are also noted. Males are more likely than females to use smokeless tobacco, engage in episodic heavy drinking, and use marijuana (CDC, 1998), but females now are equally as likely as males to use other substances. Finally, rates of tobacco and marijuana use increased substantially in the 1990s, although that increase may now have leveled off; the increases occurred across all ethnic or racial and gender groups (Johnston et al., 1998).

Sexual Behavior

Sexual behavior also has its debut in adolescence, with two out of three adolescents reporting having had sexual intercourse prior to high school graduation (CDC, 1998). This sexual activity incurs the risk of pregnancy and infectious diseases, which have significant social, economic, and physical health ramifications (Ozer et al., 1998). Overall, males are more likely to initiate sexual activity earlier than females (Ozer et al., 1998; Upchurch et al., 1998). Black adolescents are more likely than Hispanics and whites to have initiated sexual intercourse, to have had more sexual partners, and to have had begun sexual activity at a younger age (Ozer et al., 1998). Asian adolescents appear to begin sexual activity later (Upchurch et al., 1998; Bell et al., 1999) and American Indian adolescents earlier, than do whites (Gruber et al., 1996; Neumark-Sztainer et al., 1996), but these were not nationally representative samples.

In contrast with drug use behavior, sexual behaviors have declined in prevalence since the early 1990s. This decline occurred after a steady two-decade increase in the percentage of adolescents engaging in sexual activity. The decline is associated with changes in related sexual behaviors. About 75% of teens report using contraceptives at first intercourse (up from 62% in 1988) and 54% report using condoms (Ozer et al., 1998). Condom use is more prevalent among younger adolescents, while the use of birth control pills increases with age (Kann et al., 1996). Whites are more likely than blacks or Hispanics to use contraception at first intercourse (Ozer et al., 1998).

Similarly, rates of pregnancy also appear to be declining after dramatic increases since the 1970s. Still, 12% of all females ages 15–19 become pregnant each year—19% of black females, 13% of Hispanic females, and 8% of white females. Notably, of the 1 million adolescents who become pregnant each year, most (85%) report that their pregnancy was unintended (Ozer et al., 1998). More than half of these pregnancies result in births and more than a third result in abortion (Ozer et al., 1998). The birth and abortion rates among black and Hispanic adolescent females is about double that of white females. About 70% of these births occur out of wedlock. And, unfortunately, for the children of teenage mothers, there are also consequences—lower birth weight, lower cognitive and socioemotional functioning, and greater likelihood of death during the first year of life. These outcomes are linked to lower socioeconomic status, which is both a predictive factor for teenage pregnancy and an outcome of the limited opportunities and instability that are associated with being a teenage mother (Irwin and Shafer, 1992).

Sexual behavior may also result in sexually transmitted diseases, with adolescents at greater risk for these infectious diseases than any other age group (Irwin and Shafer, 1992). Chlamydia is most prevalent, affecting about 2% of female adolescents ages 15–19 (CDC, 1997). Gonorrhea and syphilis decreased in the 1990s; both of these infectious diseases are most prevalent among black adolescents (Ozer et al., 1998). Finally, although AIDS cases among adolescents are rare because of the 10-year incubation period, many adolescents become infected with HIV that will become manifest when they are in their 20s. Young adults, ages 20–29, comprise nearly one-fifth of the AIDS cases in the United States. Thus, teenage sexual behavior, while now appearing to decline, has increased dramatically in the past 25 years. The outcomes—teenage pregnancy, abortion, out-of-wedlock births, sexually transmitted diseases, and HIV—have significant implications for the future for these young people as well as for the next generation of young people in the United States.

Eating Behaviors and Physical Activity

In comparison with drug use, violence, and sexual behavior, eating and exercise may seem like relatively benign behavioral areas for adolescents. Yet eating behaviors significantly affect growth during adolescence (Story, 1992), are the second leading cause of cancer (World Cancer Research Fund, 1997), and track from adolescence to adulthood (Perry et al., 1997). Sedentary behavior contributes to obesity and chronic diseases, with activity patterns forming and tracking in childhood and adolescence (Kelder et al., 1994; U.S. DHHS, 1996; Troiano and Flegal, 1998).

The primary diet-related concerns among adolescents involve overconsumption of fat, overweight and obesity, unsafe weight-loss methods, eating disorders, and insufficient intake of fruits, vegetables, and calcium. Most adolescents do not eat a diet that meets the U.S. Department of Agriculture's (1995) *Guidelines for Americans* (Perry et al., 1997). National data show that children and adolescents, more than any other age group, are more likely to exceed the recommendations for fat and saturated fat, with more than 90% of adolescent males consuming more than 30% of their calories from fat (Kennedy and Goldberg, 1995). Black adolescents are more likely than Hispanic and white adolescents to eat more servings of high-fat food per day (CDC, 1998).

On the other hand, adolescents are not eating sufficient fruits and vegetables—only 29% eat the recommended five servings per day. Males are more likely to eat five or more servings per day than females (32% vs. 26%). In addition, the low intake of calcium is of special concern to female adolescents. Females ages 12–19 consume only 68% of the recommended amount of calcium, making it unlikely that many adolescent females will reach their full biological potential for bone mass development and making it more likely they will experience osteoporosis later in life (Kennedy and Goldberg, 1995).

Obesity is now considered the most prevalent nutrition-related health problem of children and adolescents in the United States. (Dietz, 1998). The current generation of children and adolescents will grow up to be the most obese adults in American history (Hill and Trowbridge, 1998). Although many of the outcomes of being obese or overweight during adolescence are social, such as discrimination and more negative self-images, there is now evidence that being obese contributes to earlier physical maturation, increased blood lipid levels, and diabetes among adolescents (Dietz, 1998). The Third National Health and Nutrition Examination Survey (NHANES III) data indicate that about 11% of children and adolescents ages 6–17 are overweight, compared with a 5% expected prevalence (Troiano et al., 1995; Troiano and Flegal, 1998). In other words, the prevalence of overweight children and adolescents has doubled in the past 20 years. About one-quarter of children and adolescents are in the upper 85th percentile for weight, compared with the expected prevalence of 15%, placing them at risk for continued overweight and obesity into adulthood. Black and Hispanic females were more likely to be overweight than white females (Troiano and Flegal, 1998). However, females were not more likely to be overweight than males, except among African Americans (Troiano and Flegal, 1998). In the 1997 Youth Risk Behavior Survey, 27% of high school students reported they were overweight (CDC, 1998). Females were more likely to report being overweight than males; and Hispanic students were more likely than black students to report being overweight (CDC, 1998). Notably, perceptions of being overweight did not necessarily correspond with objective measures, particularly between the genders.

Correspondingly, about 40% of high school students report trying to lose weight in the past month—60% of females and 23% of males. Healthy weight loss behaviors (such as moderate exercise, decrease in snacks, decrease in fat intake) are more prevalent than unhealthy practices (such as fasting, diet pills, laxatives, vomiting; French et al., 1995). Still, nearly 5% of students reported taking laxatives or vomiting, and 5% had taken diet pills, to control weight in the month prior to the survey (CDC, 1998); 30% of students dieted and 52% exercised to control their weight. Females were significantly more likely to use all forms of dieting methods than males. The Hispanic and white students were more likely than black students to diet or exercise to lose weight; Hispanic students were more likely than white students to use laxatives or vomiting to control weight (CDC, 1998). In one study, American Indian females were more likely to engage in unhealthy weight loss practices than whites, while Asians were less likely (Neumark-Sztainer et al., 1996) Despite some evidence that African American females are heavier than Hispanic and white females, they are more likely to be satisfied with their weight and body image, and have a lower prevalence of eating disorders (Resnicow et al., 1997). The prevalence of eating disorders ranges from 1 to 5% among adolescent females and is associated with serious outcomes (Perry et al., 1997).

Physical activity significantly declines during adolescence for both males and females, despite the benefits of regular exercise for weight control, mental health, and the prevention of osteoporosis, cardiovascular diseases, and cancer (Kelder et al., 1995; U.S. DHHS, 1996; CDC, 1998; Kohl and Hobbs, 1998). Overall, 64% of high school students participate in vigorous physical activities on three or more days each week, with male students (72%) more likely to exercise than female students (54%), and white students (67%) more likely than Hispanic (60%) or black (54%) students to participate in vigorous physical activity (CDC, 1998). Still, 14% of young people reported no recent physical activity.

Violence and Other Risky Behaviors

Violent behavior by adolescents both on school property and in the community has been a topic of national discussion and debate for the past few years, prompted by several tragic school shootings. In fact, adolescents in the United States have relatively easy access to weapons and guns (Komro, 1999); overall, 18% of high school students reported having carried a weapon during the month prior to the survey and 6% reported having carried a gun (CDC, 1998). Males (28%) were more likely than females (7%) to have carried a weapon and a gun; black (9%) and Hispanic (10%) students were more likely than white (4%) students to have carried a gun (CDC, 1998). Nearly half of male students and one-fourth of female students had been in a physical fight during the year prior to the survey. Black, Hispanic, and Asian students were more likely than white students to have been in a physical fight on school property (Hill and Drolet, 1999). Reported physical fighting decreases as students get older (CDC, 1998). Still, among older males ages 18–21, about one-third reported carrying a gun in the month prior to the survey (Ozer et al., 1998).

Adolescents engage in other behaviors that put them at risk for unintentional injury, including driving after drinking, driving at high speeds, riding with a driver who has been drinking, and not using seat belts, motorcycle helmets, or bicycle helmets. Since motor vehicle collisions are the primary cause of death for adolescents, these behaviors are of considerable concern during this period. For example, 37% of high school students reported having ridden in the past month with a driver who had been drinking; the percentage increased as students got older (CDC, 1998). Nearly 17% of students reported that they had driven a vehicle after drinking in the prior month; this was more likely for male students (21%), white (19%) and Hispanic (18%) students, and older students (CDC, 1998). Among students who rode motorcycles and bicycles, 36 and 88%, respectively, had never or rarely worn a helmet. And nearly 20% of students rarely or never use their seat belts when riding in a vehicle driven by someone else. All of these behaviors increase the risk of injury or death by motor vehicle collision.

This collection of health-related adolescent behaviors is not exhaustive. Other behaviors such as skin tanning, body piercing, prolonged listening to loud music, shoplifting, joining gangs, watching television, and playing video games, are engaged in by adolescents and may influence their short-term or long-term health. Still other behaviors, such as attending school and church, participating in extracurricular activities, helping at home, and doing volunteer work, are not usually considered "health related" yet may have a substantial influence on these behaviors. Other areas of adolescent health, such as the quality of health care for adolescents and adolescent mental health issues, are now beginning to be explored. National data on a range of other adolescent behaviors by gender and racial or ethnic subgroups, particularly with sufficient samples of Asian and American Indian adolescents, would be useful and important in order to provide a more complete picture of what adolescents are "doing."

In fact, the types of behaviors "of concern" vary across time, place, and culture. Some of the behaviors are most problematic during adolescence and would be "normal" for adults, such as moderate alcohol use and sexual behavior. Other behaviors are problematic at any age, yet have their onset or have a higher prevalence during adolescence, such as tobacco and marijuana use, violence, and eating disorders. Still other behaviors, such as eating and activity patterns, truly reflect the society at large and are problematic because of their long-term health consequences. Still, the behaviors have meaning to young people and represent adolescents' response to what the society-at-large "teaches" them to become to fit into adult society. Thus, the focus in etiology is on the social environment, rather than the adolescents themselves, because it is within the social context that behavior change can take place and interventions appear to be most efficacious.

The Etiology of Health Behaviors in Adolescence

The reasons American adolescents engage in health-compromising behaviors have been the focus of several academic and popular books, as well as hundreds of journal articles, over the past several years (DiClemente et al., 1996; Schulenberg et al., 1997; Jessor, 1998; Brownlee, 1999; Hine, 1999; Vida, 1999). Factors that influence adolescent behavior have been examined within and between multiple domains, including genetic and biological factors, social and environmental factors, and personal factors (Flay and Petraitis, 1994; Pe-

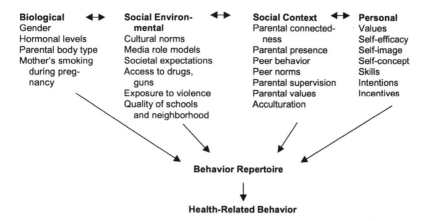

FIGURE 1. The etiology of adolescent health behavior: Examples of predictive factors. SOURCE: Adapted from Petraitis et al. (1995), Flay and Petraitis (1994), and Perry (1999b).

traitis et al., 1995; Jessor, 1998; Perry, 1999b), as shown in Figure 1. Recently, several researchers have begun to use the terms "risk" and "protective" factors within these domains to define those etiological factors that increase or decrease, respectively, the occurrence of health-compromising behavior (or, conversely, health-enhancing behavior; Catalano et al., 1999). Still, what is most important for subsequent intervention development is the identification of factors that are predictive of adolescent health-related behaviors, because those factors, whether they increase risk or are protective, explain why adolescents engage in particular behavior(s) and become the foundation for intervention design (Perry, 1999b). In particular, it is important to identify factors that are strongly predictive of subsequent behavior; that is, they account for a large proportion of the variance in health-related behavior (Baranowski et al., 1999). The factors also need to be amenable to intervention: they should be able to be promoted, changed, reduced, or eliminated through social, educational, political, and/or public health efforts.

A common thread in the recent etiological research, which parallels the trend in intervention development, is increased attention to the social environment and social context of adolescents. This has not been the exclusive focus of recent etiological research; some very interesting genetic and individual-level work has also been done (Kandel, 1998). Still, since adolescents are in a state of social transition, their social contexts acquire new and important meanings and influence. Adolescents are searching the social environment for clues on how to accomplish their developmental tasks, and peers, family members, other adults, and media all become "mentors" in the quest for development. How the environment "fits" the needs of adolescents becomes critical to successful development (Eccles et al., 1993). Thus, important concerns in analyzing adolescent health behavior are the type, frequency, and source of messages and opportunities that young people are exposed to, particularly as these relate to decisions about becoming an adult in this society. Aspects of the social environment that have received new or renewed research attention in the past decade, and have important implications for intervention design, include the role of social capital, poverty, media and advertising, family relations, work, school, and peers in the health behaviors of young people.

Social Capital

One of the most important new perspectives on adolescent behavior is the notion of social capital (Coleman, 1988). Similar to financial capital (wealth) and human capital (skills and knowledge), which are quantifications of personal acquisitions (or access) associated with more successful development, social capital is "accrued" by the types of available relationships in a young person's community, neighborhood, school, or family (Coleman, 1988; Furstenberg and Hughes, 1995; Runyan et al., 1998). Important components of social capital are social structures that effectively promote positive social norms and appropriate role models, provide useful information, are trustworthy in meeting obligations, and have definite expectations (Coleman, 1988). Runyan and colleagues (1998) demonstrated that social capital, in particular church affiliation, the perception of personal social support, and neighborhood support, was strongly associated with children's well-being. Furstenberg and Hughes (1995) found, in a longitudinal study of higher-risk adolescents, that most measures of social capital during adolescence were predictive of success in young adulthood. Significant predictors included having support from one's mother, living with one's biological father, having parents' help with homework, having a strong helping network in the community, frequently visiting with close friends, and the quality of the school (Furstenberg and Hughes, 1995). Social capital was also found to be a significant macrolevel predictor of firearm homicide rates at the state level (Kennedy et al., 1998), even when controlling for other factors. Thus, the social context and social environment, as measured by particular attributes within the family, neighborhood, school, and community, can facilitate healthy development of adolescents by providing greater opportunities, more stability, consistent norms, access to human capital, and social support.

As an example of the influence of social capital at the community level, we assessed social environmental factors related to young adolescents' alcohol use as part of a 20-community prevention trial, Project Northland (Perry et al., 1996). It was interesting to us that there was such a large amount of variability in alcohol use among eighth grade students among the 20 communities, since they appeared very homogeneous—small rural and mostly white communities in northeastern Minnesota. The prevalence of past-month alcohol use among eighth grade students, however, ranged from 16 to 43% in these communities. By creating scales with indicators of norms, role models, opportunities, and social support that were aggregated at the community level, we found that community-level norms and role models accounted for nearly 50% of the variance in eighth grade alcohol use rates (Roski et al., 1997). This guided our efforts during the second phase of Project Northland: to create appropriate community norms concerning high schools students' alcohol use (Perry, Williams et al., 2000).

Poverty

Social capital may be able to mediate some of the effects that poverty and the lack of financial resources have on young people's health (Kennedy et al., 1998). But the effects of poverty are still far-reaching in our society. In 1998, children made up 39% of the poor but only 26% of the total population. The poverty rate for children (18.9% in 1998) is higher than for any other age group, although lower than its recent peak of 22.7% in 1993. In 1998, 13.5 million children were poor. Black and Hispanic households were twice as likely to live in poverty than were white households (U.S. Census Bureau, 1999), although socioeconomic status does not explain all racial or ethnic group differences in health status (Lillie-Blanton and Laveist, 1996).

Poverty exerts its influence as an environmental and social factor in many aspects of young people's health behavior. Poor, urban youth are exposed to high rates of community violence that influence subsequent aggressive and violent behaviors and depression (Farrell and Bruce, 1997; Gorman-Smith and Tolan, 1998). Young people who are poor are less likely to finish school and are more likely to experience conduct problems and conflicts with peers (Lerner and Galambos, 1998). Young people living in poverty are more likely to experience hunger, fewer food options, and less fresh produce (Crockett and Sims, 1995), undermining their nutritional health. Thus, adolescents who live in poverty often live in poor communities, where exposure to drugs and violence is high and where access to healthful resources also may be limited. Thus, the elimination of poverty for children and adolescents must be an important goal for those involved in improving the health of young people. Secondarily, efforts should be directed toward alleviating those influences within poor communities that exacerbate health problems for young people, such as by providing more-than-adequate educational opportunities, restricting access to weapons, and offering supervised afterschool and weekend activities, free and reduced-fat meals at schools, and mentoring programs.

Media and Advertising

Among young people of all socioeconomic strata, the increase in exposure to electronic communications has been a notable characteristic of the past decade, and its effects on adolescent behavior are beginning to be documented. Media that have been studied include television, radio, movies, and music videos. Less is known about the effects of video games and Internet exposure. One problem in assessing the impact of media has been that it is both distal and all pervasive—very few young people are not exposed, so there are often inadequate samples of "controls." Thus, studies have examined levels or types of media use and may underestimate the total effect of media on behavior.

The most widely evaluated relationship is between various forms of media and subsequent or concurrent aggressive or violent behavior, although media has been shown to be associated with a range of health-risk behaviors (Wood et al., 1991; Klein et al., 1993; Strasburger, 1997; Willis and Strasburger, 1998). On average, adolescents watch about 3–6 hours of television and listen to the radio about 6 hours each day (Klein et al., 1993; Strasburger, 1997). Strasburger (1997) notes that during an average year, an adolescent is exposed to "10,000 acts of violence, 15,000 sexual innuendoes, jokes, and behaviors, and 20,000 commercials, including 1,000–2,000 beer and wine advertisements" on television (p. 404). For example, 22.4% of music television videos (MTVs) and 20.4% of rap videos portrayed violence (DuRant et al., 1997). And the result of these portrayals is clear: the greater the exposure to media violence, the more likely is subsequent aggressive behavior among adolescents (Committee on Communications, 1995; Strasburger, 1997; Strasburger, 1998; Willis and Strasburger, 1998).

There is increasing evidence of the effects of advertising on young people's behavior (U.S. DHHS, 1994; Committee on Communications, 1995; Perry, 1999a). In the last decade, substantial research has focused on the relationship between cigarette advertising or promotional activities and smoking by young people, which became very important in the tobacco litigations in states around the country (Perry, 1999a): 86% of adolescents smoke the most advertised brands of cigarettes—Marlboro, Camel, and Newport—while they are smoked by only 32% of adults (CDC, 1994). Adolescents, much more than adults, respond to new advertising campaigns, such as the introduction of women's brands in the late 1960s (Pierce et al., 1994) and Joe Camel in the early 1990s (CDC, 1994). The themes of advertising correspond with the tasks of adolescence, displaying images of independence, peer approval, and sexuality (U.S. DHHS, 1994). It is not a coincidence that the cigarette brands smoked by adolescents are significantly more likely to be in magazines with relatively high youth readership (King et al., 1998). Youth have high exposure to cigarette advertising and the greater the exposure, the more likely that the adolescent is a smoker (Schooler et al., 1996). One study found that adolescents were three times more sensitive to cigarette advertising than adults and, that a 10% increase in advertising dollars resulted in a 3% increase in market share among adults and a 9.5% increase among adolescents (Pollay et al., 1996). Finally, Pierce and colleagues (1998) found that when nonsmoking, not-susceptible adolescents had a favorite cigarette advertisement or said they would be willing to use a promotional item, they were two to three times more likely to progress to smoking 3 years later, accounting for 34% of the reason that adolescents began to smoke. Perhaps the relationship between the tobacco industry and adolescents is best summarized by an R.J. Reynolds researcher who wrote: "Realistically, if our company is to survive and prosper, over the long term, we must get our share of the youth market" (Teague, 1973).

The influence of media and advertising on adolescent behavior warrants further research, especially as the forms of electronic media change rapidly and as young people continue to be the targets of advertising. The recent removal of cigarette billboards is one example of an intervention to reduce exposure to health-compromising media messages. Similarly strong action might be warranted with violent portrayals on television (Strasburger, 1997). Children and adolescents might also benefit by learning media literacy skills to identify, analyze, investigate, and refute what is being portrayed in media and advertising (Kubey and Baker, 1999).

Family Relationships

The families of the twenty-first century bear little resemblance to those 100 years ago. It is now normative for adolescents to have experienced the separation or divorce of their parents, to have both parents working outside the home, to prepare meals for themselves, and to have several hours of unsupervised time after school (Fuchs and Reklis, 1992; Crockett and Sims, 1995). These changes, among others, provide considerable new challenges for healthy development among adolescents.

The National Longitudinal Study on Adolescent Health (Resnick et al., 1997) provides important quantification of the ways families influence adolescent behavior. Adolescents were found to be less at risk for emotional distress, violence, and drug use if they perceived themselves as connected to their parents: that is, they experienced feelings of warmth, love, and caring from their parents. This was more important than the actual presence of parents during key times of the day, although that was a significant factor as well. Parents having high expectations for their adolescents concerning school attainment was also associated with healthier and less risky behavior. On the other hand, adolescents in homes with easy access to tobacco, alcohol, drugs, and guns were more likely to be involved in violence and drug use themselves (Resnick et al., 1997).

The notion of "family capital" was developed by assessing parents' human, social, and education capital (Marjoribanks, 1998). Family capital included parents' own educational attainment, parent–child activities and homework time together, parents' aspirations for their children in terms of education and work, and parents' values on independence and learning. Family capital was found to have a moderate to large association with adolescents' academic performance and aspirations for the future (Marjoribanks, 1998).

Several researchers have examined the changes in family relationships in the context of adolescent development and developmental tasks. Associated with the task of striving for autonomy, parent-adolescent conflict has received considerable attention, although most empirical examinations show little evidence of increased conflict after early adolescence, even though there may be more emotional intensity in the conflict from early to middle adolescence (Laursen et al., 1998). When conflict exists, it is primarily concerning mundane issues such as cleaning one's room or curfew, which may be attempts by adolescents to define themselves or make their own decisions (Eccles et al., 1993). Adolescents express a desire for more participation in the decisions made in the family, and when allowed to participate more fully, there were positive results in school motivation and self-esteem (Eccles et al., 1993). Likewise, adolescents who received support from their parents to be more autonomous were less likely to initiate sexual intercourse; those who were more emotionally attached to their parents were less likely to engage in fighting and drug use (Turner et al., 1993). Finally, adolescents who perceived that their parents knew their friends, where they went at night, how they spent their money, what they did with their free time, and where they were most afternoons, were less likely to begin to use drugs (Steinberg et al., 1994).

Fostering competence and positive connections between adolescents and their parents seems critical to promoting healthy development (Resnick et al., 1997; Masten and Coatsworth, 1998). These connections may include involvement in activities together, having clear expectations about school performance, allowing greater decision making for the adolescent within the family, and communicating about how, where, and with whom the adolescent is spending time. As available time becomes an issue, these connections may need to be provided by the larger community of caring adults.

Schools, Work, and Peers

Adolescents usually progress from the relatively protected and connected environment of the elementary school to the more impersonal middle or junior high school and then to the larger high school in their communities. During this time, they also begin to work for income, and most have some formal paid work experience by the end of high school (Mortimer and Johnson, 1998). In both of these environments, same-age peers are found, and relationships are formed that carry increasing influence on adolescents' behavior. Thus, understanding how to create school and work environments that foster positive behavior among adolescents is an important area of research (Dryfoos, 1994; 1998).

Eccles and colleagues (1993) argue that the transition to middle or junior high school and the new school environment do not "fit" the developmental needs of young adolescents. They point out that in contrast to the young adolescent's need for greater participation in decision making, junior high classrooms have increased emphasis on teacher control and discipline, and fewer opportunities for decision making than did elementary school classrooms. The junior high classrooms also were less personal and had more negative teacher-student relationships; they tended to teach whole-class tasks rather than small groups; the teachers felt less effective and taught at a lower cognitive level yet they judged students' competence at a higher standard, compared with elementary schools. Thus, the junior high environment is likely, by its structure, to adversely impact the motivation and connectedness that young adolescents have for school (Eccles et al., 1993). Simmons and Blyth (1987) found a greater drop in grades among those who made the transition to a junior high school than among those who remained in a K–8 school.

Connectedness to school is critical since it is the major formal socializing institution in the United States. In the National Longitudinal Study on Adolescent Health, connectedness to school was a primary protective factor for adolescents for a variety of risk-related behaviors (Resnick et al., 1997). School can serve as a major protective factor because adolescents who are involved with school spend much of their time and attention on schoolwork and extracurricular activities, plus associate with peers who are also involved with school, and thus have fewer opportunities to engage in other health-compromising behaviors (Steinberg and Avenevoli, 1998). Disengagement from school may also lead to more intensive involvement in the workplace (Steinberg and Avenevoli, 1998), with its own implications for health behaviors. The development of a positive, caring school setting has been shown to be associated with a more positive school climate, better student behavior, and higher overall academic achievement (Haynes and Comer, 1990).

Although most adolescents work part-time during high school, Steinberg et al. (1993) found that those who worked more than 20 hours a week were more likely to become disengaged from school, engaged in delinquency and drug use and more disengaged from parents and to have decreased self-reliance. Most of these effects remained even after they stopped working. However, Mortimer and Johnson (1998) point out that work experiences during high school are a preparation for later work involvement and can be seen as a transition between school and work, with the formation of important attitudes and orientation about work. Employed adolescents learn new skills in their jobs, their income increases in the years following high school, and the experiences expand the adolescents' repertoire to manage the demands of home, school, work, and others (Mortimer and Johnson, 1998). For adolescents working less than 20 hours a week, grades and school dropout rates were improved by their involvement with a job. In their thoughtful review of long-term outcomes of working by adolescents, Mortimer and Johnson (1998) conclude that working is associated with drinking during high school (for both males and females) and smoking during high school and later (for females), but with very few other negative outcomes and with positive outcomes related to later employment.

In the context of school, work, and community, peer relationships are formed and assume an important if not central role in adolescents' social world. Peer relationships that are positive are associated with achievement, job competence, and higher sense of self-worth (Masten et al., 1995). Peer rejection is associated with aggressive behaviors and maladjustment (Masten and Coatsworth, 1998). In adolescence, peers can exert influences that can be positive rather than negative, such as encouraging academic achievement or participation in extracurricular activities (Komro et al., 1994). Peers may also encourage deviant or risky behaviors; adolescents who begin to associate with drug-using peers, for example, increase their drug use to match their peers (Steinberg et al., 1994).

Thus, the inclusion of the peer group as a part of health behavior interventions may be crucial for their success (Perry et al., 1989; Komro et al., 1996).

This brief review of some recent work in the etiology of adolescent health behaviors has focused on the social environment and social context of adolescents because of the great amount of research that is taking place in this area and because changes in the social environment are generally possible through intervention and may be critical for behavior changes of adolescents (Perry, 1999b). On one hand, the review indicates the need to "capitalize"—to improve the social, family, financial, and access-to-human capital for adolescents. However, although etiological research is the basis of intervention, intervention research demonstrates what is possible and how change can be achieved. Thus, larger changes need to be balanced by the reality of what can be accomplished in each domain of an adolescent's life and concerning which behaviors. The past two decades have provided considerable insight into these questions.

MAJOR INTERVENTION POINTS: CHANGING THE SOCIAL ENVIRONMENT

Intervention research has made considerable progress in the last quarter century. In 1975, for example, there were no school-based smoking prevention programs that had demonstrated reductions in smoking onset among adolescents (U.S. DHHS, 1994; Perry, 1999b). By 1994, meta-analyses had been written involving hundreds of studies and identifying which components of smoking prevention programs were associated with greater effectiveness in reducing onset and prevalence rates (U.S. DHHS, 1994). The expansion in prevention and intervention research involved the consistent use of theory to guide program development, process evaluation and measures of mediating variables to determine which components were most critical, and increasingly sophisticated research designs and methodologies to examine the effects of these programs. Prevention and intervention research is now considered a scientific inquiry that is independent from etiology, health education, community psychology, or social psychology, yet builds on the findings from these disciplines (and others). While epidemiological, biological, and etiological research on adolescence has a rich history and serves as a foundation for intervention programs, intervention research is concerned with trying to define, measure, and analyze changes in behavior, with its own unique set of methodological challenges (Eddy et al., 1998).

This section reviews examples of prevention-intervention research on how changes in the social environment or social context of adolescents were made. These recent intervention experiences provide models for how more general adolescent health behavior change might be approached, even when the intervention addresses only a particular behavior. Some intervention approaches may be relevant for improving a range of adolescent behaviors, and these include strategies such as changing community educational policies, improving the school environment, providing after school activities, or increasing the general social or life skills of adolescents (Botvin et al., 1995; Dryfoos, 1998). Other interventions need to be behavior specific, such as reducing access to tobacco or alcohol, providing opportunities for physical activity, or increasing the choices of foods that are served at school. What is notable about recent adolescent health behavior intervention research is that the interventions tend to be multicomponent, with changes in several social contexts; multiyear, theory driven; and evaluated using sophisticated research designs and analysis methodologies. Thus, intervention research is where the answer to, How? can truly be addressed.

Increasing Social Capital—The Seattle Social Development Project

The question of when to begin to intervene to reduce health-compromising behaviors in adolescence has not been thoroughly investigated, even though developmental research suggests continuity from childhood for several domains of concern (Masten et al., 1995). Hawkins and colleagues (1999) reported the effects at age 18 of a multicomponent, multiyear intervention with 18 urban public elementary schools, which took place when the targeted cohort was in the first through sixth grades. The intervention consisted of (1) annual in-service training with teachers on proactive classroom management, interactive teaching, and cooperative learning; (2) social competence training for students when they were in first and sixth grades; and (3) parent training classes when students were in first through third and fifth through sixth grades to provide skills to promote academic achievement of their children and reduce their risk of drug use. These interventions were intended to increase the social bonds that children had to school and their families.

At age 18, students exposed to the entire intervention reported less involvement in violence, sexual intercourse, and heavy drinking, and greater commitment to school and better academic achievement (Hawkins et al., 1999). Students exposed to the intervention only in fifth and sixth grades did not demonstrate these long-term outcomes, suggesting that an intervention embedded in the entire elementary school experience can have significant and lasting effects on adolescent behavior. However, the intervention had the greatest effects on school-related and sexual behaviors. There were no effects on criminal behavior, smoking, alcohol use, marijuana use, or other drug use (except heavy drinking). This suggests that the social development approach might serve as a preliminary and even necessary step in promoting health among adolescents by creating an appropriate, positive, and consistent orientation toward schooling and achievement prior to and during adolescence (Catalano et al., 1999). But additional interventions appear to be needed to delay or prevent the onset of tobacco, alcohol, and other drug use.

Marketing Health—Prosocial Media, Counterads, and the Truth Campaign

The significant influence of media and marketing on adolescent consumer behavior suggests that these approaches might be used to improve health behavior as well. Flynn and colleagues (1992) demonstrated long-term reductions in smoking onset with adolescents when television and radio messages supplemented a school-based program. It is interesting that although the school and media programs shared similar themes, they were developed independently, so they were perceived by the students to be messages from multiple sources and reinforced the notion that smoking was not normative (U.S. DHHS, 1994).

Dorfman and Wallack (1993) point out that advertising strategies for health promotion include a range of strategies from person- to policy-oriented media, with public service announcements generally aimed at individual behavior change and counterads aimed at larger environmental or policy changes. The latter often suggest political action and are more likely to generate controversy. Ads that specifically targeted the tobacco industry executives, and questioned the marketing of a deadly product, were designed in California to change the perception that smoking is normative and acceptable, and to turn the public's attention to the tobacco industry, rather than smokers, as the cause of problems related to tobacco (Dorfman and Wallack, 1993). Targeting industry manipulation was also suggested by youth as being one of the most effective strategies for making smoking less normative (Goldman and Glantz, 1998).

This approach was taken one step further in Florida in an effort to reduce teen smoking. Using funds from its settlement with the tobacco industry, the "Truth" campaign was developed by Florida's teens during the Governor's Teen Tobacco Summit in March 1998. This was part of the larger Florida Tobacco Pilot Program, which had as one of its main goals to empower youth to lead community involvement against tobacco (Holtz, 1999). The advertising campaign focused on the tobacco industry, with teens demanding more honesty from the industry, including tobacco distributors, retailers, advertising agencies, and media associated with the industry. The Truth campaign included print and broadcast ads, a teen grassroots movement against tobacco use, school curricula, enforcement of retail sales restrictions, and the creation of a web site (www.wholetruth.com; Florida Department of Health, 1999). The ads used quotes or situations with tobacco executives and others to create rebellion among youth against the tobacco industry. For example, one ad portrayed an Academy Awards-like event "in downtown Hades" where an award was to be given for the most deaths in a single year (News America Digital Publishing, 1999). Suicide, illicit drugs, tobacco, and murder were contestants, and known mass killers such as Adolf Hitler were in the audience. Tobacco wins the award, and it is accepted by a clean-cut tobacco executive, who exclaims, "I want to thank all you smokers out there. This one is for you."

The Truth campaign resulted in significant declines in smoking among middle, junior high, and high school students from February 1998 to February

1999—a larger decrease than has been documented with any of the other large statewide campaigns and in sharp contrast to the level or increasing rates of smoking among adolescents nationwide (Clary, 1999; News America Digital Publishing, 1999). The combination of hard-hitting media—which some have argued is of questionable taste—extensive youth involvement, higher cigarette prices, and enforcement of youth access laws may all have contributed to the success of the campaign. Unfortunately, funding for the campaign was significantly reduced during its second year by the Florida legislature (Clary, 1999). Still, the campaign results suggest that media and advertising that is designed to attract the attention of youth, and uses some of the same methods as commercial advertising may have a significant impact on adolescent behavior.

Changing Community Norms—
The Tobacco Policy Options Program

Obtaining community involvement and changing community norms are critical to providing a social environment that supports the healthy development of adolescents (Hansen and Graham, 1991; Glanz et al., 1995; Perry et al., 2000). The short-term effects of school-based programs, for example, may be the result of behavior change that is inconsistent with the larger community norms, so that healthy behavior is not supported and reinforced after the program is completed. Longer-term effects for smoking prevention have generally involved changes in the larger community (Flynn et al., 1992; Perry et al., 1992; U.S. DHHS, 1994). However, a more systematic approach to community organizing around adolescent health has emerged in the past few years.

In the Tobacco Policy Options Program, 14 communities were randomly assigned to receive the intervention or to serve as a control (Forster et al., 1998). The goal of the intervention program was to reduce teenage access to tobacco, from stores and vending machines, by using a direct action community organizing model (Blaine et al., 1997). Community organizers were hired in each of the seven intervention communities and trained in organizing methods. These included doing extensive interviews ("one-on-ones") with community citizens representing a variety of sectors such as business, education, religion, government, service, and so forth. Each organizer conducted one-on-ones until there were no more nominations from those interviewed; this resulted in hundreds of interviews. Then, an "action team" was organized of people, with a personal commitment to do something about teenage smoking, who represented a variety of community sectors; the teams also had youth representatives. These action teams created action plans that involved policy changes at the community level concerning how to deal with commercial access to tobacco. The resulting actions included purchase attempts by adolescents to demonstrate ease in access, local media, presentations at meetings, and ordinance changes in all of the intervention communities over a period of 2–3 years. The intervention resulted in significant reductions in youth smoking over the period of the project and suggests the power of community normative change, since actual access to tobacco was not changed by the intervention (Forster et al., 1998). Direct action community organizing has been adapted for use in other interventions involving alcohol use and nutrition policies, as well as social access to tobacco (Perry et al., 2000; Wagenaar et al., 2000).

Connecting with Parents—The Adolescent Transitions Program

While parenting practices have repeatedly been identified as key etiological factors in adolescent health behavior development, effective interventions have only recently been forthcoming that are applicable to most or all parents. Parents are difficult to reach, since their involvement is voluntary and participation rates in organized activities tend to be low (Perry, 1999b). Still, when the topic is one that many parents are concerned about, such as drug use, or if their adolescent is involved in the presentation, or if young people bring activities home to complete with their parents, higher participation rates and more positive outcomes have been achieved (Williams and Perry, 1998).

The Adolescent Transitions Program (ATP) was a multicomponent program for parents of high-risk young adolescents (Andrews et al., 1995; Dishion and Andrews, 1995). ATP included a parent program that targeted family management practices and communication skills, and a teen program that targeted self-management and prosocial behavior. The parent program involved 12 weekly 90-minute sessions that were conducted by trained therapists and assisted by parents who had taken part in the program. Three additional sessions took place individually with each family. The parent program had a structured curriculum that focuses on skills related to monitoring their adolescent, positive reinforcement, limit setting, and problem solving, based on Patterson's (1982) research. The teen program provided skill development in self-monitoring and tracking, prosocial goal setting, developing positive peer environments, problem solving, and communications with peers and parents. The results of the parent program showed considerable promise—parent–child conflict was reduced as well as problem behaviors in school (Andrews et al., 1995). However, the teen program had long-term untoward effects of increasing tobacco use and problem behaviors, probably due to the closer associations among high-risk adolescents that the groups provided (Dishion and Andrews, 1995; Eddy et al., 1998).

Promoting Positive Peer Involvement—Project Northland

Project Northland was a randomized community trial to reduce the onset and prevalence of alcohol use among young adolescents in 24 school districts and surrounding communities (Perry et al., 1993). The three-year intervention program consisted of classroom-based curricula in sixth through eighth grades, parental education and involvement activities, peer leadership opportunities, and community-wide task force activities. Each year had a specific theme that corresponded to the developmental stage of the students, and brought together the four components of the intervention. In the first year, the focus was on parental involvement and parent–child communication (the Slick Tracy Program); the second-year focus was on peer influence and alternative activities (Amazing Alternatives!); the third-year focus was on community influence and involvement (PowerLines). At the end of eighth grade, students in the intervention communities had significantly reduced their alcohol use. Baseline nondrinkers, about two-thirds of the sample, additionally reported significant reductions in cigarette smoking and marijuana use (Perry et al., 1996).

Recent mediation analyses show that the important mediators of Project Northland's effect on alcohol use were changes in peer norms, peer influences to use alcohol, functional meanings of alcohol use, and risk-related attitudes and behaviors. Project Northland appears to have been most effective in changing the peer groups to be more prosocial and less supportive of alcohol use (Komro et al., in press).

Peer leadership permeated the Project Northland intervention, with increasing opportunities for involvement from young people over the course of the three years. In the sixth grade, the Slick Tracy Program was facilitated by the students both in the classrooms and at home. The students created and presented their projects at Slick Tracy Night, so the evening revolved around their ideas (Williams et al., 1995). In the seventh grade, elected students in each classroom were trained to conduct the eight-session classroom program. Having peers teach the Amazing Alternatives! curriculum had previously been shown to be critical to its success (Perry et al., 1989). Student volunteers also participated in teams that designed, developed, and implemented extracurricular social activities for their peers (Komro et al., 1994). The involvement of students in planning activities was shown to significantly reduce their alcohol use (Komro et al., 1996). In the eighth grade, students again acted as group leaders in the classroom and continued planning social activities. They also participated in producing a play in each of the communities and performed the play for other students, their parents, and community members (Perry et al., 1996). The active involvement of sixth through eighth grade students, then, was central to the design and implementation of Project Northland; the results demonstrate that such involvement can affect peer norms and behaviors, as well as associated problem behaviors, which is consistent with a recent meta-analysis of prevention programs (Black et al., 1998). Thus, in changing the social context for adolescents, we need to consider their roles and leadership in their own educational and social endeavors.

More comprehensive reviews of recent interventions around each of the adolescent health behaviors have been undertaken by the Centers for Disease Control and Prevention and others (Drug Strategies, 1996, 1998; Catalano et al., 1999; Perry, 1999b; U.S. DHHS, 1999; Komro and Stigler, in press). In addition, the science of intervention development has evolved considerably, so that there are now available resources to guide program design that is based on research, theory, and creativity (Cullen et al., 1998; Perry, 1999b). These five examples of interventions are a sampling of the types of recent research that seems particularly promising—interventions that significantly change the social context of adolescents to be supportive of their development and reduce their opportunities for health risk behaviors.

New Opportunities for Research and Intervention

Despite the successes noted above, there still exists a dire need for more large-scale intervention research to demonstrate that healthful behavior among adolescents can be achieved. There is much more that we know about the etiology of adolescent behavior than what we have been able to translate into effective intervention strategies. Thus, one opportunity that exists is to fund well-designed, large-scale, longitudinal intervention research that includes careful delineation and assessment of process, mediating, and outcome variables. This can lead to intervention research that serves three purposes: (1) the research can demonstrate whether or not a particular strategy or set of strategies is effective in changing targeted behaviors; (2) it can demonstrate how the changes were achieved, through mediation analyses; and (3) it can chart the course of development of the behaviors with and without intervention, so that etiological research becomes embedded in intervention. Intervention research, across the range of behaviors and social contexts of adolescents, should be given high priority to more quickly and efficiently move ahead the knowledge of how to achieve changes in the health and social behaviors of adolescents.

This review has revealed a significant mismatch in our society between the social contexts in which adolescents often find themselves and what they need to develop healthfully. Overall, adolescents need greater opportunities to learn social, emotional, and educational skills; more support and collaboration with adults; fewer hours spent unsupervised, alone, or in a place where they must be sedentary; less access to harmful substances, weapons, and images; and more access to positive, active, and healthful role models. This may require a national-level commitment to, and policies for, healthy youth development, so that schools have the resources to stay open and provide opportunities in the evenings and weekends; so that communities can provide safe transportation for adolescents if they do stay after school; so that all parents have the opportunity to learn how best to deal with their adolescents; so that youth have the mentors and opportunities to take increasing leadership roles in their communities; so that access for adolescents to drugs and weapons is eliminated; so that the national media are required to consider the violence of the messages they send; and so that schools or other groups who want to implement successful targeted programs have the financial resources to do so. Despite all the research on the "capital" of youth, it seems that not enough actual capital has been spent on increasing the social, educational, human, and family capital of adolescents in the United States.

Given the backdrop of greater attention to youth development, beginning early in children's lives and extending through adolescence, with strong federal and state support, there are specific areas of intervention research that are important to continue to guide this process. First, there needs to be more research on interventions with varied cultural and ethnic groups, and by gender, specifically concerning behaviors where they are at greater risk. This has already been forthcoming from various funding agencies, but needs to be underscored, given the high rates of some risk behaviors in these groups. Second, there needs to be research on timing of interventions. For example, long-term outcomes were observed for an eating pattern intervention that was implemented with third through fifth graders, but such outcomes have not been observed with drug use interventions (Nader et al., 1999). There may be targeted programs that will be most efficacious at particular times in a young person's life. Third, the types of competencies, skills, or opportunities for adolescents that might influence their behavior need to be more fully explored and expanded and included in intervention research, and might include self-management, communication, academic planning, character building, community organizing, and even spiritual skills. For example, in Project Northland, students' self-evaluation of their own wisdom (including harmony and warmth, intelligence, and spirituality scales) was significantly predictive of their alcohol, tobacco, and marijuana use and their violence at 12th grade (Jason et al., in press). These new areas may be alternative avenues or skills for adolescents, with multiple potential outcomes. Fourth, we must have greater knowledge of the needed competencies for schools, neighborhoods, families, clinics, and communities that work with and serve adolescents, and importantly, how these competencies can be taught, promoted, or disseminated. This is particularly critical for communities with varied ethnic or racial groups or with recent immigrants. Fifth, dissemination research should be supported, since outcomes found in controlled trials often cannot be replicated when more broadly implemented (DiClemente and Wingood, 1998; Perry, 1999b). Finally, policy research, where changing public policy is the goal, should be encouraged, to learn about the process and outcomes of policy changes that affect adolescents. It is clear that we need much more than competent adolescents—we need to create and provide a social environment for them that is competent and compassionate as well.

The American experiment has had some side effects in the latter part of the twentieth century. While countries such as India, China, Japan, and Singapore have relatively few problems with their adolescents, the United States continues to have significant and, in some cases, growing problems among its youth. While turning the clock back a century, or adopting social policies from Asia, are not feasible solutions to these concerns, it might be useful to examine social contexts in which the overwhelming majority of youth are healthful, productive, and content. How many hours do they spend in school? Do they spend significant time unsupervised? Are they involved in food preparation? Are there safe places to walk or bicycle to be with friends? Is academic achievement rewarded throughout the community? And so forth. This might lead to broader societal changes, alternative solutions, or creative options that may have salutary effects on adolescents and their health behaviors in the twenty-first century.

REFERENCES

Andrews, D.W., Soberman, L.H., and Dishion, T.J. (1995). The Adolescent Transitions Program for high-risk teens and their parents: Toward a school-based intervention. *Education and Treatment of Children*, 18, 478–498.

Arnett, J. (1992). Reckless behavior in adolescence: A developmental perspective. *Developmental Review*, 12, 339–373.

Arnett, J.J. (1999). Adolescent storm and stress, reconsidered. *American Psychologist*, 54(5), 317–326.

Baranowski, T., Cullen, K.W., and Baranowski, J. (1999). Psychosocial correlates of dietary intake: Advancing dietary intervention.. *Annual Review of Nutrition*, 19, 17–40.

Beauvais, F. (1992).Trends in Indian adolescent drug and alcohol use. *Journal of the National Center for American Indian and Alaskan Native Mental Health Resources*, 5, 1–12.

Bell, D.L., Ragin, D.F., and Cohall, A. (1999). Cross-cultural issues in prevention, health promotion, and risk reduction in adolescence. *Adolescent Medicine: State of the Art Reviews*, 10(1), 57–69.

Black, D.R., Tobler, N.S., and Sciacca, J.P. (1998). Peer helping/involvement: An efficacious way to meet the challenge of reducing alcohol, tobacco, and other drug use among youth? *Journal of School Health*, 68(3), 87–93.

Blaine, T.M., Forster, J.L., Hennrikus, D., O'Neil, S., Wolfson, M., and Pham, H. (1997). Creating tobacco policy control at the local level: Implementation of a direct action organizing approach. *Health Education and Behavior*, 24, 640–651.

Blum, R. (1998). Adolescent health: Priorities for the next millennium. *Maternal and Child Health Journal*, 22, 368–375.

Blum, R.W., and Stark T. (1985). Cognitive development in adolescence. *Seminars in Adolescent Medicine*, 1(1), 25–32.

Botvin, G.J., Baker, E., Dusenbury, L., Botvin, E.M., and Diaz, T. (1995). Long-term follow-up results of a randomized drug abuse prevention trial in a white middle-class population. *Journal of the American Medical Association*, 273, 1106–1112.

Bronfenbrenner, U., and Morris, P.A.(1998). The ecology of developmental processes. In W. Damon and R.M. Lerner (Eds.), *Handbook on Child Psychology: Vol.1. Theoretical Models of Human Development* (5th ed., pp. 993–1028). New York: John Wiley and Sons,.

Brooks-Gunn, J. (1988). Commentary: Developmental issues in the transition to early adolescence. In M.R. Gunnar and W.A. Collins (Eds.), *Minnesota Symposia on Child Psychology: Vol. 21. Development During the Transition to Adolescence* (pp. 189–208). Hillsdale, NJ: Lawrence Erlbaum Associates.

Brooks-Gunn, J., and Warren, M.P. (1989). Biological and social contributions to negative affect in young adolescent girls. *Child Development*, 60, 40–55.

Brooks-Gunn, J., Graber, J.A., and Paikoff, R.L. (1994). Studying links between hormones and negative affect: Models and measures. *Journal of Research on Adolescence*, 4(4), 469–486.

Brownlee, S. (1999). Inside the teenage brain. *U.S. News and World Report*, 45–54.

Buchanan, C.M., Eccles, J.S., and Becker, J.B. (1992). Are adolescents the victims of raging hormones: Evidence for activational effects of hormones on moods and behavior at adolescence. *Psychological Bulletin*, 111(1), 62–107.

Catalano, R.F., Berglund, M.L., Ryan, J.A.M., Lonczak, H.S., and Hawkins, J.D. (1999). *Positive Youth Development in the United States: Research Findings on Evaluations of Positive Youth Development Programs*. Washington, DC: U.S. DHHS, NICHHD.

Centers for Disease Control and Prevention (CDC). (1993). Mortality trends, causes of death, and related risk behaviors among U.S. adolescents. *Adolescent Health: State of the Nation Monograph Series #1* (CDC Pub No 099-4112). Atlanta: CDC.

Centers for Disease Control and Prevention (CDC). (1994). Changes in cigarette brand preferences of adolescent smokers—United States, 1989–1993. *Morbidity and Mortality Weekly Report,* 43(32), 577–581.

Centers for Disease Control and Prevention (CDC). (1997). *Sexually Transmitted Disease Surveillance 1996*. Atlanta: CDC.

Centers for Disease Control and Prevention (CDC). (1998). Youth risk behavior surveillance—United States, 1997. *Morbidity and Mortality Weekly Report,* 47, SS-3.

Chen, X., Unger, J.B., Cruz, T.B., and Johnson, C.A. (1999). Smoking patterns of Asian-American youth in California and their relationship with acculturation. *Journal of Adolescent Health*, 24, 321–328.

Clary, M. (1999). Lawmakers try to get apparently successful anti-smoking campaign. *Los Angeles Times*, A14.

Clausen, J.A. (1975). The social meaning of differential physical and sexual maturation. In S.E. Dragastin and G.H. Elder (Eds.), *Adolescence in the Lifecycle* (pp. 25–47). New York: Halsted.

Coleman, J.S. (1988). Social capital in the creation of human capital. *American Journal of Sociology*, 94, S95–S120.

Committee on Communications. (1995). Children, adolescents, and advertising. *Pediatrics*, 95(2), 295–297.

Crockett, L.J., and Petersen, A.C. (1993). Adolescent development: Health risks and opportunities for health promotion. In S.G. Millstein, A.C. Petersen, and E.O. Nightingale (Eds.), *Promoting the Health of Adolescents* (pp. 13–37). New York: Oxford University Press.

Crockett, S.J., and Sims, L.S. (1995). Environmental influences on children's eating. *Journal of Nutrition Education*, 27(5), 235–249.

Cullen, K.W., Bartholomew, L.K., Parcel, G.S., and Kok, G. (1998). Intervention mapping: Use of theory and data in the development of a fruit and vegetable nutrition program for Girl Scouts. *Journal of Nutrition Education*, 30, 188–195.

Dietz, W.H. (1998). Health consequences of obesity in youth: Childhood predictors of adult disease. *Pediatrics*, 101, 518–525.

DiClemente, R.J., Hansen,W.B., and Ponton, L.E. (1996). *Handbook of Adolescent Health Risk Behavior*. New York: Plenum Press.

DiClemente, R.J., and Wingood, G.M. (1998). Monetary incentives: A useful strategy for enhancing enrollment and promoting participation in HIV/STD risk reduction interventions. *Sexually Transmitted Infections*, 74, 239–242.

Dishion, T.J., and Andrews, D.W. (1995). Preventing escalation in problem behaviors with high-risk young adolescents: Immediate and 1-year outcomes. *Journal of Consulting and Clinical Psychology*, 63, 538–548.

Dorfman, L., and Wallack, L. (1993). Advertising health: The case for counter-ads. *Public Health Reports*, 108(6), 716–726.

Drug Strategies (1996). Making the grade: A guide to school drug prevention programs. Washington, DC, Drug Strategies.

Drug Strategies (1998). Safe schools, safe students: A guide to violence prevention strategies. Washington, DC: Drug Strategies.

Dryfoos, J.G. (1994). *Full-Service Schools*. San Francisco: Jossey-Bass.

Dryfoos, J.G. (1998). *Safe Passage: Making It Through Adolescence in a Risky Society*. New York: Oxford University Press.

DuRant, R.H., Rich. M., Emans, S.J., Rome, E.S., Allred, E., and Woods, E.R. (1997). Violence and weapon carrying in music videos. *Archives of Pediatrics and Adolescent Medicine*, 151, 443–448.

Eccles, J.S., Midgley, C., Wigfield, A. Buchanan, C.M., Reuman, D., Flanagan, C., and Iver, D.M. (1993). Development during adolescence: The impact of stage-environment fit on young adolescents' experiences in schools and in families. *American Psychologist*, 48(2), 90–101.

Eddy, J.M. Dishion, T.J., and Stoolmiller, M. (1998). The analysis of intervention change in children and families: Methodological and conceptual issues embedded in intervention studies. *Journal of Abnormal Child Psychology*, 26(1), 53–69.

Elder, G.H. (1974). *Children of the Great Depression*. Chicago: University of Chicago Press.

Elkind, D. (1967). Egocentrism in adolescence. *Child Development*, 38, 1025–1034.

Epstein, J.A., Botvin, G.J., Baker, E., and Diaz, T. (1998). Patterns of alcohol use among ethnically diverse black and Hispanic urban youth. *Journal of Gender, Culture, and Health*, 3(1), 29–39.

Epstein, J.A., Botvin, G.J., and Diaz, T. (1998). Ethnic and gender differences in alcohol use among a longitudinal sample of inner-city adolescents. *Journal of Gender, Culture, and Health*, 3(4), 193–207.

Farrell, A.D., and Bruce, S.E. (1997). Impact of exposure to community violence on violent behavior and emotional distress among urban adolescents. *Journal of Clinical Child Psychology*, 26(1), 2–14.

Flavell, J.H. (1985). *Cognitive Development (2nd ed)*. Englewood Cliffs, NJ: Prentice-Hall.

Flay, B.R., and Petraitis, J. (1994). The theory of triadic influence: A new theory of health behavior with implications for preventive interventions. *Advances in Medical Sociology*, 4, 19–44.

Florida Department of Health. (1999). *Tobacco Prevention and Control: Resources for a Comprehensive Plan for Florida*. Florida Leadership Council for Tobacco Control. Tallahassee, FL: Florida Department of Health.

Flynn, B.S., Worden, J.K., Secker-Walker, R.H., Badger, F.J., Geller, B.M., and Costanza, M.C. (1992). Prevention of cigarette smoking through mass media intervention and school programs. *American Journal of Public Health*, 82(6), 827–834.

Forster, J.L., Wolfson, M., Murray, D.M., Blaine, T.M., Wagenaar, A.C., and Hennrikus, D.J. (1998). The effects of community policies to reduce youth access to tobacco. *American Journal of Public Health*, 1193–1196.

French, S.A., Perry, C.L., Leon, G.R., and Fulkerson, J.A. (1995). Dieting behaviors and weight change history in adolescent females. *Health Psychology*, 14(6), 548–555.

Fuchs, V., and Reklis, D. (1992). The status of American children. Science, 255, 41–46.

Furstenberg, F.F., and Hughes, M.E. (1995). Social capital and successful development among at-risk youth. *Journal of Marriage and Family*, 57, 580–592.

Glanz, K., Lankenau, B., Foerster, S., Temple, S., Mullis, R., and Schmid, T. (1995). Environmental and policy approaches to cardiovascular disease prevention through nutrition: Opportunities for state and local action. *Health Education Quarterly*, 22(4), 512–527.

Goldman, L.K., and Glantz, S.A. (1998). Evaluation of antismoking advertising campaigns. *Journal of the American Medical Association*, 279 (10), 772–777.

Gorman-Smith, D., and Tolan, P. (1998). The role of exposure to community violence and developmental problems among inner-city youth. *Development and Psychopathology*, 10, 101–116.

Gruber, E., DiClemente, R.J., and Anderson, M.M. (1996). Risk-taking behavior among Native American adolescents in Minnesota public schools: Comparisons with black and white adolescents. *Ethnicity and Health*, 1(3), 261–267.

Hall, G.S. (1904). *Adolescence: Its Psychology and Its Relation to Physiology, Anthropology, Sociology, Sex, Crime, Religion, and Education (Vols. I and II)*. Englewood Cliffs, NJ: Prentice-Hall.

Hamburg, B. (1986). Subsets of adolescent mothers: Developmental, biomedical, and psychosocial issues. In J.B. Lancaster and B.A. Hamburg (Eds.). *School-Age Pregnancy and Parenthood: Biosocial Dimensions* (pp. 115–145). New York: Aldine de Gruyter.

Hansen, W.B., and Graham, J.W. (1991). Preventing alcohol, marijuana, and cigarette use among adolescents: Peer pressure resistance training versus establishing conservative norms. *Preventive Medicine*, 20, 414–430.

Havighurst, R.J. (1972). *Developmental Tasks and Education (3rd ed.)*. New York: David McKay.

Hawkins, J.D., Catalano, R.F., Kosterman, R., Abbott, R., and Hill, K.G. (1999). Preventing adolescent health-risk behaviors by strengthening protection during childhood. *Archives of Pediatrics and Adolescent Medicine*, 153, 226–234.

Haynes, N.M., and Comer, J.P. (1990). The effects of a school development program on self-concept. *Yale Journal of Biology and Medicine*, 63, 275–283.

Herman-Giddens, M.E., Slora, E.J., and Wasserman, R.C. (1997). Secondary sexual characteristics and menses in young girls seen in office practice: A study from the pediatric research in office settings network. *Pediatrics*, 99, 505–512.

Hill, J.O., and Trowbridge, F.L. (1998). Childhood obesity: Future directions and research priorities. *Pediatrics*, 101, 570–574.

Hill, J.P. (1980). *Understanding Early Adolescence: A Framework*. Center for Early Adolescence. Durham, NC: Wordworks.

Hill, J.P., and Holmbeck, G.N. (1986). Attachment and autonomy during adolescence. *Annals of Child Development*, 3, 145–189.

Hill, S.C., and Drolet, J.C. (1999). School-related violence among high school students in the United States, 1993–1995. *Journal of School Health*, 69(7), 264–272.

Hine, T. (1999). *The Rise and Fall of the American Teenager*. New York: Avon Books.

Holtz, A. (1999). Turning the rebellion: How Florida is trying to incite teens against tobacco. *Holtz Report* [on line]. Available: nasw.org/users/holtza/FL_paper.htm; accessed 11/12/99.

Hopwood, N.J. Kelch, R.P., Hale, P.M., Mendes, T.M., Foster, C.M., and Beitins, I.Z. (1990). The onset of human puberty: Biological and environmental factors. In J. Bancroft, J.M. Reinisch (Eds.), *Adolescence and Puberty* (pp. 29–49). New York: Oxford University Press.

Irwin, C.E., and Shafer, M.A. (1992). Adolescent sexuality: Negative outcomes of a normative behavior. In D.E. Rogers and E. Ginzbert (Eds.), *Adolescents at Risk: Medical and Social Perspectives* (pp. 35–79). Boulder, CO: Westview Press.

Jason, L.A., Reichler, A., King, C., Madsen, D., Camacho, J., and Marchese, W. (in press). The measurement of wisdom: A preliminary effort. *Journal of Community Psychology*.

Jessor, R. (1993). Successful adolescent development among youth in high-risk settings. *American Psychologist*, 48(2), 117–126.

Jessor, R. (1998). *New Perspectives on Adolescent Risk Behavior.* Cambridge, UK: Cambridge University Press.

Jessor, R., and Jessor, S.L. (1977). *Problem Behavior and Psychosocial Development: A Longitudinal Study of Youth.* New York: Academic Press.

Johnston, L.D., O'Malley, P.M., and Bachman, J.G. (1998). *Drug Use by American Young People* [on line]. Available: www.isr.umich.edu/src/mtf; accessed 11/10/99.

Kandel, D.B. (1998). Persistent themes and new perspectives on adolescent substance use: A lifespan perspective. In R. Jessor (Ed.), *New Perspectives on Adolescent Risk Behavior* (pp. 43–89). Cambridge, UK, Cambridge University Pres.

Kann, L., Warren, C.W., Harris, W.A., Collins, J.L., Douglas, K., Collins, B., Williams, B., and Kolbe, L.J. (1996). *Youth Risk Surveillance, 1995.* Division of Adolescent and School Health. Atlanta: CDC.

Kaplowitz, P.B., and Oberfield, S.E. (1999). Reexamination of the age limit for defining when puberty is precocious in girls in the United States: Implications for evaluation and treatment. *Pediatrics*, 104(4), 936–941.

Kelder, S.H., Perry, C.L., Klepp, K-I., and Lytle, L.A. (1994). Longitudinal tracking of adolescent smoking, physical activity, and food choice behaviors. *American Journal of Public Health*, 84, 1121–1126.

Kelder, S.H., Perry, C.L., Peters, R.J., Lytle, L.A., and Klepp, K-I. (1995). Gender differences in the Class of 1989 Study: The school component of the Minnesota Heart Health Program. *Journal of Health Education,* 26(2), S36–S44.

Kennedy, B.P., Kawachi, I., Prothrow-Stith, D., Lochner, K., and Gupta, V. (1998). Social capital, income inequality, and firearm violent crime. *Social Science and Medicine*, 47(1), 7–17.

Kennedy, E., and Goldberg, J. (1995). What are American children eating? Implications for public policy. *Nutrition Reviews*, 53, 111–126.

King, C., Siegel, M., Celebucki, C., and Connolly, G.N. (1998). Adolescent exposure to cigarette advertising in magazines. *Journal of the American Medical Association,* 279(7), 516–520.

Klein, J.D., Brown, J.D., Childers, K.W., Oliveri, J., Porter, C., and Dykers, C. (1993). Adolescents' risky behavior and mass media use. *Pediatrics*, 92(1), 24–31.

Kohl, H.W., and Hobbs, K.E. (1998). Development of physical activity behaviors among children and adolescents. *Pediatrics,* 101, 549–554.

Komro, K.A. (1999). Adolescents' access to firearms: Epidemiology and prevention. *Journal of Health Education,* 30(5), 290–296.

Komro, K.A. and Stigler, M.H. (In press). *A Community Road Map to Healthy Youth Development: Vehicles for Success.* University of Minnesota, Konopka Institute for Best Practices in Adolescent Health.

Komro, K.A., Perry, C.L., Murray, D.M., Veblen-Mortenson, S., Williams, C.L., and Anstine, P.S. (1996). Peer planned social activities for the prevention of alcohol use among young adolescents. *Journal of School Health*, 66(9), 328–336.

Komro, K.A., Perry, C.L., Veblen-Mortenson, S., and Williams, C.L. (1994). Peer participation in Project Northland: A community-wide alcohol use prevention project. *Journal of School Health,* 64(8), 318–322.

Komro, K.A., Perry, C.L., Williams, C.L., Stigler, M.H., Farbakhsh, K., and Veblen-Mortenson, S. (In press). How did Project Northland reduce alcohol use among young adolescents? Analysis of mediating variables. *Health Education Research.*

Kubey, R., and Baker, F. (1999). Has media literacy found a curricular foothold? *Education Week* [on line]. Available: www.edweek.org/ew/ewstory.cfm?slug=09ubey2.h19; accessed 11/11/99.

Laursen, B., Coy, K.C., and Collins, W.A. (1998). Reconsidering changes in parent–child conflict across adolescence: A meta-analysis. *Child Development*, 69(3), 817–832.

Lerner, R.M., and Galambos, N.L. (1998). Adolescent development: Challenges and opportunities for research, programs, and policies. *Annual Review of Psychology*, 49, 413–446.

Lillie-Blanton, M., and Laveist, T. (1996). Race/ethnicity, the social environment, and health. *Social Science and Medicine*, 43(1), 83–91.

Lytle, L.A., Kelder, S.H., Perry, C.L., and Klepp K-I. (1995). Covariance of adolescent health behaviors: The Class of 1989 Study. *Health Education Research*, 10, 133–146.

Marjoribanks, K. (1998). Family capital, children's individual attributes, and adolescents' aspirations: A follow-up analysis. *Journal of Psychology,* 132(3), 328–336.

Marshall, W.A., and Tanner, J. (1970). Variations in the pattern of pubertal changes in boys. *Archives of Diseases in Childhood*, 45, 13–23.

Masten, A.S., and Coatsworth, J.D. (1995). Competence, resilience, and psychopathology. In D. Cicchetti and D. Cohen (Eds.), *Developmental Psychopathology: Vol 2. Risk, Disorder, and Adaptation* (pp. 715–752). New York: John Wiley and Sons.

Masten, A.S., and Coatsworth, J.D. (1998). The development of competence in favorable and unfavorable environments: Lessons from research on successful children. *American Psychologist,* 53(2), 205–220,.

Masten, A.S., Coatsworth, J.D., Neemann, J., Gest, S.D., Tellegen, A., and Garmezy, N. (1995). The structure and coherence of competence from childhood through adolescence. *Child Development*, 66, 1635–1659.

Moffitt, T.E. (1993). Adolescence-limited and life-course-persistent antisocial behavior: A developmental taxonomy. *Psychological Review*, 100(4), 674–701.

Money, J. (1980). *Love and Love Sickness: The Science of Sex, Gender Difference, and Pair-Bonding*. Baltimore: Johns Hopkins University Press.

Mortimer, J.T., and Johnson, M.K. (1998). New perspectives on adolescent work and the transition to adulthood. In R. Jessor (Ed.), *New Perspectives on Adolescent Risk Behavior* (pp. 425–496). Cambridge, UK: Cambridge University Press.

Nader, P.R., Stone, E.J., Lytle, L.A., Perry, C.L., Osganian, S.K., Kelder, S., Webber, L.S., Elder, J.P., Montgomery, D., Feldman, H.A., Wu, M., Johnson, C., Parcel, G.S., and Luepker, R.V. (1999). Three-year maintenance of improved diet and physical activity: The CATCH cohort. *Archives of Pediatrics and Adolescent Medicine*, 153, 695–704.

Neumark-Sztainer, D., Story, M., French, S., Cassuto, N., Jacobs, D.R., and Resnick, M.D. (1996). Patterns of health-compromising behaviors among Minnesota adolescents: Sociodemographic variations. *American Journal of Public Health,* 86(11), 1599–1606.

News America Digital Publishing. (1999). CDC: Anti-smoking campaign in Florida shows solid results. *Fox Market Wire* [on line]. Available: www.foxwire.com; accessed 11/4/99.

Nottelmann, E.D., Inoff-Germain, G., Susman, E.J., and Chrousos, G.P. (1990). Hormones and behavior at puberty. In J. Bancroft and J.M. Reinisch (Eds.), *Adolescence and Puberty* (pp. 88–123). New York: Oxford University Press.

Olweus, D., Mattsson, A., Schalling, D., and Low, H. (1998). Circulating testosterone levels and aggression in adolescent males: A causal analysis. *Psychosomatic Medicine*, 50, 261–272.

Ozer, E.M., Brindis, C.D., Millstein, S.G., Knopf, D.K., and Irwin, C.E. (1998). *America's Adolescents: Are They Healthy?* San Francisco: National Adolescent Health Information Center, University of California, San Francisco.

Patterson, G.R. (1982). *Coercive Family Process.* Eugene, OR: Castalia.

Perry, C.L. (1999a). The tobacco industry and underage youth smoking: Tobacco industry documents from the Minnesota litigation. *Archives of Pediatrics and Adolescent Medicine,* 153, 935–941.

Perry, C.L. (1999b). *Creating Health Behavior Change: How to Develop Communitywide Programs for Youth.* Thousand Oaks, CA: Sage.

Perry, C.L., Grant, M., Ernberg, G., Florenzano, R.U., Langdon, M.D., Blaze-Temple, D., Cross, D., Jacobs, D.R., Myeni, A.D., Waahlberg, R.B., Berg, S., Andersson, D., Fisher, K.J., Saunders, B., and Schmid, T. (1989). WHO collaborative study on alcohol education and young people: Outcomes of a four-country pilot study. *International Journal of Addictions,* 24(12), 1145–1171.

Perry, C.L., Kelder, S.H., Murray, D.M., and Klepp K-I. (1992). Community-wide smoking prevention: Long-term outcomes of the Minnesota Heart Health Program and the Class of 1989 Study. *American Journal of Public Health,* 82(9), 1210–1216.

Perry, C.L., Story, M., and Lytle, L.A. (1997). Promoting healthy dietary behaviors. In R.P. Weissberg, T.P. Gullotta, G.R. Adams, R.L. Hampton, and B.A. Ryan (Eds). *Healthy Children 2010: Enhancing Children's Wellness, Volume 8: Issues in Children's and Families' Lives.* Thousand Oaks, CA: Sage.

Perry, C.L., Williams, C.L., Forster, J.L., Wolfson, M., Wagenaar, A.C., Finnegan, J.R., McGovern, P.G., Veblen-Mortenson, S., Komro, K.A., and Anstine, P.S. (1993). Background, conceptualization, and design of a communitywide research program on adolescent alcohol use: Project Northland. *Health Education Research: Theory and Practice,* 8(1), 125–136.

Perry, C.L., Williams, C.L., Komro, K.A., Veblen-Mortenson, S., Forster, J., Bernstein-Lachter, R., Pratt, L.K., Dudovitz, B., Munson, K.A., Farbakhsh, K., Finnegan, J., and McGovern, P. (2000). Project Northland high school interventions: Community action to reduce adolescent alcohol use. *Health Education and Behavior.* 27(1), 29–49.

Perry, C.L., Williams, C.L., Veblen-Mortenson, S., Toomey, T., Komro, K.A., Anstine, P.S., McGovern, P.G., Finnegan, J.R., Forster, J.L., Wagenaar, A.C., and Wolfson, M. (1996). Project Northland: Outcomes of a community-wide alcohol use prevention program during early adolescence. *American Journal of Public Health,* 86(7), 956–965.

Petersen, A.C., and Taylor, B. (1980). The biological approach to adolescence: Biological change and psychological adaptation. In J. Adelson (Ed.), *Handbook of Adolescent Psychology* (pp. 117–155). New York: John Wiley and Sons.

Petraitis, J., Flay, B.R., and Miller, T.Q. (1995). Reviewing theories of adolescent substance use: Organizing pieces of the puzzle. *Psychological Bulletin,* 117(1), 67–86.

Pierce, J.P., Lee, L., and Gilpin, F.A. (1994). Smoking initiation by adolescent girls; An association with targeted advertising. *Journal of the American Medical Association,* 271(8), 608–611.

Pierce, J.P., Choi, W.S., Gilpin, E.A., Farkas, A.J., and Berry, C.C. (1998). Tobacco industry promotion of cigarettes and adolescent smoking. *Journal of the American Medical Association,* 279 (7), 511–515.

Pollay, R.L., Siddarth, S., Siegel, M., Haddix, A., Merritt, R.K., Giovino, G.A., and Eriksen, M.P. (1996). The last straw? Cigarette advertising and realized market shares among youths and adults. *Journal of Marketing,* 60, 1–16.

Resnick, M.D., Bearman, P.S., Blum, R.W., Bauman, K.E., Harris, K.M., Jones, J., Tabor, J., Beuhring, T., Sieving, R.E., Shew, M., Ireland, M., Bearinger, L.H., and Udry, J.R. (1997). Protecting adolescents from harm: Findings from the National Longitudinal Study on Adolescent Health. *Journal of the American Medical Association*, 278(10), 823–832.

Resnicow, K., Braithwaite, R.L, and Kuo, J.A. (1997). Interpersonal interventions for minority adolescents. In D.K. Wilson, J.R. Rodrigue, and W.C. Taylor (Eds.), *Health-Promoting and Health-Compromising Behaviors Among Minority Adolescents* (pp. 201–228). Washington, DC: American Psychological Association.

Roski, J., Perry, C.L., McGovern, P.G., Williams, C.L., Farbakhsh, K., and Veblen-Mortenson, S. (1997). School and community influences on adolescent alcohol and drug use. *Health Education Research: Theory and Practice*, 12(2), 255–266.

Runyan, D.K., Hunter, W.M., Socolar, R.R.S., Amaya-Jackson, L., English, D., Landsverk, J., Dubowitz, H., Browne, D.H., Bangdiwala, S.L., and Mathew, R.M. (1998). Children who prosper in unfavorable environments: The relationship to social capital. *Pediatrics*, 101(1), 12–18.

Scheer, S.D., Unger, D.G., and Brown, M.B. (1996). Adolescents becoming adults: Attributes for adulthood. *Adolescence*, 31(121), 127–131.

Schooler, C., Feighery, E., and Flora, J.A. (1996). Seventh graders' self-reported exposure to cigarette marketing and its relationship to their smoking behavior. *American Journal of Public Health,* 86(9), 1216–1221.

Schulenberg, J. Maggs, J., and Hurrelmann, K. (1997). *Health Risks and Developmental Transitions During Adolescence*. Cambridge, UK: Cambridge University Press.

Silbereisen, R.K. and Kracke, B. (1993). Variation in maturational timing and adjustment in adolescence. In S. Jackson and H. Rodriguez-Tome (Eds.), *Adolescence and Its Social Worlds* (pp. 67–94). East Sussex, UK: Erlbaum.

Silbereisen, R.K., Petersen, A.C., Albrecht, H.T., and Kracke, B. (1989). Maturational timing and the development of problem behavior: Longitudinal studies in adolescence. *Journal of Early Adolescence*, 9, 247–268.

Simmons, R.G., and Blyth, D.A. (1987). *Moving into Adolescence: The Impact of Pubertal Change and School Context*. Hawthorne, NY: Aldine de Gruyter.

Steinberg, L.D. (1989). Pubertal maturation and parent-adolescent distance: An evolutionary perspective. In G.R. Adams, R. Montemayor and T.P. Gulotta (Eds.), *Biology of Adolescent Behavior and Development* (pp. 71–97). Newbury Park, CA: Sage.

Steinberg, L., and Avenevoli, S. (1998). Disengagement from school and problem behavior in adolescence: A developmental-contextual analysis of the influences of family and part-time work. In R. Jessor (Ed.), *New Perspectives on Adolescent Risk Behavior* (pp. 392–424). Cambridge, UK: Cambridge University Press.

Steinberg, L., Fegley, S., and Dornbusch, S.M. (1993). Negative impact of part-time work on adolescent adjustment: Evidence from a longitudinal study. *Developmental Psychology*, 29(2), 171–180.

Steinberg, L., Fletcher, A., and Darling, N. (1994). Parental monitoring and peer influences on adolescent substance use. *Pediatrics*, 93(6), 1060–1064.

Story, M. (1992). Nutritional requirements during adolescence. In E.R. McAnarney, R.E. Kreipe, D.P. Orr, and G.D. Comerci (Eds.), *Textbook of Adolescent Medicine* (pp. 75–84). Philadelphia: W.B. Saunders.

Strasburger, V.C. (1997). "Sex, drugs, rock 'n' roll" and the media—Are the media responsible for adolescent behavior? *Adolescent Medicine: State of the Art Reviews*, 8(3), 403–414.

Strasburger, V.C. (1998). Is it only rock 'n' roll? The chicken-and-the-egg dilemma. *Journal of Adolescent Health,* 23(1), 1–2.

Surbey, M.K. (1990). Family composition, stress, and the timing of human menarche. In T.E. Ziegler and F.B. Bercovitch (Eds.), *Socioendocrinology of Primate Reproduction* (pp. 11–32). New York: John Wiley and Sons.

Susman, E.J. (1997). Modeling developmental complexity in adolescence: Hormones and behavior in context. *Journal of Research on Adolescence,* 7(3), 283–306.

Tanner, J.M. (1978). *Fetus into Man: Physical Growth from Conception to Maturity.* Cambridge, MA: Harvard University Press.

Teague, C.E. (1973). *Some Thoughts About New Brands of Cigarettes for the Youth Market, RJ Reynolds' research planning memorandum. RJR Bates # 50298 7357.* Minnesota documents depository.

Troiano, R.P., and Flegal, K.M. (1998). Overweight children and adolescents: Description, epidemiology, and demographics. *Pediatrics,* 101(3), 497–504.

Troiano, R.P., Flegal, K.M., Kuczmarski, R.J., Campbell, S.M., and Johnson, C.L. (1995). Overweight prevalence and trends for children and adolescents. *Archives of Pediatrics and Adolescent Medicine,* 149, 1085–1091.

Turner, R.A., Irwin, C.E., Tschann, J.M., and Millstein, S.G. (1993). Autonomy, relatedness, and the initiation of health risk behaviors in early adolescence. *Health Psychology,* 12(3), 200–208.

Udry, J.R. (1988). Biological dispositions and social control in adolescent sexual behavior. *American Sociological Review,* 53, 709–722.

Upchurch, D.M., Levy-Storm, L., Sucoff, C.A., and Aneshensel, C.S. (1998). Gender and ethnic differences in the timing of first sexual intercourse. *Family Planning Perspectives,* 30(3), 121–127.

U.S. Census Bureau. Press briefing on 1998 income and poverty estimates. (1999) [on line]. Available: www.census.gov/hhes/income/income98/prs99acs.html; accessed 11/11/99.

U.S. Department of Agriculture (1995). *Dietary Guidelines for Americans.* Washington, DC: U.S. Department of Health and Human Services.

U.S. Department of Health and Human Services (1994). *Preventing Tobacco Use Among Young People: A Report of the Surgeon General.* Atlanta: CDC.

U.S. Department of Health and Human Services (1996). *Physical Activity and Health: A Report of the Surgeon General.* Atlanta: CDC.

U.S. Department of Health and Human Services (1998). *Tobacco Use Among U.S. Racial/Ethnic Minority Groups: A Report of the Surgeon General.* Atlanta: CDC.

U.S. Department of Health and Human Services (1999). *Understanding Substance Abuse Prevention: Toward the 21st Century: A Primer on Effective Programs.* DHHS Pub No 99–3301. Washington, DC: CSAP.

Vega, W.A. and Gil, A.G. (1998). *Drug Use and Ethnicity in Early Adolescence.* New York, Plenum Press.

Vega, W.A, Gil, A.G., and Zimmerman, R.S. (1993). Patterns of drug use among Cuban Americans, African Americans, and white non-Hispanic boys. *American Journal of Public Health,* 83, 257–259.

Vida, V. (1999). *Girls on the Verge.* New York: St. Martin's Press.

Wagenaar, A. C. Murray, D.M., Gehan, G.P., Wolfson, M., Forster, J.L., Toomey, T.L., Perry, C.L., and Jones-Webb, R. (2000). Communities mobilizing for change on alcohol: Outcomes from a randomized community trial. *Journal of Studies on Alcohol,* 61, 85–94.

Williams, C.L., and Perry, C.L. (1998). Design and implementation of parent programs for a community-wide adolescent alcohol use prevention program. *Journal of Prevention and Intervention in the Community*, 17, 65–80.

Williams, C.L., Perry, C.L., Dudovitz, B., Veblen-Mortenson, S., Anstine, P.S., Komro, K.A., and Toomey, T. (1995). A home-based prevention program for sixth grade alcohol use: Results from Project Northland. *Journal of Primary Prevention,* 16(2), 125–147.

Willis, E., and Strasburger VC. (1998). Media violence. *Pediatric Clinics of North America*, 45(2), 319–331.

Wood, W., Wong, F.Y., and Chachere J.G. (1991). Effects of mass media on viewers' aggression in unconstrained social interaction. *Psychological Bulletin,* 109(3), 371–383.

World Cancer Research Fund. (1997). *Food, Nutrition and the Prevention of Cancer: A Global Perspective.* Washington, DC: American Institute for Cancer Research.

Wyshak, G., and Frisch, R.E. (1982). Evidence for a secular trend in age of menarche. *New England Journal of Medicine*, 306, 1033–1035.

PAPER CONTRIBUTION F

Behavioral and Social Science Contributions to the Health of Adults in the United States

Karen M. Emmons, Ph.D.

The purpose of this paper is to briefly review the major causes of morbidity and mortality during adulthood and to provide a selected review of the literature that addresses efforts to reduce the prevalence of preventable disease among adults in the United States. Substantial progress has been made in reducing risk factor prevalence among adults. The premise of this paper is that the social and behav-

Dr. Emmons is associate professor, Department of Adult Oncology, Dana-Farber Cancer Institute, Dana-Farber/Harvard Cancer Center, and associate professor, Department of Health and Social Behavior, Harvard School of Public Health. This paper was prepared for the symposium, "Capitalizing on Social Science and Behavioral Research to Improve the Public's Health," the Institute of Medicine and the Commission on Behavioral and Social Sciences and Education of the National Research Council, Atlanta, Georgia, February 2–3, 2000.

The author would like to thank Edwin Fisher, Russ Glasgow, Ellen Gritz, David Hemenway, Bernard Glassman, Sue Curry, Barbara Rimer, Tracy Orleans, and Judy Ockene for their thoughts on the topic of this paper and the future directions of the field. The author would also like to thank Glorian Sorensen for her contributions to the conceptualization of this manuscript and her ongoing contributions to the author's research. Jocelyn Pan contributed significantly to reviewing the literature discussed in this paper, and Mary Eileen Twomley provided editorial and manuscript preparation assistance. Portions of this paper are drawn from the author's previous writings (Sorensen et al., 1998, 1999; Emmons, in press).

This work was supported by grants from the Liberty Mutual Insurance Group, NYNEX, Aetna, the Boston Foundation, and NIH Grants 1RO1CA73242 and 1RO1HL50017 Best Beginnings: 5RO1 CA73242-04; PO1: 1 PO1CA75308-01A2; Polyp: 5RO1CA74000-02; CCSS: 1 R01 CA77780-02.

ioral sciences have made a significant contribution to these improvements. These contributions include providing a broader perspective on disease causation that goes beyond biomedical approaches, utilizing theory-based interventions, evaluating intervention strategies that vary in intensity and cost, and utilizing population-based approaches that extend intervention research beyond high-risk populations. A great deal of what we have learned has considerable potential for yielding greater intervention outcomes than have been achieved to date. A number of issues will be discussed that need to be considered in the design and evaluation of health behavior interventions in order to further advance our progress. These issues are presented briefly here and discussed in further detail later in the paper.

First, research is needed that connects and bridges individual, community, environmental, and policy-level interventions. Second, more research is needed in how to effectively target multiple risk factors for chronic disease and to take advantage of naturally occurring relationships between health behaviors. Third, behavioral scientists need to anticipate the impact that advances in computer technology may have on intervention development and delivery, and to be prepared to take advantage of the resources that this technology has to offer. Fourth, it is argued that while there have been a number of innovations emanating from the behavioral and social sciences related to intervention design and delivery, such strategies are not typically implemented outside the research setting. Significant attention needs to be given to the issues of sustainability and dissemination because current efforts to disseminate effective interventions are poor. Finally, increased attention to social contextual factors that influence the development and maintenance of health behaviors is needed.

Major Risks to Health During Adulthood

Leading causes of morbidity and mortality among adults vary by age and gender, but are largely preventable. A brief review follows of the three leading causes of morbidity and mortality during early to middle and middle to older adulthood (see Table 1).

Leading Causes of Mortality in Early to Middle Adulthood (Ages 20–45)

In early to middle adulthood, the leading cause of mortality is unintentional injuries. Among very young adults (≤24 years), injuries account for 77% of all deaths. The homicide rate among young males is almost 20 times higher than that found in most other industrialized nations (*MMWR*, 1993; Rachuba et al., 1995; Rosenburg, 1995). Across all age groups during adulthood, motor vehicle accidents account for the majority of deaths due to injury, although the death rate per miles driven has been reduced substantially in the past three decades (Bonnie, et al., 1999). Death rates for motor vehicle accidents are nearly equi-

TABLE 1. Leading Causes of Death and Numbers of Death, According to Age and Gender, United States, 1996

Cause of Death	Age 25–44[a]		Age 45–64[b]		Males[c]		Females[d]	
	Deaths	Rank	Deaths	Rank	Deaths	Rank	Deaths	Rank
Unintentional injuries	27,092	1	16,717	3	61,589	4	33,359	7
Malignant neoplasms	21,894	2	131,455	1	281,898	2	257,635	2
HIV	21,685	3	8,053	8	25,227	8		
Heart disease	16,567	4	102,369	2	360,075	1	373,286	1
Suicide	12,602	5	7,762	9	24,998	9		
Homicide and legal intervention	9,322	6						
Chronic liver disease and cirrhoses	4,210	7	10,743	7	16,311	10		
Cerebrovascular diseases	3,442	8	15,468	4	62,475	3	97467	3
Diabetes	2,526	9	12,687	6	27,646	7	34,121	6
Pneumonia and influenza	2,029	10	5,706	10	37,991	6	45,736	5
Chronic obstructive pulmonary disease			12,847	5	54,485	5	51,542	4
Alzheimer's disease							14,426	8
Nephritis							12,662	9
Septicemia							12,177	10

[a] All cause mortality = 147,180.
[b] All cause mortality = 378,054.
[c] All cause mortality = 1,163,569.
[d] All cause mortality = 1,151,121.

valent for black, white, and Hispanic men, although much lower for Asian men. Motor vehicle death rates among women are about one-third of those found in men. Fires also cause a substantial proportion of unintentional injuries; cigarettes are a major cause of residential fires (Baker et al., 1992). On average, one out of every 200 households experiences a fire each year; this rate is greater among poor households (National Center for Health Statistics, 1996b).

Cancer is the second leading cause of death in early to middle adulthood. The death rate due to cancer among men and women is roughly equivalent for whites, Hispanics, and Asians; it is significantly higher among black men than black women, and is higher among Native American women than Native American men (USDHHS, 1998). In this age range, cancer morbidity is greater among women, especially those ages 35–44, and is most common among blacks, followed by whites. Similar patterns in morbidity rates by race or ethnicity are found among men. Cancer morbidity has also consistently been found to have an inverse relationship with socioeconomic status (SES) (Devesa and Diamond, 1980, 1983; McWhorter et al., 1989; Morton et al., 1983; Tomatis, 1992; Williams and Horm, 1977). The third leading cause of death in early to middle adulthood is HIV; incidence is clustered in large metropolitan areas. Gay and bisexual men still represent most prevalent HIV infections; although overall incidence is significantly lower now than in the 1980s; incidence among young and minority gay men remains high (Holmberg, 1996). Roughly half of all new infections occur among injection drug users (IDUs). Black and Hispanic IDUs are more likely to be HIV infected than are white IDUs (Friedman et al., 1999). In 1997, 22% of all new adult AIDS cases were in women. In the United States, AIDS cases among women have been concentrated in blacks and Hispanics (Kamb and Wortley, 2000). The primary routes of transmission among women are injection drug use and heterosexual contact with an HIV-infected male sex partner.

Leading Causes of Mortality in Middle to Older Adulthood (ages 45–64)

The leading cause of death from ages 45 to 64 is cancer. Heart disease is the second leading cause of death in this age group; death rates are three times greater in men than women. Death rates due to heart disease are twice as high in black men as in white men, and slightly higher for Native American men than white men. Unintentional injury is the third leading cause of death in this age range (USDHHS, 1999).

Leading Causes of Morbidity in Adulthood

Morbidity related to a number of chronic conditions can cause substantial reductions in quality of life and contribute significantly to medical care costs. In the United States, 24% of adults have been diagnosed with hypertension (Burt et al., 1995); prevalence increases with age and is slightly higher among men than women (He and Whelton, 1997); age-adjusted prevalence is higher in non-Hispanic blacks than non-Hispanic whites (Burt et al., 1995; Hall et al., 1997). Among both blacks and whites, hypertension is higher among men than women. The prevalence of hypertension in Mexican Americans is lower than in non-Hispanic whites. Asian Americans have lower prevalence of hypertension compared to other ethnic groups. The severity of hypertension is greater among those of low SES (Moorman et al., 1991).

The prevalence of diabetes has increased over the past decade (USDHHS, 1996a). It is estimated that 15.7 million persons in the United States have diabetes (*MMWR,* 1997; National Diabetes Information Clearinghouse, 1999). The overall prevalence of diabetes increases with age. The prevalence rate among blacks is more than 80% higher than for the total population; rates among American Indians or Alaskan Natives and Mexican Americans are also quite elevated, compared to the total population (Harris, 1998; *MMWR,* 1997). Heart disease is the leading cause of diabetes-related deaths. Type 2 diabetes, which accounts for more than 90% of all diagnosed diabetes, is associated with modifiable risk factors (e.g., obesity, physical inactivity) and nonmodifiable risk factors (e.g., genetic factors or family history, age, and race or ethnicity).

Mental health problems are a major concern in adulthood. Between 10 and 15% of adults in the United States have a diagnosable mental disorder, and up to 24% of adults have experienced a mental disorder during the preceding year (*MMWR,* 1998; Regier et al., 1993a; Robins et al., 1981). The impact of mental health problems on functional disability and quality of life is profound (Wells et al., 1989a). Marital status (being divorced or separated) and having low SES are powerful correlates of mental health problems (Bebbington et al., 1981; Henderson et al., 1979; Hodiamont et al., 1987; Mavreas et al., 1986; Regier et al., 1993a; Surtees et al., 1983; Vazquez-Barquero et al., 1987). After controlling for other factors, there are no racial or ethnic differences in mental health disorders (Regier et al., 1993a). Substance use disorders are most common among very young adults, while affective disorders are elevated in early to middle adulthood; all mental disorders are less common during older adulthood than in the younger age group. Men are more likely to have substance use disorders and personality disorders; women are more likely to have affective and anxiety disorders (Kessler et al., 1994).

Unintentional injuries are also the cause of significant morbidity during adulthood, as well as mortality as noted above. In addition to the morbidity associated with motor vehicle and other types of accidents, occupational injuries and exposures cause 13.2 million nonfatal injuries and 862,200 illnesses occurring among the American workforce annually (Leigh et al., 1997).

Risk Factors for Primary Causes of Morbidity and Mortality During Adulthood

Over the past three decades there has been extensive research into the causes of heart disease, cancer, and other chronic diseases. As noted above, age and gender are nonmodifiable risk factors for certain diseases, although the direction of this effect varies considerably across diseases. Genetic causes of chronic disease have become the focus of intense research attention in the past decade. Genetic factors have been implicated in certain forms of diabetes (Kahn et al., 1996), cancer (Easton and Peto, 1990), stroke (Rastenyte et al., 1998), and myocardial infarction (Marian, 1998). However, in most cases the overall contribution of genetics to disease incidence is likely to be relatively small compared to behavioral or environmental factors (Lerman, 1997).

Social epidemiology has demonstrated the profound effect that social class has on health (Emmons, 2000). Although SES is typically thought of as a nonmodifiable modifying condition in epidemiological and behavioral research, a growing body of work suggests that if we are ever to make a significant impact on economic disparities in health, we need to begin efforts in which we reconceptualize socioeconomic status as a modifiable variable, both in our research efforts and in political dialogue.

Modifiable risk factors for chronic disease morbidity and mortality include individual and environmental-level exposures. Strong relationships exist between health behaviors and risk for all of the leading causes of morbidity and mortality during adulthood. For example, heart disease, stroke, and cancer have been linked to a number of modifiable risk factors, including physical inactivity, obesity, hypertension, cholesterol level, diet, smoking, and sun exposure (He and Whelton, 1997; Wilson and Culleton, 1998). For many diseases, screening and early detection strategies are available that can reduce the severity of disease and substantially increase survival time. Environmental or organizational-level risk factors include occupational exposure and work practices, motor vehicle and other product design, and environmental design (e.g., highway redesign).

A number of recommendations have been put forth for the adoption of health-promoting behaviors in order to reduce the incidence of chronic disease morbidity and mortality (Greenwald et al., 1995; U.S. Preventive Services Task Force, 1996; USDHHS, 1996b, 1996c). The latest health promotion guidelines related to the primary causes of morbidity and mortality among adults are outlined in Box 1.

WHERE DO WE STAND?

There have been some significant improvements in morbidity and mortality rates over the past several decades; deaths from cardiovascular disease have declined dramatically (Cole and Rodu, 1996; USDHHS, 1996c), and cancer mortality has recently declined for the first time since such records have been kept (Heath et al., 1995). Recent data from the Framingham Heart Study suggest that there have been secular changes toward a less disabled and generally healthier population among adults aged 55 to 70 (Allaire et al., 1999). Of note, there have been improvements on 59% of the Healthy People 2000 target objectives (National Center for Health Statistics, 1996b). These successes should be celebrated, and social and behavioral scientists should be recognized for their contributions to these gains and to our understanding of the factors that influence health behaviors among diverse populations (Airhihenbuwa et al., 1996; Braithwaite et al., 1994; Kirsch et al., 1993; Kumanyika and Morssink, 1997; Kumanyika and Charleston, 1992; Pasick et al., 1996; Resnicow et al., 1999; Snow, 1974; Weiss et al., 1992). However, despite these gains, many diseases continue to have disproportionately high prevalence among minority groups. In addition, a number of studies highlight the importance of further improving behavioral risk factor prevalence on a population level, across all race, ethnicity, and gender groups. It has been estimated that community-based cholesterol interventions are cost-effective if cholesterol is reduced by as little as 2% (Tosteson et al., 1997). Other estimates suggest that implementation of currently available cancer prevention and early detection strategies at the population level could reduce U.S. cancer mortality by approximately 60% (Colditz et al., 1996; Willett et al., 1996).

Given the encouraging estimates of the additional health gains that could be achieved from population-level adoption of recommended health behaviors, and the fact that many gains have been made, it is still disheartening that more than 50 years after the Framingham Heart Study demonstrated that behavioral risk factors greatly increase the risk of developing coronary heart disease, the prevalence of risk factors for this and many other diseases remains high. Only 24% of Americans engage in light to moderate physical activity at recommended levels (National Center for Health Statistics, 1996b). Racial and ethnic minority populations are less active than white Americans, with the largest differences found among women (Caspersen et al., 1986; Caspersen and Merritt, 1992; DiPietro and Caspersen, 1991). Physical activity patterns are also directly related to educational level and income (Caspersen et al., 1986; Centers for Disease Control and Prevention, 1990; Folsom et al., 1985; Siegal et al., 1993). Obesity is considered by some to be reaching epidemic proportions in the United States, with 18% of the U.S. adult population being obese and almost 60% being overweight (Must et al., 1999). Of particular concern is the recent finding that across most population groups, the prevalence of obesity and overweight is increasing rapidly (Mokdad et al., 1999).

Significant improvements have been made in dietary habits over the past several years. Although the median intake of fruits and vegetables among adults is still less than five servings per day (Subar et al., 1995), intake has increased significantly since 1989 (National Cancer Institute, 1997). Consumption of red meat has also decreased substantially (U.S. Department of Agriculture, 1991). Fruit and vegetable consumption is higher among women than men at all ages, although the gender difference appears to increase with age. Lower-income households have significantly lower consumption of fruits and vegetables (Krebs-Smith et al., 1995), and have experienced less reduction in red meat consumption compared to higher-income households (Interagency Board for Nutrition Monitoring and Related Research, 1993). Recent data indicate that 24.7% of adults smoke in the United States (*MMWR*, 1999), which represents a dramatic reduction in smoking prevalence over the past 30 years (Centers for Disease Control and Prevention, 1996). However, overall smoking prevalence has been virtually unchanged in the past 5 years. Educational status remains the strongest predictor of smoking status (Novotny et al., 1988; Pierce et al., 1989). Of particular concern is the recent finding that smoking prevalence among very young adults (ages 18–24) has increased substantially.

Although there have been many increases in the prevalence of safety and injury prevention behaviors, only 61% of people in the United States wear seat belts (Bonnie et al., 1999). Although 49 states have seat belt laws, such regulations are rarely enforced. Other areas where injuries remain high, such as injuries involving firearms, have been the subject of little regulatory action (Freed et al., 1998).

Unfortunately, the higher-than-ideal prevalence of modifiable risk factors is not limited to disease-free groups. There is an astonishingly low rate of action taken to control disease among those who have already been diagnosed with a chronic disease. For example, only 30% of white hypertensive men and 50% of black hypertensive men take action to control their blood pressure (USDHHS, 1999). Only 50% of people who have undergone angioplasty comply with postsurgical regimens for diet and exercise. Among diabetics, only 43% attend diabetes management classes, although significant progress has occurred among blacks in the past several years, with 50% of black diabetics now receiving this type of education (National Center for Health Statistics, 1996a).

The data presented in this section illustrate that clear progress has been made on many risk factors for chronic disease as well as morbidity and mortality among adults. Effective strategies are available for reducing most risk factors. If applied effectively at the population level, such strategies could substantially reduce risk and improve disease outcomes. However, population-level interventions have been limited, and preventable risk factors remain the primary cause of morbidity and mortality.

INTERVENTION OUTCOMES—EXAMPLES OF EFFECTIVE INTERVENTIONS

The next section of this paper provides a brief discussion of outcomes for selected interventions targeting the causes of morbidity and mortality in adults. In particular, examples of intervention outcomes in key channels (e.g., communities, work sites, churches) that may exert influence on adults' health are provided. The social ecological model offers a framework for much of the discussion in this section (Stokols et al., 1996b). An ecological framework recognizes that behavior is affected by multiple levels of influence, including *intrapersonal* factors (e.g., motivation, skills, knowledge); *interpersonal* processes (e.g., social support, social network, social norms); *institutional or organizational* factors (e.g., company management characteristics, workplace policies); *community* factors (e.g., social capital, neighborhood effects); and *public policy* (e.g., regulatory laws, tobacco taxes). A number of intervention studies have been conducted targeting health behaviors, occupational health, and injury prevention; the available literature for these targets varies by intervention level. For example, health behavior interventions often address intrapersonal and interpersonal levels, while occupational health and injury prevention interventions typically address policy and regulatory levels. Examples of interventions at each of the levels in the social ecological model are provided in Box 2. Examples of strategies for operationalizing the principles of the social ecological model at each level of influence are provided in Table 2.

Reviews of behavior change interventions suggest that more intensive programs and those targeted at high-risk populations have the strongest outcome effects (Bowen and Tinker, 1995; Bowen et al., 1994; Sorensen et al., in press). These intervention strategies typically focus on intrapersonal factors and are studied in a reactive model, where participants who are ready to change are more likely to approach a specialty clinic or respond to advertisements for study programs. However, more recently many individual-level interventions have proactively recruited participants from a de- fined population. Common intervention modalities that have been utilized across a variety of intervention channels include individual counseling, group programs, telephone, computer-based interventions, and self-help or other mailed materials. These modalities vary in terms of their intensity, level of interpersonal interaction, and cost.

Individual-level counseling interventions have come out of the medical model and psychological traditions, and generally have been found to be highly effective, while at the same time quite costly (Compas et al., 1998; Fisher et al., 1993). Individual counseling is limited in terms of its reach, and public health models are being developed that provide alternative strategies to intensive one-to-one counseling (Emmons and Rollnick, in press). Efforts to reach individuals who are at especially high risk have increasingly used home visitation models to deliver individualized counseling (Olds et al., 1986, 1997). One strategy is to combine a very limited number of counseling sessions with less costly intervention modalities (e.g., mailed materials, telephone counseling).

Group sessions are also utilized as a way to deliver interpersonal counseling at a reduced cost. For some health behaviors, such as smoking and obesity, group programs have been found to outperform self-help materials, although their effectiveness relative to individual counseling has not been well evaluated (Hayaki and Brownell, 1996; Stead and Lancaster, 1999). Further, group approaches share the concerns about reach and generalizability that have been raised about individual counseling. Incorporating group sessions into community-based channels that attend to social contextual factors may be one way of improving generalizability. Telephone counseling has also become increasingly utilized as a modality for individual counseling (Ferguson, 1996; Glasgow et al., in press-b; Street et al., 1997). The impact of telephone-based interventions

TABLE 2. Health Recommendations Related to Primary Causes of Morbidity and Mortality Among Adults

Health Promotion
- accumulation of at least 30 minutes of moderate physical activity on most days of the week
- consumption of a prudent diet

  ⇒ 30% or less of calories from fat
  ⇒ 20–30 grams or more of fiber per day
  ⇒ five or more servings of fruits and vegetables per day
  ⇒ daily multivitamin
  ⇒ limit alcohol intake

- avoidance of unprotected sun exposure
- avoidance of weight gain
- practice of safe sex

Health Protection
- use seat belts and other safety equipment
- minimize exposure to occupational hazards
- use of smoke detectors

Screening
- comply with age-appropriate guidelines and health care provider's recommendations for the following screening tests:

  ⇒ cholesterol, blood pressure
  ⇒ pap tests
  ⇒ mammography
  ⇒ colon cancer screening
  ⇒ prostate cancer screening
  ⇒ depression

SOURCE: Adapted from U.S. Preventive Services Task Force Guidelines, Healthy People 2000 Objectives, and Healthy People 2010 Objectives.

on long-term behavior change is somewhat equivocal, although continued evaluations of its impact are needed (Bastani et al., 1999; Lichtenstein et al., 1996). Research is also needed on the effectiveness of telephone counseling with underserved and low-income populations, because this group is less likely to have telephones and thus may be more difficult to reach effectively with this strategy. It is also unclear whether removal of the face-to-face contact diminishes the impact of telephone intervention, especially among lower-income populations that may already be somewhat disenfranchised.

Self-help materials are another strategy for reaching large numbers of people. With most health behaviors, self-help interventions are more effective than no-intervention controls, although the overall intervention effects seen with self-help materials are generally small (Curry, 1993; Fiore et al., 1996; Glanz, 1997; Lancaster and Stead, 1999). However, the cost of self-help materials is low and the potential reach is high, which makes self-help an important component of many intervention programs.

There is evidence for the contribution made by individual approaches to health behavior change. For example, Orleans and colleagues (Orleans et al., in press) evaluated interventions for six health-damaging behaviors, including tobacco use, alcohol abuse, drug abuse, unhealthy diet, sedentary life-style, and risky sexual practices. They conclude that at the individual level, there are reasonably effective interventions for these six risk factors. Minimal intervention strategies for several risk factors have produced clinically meaningful changes when extrapolated to the population level (Abrams et al., 1996; Calfas et al., 1996; Jeffrey, 1989; McLeroy et al., 1988; O'Malley et al., 1992; Velicer et al., 1999; Warner et al., 1997). However, there is also increasing recognition of the limitations of the individual perspective. Such approaches have contributed enormously to our understanding of health behavior, and they play an important role in a comprehensive approach to public health. However, individual-level approaches are limited in their potential for health behavior change if they are conducted in isolation without the benefit of interventions and policies that also address interpersonal and societal factors that influence health behaviors.

McKinlay (1995) argued for the adoption of a population perspective to health promotion. He has proposed that effective behavior change at the population level requires concerted effort across the full spectrum of intervention levels posited by the social ecological model, which would include *downstream* interventions (e.g., individual-level interventions for those at risk or already affected); *mainstream* interventions (e.g., population-level or channel-based interventions that target defined populations for prevention); and *upstream* interventions (e.g., macro-level public policy and environmental interventions to create and strengthen social norms for healthy behaviors to reduce access to unhealthy products, and provide incentives for engaging in healthy behaviors).

Population-based approaches to health promotion have arisen out of an interest in broadening the reach of prevention interventions. The work of Rose (1992) provided a particularly good illustration of the paradox of health promotion and prevention efforts. Individually based interventions may be more effective for the individual participants, particularly those at high risk, but have limited population coverage. In contrast, population-based efforts target a large percentage of the population, but typically have lower levels of effectiveness compared to individually based intervention approaches. However, as noted earlier, small changes at the population level can lead to large effects on disease risk. In evaluating health promotion interventions, the level of intervention impact must be judged as a function of the intervention's efficacy in terms of producing individual change, as well as its reach or penetration within the population (Abrams et al., 1996; Glasgow et al., 1999; Sorensen et al., in press). Focusing on impact and reach is a more useful dialogue than the increasingly common arguments pitting individual and population approaches against each other and would argue for interventions that bridge intervention levels, thus taking advantage of higher change levels found in individual intervention, while simultaneously expanding reach into the population.

The next section provides a brief review of outcomes for selected interventions targeting the causes of morbidity and mortality in adults. In particular, examples of intervention outcomes in key channels (e.g., communities, work sites, health care settings, churches) that may exert influence on adults' health are provided. In summarizing the work done in each channel, the review criteria suggested by Hancock and colleagues (Hancock et al., 1997) have been considered. Their criteria for rigorous scientific evaluation of community intervention trials include four domains: (1) design, including the randomization of communities or organizations to condition; (2) measures, including the use of outcome measures with demonstrated validity and reliability, and use of intervention process measures; (3) analysis, including consideration of both individual- and community-level variation within each treatment condition; and (4) specification of the intervention in enough detail to allow replication. Although this paper is not intended to be a thorough review of each channel, a summary statement will be provided regarding the extent to which research within each channel meets these criteria.

COMMUNITY-BASED TRIALS

Community-based health promotion interventions were first studied in the late 1970s and early 1980s, as a result of the increased recognition that coronary heart disease prevention requires efforts beyond the individual level (Farquhar, 1978; Farquhar et al., 1977, 1985; Kottke et al., 1985; Puska et al., 1983; Rose, 1982). The behavioral sciences made key contributions to the development and evaluation of these trials and to the movement of chronic disease prevention and management out of the medical model. Community-based population-level approaches do have much greater potential for impacting behavior among a larger number of people, although these interventions are typically much less intensive than individually targeted interventions and therefore the intervention effects for the individual tend to be much smaller. Some of the community-based studies conducted to date have found no intervention effects across all studied risk factors (Glasgow et al., 1995); others have found effects on some of the targeted behaviors (Carleton et al., 1987; Luepker et al., 1994; Sorensen et al., 1996a). Overall, community interventions have yielded many significant effects. Further, economic policy models suggest that population-level application of the results found in community trials (Winkleby et al., 1996) would be highly cost-effective when compared with most accepted medical interventions (Tosteson et al., 1997).

Unlike the heart disease prevention trials that targeted a specific disease, other community-based trials have targeted specific health behaviors that confer risk for a number of diseases. In 1989, the National Cancer Institute (NCI) launched the Community Intervention Trial for Smoking Cessation (COMMIT) (COMMIT, 1991, 1995a, 1995b) in an effort to increase smoking cessation rates, using methods similar to those utilized in the heart disease prevention programs. COMMIT utilized a randomized control design, with 11 matched pairs of communities. A significant intervention effect was found among light-to-moderate smokers, and quit rates were higher among less educated smokers in the intervention group (COMMIT, 1995a); no intervention effect was found among heavy smokers (COMMIT, 1995a, 1995b). There is mixed support for community-based nutrition interventions with adults, although there have been promising findings related to point-of-choice information, risk reduction for coronary heart disease in medical settings, and work sites (Glanz et al., 1992, 1996; Levy et al., 1985; Sorensen et al., 1992, 1996a).

It should be noted that few community-based studies meet the criteria specified by Hancock and colleagues (Hancock et al., 1997) for rigorous scientific evaluation (Sorensen et al., in press). The community is rarely used as the unit of analysis, and response rates are often low. Because of cost, outcomes are typically self-report and not validated. Thus, even though there have been some positive outcomes from community trials, our ability to draw firm conclusions on the basis of the existing trials is limited.

CHANNELS WITHIN THE COMMUNITY

The community trials have focused on community-level effects, randomizing communities instead of individuals. Other studies within the community have utilized a range of different intervention modalities and different units of analysis (e.g., individuals, workplaces, and health care settings). Channel-based interventions have the advantage of having defined populations that can be reached through direct contact, environmental-, organizational-, and policy-level interventions. They also provide the opportunity for delivery of a more intensive intervention dose. Although all studies have not uniformly had significant results, social and behavioral scientists have made significant progress in identifying a number of key channels in which prevention interventions can be effectively and efficiently delivered.

Work Site Interventions

There is a relatively large body of work site health promotion research; work sites are now considered key channels for disease prevention among adults (Abrams, 1991; Abrams et al., 1994a; Fielding, 1984; Heimendinger et al., 1990). Work site interventions have the advantage of being able to reach across intervention levels and include interventions targeting individuals, the organization, and the environment. A number of risk factors have been targeted through the workplace, including smoking (Jeffery et al., 1993; Sorensen et al., 1993, 1996b), nutrition (Byers et al., 1995; Sorensen et al., 1996a, 1999), cholesterol

(Byers et al., 1995; Glasgow et al., 1995, 1997b), physical activity (Shepard, 1996), and alcohol (Roman and Blum, 1996), HIV (Wilson et al., 1996b), colorectal cancer screening (Tilley et al., 1999b), and occupational exposures (Ellenbecker, 1996; Heaney and Goldenhar, 1996; Sorensen et al., 1995). Sorensen et al. (in press) recently reviewed the results of 15 representative, randomized control work site studies that targeted smoking, nutrition, weight management, physical activity and/or cholesterol reduction (Byers et al., 1995; Dishman et al., 1998; Emmons et al., 1999b; Glasgow et al., 1995, 1997b; Heirich et al., 1993; Jeffery et al., 1993, 1994; Salina et al., 1994; Sorensen et al., 1992, 1993, 1996a, 1999). At least half of the studies reviewed achieved significant effects on the target behavioral outcomes (Glasgow et al., 1997b; Jeffery et al., 1993; Salina et al., 1994; Sorensen et al., 1992, 1993, 1996a, 1996b; Tilley et al., 1999a). The studies that included extended follow-up periods found that intervention effects were maintained or increased beyond the postintervention follow-up (Byers et al., 1995; Salina et al., 1994; Sorensen et al., 1993). Studies of workplace physical activity interventions have found increased physical activity levels and favorable changes in body mass index (BMI) and fitness levels, as well as improved illness and injury rates (Evans et al., 1994; Farquhar et al., 1985; Peterson and Aldana, 1999; Shepard, 1996), although a recent review of work site physical activity interventions concluded that the generally poor scientific quality of these studies limits the conclusions that can be drawn (Dishman et al., 1998). Concerns about quality of study designs have been raised about other areas of work site research (Glanz ct al., 1996; Hennrikus and Jeffery, 1996; Wilson et al., 1996a), although Sorensen et al. (Sorensen et al., in press) conclude that the majority of work site intervention trials do meet many of the criteria for scientific quality outlined by Hancock et al. (1997).

Although few work site health promotion interventions effectively include multiple levels of intervention over a sustained period of time, those that do have improved outcomes and have shown effects for more difficult-to-reach subgroups (Sorensen et al., 1998c; Willemsen et al., 1998). Patterson et al. (1997) demonstrated that longer, interactive interventions in the workplace result in more positive outcomes. Given the number of work site health promotion intervention studies that have been conducted, it is surprising that so few studies have provided data on the impact of the intervention on the environmental- or organizational-level outcomes. One of the few such evaluations used data from the Working Well Trial (Biener et al., 1999). This multilevel intervention led to significant increases in the availability of fruit and vegetables, access to nutrition information at work, and positive social norms regarding dietary choice; no effects were observed for smoking policies. The impact of the intervention on the environment tracked well with employee behavior changes, in which significant improvements were observed for dietary outcomes but not for smoking (Sorensen et al., 1996c).

The most substantial study of regulatory and policy interventions in the workplace has been in occupational health (Wilson et al., 1996a). Much of the emphasis in comprehensive approaches to occupational health is to be as far upstream in the causal pathway as possible (e.g., preventing exposure and injury is the optimal strategy) (LaMontagne and Christiani, in press). This emphasis is in part driven by the Occupational Safety and Health Act of 1970, which requires employers to provide employees a workplace that is free from recognized hazards that can lead to death or serious physical harm (NIOSH, 1996). A continuum of strategies, known as the "hierarchy of controls," is a comprehensive set of exposure prevention and control measures used by occupational health professionals to reduce exposures at the organizational and individual levels (Wegman and Levy, 1995). Hazard elimination or substitution is the first step in the hierarchy. There are a number of examples where hazards testing led to elimination or substitution of processes that were known to be carcinogenic (LaMontagne and Christiani, in press). Other upstream interventions that have been effective in reducing occupational hazards include installation of effective ventilation systems, substitution of toxic chemicals, and job redesign (Becker, 1990; Erfurt et al., 1991; Sundstrom, 1986; Williams, 1982). Several states have also passed toxics use reduction laws that integrate reduction of occupational exposures to hazardous chemicals with reduction of environmental exposures in surrounding communities. Such laws have been associated with substantial reduction in the use of toxic chemicals in affected industries (LaMontagne and Christiani, in press).

Integration of Office Practice Systems and Health Care Provider Training in Prevention into the Standard of Health Care Delivery

The health care system provides an important channel for prevention interventions. Several national and clinical care guidelines recommend that physicians routinely advise their patients regarding behavioral risk factors for chronic disease (American Cancer Society, 1980; National Cancer Institute, 1987; USDHHS, 1991) and screen for mental health problems such as depression (Elkin et al., 1989; U.S. Preventive Services Task Force, 1996). A substantial number of controlled clinical trials have shown that brief physician counseling is effective in changing a number of patients' health behaviors (Adams et al., 1998; Calfas et al., 1997; Dietrich et al., 1992; Friedman et al., 1994; Hunt et al., 1995; Kottke et al., 1988; Levine, 1987; Lewis, 1988; Manley et al., 1992; Marcus et al., 1997; Ockene et al., 1991, 1999), and proactive depression screening results in improved recognition of and treatment for depression (Elkin et al., 1989; Regier et al., 1993b). However, in clinical practice it is difficult for primary care physicians to accomplish recommended activities. The rates of physician interventions for key preventive interventions are quite low; 20–50% of patients are given dietary advice (Dietrich et al., 1992; Hunt et al., 1995; Lewis, 1988; Orleans et al., 1985; Wells et al., 1986; Wells and Lewis, 1984); only 15% of patients are given advice to be more active (Friedman et al., 1994); only 42% of obese patients report that their health care provider has advised them to lose weight (Galuska et al., 1999); and only 50% of physicians report providing smoking cessation counseling to their patients who smoke (Thorndike et al., 1998). Mental health problems are also unrecognized and undertreated in the primary care setting; primary care providers do not recognize major depression in approximately 50% of their patients with this disorder (Attkisson et al., 1990; Borus et al., 1988; Coyne et al., 1991; Panzarino, 1998; Schulberg et al., 1985; Wells et al., 1989b). Further, in community settings, health care providers demonstrate relatively low levels of competence in many prevention topics as well as chronic disease management (Griffin and Kinmonth, 1999; Levine et al., 1993; Velasquez et al., in press).

It has been shown that structured office systems that include physician reminders to conduct counseling and brief screenings are a critical component of provider-based interventions (e.g., computerized reminders, chart stickers, chart checklists, nurse-initiated reminders). Such office system interventions have been found to significantly increase the rate of several health promotion or prevention interventions among community physicians (Dietrich et al., 1992; Harvey et al., 1999). Although provider education is also important, education alone does not increase provider's provision of prevention counseling, but education plus office systems do (Ockene et al., 1995, 1996, 1999; Wilson et al., 1988).

The quality of the provider-delivered intervention studies has generally been high, with a majority of studies meeting the criteria outlined by Hancock et al. (1997), including inclusion of the provider as the unit of randomization, adequate response rates, and validation of outcomes related to provider counseling.

Family-Based Intervention

The important role that families play in determining health behaviors among both children and adults has been well documented (Baranowski, 1997; Kintner et al., 1981; Schafer, 1978; Schafer and Keith, 1982). However, most family interventions have targeted health behaviors in children, and thus there has been relatively little behavioral intervention work utilizing family interventions to impact on health behaviors among adults (Baranowski, 1997). There is a relative scarcity of studies on health behavior that specify the sequence or causal linkages by which individuals influence and are influenced by the larger social context, including the family (Altman and King, 1986; Sorensen et al., 1998b; Winett et al., 1989). One exception is the evaluation of a family and work site intervention conducted by Sorensen et al. (1999). The work site plus family intervention lead to a 19% increase in total fruit and vegetable increase, compared to a 7% increase found in a work site intervention-only group; there was no change in the control group. This is an excellent example of the synergy in intervention channels and the potentially powerful impact that family interventions may play in improving the health of adults.

Church-Based Interventions

With increasing disparities in chronic disease morbidity and mortality between black and white Americans (Lundberg, 1991; McBeath, 1991; National Research Council, 1989; Thomas et al., 1994), public health researchers have begun to investigate alternative strategies for delivering health interventions to black communities. The church has a long history of addressing unmet health and human service needs of the black community, and therefore health behavior interventions are likely to fit well within the church's priorities (Eng et al., 1985; Levin, 1984; Thomas et al., 1994; Wiist and Flack, 1990). Several recent studies suggest that church-based interventions are an important strategy for contextualizing health behavior interventions (Davis et al., 1994; DePue et al., 1990; Eng et al., 1985; Levin, 1984; Thomas et al., 1994; Voorhees et al., 1996; Wiist and Flack, 1990). Becker and colleagues have conducted a number of church-based interventions as part of a model partnership program between the Johns Hopkins Academic Health Center and the East Baltimore community, within which organizations such as Clergy United for Renewal of East Baltimore and other community organizations play key leadership roles (Becker et al., 1999; Levine et al., 1994; Voorhees et al., 1996). Much of this work has utilized spiritually based "environmental" interventions (e.g., pastoral sermons on smoking, testimony during church services, training of volunteers as lay smoking cessation counselors) and individually oriented interventions (individual and group support supplemented with spiritual audiotapes containing gospel music, day-by-day scripturally guided behavior change booklets, and health fairs targeting cardiovascular risk and personalized health feedback). A spiritually based smoking intervention yielded impressive quit rates but was not significantly different from an American Lung Association program that was also delivered in the church setting (Voorhees et al., 1996). A church-based obesity intervention among African-American women yielded small but significant overall changes at the 1-year follow-up in weight, waist circumference, and diastolic blood pressure. Of note, 20% of participants achieved highly significant long-term reductions in these outcomes (Becker et al., 1999). Campbell and colleagues (Campbell et al., 1999) conducted an intervention focused on increasing fruit and vegetable consumption among members of rural African-American churches. Ten counties comprising 50 churches were matched and assigned to 20-month intervention or delayed intervention. At the 2-year follow-up, the intervention group consumed 0.85 servings per day more than the comparison group; effects were even greater among subgroups.

These studies demonstrate that the church is a viable setting for conducting health interventions and that substantial effects can be achieved. Interventions that place health in the context of religion and emphasize the church's religious values have been particularly effective. Utilization of peer health advisers and church volunteers for intervention design and delivery is particularly promising because these strategies not only help to contextualize the intervention messages, but also increase the likelihood of program institutionalization within both the church culture and its ministry. Evaluations of organizational characteristics of churches suggest that larger churches with more educated clergy are most likely to offer church-based health promotion programs (Thomas et al., 1994). Although response rates of church-based studies have been variable, many studies have used the church as the unit of analysis, and validated measures are typically included. There is excellent process data available regarding church-based interventions, and intervention details are well specified (Emmons, 2000).

Regulatory Channels

There have been some examples of regulatory action to promote preventive health behaviors, although the potential of regulatory interventions has not nearly been realized. For example, legislative and policy efforts that create a safe physical environment and incentives for increased activity have been virtually untested in the United States (Bauman et al., in press; King et al., 1995). The recent federal nutrition labeling laws represent important progress at the regulatory level in terms of diet. Labeling is an important innovation because the use of food nutrition labels is associated with lower fat intake (Guthrie et al., 1995; Kreuter and Brennan, 1997; Neuhouser et al., 1999). There are many other potentially effective regulatory strategies that have not been adopted (e.g., price supports for healthy foods, taxes on unhealthy foods). In addition, there are virtually no data about the effects of combining regulatory approaches with dietary counseling (Glanz et al., 1995; Glanz, 1997). Tobacco control is one health behavior in which there has been considerable use of upstream interventions (e.g., tobacco taxes, access policies to prevent minors from buying cigarettes, workplace smoking policies) (Emmons et al., 1997), with significant effects observed on smoking prevalence (Glasgow et al., 1997a). It has been estimated that requiring all work sites to be smoke-free would reduce smoking prevalence by at least 10% (see Paper Contribution K for further discussion of tobacco control policies) (Farrelly et al., 1999).

Two areas in which considerable progress has been made at the policy and regulatory levels are injury prevention and occupational health. Legislation to reduce driving under the influence of alcohol is credited in part with the 26% reduction observed in deaths from alcohol-related crashes between 1983 and 1993 (National Highway Traffic Safety Administration, 1996b). Introduction of lap and shoulder restraints and car seats is estimated to have reduced the risk of death or serious injury by 45% and 70%, respectively (Johnson and Walker, 1996; *MMWR*, 1991; National Highway Traffic Safety Administration, 1996a). Laws requiring installation of smoke detectors are common, and it is estimated that they have resulted in an 80% decrease in fire-related mortality and similar levels of decrease in injury (Mallonee et al., 1996). A number of laws (e.g., Occupational Safety and Health Act of 1970, Toxic Substances Control Act of 1976) have led to reduced occupational hazards at the workplace, although there have been a number of court challenges to efforts to strengthen regulatory control over occupational hazards that have significantly reduced and/or delayed adoption of important controls at the regulatory and policy levels (LaMontagne and Christiani, in press).

HOW CAN SOCIAL AND BEHAVIORAL SCIENCES EXPAND ON PROGRESS TO DATE?

One of the key goals of this IOM committee is to explore the untapped potential of social and behavioral sciences to improve health, and to determine how to build on the current knowledge base to achieve this goal. Despite the relatively limited resources available for widespread population-level public health endeavors, there have been a number of successes in specific intervention channels. Some might argue that more progress should have been made to date. However, in evaluating the contributions of the social and behavioral sciences to health promotion, there are a number of factors that must be considered. First, the history of involvement of the social and behavioral sciences in prevention is relatively limited. For example, this history spans only about four decades, compared to the lengthy history of work conducted in the medical sciences. Second, treatment advances in medicine have been developed in large part as the result of the very large investments that drug companies and the federal government have made in the development of drugs. Although there have been substantial government resources available in the past decade for social and behavioral science research, there is no funding stream for the behavioral and social sciences parallel to that seen in drug development. Third, there has been considerable success in developing behavioral interventions to improve health at the individual level. The upstream approaches that are a central part of efforts to make an impact at the population level require coordinated, sustained effort, and lobbying for policy and legislative changes at the local, state, and national levels. Although advocacy is an established tradition within public health, the available resources are typically swamped in comparison to those available to businesses and corporations. The best example of what is possible within public health is the case of tobacco, in which the coordinated efforts of scientists, public health advocates, teachers, parents, and the legal system came together to force change on an industry that had spent tremendous resources on making itself invulnerable. States that have used tobacco taxes to organize and fund comprehensive tobacco control programs have had significant reductions in smoking prevalence, while prevalence has remained relatively stable in states without such comprehensive programs (*MMWR*, 1999). This is a wonderful example of what can be done if resources are available and coordinated.

This section of the paper focuses on a discussion of factors that have an impact on the success of health behavior change interventions, including the need to link multiple levels of intervention, development of effective strategies for targeting multiple risk factors, anticipation of the impact that advanced computer technology may have on intervention design and delivery, a focus on sustainability and dissemination, and consideration of the social context of health behaviors. These issues will be discussed and examples of interventions

provided that show promise for making further progress on risk factor prevalence. It should be noted that while the majority of studies discussed in the remainder of this paper are randomized controlled trials, examples of demonstration projects or quasi-experimental studies are utilized where such work
demonstrates promise and further exploration is warranted.

LINKAGES BETWEEN MULTIPLE LEVELS OF INTERVENTION

One key contribution of social and behavioral sciences has been to broaden
the perspectives that are used to study and improve health beyond biomedical
approaches to disease causation, as illustrated in Figure 1. As this figure illustrates, different disciplines have different "lenses" through which the mechanisms of disease causation are viewed. The broadened focus contributed by the
social and behavioral sciences has led to increased interdisciplinary research and
the development of frameworks such as the social ecological model that consider the domains of interest across disciplines. Proponents of the social ecological model strongly emphasize the importance of conducting cross-level interventions (Stokols et al., 1996b). The injury prevention area has provided some
good examples of efforts to link upstream or regulatory interventions with those
targeting other levels of the social ecological model (Bonnie et al., 1999). Perhaps the most compelling example is the prevention of motor fatalities. Although educational campaigns to encourage increased use of safety belts by individuals are important, air bags, minimum legal drinking age laws, redesign of
cars to include safety features, and redesign of highways have been credited
with making the greatest contribution to reduced fatality rates per mile driven
(Henry et al., 1996; Rivara et al., 1997; Womble, 1988). Another example of
multilevel injury prevention is the use of smoke detectors (Bonnie et al., 1999).
Passage of legislation that requires installation and/or inspection of smoke detectors at the time of home sales increases the likelihood that homes will have
smoke detectors; educational campaigns reminding people to test their smoke
detectors and change their batteries every year on their birthday increase the
likelihood that homes will have *functioning* smoke detectors. There are also a
number of examples of effective multilevel interventions in occupational health.
For example, exposure to occupational carcinogens has been reduced by implementing engineering solutions to limit the source of exposure and conducting
training sessions to improve worker awareness and efforts to reduce personal
exposure (LaMontagne et al., 1992).

In the health promotion area, there have been efforts to link access and policy-level interventions with individual-level interventions, although this is rarely

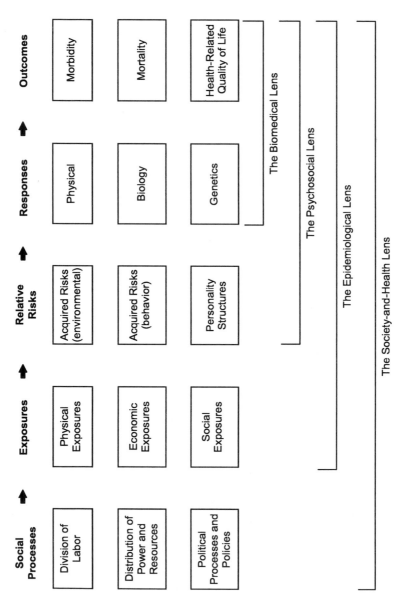

FIGURE 1. The Contribution of Social and Behavioral Sciences to the Biomedical Perspective on Disease Causation. SOURCE: Adapted from Walsh, Sorensen, and Leonard in Amick BC, Levin S. Tarlov AR, and Walsh DC (eds), Society and Health, Oxford University Press, Oxford, 1995.

done in the context of randomized studies. The Massachusetts farmer's market coupon program for low-income elders (Webber et al., 1995) is an excellent example of an intervention designed to increase individual fruit and vegetable consumption by increasing access. Through collaboration between the Massachusetts Department of Public Health and Department of Food and Agriculture, farmer's market coupons were distributed through elderly nutrition projects throughout the state. In 1992, almost $86,000 in coupons was distributed by 23 agencies to 17,200 older adults; 73% of the coupons were redeemed, and 32% of the seniors reported buying significantly more fruit and vegetables since receiving the coupons. Coupons distributed through this program brought an additional $62,000 in revenue to the markets, in addition to money spent at the markets after the coupons had been spent. This is an excellent example of an access-oriented intervention that targets both individual behavior and organizational- and policy-level change, building on an interagency collaboration that addresses separate and overlapping goals of each agency.

Environmental- or policy-level changes also can provide improved access to health promotion opportunities. Linenger et al. (1991) used a quasi-experimental design to evaluate the impact of an environmental intervention for physical activity on fitness levels among two naval communities and a Navy-wide sample. The environmental intervention included building bicycle paths along roadways, extending hours at recreation facilities, purchasing new exercise equipment for gyms, holding basewide athletic events, organizing running and bicycling clubs, opening women's fitness centers, and marking running courses at various sites. This comprehensive environmental and norm-based intervention led to significantly greater improvements in fitness in the intervention community. Although policy interventions on physical activity may be somewhat easier to implement in the context of the military, there are many environmental approaches to physical activity in civilian communities that could be relatively easy to implement. Passive approaches to promoting physical activity (e.g., restricting downtown centers for foot or bicycle traffic, placing parking lots at a distance from buildings, and making stairways more convenient and safe) have important potential for achieving widespread increases in physical activity at the population level (King et al., 1995).

Linkages between channels are also important. Wang et al. (1999) evaluated the impact of a recommendation to see one's physician as part of a work site cholesterol screening program on compliance with the recommendation and on change in risk factors for heart disease. Only 35% of participants with an elevated cholesterol level saw their provider following receipt of a recommendation for follow-up. This fact illustrates the importance of finding better ways to link such key intervention channels.

There is growing evidence that full-spectrum interventions (McKinlay, 1995) show substantial promise for improving the effectiveness of behavior change interventions related to health promotion topics, although few interventions targeting adults have provided a substantial intervention dose across all levels of the social ecological model. At the population level, stepped-care approaches, in which increasingly intense strategies are applied only after a person has been unsuccessful with less intense approaches, have been recommended as one way to improve intervention delivery across levels (Abrams et al., 1996). While stepped-care models do provide an important means of insuring the availability of a broad range of services, they do not necessarily provide linkages across levels of the social ecological model. Strong interventions across all levels are needed in order to consistently outperform secular trends (Bauman et al., 1999; Glasgow et al., 1995; Sorensen et al., 1998a; Winkleby et al., 1997). In their "report card" on progress in population health promotion, Orleans and colleagues (Orleans et al., in press) concluded that the ideal of a "full court press" involving interventions across levels is seldom met.

Glasgow and colleagues (1999) have taken an important step toward developing a theoretically driven framework for use in multilevel community-based and public health interventions. In particular, they argue that many multilevel interventions are not amenable to classic evaluation strategies (e.g., randomized controlled, double-blind trials) and thus require alternative evaluation approaches. The goal of identifying interventions that have significant effects often is met at the expense of developing interventions that can be institutionalized (Bandura, 1977; Flora et al., 1993; Lefebvre and Flora, 1988; Rogers, 1983). Even when interventions are found to be cost-effective, structural and political issues can delay or impede implementation (Glasgow et al., in press-a; Vogt et al., 1998). The RE-AIM evaluation framework proposed by Glasgow is designed to be compatible with social ecological approaches to promoting health in communities. Central to the RE-AIM framework is that the public health impact of an intervention is a function of the interaction of a program's performance on five separate evaluative dimensions, including (1) *Reach* into the population of interest; (2) *Efficacy* of the intervention; (3) *Adoption* by representative organizations; (4) *Implementation* under real world conditions; and (5) *Maintenance* over time (see Table 3). This framework allows for the calculation of a "public health impact summary score," which is a multiplicative combination of the component dimensions. The RE-AIM model highlights the limitations of the classic randomized controlled trial methodology that is frequently applied to community-based intervention trials and particularly points out the insufficiencies of the exclusive emphasis on efficacy inherent in this latter approach. Assessing intervention outcomes across multiple levels of influence can make it possible to determine what programs are worth sustained investment.

COLLABORATION BETWEEN ACADEMIC AND COMMUNITY PARTNERS

It has become clear that there is a great need for community-based research efforts that are not conducted *on* communities, but that are conducted *by* communities. In the past several years there has been an increased emphasis on the importance of greater community involvement and control through partnerships

TABLE 3. Social Ecological Model: Examples of Interventions at
Each Level of Influence

Intrapersonal Level
⇒ motivational interventions
⇒ skills building opportunities
⇒ tailored intervention materials

Interpersonal Level
⇒ interventions targeting social norms and social networks

Organizational/Environmental Level
⇒ interventions in health care system
⇒ interventions in workplaces
⇒ interventions in schools

Community Level
⇒ networking with community resources
⇒ social service advocacy
⇒ structural/environmental interventions in communities
⇒ community-based interventions

Policy Level
⇒ local, state, and federal laws
⇒ intervention with federal regulatory agencies

---

among academic, health, and community organizations (Clark and McLeroy, 1995; Israel et al., 1995; Minkler and Wallerstein, 1997; Novotny and Healton, 1995; Sorensen et al., in press). Israel distinguishes between community-*based* research, which is characterized by community members being actively engaged and having influence and control in all aspects of the research process, and community-*placed* research, in which research is conducted in a community as a place or setting, but the role of community members is restricted to that of study participants. Community-placed research is not usually the result of an interest to exclude the community from the research planning process, but more likely a function of researchers finding themselves in the situation of having an idea for a study or a funding opportunity with a very tight time line and then approaching community organizations or members with the agenda well formulated. Although many trials have been conducted under these circumstances, such an approach often ignores the agenda and context of the community and thus is likely to lead to difficulties in implementation and/or suboptimal outcomes.

The Centers for Disease Control and Prevention's (CDC's) Prevention Research Centers (PRCs) are an excellent example of academic-community partnerships. Twenty-three centers were recently funded to conduct community-based prevention research. A variety of health and social problems are targeted in diverse populations (CDC, 1999). This funding mechanism is designed to support interdisciplinary research on risk conditions and social determinants of health, and to focus on sustainability and dissemination (CDC, 1997). The centers are also charged with enhancing the process by which communities become equal partners in all phases of research. The PRC program holds great promise for larger-scale collaboration with communities and the development of effective strategies for sustaining and disseminating research programs.

Increased Emphasis on Multiple Risk Factor Interventions

It is clear that risk increases proportionally with the number of risk factors an individual has (Anderson et al., 1991; Berglund et al., 1996; Sebastian et al., 1989; Taylor, Robson, and Evans, 1992). Reduction of multiple risk factors leads to substantial increases in cost-effectiveness (Tosteson et al., 1997). Multiple behavioral risk factors are prevalent across the life span (Emmons et al., 1994; French et al., 1996; Neumark Sztainer et al., 1996; Pate et al., 1996); between 40% and 60% of adults have more than one risk factor for chronic disease (Emmons et al., 1994, 1999a; Greenlund et al., 1998). Certain risk factors have been found to cluster, and there are important relationships in how people think about their different health behaviors. For example, there are inverse relationships between expected consequences for exercise and smoking; individuals who rate the *negative* consequences of smoking highly are also more likely to rate the *positive* benefits of exercise highly (King et al., 1996). Self-efficacy levels for these two behaviors are also positively related. Development of effective interventions for changing multiple risk factors is important for a number of reasons. First, the clustering of risk factors and the interrelationships in cognitive mediators across health behaviors suggest that there may be some efficiency in targeting more than one risk factor at a time. Second, prevalence of multiple risk factors is high. Third, there is some evidence available to suggest that change on one behavioral risk factor may serve as a stimulus or gateway for change in other health behaviors. Recent studies suggest that leisure time activity may increase among smokers who quit (French et al., 1996; Gomel et al., 1997), and combined exercise and smoking cessation interventions have led to increased smoking cessation rates (Marcus et al., 1991, 1995, 1999). Changes in smoking prevalence and smoking behavior have been found in a number of studies following introduction of workplace physical activity interventions (Shepard, 1996). Intentions to become more physically active and to limit alcohol consumption have been found to be higher among recent quitters than among continuing smokers (Unger, 1996), and there is increasing evidence that smoking cessation may benefit alcohol relapse prevention among alcoholic smokers (Abrams et al., 1994b; Sobell et al., 1990).

Despite the relationships that have been found across multiple risk factors, not all investigations of multiple risk factor interventions have been positive (Hall et al., 1992). A recent review of multiple risk factor interventions for primary prevention of coronary heart disease concluded that multiple risk factor changes in such trials are modest (Ebrahim and Davey Smith, 1999). Thus, the authors conclude that multiple risk factor interventions have limited value. However, the trials reviewed were primarily individual risk factor interventions that did not utilize multiple levels of intervention. Further, multiple risk factor interventions typically have been several different individual risk factor interventions delivered simultaneously. Rarely have multiple risk factor interventions paid attention to the methodology of implementing changes on more than one risk factor at a time. Rather, such interventions typically target several risk factors in a single population, but do not link the process of changing the target behaviors. Little is known about how to best approach multiple risk factor change, and thus it is premature to dismiss this approach. The interrelationships among risk behaviors cannot be ignored and may provide an important opportunity to maximize the potency of health promotion interventions. Key questions that need to be addressed include at what point multiple risk factor approaches are overwhelming to participants and thus affect recruitment and retention rates, which risk factors are most facilitative for change in other risk factors (c.g., What risk factors should be targeted together and in what sequence?), the optimal intervention dose needed to accomplish change in more than one behavior, and whether multiple risk factor approaches are cost-effective. Efforts to develop and evaluate strategies for reducing multiple risk factors simultaneously are an important part of efforts to improve the outcome of health promotion interventions.

Use of Computer Technology for Intervention Development and Delivery

Computer technology offers several new options for intervention development and delivery. It is estimated that 33% of all U.S. adults have on-line access, and 38% of these adults have used the Internet for health and medical information in the past 12 months (American Internet User Survey, 1999); use rates are increasing dramatically each year. Computers are also playing an increasingly important role in health care practice, and computer-based integrated practice systems are becoming key tools to help health care providers effectively manage the time and administrative burdens of today's health care system. For example, WebMD is an Internet-based health care service system that currently has more than 35 major health care system members (representing 42,000 physicians). Such integrated systems may include use of the Internet for prescription refills and ordering lab tests, on-line drug interaction services, increased e-mail correspondence between patients and providers, customized websites for patient education, use of the Internet for referral and patient information services, and provision of on-line continuing medical education courses. These are trends that behavioral scientists must be keenly aware of, because they provide new and unique opportunities for delivery of health promotion and protection interventions.

There is also an increasing emphasis on the use of computer technology to improve the effectiveness and reach of behavior change interventions. Computers offer the opportunity for computer-assisted learning, which can teach prevention and self-management skills in an interesting and standardized manner (Lehmann and Deutsch, 1995; Marrero, 1993). For example, diabetes simulations have been developed that allow diabetics to explore various therapeutic options with a physiologically appropriate computer-based model (Glasgow et al., in press-b). Such an approach allows participants to learn how to manage error and build their self-management skills without the real health risks that are associated with real-life trial and error.

Another technology-based innovation is telephone-linked care (TLC), which is computer-controlled telephone counseling of patients in their homes (Friedman, 1998; Ramelson et al., 1999). TLC uses a digitized human voice that delivers counseling based on theoretically determined algorithms. A randomized trial of TLC applied to medication adherence resulted in significantly increased adherence in the intervention group at the 6-month follow-up (Friedman, 1998). Importantly, the intervention group experienced a substantial reduction in diastolic blood pressure, while the control group experienced an increase. A TLC intervention for dietary modification in hypercholesterolemic patients led to significant intervention effects for cholesterol level (Dutton et al., 1995), and a TLC intervention for exercise resulted in large intervention effects differences that reached marginal levels of significance (Cullinane et al., 1994). Delivery of TLC interventions is low cost; for example, the cost of the TLC adherence intervention was $32.50 per patient, for a cost-effectiveness ratio of $5.42 per 1% improvement in adherence (Friedman et al., 1996). These results suggest that this approach has great promise as a tool that can be integrated into the health care delivery system.

A growing body of research has been conducted on tailored interventions that use computer algorithms to prepare intervention materials in which messages are designed especially for a particular individual based on relevant and important personal information (Crane et al., 1998; Curry et al., 1995; King et al., 1994; Rimer and Glassman, 1997; Rimer et al., 1994; Velicer et al., 1993). Tailored interventions typically utilize computer-based "expert systems" programs that match a large library of messages to patient information needs, combining specific statements and graphics into a personalized intervention at relatively modest cost (Skinner et al., 1993). These are often proactive interventions that deliver tailored materials to a defined population (e.g., health maintenance organizations [HMO] members), regardless of whether or not the individuals are seeking to change.

Many tailored interventions have been found to increase short- and long-term behavior change rates (Bastani et al., 1999; Brug et al., 1998, 1996; Curry et al., 1995; King et al., 1994; Koffman et al., 1998; Rakowski et al., 1998; Rimer and Glassman, 1997; Rimer et al., 1994; Strecher et al., 1994), although other studies have not yielded significant results across all (Bull et al., 1999; Crane et al., 1998; Kreuter and Strecher, 1996; Lutz et al., 1999; Rimer et al.,

1999). There is some evidence that iterative tailored communications can increase behavior change over single tailored communications (Brug et al., 1998). A recent review by Skinner and colleagues (1999) reached the conclusion that tailored print materials have been demonstrated to attract notice and readership and to influence behavior change. The impact of tailored interventions on long-term behavior change requires further evaluation (Bastani et al., 1999).

Tailored intervention strategies could be an effective means of targeting the pockets of heightened prevalence in which disease risk is clustered (Feinleib, 1996; Fisher, 1995b); however, unless such interventions are perceived as relevant to the issues faced on a daily basis by the target population, the likelihood of achieving either short-term or sustained intervention impact is greatly diminished. Interventions may be tailored to the unique needs and cultures of communities and could include factors such as social class, literacy level, culture, or neighborhood of residence (Rothman, 1970; Sorensen et al., in press). One example of an excellent effort to address contextual factors utilized a combination of a tailored health care provider prompting intervention (tailored to patients' stage of change) with tailored interventions to promote smoking cessation among low-income African Americans who were patients in a community health center (Lipkus et al., in press). Participants were randomly assigned to receive the provider prompting intervention only, the provider intervention plus tailored print materials (birthday cards and birthday newsletters); or the provider intervention, tailored print materials, and tailored telephone counseling (tailored variables included reasons for quitting, nicotine dependence, and previous quit attempts). Of note, the tailored print materials reflected the context of participants' lives (e.g., a section on transportation barriers included information about bus routes; messages about life stresses reflected participants' low-income status; art and graphics were designed by a local African-American artist and tailored by gender). Smoking cessation rates at the 16-month follow-up were significantly greater among those who received provider prompting plus tailored print materials, compared to both those who received all three levels of intervention and those who received provider prompting alone.

It is important to recognize that there may be some limits to the use of tailored interventions with lower-income populations. For example, tailored interventions typically rely upon completion of extensive questionnaire batteries, either by telephone or in person (Velicer et al., 1993). Lower-income individuals are less likely to be accessible by telephone (Resnicow et al., 1996) and are more likely to have low literacy skills that can limit the length of assessments that are feasible (Kirsch et al., 1993; Williams et al., 1995). Interactive computer-assisted videos have been developed and may be one alternative for delivering tailored interventions that addresses some of these constraints (USDHHS, 1994).

Sustainability

There is ample evidence from a number of community intervention trials demonstrating that community-wide behavior change is possible (Farquhar et al., 1990; Pietinen et al., 1996, 1983). These studies clearly state that health education, social policies, and economic conditions cause risk factor change (Fortmann et al., 1993a, 1993b, 1990). However, too often there is insufficient community-level buy-in to sustain interventions, and thus they typically end when the research is over. Sustainability refers to the infrastructure that remains in a community after a research project ends and includes consideration of interventions that are maintained; organizations that modify their behavior as a result of participation in research; and individuals who, as part of their involvement in the research process, gain knowledge and skills that are used in other life domains (Altman, 1995; Bracht et al., 1994; Goodman and Steckler, 1989; Jackson et al., 1989). There has generally been limited emphasis on assessing intervention sustainability, and when it has been measured, there has been limited success. Sorensen et al. (1998d) found that 2 years following completion of a work site intervention, the infrastructure for continuing the program was in place (e.g., committees existed that had responsibility for health promotion planning, specific individuals had job responsibilities that included health promotion planning). However, program sustainability was poor, with intervention activities at the 2-year follow-up almost returning to baseline levels. Altman (1995) recommended several types of policy interventions that could facilitate infrastructure support for sustainability, including use of revenues from tobacco or alcohol taxes to fund community interventions on an ongoing basis, requiring federally funded researchers to have a plan for sustainability in all research proposals, including community workers in the review process for research grants to help evaluate the sustainability plan, and supporting research on methods to enhance sustainability. More attention is needed to the development of community relationships if we are to maximize efforts to transfer innovations from the experimental context to community systems (Altman, 1995).

The community capacity-building (CCB) approach used following the original research phase of the Stanford Five-City Project is a good example of how the sustainability process can work (Jackson et al., 1994). The emphasis of the CCB approach was on strengthening community resources related to intervention development, evaluation, and maintenance, working within existing community organizations, and developing skills to adapt and innovate interventions. Technical assistance, training, and professional development were provided, and the benefits of participation in research were shared among both community and academic partners. As a result of this collaborative, a local health department became the community focal point for the sustainability efforts, and a Division of Health Promotion was created within the health department to support these efforts.

Social Context

Work in the social and behavioral sciences has led to increased recognition of the impact that social contextual factors have on health behaviors and chronic disease morbidity and mortality (Adler et al., 1994; Kennedy et al., 1996; Krieger et al., 1993; Marmot et al., 1978, 1996; Marmot and Davey Smith, 1997; Wilkinson, 1992). Social context is comprised of factors in one's physical, social, and cultural environment that influence health (e.g., access to health-promoting opportunities; social support, social networks, social norms, cultural beliefs, language, SES, stressors of having a low income, multiple roles, or role strain). Distal social structural forces clearly shape people's day-to-day experiences in ways that are typically not considered by health promotion interventions (Amick et al., 1995; Kaplan, 1995; Sorensen et al., in press). For example, it may be much more difficult for low-income individuals to change their health behaviors, compared to their middle-income counterparts, because of the social forces surrounding them. The population density per food market is much greater in poor neighborhoods, compared to middle- and upper-class neighborhoods; the typical cost of food is approximately 15–20% higher in poor neighborhoods, while the quality of food available is poorer (Troutt, 1993). Thus, an individual in a low-income neighborhood who wishes to improve his or her diet may find many fewer local resources to support this goal. Many low-income neighborhoods are unsafe, with parks and local areas in which physical activity could occur being sources of criminal activity. As a result, people living in low-income areas are much less able to access opportunities to participate in healthful activities in their own neighborhoods. Further, children growing up in these neighborhoods are regularly exposed to cues supporting development of norms that support unhealthy life-styles. If we are to achieve significant improvements in the health of the nation, these factors must begin to play more of a central role in the development and evaluation of public health-oriented health promotion efforts.

Several models have been proposed that nicely illustrate the contributions that the social and behavioral sciences have had in expanding our view of disease causation. Figure 2 illustrates the context of health related to intervention delivery in cross-cultural and multicultural settings (Kumanyika and Morssink, 1997). This model illustrates the importance of factors at all levels of the social ecological model on health and well being. Figure 3 illustrates a conceptual model of the ecology of urban violence in low-income minority communities that addresses the impact that exposure to violence may have on health promotion behaviors (Sanders-Phillips, 1996). This model illustrates that the relationship between income level and health behaviors goes well beyond access and knowledge, but may be a function of the impact of increased exposure to violence, which significantly affects an individual's ability to respond to other barriers effectively.

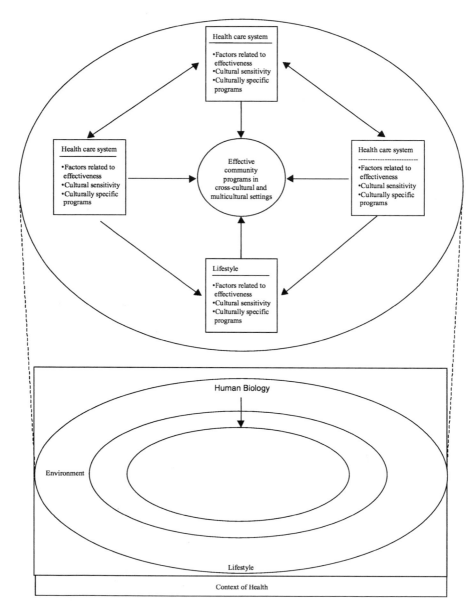

FIGURE 2. The context of health. SOURCE: Adapted from Kumanyik and Morrsink (1993).

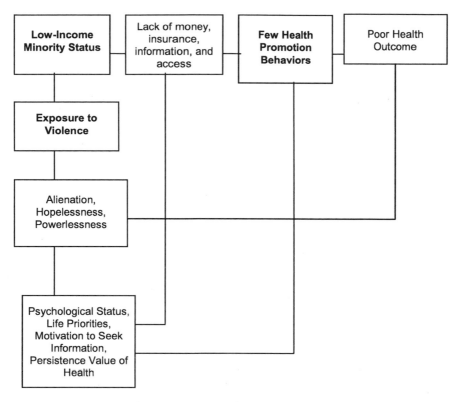

FIGURE 3. A conceptual model of the relationship between exposure to violence and health promotion behaviors among low-income, minority groups. Adapted from Sanders-Phillips, 1996.

Other studies have found that the social context plays a key role in driving the smoking habits of low-income women (Graham, 1994) and that the overall pattern of difficulties and disadvantage faced by low-income women who smoke suggests that their adaptive capacity may be taxed to the limit. Interventions that acknowledge the experiences that come with having a low income (e.g., exposure to violence, frequent housing disruption), that help to reduce the burden of heavy caring responsibilities, and that improve participants' social material circumstances may be a step toward lifting the barriers that prevent low-income individuals from focusing on health behaviors.

An example of work focused on addressing social contextual factors is Fisher et al.'s (1993)evaluation of the role of community health workers as "asthma coaches" for parents of low-income African-American children who have been hospitalized for asthma. The coach's role is to promote coordinated preventive care, reduce hospitalizations and acute care visits, reduce exposure to asthma triggers (e.g., environmental tobacco smoke and cockroach allergen), encourage adherence to asthma management practices, and provide support for the families. The coaches interact with parents via face-to-face and telephone contact on a flexible schedule determined by the parents' needs, circumstances, and preferences. Process evaluations of the asthma coaches' intervention have demonstrated that the coaches can establish and maintain effective working relationships with parents, improve avoidance of environmental triggers, and promote adherence to asthma management practices (Tarr et al., 2000). Use of community health workers (CHWs) such as the coaches is an important strategy for developing more contextually based interventions. CHWs typically live in the target neighborhoods, are embedded and active members of their social networks, and have a basic philosophy and values that are consistent with those of the program. Because of shared experiences, CHWs can translate or contextualize interventions in a way that increases their relevance to participants (Eng, et al., 1997; Eng and Smith, 1995; Eng and Young, 1992; Meister et al., 1992; Parker et al., 1998; Schultz et al., 1997). Another key to the success of the Asthma Coaches Project may be the fact that it capitalizes on an existing situation that provides a context for a focus on the health problem at hand (e.g., having a child hospitalized for asthma). Interventions that have adopted this approach in other risk factor areas, such as conducting HIV prevention programs in the context of sexually transmitted disease (STD) clinics (Kelly et al., 1994) and prenatal care (Hobfoll et al., 1994) have also found significant treatment effects.

Over the past decade, there has been increased emphasis on social contextual factors within social epidemiology, but this focus is just beginning to be considered in the behavioral sciences. Careful and thoughtful collaboration between social epidemiologists who are examining the relationship between social factors and health behaviors, and behavioral scientists who are developing interventions will increase the likelihood that health promotion interventions more systematically address these contextual factors.

Contamination

Increasingly, community-based trials have utilized communities or organizations as the unit of analysis and have utilized the intention-to-treat principle to guide outcome analysis. Although contributing to improved scientific rigor, these approaches have not been without an impact on the ability to detect intervention effects. Kalsbeek and colleagues (Kalsbeek et al., under review) recently conducted a very important analysis of the impact of "noncompliance," or exposure to the nonassigned intervention in community trials (e.g., control community members' exposure to intervention in the experimental community). This analysis used data from a study of churches in which counties were randomized, and a stratified sample of churches within each group of counties received either the intervention or the delayed intervention (Campbell et al., 1999). Based on data from the intervention process evaluation, the authors concluded that the intervention effect was underestimated by as much as 16.6%. The authors point out the importance of adjusting for the biasing effect of treatment contamination, which may lead to a serious misrepresentation of the health importance of community intervention programs. This analysis also provides a different perspective on the modest effect sizes found in many studies and highlights the importance of using standards for interpretation of community-based interventions that are based on the public health significance of the effects, rather than on clinical significance (Sorensen et al., in press).

SUMMARY

This selected review highlights the many contributions that the behavioral and social sciences have made to improving the health and health behaviors of adults. However, it is also evident that the full potential of these disciplines has not been realized. This paper has attempted to suggest several factors that may improve intervention effectiveness. This final section focuses on key research issues within each of these areas that need to be considered in the next generation of research studies.

Linked, Multilevel Interventions Should Be the Norm, Rather than the Exception

Individual-level behavior change approaches should not be abandoned in the search for an exclusive focus on societal solutions to health problems, but, rather, should become integrated within population-level approaches. Societal and policy-level changes are likely to be slow in the making, and thus exclusion of behavior change efforts at the individual level is likely to lead to generations of children being exposed to even higher prevalence of poor health behaviors in the future. Further, it is likely that there will always be population groups that need additional, individual assistance with health behavior change, and it would be unfortunate indeed if this likelihood was not considered in the development of disease prevention paradigms for entire populations.

A top research priority for behavioral and social scientists is to determine how to create better linkages between interventions at different levels of influence. By linking interventions across delivery channels, consistent intervention messages, support, and follow-up can be provided over time. For example, preventive options that are available through employee benefits programs could be actively promoted through interventions and incentive programs at the workplace. Workplace intervention efforts could be linked to local and statewide prevention efforts through departments of health. Larger employers in a community could collaborate with schools to send consistent messages to entire family systems, rather than sporadically to children or parents. Statewide services (e.g., tobacco hotlines) could be linked with both primary care and hospital-based systems, so that patients receive continuity of care and access to services on an ongoing basis.

However, at present, we know little about how best to integrate across levels in order to achieve the greatest benefit. Key empirical questions include how interventions across levels should be ordered to offer the maximal benefit. For example, should social policy interventions precede individual and social network-level interventions? At what point do multilevel interventions support change from several directions, rather than bombard an individual with unwanted messages, thus increasing resistance to change? How can organizational systems (e.g., workplaces, schools, health care providers, families) be linked to maximize intervention effectiveness? Recent studies have revealed that smokers who have household smoking bans and/or work in environments with smoking restrictions are more likely to try to quit smoking, have lower rates of relapse, and lower cigarette consumption compared to those who do not have restriction at home or work (Farkas et al., 1999). However, we don't yet know the effect of combining bans at home and work, and how the relationships between home and work can be applied to other health behaviors. Can workplace-based interventions be effectively linked with health care provider messages about health promotion? Do policy-level interventions have a consistent impact on individuals and networks, or does the effect vary over time? Further study is needed of the impact of combined interventions, across levels, including policy interventions, on the initiation and maintenance of behavior change. It is critical that the next generation of health promotion research begin to address the need to develop truly integrated, multilevel interventions that provide continuity of intervention, so that societal influences reinforce healthy behaviors and serve to shift population norms in a healthful direction.

More Regulatory and Policy Research Is Needed in Key Areas

A number of regulatory interventions could contribute to improved health outcomes, including increased availability of mental health services, price supports for healthy foods, legislative efforts to mandate the manufacture of fire-safe cigarettes, firearms design requirements that would prevent unauthorized use of guns, incorporation of an assessment of physical activity opportunities into building permits for public buildings, legislative or incentive programs for walk- or bike-to-work programs, and price supports for sun protection products that meet SPF standards.

Computer Technology Can Enhance Intervention Design and Delivery

As more behavioral and social scientists turn to the Web or Internet to deliver health-related interventions, careful attention must be given to the issue of the "digital divide" so that interventions are not developed that exclude certain population subgroups. Although there have been unprecedented increases in Internet access, the disparities in penetration levels between upper- and lower-income households, and among racial groups, have also increased in the past 5 years (McConnaughy et al., 1997). There is currently no infrastructure for access to computer-based resources for health information in the public sector. Although health departments and community health centers may be in an excellent position to adapt research-based tailored algorithms for use in routine care delivery, this will not be possible unless such settings have access to the equipment needed to deliver these interventions. As technology improves and equipment costs decrease, there should be increased emphasis on providing the computer infrastructure to disseminate tailored interventions through public health channels.

Tailoring shows significant promise as a means for increasing intervention reach and impact, but there is a clear need to increase our understanding about the specific mechanisms that drive the effectiveness of tailoring (Abrams et al., in press; Rimer and Glassman, 1999; Skinner et al., 1999). Research must address mechanistic questions such as how best to operationalize theoretical variables within tailored communications, whether tailoring is more effective for some behaviors than others or more effective in certain settings than others, what optimal types and number of variables should be included in tailored communications, and how to use advanced computer technologies to enhance the effectiveness of tailoring (Dijkstra et al., 1998; Kreuter et al., 1999). Other technologies that deserve further exploration include computer-based risk assessment and behavior change programs that can be incorporated into primary care practice (Emmons et al., in press) and use of computer-assisted telephone technologies for intervention delivery (Friedman, 1998; Ramelson et al., 1999). Research on health and risk communication will likely play a central role in tailored interventions that address primary prevention of chronic disease (Lipkus et al., in press; Weinstein, 1988).

Dissemination Must Become a Central Focus

Given the relatively large amount of money that has been spent on clinical research, very little attention has been paid to means for translating effective strategies into routine clinical practice (Bero et al., 1998). Overall, there is relatively little guidance in the literature related to effective dissemination, and what little dissemination has occurred has been uncoordinated (Brunner et al., 1997; Glanz, 1997a, in press; Sorensen et al., in press); a strong emphasis on dissemination research is clearly needed. It is tempting to focus primarily on efforts to work with existing interventions to increase their effectiveness. However, Rose (1992) and others (Tosteson et al., 1997) have clearly demonstrated that at the population level, even small to moderate effects can shift population distributions of health behavior and health outcomes. In addition, if currently available intervention strategies are disseminated effectively, population-level shifts in social norms about health behaviors may also occur, which may lead to larger effect sizes than seen within the context of a single research project.

Although there is an increasing amount of research focusing on dissemination, the most common strategies—passive dissemination approaches (e.g., publication of consensus conferences, mailing of educational materials)—are least effective (Bero et al., 1998; Freemantle et al., 1999). Following completion of the Working Well Trial, intervention materials were disseminated to the 42 control work sites; no increase in the number of tobacco control activities offered was observed by the 2-year follow-up (Sorensen et al., 1998d). Bero and colleagues emphasize the importance of conducting studies that will help to clarify the circumstances that are likely to modify intervention effectiveness and the importance of economic evaluations of dissemination efforts. Careful thought about appropriate evaluation approaches is also needed. In the context of dissemination, impact and outcome evaluations are less relevant, but increased emphasis on process evaluation is critical and could provide important clues as to how successfully an intervention is disseminated. Process evaluation focusing on dissemination would include evaluation of program reach, the development of effective relationships to support and implement the program's dissemination (Israel et al., 1995), the percentage of organizations or settings that try to implement the intervention, the consistency and quality of the intervention delivery, and the extent to which the intervention continues to be delivered over time (Glasgow et al., in press-a).

Best et al. (unpublished) and others (Orleans et al., in press; Seetharam, 1999) have advocated the use of a "best-practices" model in tobacco control as one part of the diffusion process. In this approach, a common definition of effectiveness is identified for different levels of practice (e.g., individual, population), channel, and target population. Rules for evaluating the evidence in determining best practices need to be articulated (Best et al., unpublished). This recommendation is exceedingly complex since there are many examples of different disciplines reviewing the same evidence and reaching different conclusions. However, achieving multidisciplinary consensus on best practices is a key part of dissemination efforts and should be a priority. The National Cancer Institute has undertaken an effort to identify the evidence base in cancer control and is posting a review of evidence in selected areas on its website (http://dccps.nci.nih.gov/DECC). This is an important effort that can build the foundation from which best practices can be identified and dissemination can occur.

Infrastructures for Dissemination Are Needed

Another central issue is how to develop an infrastructure for disseminating effective interventions. One way to do this may be to form effective partnerships with key organizations and corporations that share common goals. There are excellent models for such efforts at both the local and the national levels that were the result of effective partnerships between public health organizations and the private sector. For example, the 5-a-Day for Better Health program has resulted in there being persistent and inescapable cues regarding fruits and vegetables in most supermarkets in the United States (e.g., produce bags with the 5-a-Day logo, recipe card, posters, and other signage in grocery stores). A similar model is being used by the American Sun Protection Association, a trade association comprised of public health experts and sun protection manufacturers with the goal of improving skin cancer prevention in the United States (Buller, August 30, 1999). The mission of this association is to join skin cancer prevention advocates and all businesses in the sun protection industry under one umbrella organization and to raise funds through product certification that will be used for public education, point-of-purchase campaigns, and legislative initiatives.

We have only begun to tap the potential of such public-private partnerships. Although caution is certainly warranted, utilizing the resources of private sector enterprises that manufacture or market health-promoting products may be an effective way to increase the reach of intervention messages and to sustain interventions outside of research settings. Further, corporate leaders can disseminate effective interventions, which can further increase the penetration and reach. An upstream approach to selecting partners for dissemination may be most fruitful. For example, efforts to increase physical activity would be greatly aided by involving architects, engineers, and city planners. If the key groups that design our physical environments became invested in the role that their work could have in improving the health of the nation, they might be better positioned to advocate design of buildings and city spaces that maximize opportunities for physical activity. Product designers and engineers have a long history of developing products to reduce and prevent injury. Extending this focus to include prevention of chronic disease and developing strong collaborations with building design and trade organizations might form the infrastructure from which more widespread design of health-promoting environments is possible (Christoffel and Gallagher, 1999). This discussion also emphasizes the need for social and behavioral scientists to collaborate with other disciplines in identifying solutions to improve population health.

A System for Disseminating Office Systems Interventions to Health Care Providers Is Essential

Particular consideration should be given to building an infrastructure for institutionalization and dissemination of effective programs in the health care setting. Health care providers are effective at providing prevention interventions, and office systems greatly increase the likelihood that providers will address health behaviors. However, the mounting fiscal pressures within the health care delivery system are eroding physicians' capabilities to deliver any health behavior interventions. Efforts are needed to develop physician extender strategies that are feasible within today's health care climate. Further, technologic strategies that are known to facilitate provision of counseling (e.g., computer-based office reminder systems) are imperative. Cooley et al. (1999) demonstrated that *4 years* after implementation of a computer-based office systems intervention, provider compliance and use of the system were very high (80%), yet there is no systematic structure for incorporating these systems into the standard of care. Consideration should be given regarding how to build the infrastructure to make such systems available to providers in all types of delivery systems (e.g., group practices, neighborhood health centers, IPAs). Partnerships with Internet health care systems may be one strategy for systematically incorporating prevention topics into office management systems. NCQA and other oversight bodies provide incentives for providers in some health care environments to implement office systems, although incentives for prevention are limited in many settings.

One way to increase provider interest in adopting office systems for prevention might be to incorporate multiple risk factors and screening, so that the systems can be utilized with all patients, and to also incorporate strategies for addressing adherence to treatment recommendations. Poor compliance with recommendations for secondary prevention is of considerable concern, and has substantial cost implications for providers in capitated systems. Health care providers need to be linked into existing mechanisms and delivery structures for disease prevention (e.g., tobacco control hotlines) that can be used as referral sources; provider influence could connect people with resources and thus extend physician involvement as well as provide follow-up services. It is critical that efforts now focus on developing an infrastructure for assisting providers in developing effective office systems. Physician groups (e.g. American College of Chest Physicians, American College of Preventive Medicine) may be particularly good partners for these efforts.

Workplace Interventions Should Be Disseminated

There is also enough evidence currently available to suggest that workplace health promotion should be an integral part of corporate activities and benefits programs (Evans et al., 1994; Farquhar et al., 1985; Glasgow et al., 1997b; Jeffery et al., 1993; Peterson and Aldana, 1999; Salina et al., 1994; Sorensen et al., 1992, 1996a). In particular, policy interventions have been found to be effective at increasing preventive health behaviors (Farrelly et al., 1999; Glasgow et al., 1997a). It is encouraging that the prevalence of workplace health promotion activities has increased considerably in the past decade, although most of the workplace programs that are offered are typically quite low intensity (e.g., self-help materials, intermittent classes) and consist of approaches that have the weakest effects. Consideration of how to disseminate what is known about effective health promotion practice and policy implementation in the workplace setting is needed, particularly in small businesses. The importance of developing an organizational infrastructure to foster and sustain comprehensive health promotion programs in workplaces has been noted (Stokols et al., 1996a). Such an undertaking is likely to require that a coordinating group or agency provide vision in order to ensure adequate planning, implementation, and sustainability. A recent study found that a management training intervention for human resource managers yielded highly significant levels of change in measures of organizational and environmental support for health promotion (Golaszewski et al., 1998). This model may be effective for increasing dissemination and impacting on organization support for health promotion. In addition, efforts to integrate health promotion and health protection interventions have shown significant promise (Sorensen et al., 1995).

Social Context Must Be Considered in Intervention Design

Much of health promotion research has been conducted in a social vacuum, with limited attention to the influence of sociopolitical and regulatory factors (Altman, 1995; Wallack and Winkleby, 1986). It is becoming increasingly clear that effective health promotion interventions can no longer ignore social contextual factors. Recent reviews of the status of health promotion interventions highlight the urgent need for treatment advances that target new insights through innovative study designs, careful qualitative and process evaluations, and partnerships with the community, rather than from incremental improvements of existing approaches (Fisher et al., 1993; Shiffman, 1993). This paper has argued that innovations in behavior change approaches must also draw upon insights from social epidemiology and integrate strategies for dealing with social factors with those developed for individual-level change. Historically, there has been a divergence between social epidemiologists, who focus on documenting the relationship between social conditions and health outcomes, and behavioral scientists, who develop health-related interventions that are often devoid of social contextual factors. Intervention research must begin to address the role of social factors in health behaviors, to expand our theoretical models to incorporate social factors, and to develop innovative intervention designs that will help to elucidate the most effective strategies for intervening within this context. Intervention research that represents a collaboration with existing community groups, social service agencies, and health care providers, and utilizes existing social networks and relationships to creatively design interventions that address social contextual factors, is critical if we are to make a significant impact on health risk factors in the United States.

As recently noted by Syme (1997) and Altman (1995), efforts to develop the next generation of prevention interventions must focus on building relationships with communities and developing interventions that derive from the communities' assessments of their needs, rather than the experts' assumptions about what is needed. Israel (Israel et al., 1998) has offered some strategies for forming effective community-based partnerships. Funders should give careful consideration to the impact that these steps have on the time lines for research development, implementation, and evaluation.

Theoretical Issues Need Further Attention in Health
Behavior Change Research

Theory may play an important role in improving the effectiveness and efficacy of prevention interventions. There has been an increased focus on theory in the past decade (Abrams et al., 1997; Glanz et al., 1997), although many studies conducted have not used well-articulated theoretical constructs to guide the intervention development or evaluation. Further, few studies have clearly articulated key hypothesized mediating variables, and fewer still have longitudinally assessed the impact of an intervention on mediating variables; those studies that have often show that interventions have not substantially effected change in those hypothesized mechanisms (Baranowski et al., in press; Hansen and McNeal, 1996). The ability of interventions to yield change in mediating variables will determine to some extent the ability of the intervention to impact on the target outcome behaviors. Baranowski et al. (in press) call for a priority to be placed on research that increases our understanding of the relationships between theoretical variables and outcomes, and the impact of community-based interventions on these mediating variables, a move that is necessary if we are to take our intervention efforts to the next level of effectiveness.

Theory is needed that is grounded in social experience and thus creates more effective practice (Altman, 1995; Israel et al., 1998; Schensul, 1985). Cultural influences on both mediating mechanisms and health behaviors are also important to consider. In some cultures, concepts such as self-efficacy do not have meaning because of the emphasis on societal well-being. In other cultural groups or communities, strong social support may come from parents or family members who are overall very supportive but do not believe that their adult children need to lose weight or watch their fat intake. Many intervention programs would recommend that the participant avoid this source of negative influence, which in some cases may be tantamount to asking people to forsake strong and positive sources of influence in their life in order to change their diet (Airhihenbuwa et al., 1996).

Expectations for Effect Sizes Need to Be Realistic

Concerns have been raised about the relatively modest magnitude of effects found in community-based and behavioral risk factor reduction interventions (Fisher, 1995a; Susser, 1985; Winkleby, 1994). It is likely that at the level of individual behavior change outcomes, community-based interventions will always have more modest effects than reactive, clinic-based interventions that rely on motivated volunteers. However, economic policy models suggest that population-level application of even the modest level of results found in community trials (Winkleby et al., 1996) would be highly cost-effective compared with

TABLE 4. The Application of the Social Ecological Model to Health Behavior Interventions

Operating Guidelines	Application in Health Behavior Interventions
Encompass multiple settings and life domains	• Provide methods/strategies to involve participants' families, friends, community • Design interventions that span multiple settings and have enduring positive effects on well-being • Integrate biomedical, behavioral, regulatory, and environmental interventions
Reinforce health-promoting social norms through existing social networks	• Provide cues for healthy behaviors throughout target community • Involve health care providers; engage family members and significant others; provide follow-up counseling • Connect participants with community organizations that support the individual's target goals
Target changes in the organization and environment in support of participant health	• Utilize input from advisory boards of constituents/representatives of target population to develop appropriate intervention methods and materials • Identify behavioral and organizational "leverage points" for health promotion • Train key community gatekeepers to deliver cancer prevention messages (e.g. healthcare providers, teachers, community leaders, preachers, camp counselors) • Provide key community leaders with materials and resources for extending their intervention efforts • In target organizational settings, review policies that can impact on norms for health behaviors (e.g., choice of foods for vending machines, smoking policies, youth access to cigarettes), and make recommendations • Utilize "other-directed," passive policy intervention strategies
Tailor programs to the setting through community participation and ownership	• Develop Community Advisory Boards, comprised of key leaders and representatives of target population • Collaborate with Community Advisory Board to develop appropriate resources and networks of community organizations that can support participants' behavior change goals • Develop interventions that enhance the fit between people and their surroundings
Empower individuals to make behavior change	• Provide motivational strategies to empower participants to make changes • Provide opportunities for making small steps toward target changes • Impact on social norms related to targeted changes
Utilize multiple delivery points for intervention messages	• Deliver interventions through multiple channels, and embed interventions into ongoing community programs and activities

TABLE 5. Characteristics of the RE-AIM Framework

Evaluation Dimension	Ecological Target Level	Units and Level of Measurement	Prevalence of Research
Reach	Individual	Percent and representativeness of members of an organization that participate	Modest
Adoption	Organization or community	Magnitude or percent of improvement on outcome(s) of concern	Substantial
Efficacy	Individual, organization, or community	Percent of organizations or settings that try an intervention	Minimal
Implementation	Individual and organization or community	Consistency and quality of intervention delivery under real world conditions	Moderate
Maintenance	Individual and organization or community	Extent to which individuals or implementation agents continue to deliver a program over time	Little
Public Health Impact		End result of interaction of factors	None

Adapted from Glasgow et al., in press.

most accepted medical interventions (Tosteson et al., 1997). This work highlights the importance of evaluating the impact of behavior change programs based on cost-effectiveness within the population, rather than based solely on absolute levels of change among individuals. Further, requirements of standard approaches to research, such as use of the randomized controlled trial, may reduce our ability to detect effects in population-level interventions. For example, Kalsbeek et al. (under review) found that contamination (e.g., control participants exposed to interventions) led to an underestimation of intervention effects in one community-based study. It is quite unusual for investigators to consider the results of as much as 16% contamination on effect sizes, and this study illustrates the importance of doing so. Other investigators have demonstrated that secular trends greatly impact the ability to detect intervention effects, with program effects being larger when secular trends were smaller in control communities (Bauman et al., 1999). Although it is unlikely that the randomized controlled trial will continue to be the gold standard for intervention research, it is increasingly being recognized that because of the dynamic nature of communities, this evaluation format has limitations in its applicability for evaluation of community-based interventions (Cummings, 1999; Sorensen et al., in press). The restricted hypotheses that the randomized controlled trial is able to test may fail to consider the complexities of communities, and this evaluation strategy may alter the interaction between the intervention and community, resulting in an attenuation of the intervention's effectiveness. McKinlay (1995) further argues that alternative evaluation strategies are needed for interventions where individual behavior change is not the target. Sorensen and colleagues (in press) propose that a fuller range of research methodologies be applied and that careful consideration be given to the conditions under which the use of randomized controlled trials is appropriate in community settings.

CONCLUSIONS

Social and behavioral sciences have added significant understanding to the factors needed to accomplish health objectives in the context of human culture, needs, and behavior (Morrow and Bellg, 1994). These disciplines have provided a solid foundation of knowledge about intervention and evaluation strategies for improving health and have contributed to an improved understanding of health at virtually every level of intervention and evaluation research. In order to continue to build on these contributions, innovations are needed that draw upon insights from social epidemiology, policy, and regulatory approaches, and interventions are needed that integrate strategies for dealing with social factors with those developed for individual-level change. Health behavior research also needs to stretch beyond the individual and interpersonal levels and continue to explore ways to work together with communities to systemically integrate social, governmental, and policy-level factors into behavior change interventions. Future studies must utilize rigorous methods that are appropriate to the study population, yet are flexible enough to address some of the inherent challenges of conducting population-based research of this nature. Public health interventions realistically may lead to small changes that, when observed at the population level, contribute to meaningful public health benefits (Rose, 1985; Rose, 1992; Tosteson et al., 1997). By adopting multilevel approaches, increasing the focus on social contextual factors, and building infrastructures for sustaining and disseminating effective interventions, we will be well-positioned to expand on the contributions to date in the next generation of social and behavioral science research.

REFERENCES

Abrams, D. (1991). Conceptual models to integrate individual and public health interventions: The example of the workplace. In M. Henderson (Ed.), *Proceedings of the International Conference on Promoting Dietary Change in Communities* pp. 173–194. Seattle: The Fred Hutchinson Cancer Research Center.

Abrams, D., Orleans, C., Niaura, R., Goldstein, M., Prochaska, J., and Velicer, W. (1996). Integrating individual and public health perspectives for treatment of tobacco dependence under managed health care: A combined stepped-care and matching model. *Annals of Behavioral Medicine, 18*(4), 290–304.

Abrams, D. B., Boutwell, W. B., Grizzle, J., Heimendinger, J., Sorensen, G., and Varnes, J. (1994a). Cancer control at the workplace: The Working Well Trial. *Preventative Medicine, 23*(1), 15–27.

Abrams, D. B., Emmons, K. M., and Linnan, L. (1997). Past, present, and future directions in health education theory and research. In K. Glanz, F. M. Lewis, and B. K. Rimer (Eds.), *Health Behavior and Health Education,* 2nd ed., pp. 453–478. San Francisco: Jossey-Bass.

Abrams, D. B., Emmons, K. M., Linnan, L., and Biener, L. (1994b). Smoking cessation at the workplace: Conceptual and practical considerations. In R. Richmond (Ed.), *International Perspective on Smoking: An International Perspective,* Section II, Chapter 7, pp. 137–169.

Abrams, D. B., Mills, S., and Bulger, D. (in press). Challenges and future directions for tailored communication research. *Annals of Behavioral Medicine, 21(4),* 299–306.

Adams, A., Ockene, J. K., Wheller, E. V., and Hurley, T. G. (1998). Alcohol counseling: Physicians will do it. *Journal of General Internal Medicine, 13*(10), 692–698.

Adler, N. E., Boyce, T., Chesney, M. A., Cohen, S., Folkman, S., Kahn, R. L., and Syme, S. L. (1994). Socioeconomic status and health. The challenge of the gradient. *American Psychologist, 49*(1), 15–24.

Airhihenbuwa, C. O., Kumanyika, S., Agurs, T. D., Lowe, A., Saunders, D., and Morssink, C. B. (1996). Cultural aspects of African American eating patterns. *Ethnicity and Health, 1*(3), 245–260.

Allaire, S., LaValley, M., Evans, S. et al. (1999). Evidence for decline in disability and improved health among persons aged 55–70 years: The Framingham Heart Study. *American Journal of Public Health, 89,* 1678–1683.

Altman, D., and King, A. (1986). Approaches to compliance in primary prevention. *Journal of Compliance in Health Care, 1*(1), 55–73.

Altman, D. G. (1995). Sustaining interventions in community systems: On the relationship between researchers and communities. *Health Psychology, 14*(6), 526–536.

American Cancer Society. (1980). Guidelines for cancer-related check-up: Recommendations and rationale. *Cancer, 30,* 194–240.

American Internet User Survey. (1999). Cyber dialogue study shows US internet audience growth slowing. *Cyberdialogue,* Internet report: www.cyberdialogue.com.

Amick, B., Levin, S., Tarlov, A., and Walsh, D. (1995). Community and Health. In D. Patrick and T. Wickizer (Eds.), *Society and Health.* Oxford: Oxford Press.

Anderson, K. M., Wilson, P. W., Odell, P. M., and Kannel, W. B. (1991). An updated coronary risk profile. A statement for health professionals. *Circulation, 83*(1), 356–362.

Attkisson, C., Zich, J., and eds. (1990). *Depression in Primary Care: Screening and Detection.* New York: Routledge.

Baker, S., O'Neill, B., Ginsburg, M., and Li, G. (1992). *The Injury Fact Book.* New York: Oxford Press.

Bandura, A. (1977). *Social Learning Theory.* Englewood Cliffs: Prentice-Hall.

Baranowski, T. (1997). Families and Health Actions. In D. S. Gochman (Ed.), *Handbook of Health Behavior Research I: Personal and Social Determinants* (pp. 179–205). New York: Plenum Press.

Baranowski, T., Lin, L., Wetter, D., Resnicow, K., and Davis Hearn, M. (in press). Theory as mediating variables: Why aren't community interventions working as desired? *American Psychologist, 51*(1), 42–51.

Bastani, R., Maxwell, A. E., Bradford, C., Das, I. P., and Yan, K. X. (1999). Tailored risk notification for women with a family history of breast cancer. *Preventative Medicine, 29*(5), 355–364.

Bauman, A., Sallis, J., and Pratt, M. (in press). Environmental/policy approaches to increasing physical activity. *American Journal of Preventative Medicine.*

Bauman, K. E., Suchindran, C. M., and Murray, D. M. (1999). The paucity of effects in community trials: Is secular trend the culprit? *Preventative Medicine, 28*(4), 426–429.

Bebbington, P., Hurry, J., Tennant, C., Sturt, E., and Wing, J. (1981). Epidemiology of mental disorders in camberwell. *Psychological Medicine, 11,* 561–579.

Becker, D., Yanek, L., Raqueno, J., Griffin, T., and Garrett, D. (1999). Changes in weight and blood pressure in African American women in a church-based risk reduction trial (Abstract); Presented at the 72nd Scientific Sessions of the American Heart Association; November 8, 1999; Atlanta. *Circulation, 18 (Suppl),* 1–219.

Becker, F. (1990). *The Total Workplace: Facilities Management and the Elastic Organization.* New York: Van Nostrand Reinhold.

Berglund, G., Eriksson, K., Israelsson, B., Kjellstrom, T., Lindegarde, F., Mattlaason, I., Nilsson, J., and Stavenow, L. (1996). Cardiovascular risk groups and mortality in an urban Swedish male population: The Malmo Prevention Project. *Journal of Internal Medicine, 239,* 489–497.

Bero, L. A., Grill, R., Grimshaw, J. M., Harvey, E., Oxman, A. D., and Thomson, M. A. (1998). Closing the gap between research and practice: An overview of systematic reviews of interventions to promote the implementation of research findings. *British Medical Journal, 317,* 465–468.

Best, J., Lovato, C., Olsen, L., and Banwell, W. (unpublished). *Tobacco prevention strategies for adolescent women: A literature review.*

Biener, L., Glanz, K., McLerren, D., Sorensen, G., Thompson, B., Basen-Engquist, K., Linnan, L., and Varnes, J. (1999). Impact of the Working Well Trial on the worksite health environment. *Health Education and Behavior, 26*(4), 478–494.

Bonnie, R., Fulco, C., Liverman, C., eds. (1999). *Reducing the Burden of Injury-Advancing Prevention and Treatment.* Washington, DC: National Academy Press.

Borus, J. F., Howes, M. J., Devins, N. P., Rosenberg, R., and Livingston, W. W. (1988). Primary health care providers' recognition and diagnosis of mental disorders in their patients. *General Hospital Psychiatry, 10*(5), 317–321.

Bowen, D., and Tinker, L. (1995). Controversies in changing dietary behavior. In F. Bronner (Ed.), *Nutrition and Health. Topics and Controversies* . Boca Raton, FL: CRC Press.

Bowen, D. J., Henderson, M. M., Iverson, D., Burrows, E., Henry, H., and Foreyt, J. (1994). Reducing dietary fat: Understanding the Success of the Women's Health Trial. *Cancer Prevention International, 1*, 21–30.

Bracht, N., Finnegan, J., Rissel, C., Weisbrod, R., Gleason, J., Corbett, J., and Velblen-Mortenson, S. (1994). Community ownership and program continuation following a health demonstration project. *Health Education and Research, 9*, 243–255.

Braithwaite, R., Bianchi, C., and Taylor, S. (1994). Ethnographic approach to community organization and health empowerment. *Health Education Quarterly, 21*(3), 407–416.

Brug, J., Glanz, K., Van Assema, P., Kok, G., and van Breukelen, G. J. (1998). The impact of computer-tailored feedback and iterative feedback on fat, fruit, and vegetable intake. *Health Education and Behavior, 25*(4), 517–531.

Brug, J., Steenhuis, I., van Assema, P., and de Vries, H. (1996). The impact of a computer-tailored nutrition intervention. *Preventative Medicine, 25*(3), 236–242.

Brunner, E., White, I., Thorogood, M., Bristow, A., Curle, D., and Marmot, M. (1997). Can dietary interventions change diet and cardiovascular risk factors? A meta-analysis of randomized controlled trials. *American Journal of Public Health, 87*(7), 1415–1422.

Bull, F. C., Jamrozik, K., and Blanksby, B. A. (1999). Tailored advice on exercise—does it make a difference? *American Journal of Preventative Medicine, 16*(3), 230–239.

Buller, M. (August 30, 1999). Personal Communication.

Burt, V., Whelton, P., Roccella, E. et al. (1995). Prevalence of hypertension in the U.S. adult population. *Hypertension, 25*, 305–313.

Byers, T., Mullis, R., Anderson, J., Dusenbury, L., Gorsky, R., Kimber, C., Krueger, K., Kuester, S., Mokdad, A., Perry, G., and Smith, C. A. (1995). The costs and effects of a nutritional education program following work-site cholesterol screening. *American Journal of Public Health, 85*(5), 650–655.

Calfas, K. J., Long, B. J., Sallis, J. F., Wooten, W. J., Pratt, M., and Patrick, K. (1996). A controlled trial of physician counseling to promote the adoption of physical activity. *Preventative Medicine, 25*(3), 225–233.

Calfas, K. J., Sallis, J., F., Oldenburg, B., and French, M. (1997). Mediators of change in physical activity following an intervention in primary care. *Preventative Medicine, 26*, 297–304.

Campbell, M. K., Demark-Wahnefried, W., Symons, M., Kalsbeek, W. D., Dodds, J., Cowan, A., Jackson, B., Motsinger, B., Hoben, K., Lashley, J., Demissie, S., and McClelland, J. W. (1999). Fruit and vegetable consumption and prevention of cancer: The Black Churches United for Better Health project. *American Journal of Public Health, 89*(9), 1390–1396.

Carleton, R. A., Lasater, T. M., Assaf, A., Lefebvre, R. C., and McKinlay, S. M. (1987). The Pawtucket Heart Health Program: I. An experiment in population-based disease prevention. *Rhode Island Medical Journal, 70*, 533–538.

Caspersen, C., Christenson, G., and Pollard, R. (1986). The status of the 1990 Physical Fitness Objectives—evidence from NHIS 1985. *Public Health Reports, 101*, 587–592.

Caspersen, C., and Merritt, R. (1992). Trends in physical activity patterns among older adults: The behavioral risk factor surveillance system. *Medical Science, Sports and Exercise, 24*(Suppl), S26.

CDC. (1999). Prevention research centers begin a new era. *Chronic Disease Notes and Reports, 12*(1).

CDC. (1997). *Linking Research and Public Health Practice: A Review of CDC's Program of Centers for Research and Demonstration of Health Promotion and Disease Prevention.* Washington, DC: National Academy Press.

Center for Disease Control and Prevention. (1990). Coronary heart disease attributable to sedentary lifestyle-selected states, 1988. *Journal of the American Medical Association, 264*, 1390–1392.

Centers for Disease Control and Prevention. (1996). Cigarette smoking among adults—United States. *Morbidity and Mortality Weekly Report, 45*(27), 588–590.

Christoffel, T., and Gallagher, S. (1999). Injury Prevention: Environmental Modification, *Injury Prevention and Public Health: Practical Knowledge, Skills, and Strategies,* pp. 161–179. Gaithersburg, MD: Aspen Publishers.

Clark, N., and McLeroy, K. (1995). Creating capacity through health education: What we know and what we don't. *Health Education Quarterly, 22*, 273–289.

Colditz, G., DeJong, W., Hunter, D., Trichopoulos, D., and Willett, W. (1996). Harvard Report on Cancer Prevention: Causes of human cancer. *Cancer Causes and Control, 1*(7), 1569–1574.

Cole, P., and Rodu, B. (1996). Declining cancer mortality in the United States. *Cancer, 78*(10), 2045–2048.

COMMIT. (1991). Community Intervention Trial for Smoking Cessation (COMMIT): Summary of Design and Intervention. *Journal of the National Cancer Institute, 83*(22), 1620–1628.

COMMIT. (1995a). Community interventional trial for smoking cessation (COMMIT): I Cohort results from a four-year community intervention. *American Journal of Public Health, 85*, 183–192.

COMMIT. (1995b). Community interventional trial for smoking cessation (COMMIT): II Changes in adult cigarette smoking prevalence. *American Journal of Public Health, 85*, 193–200.

Compas, B. E., Haaga, D. A., Keefe, F. J., Leitenberg, H., and Williams, D. A. (1998). Sampling of empirically supported psychological treatments from health psychology: Smoking, chronic pain, cancer, and bulimia nervosa. *Journal of Consulting and Clinical Psychology, 66*(1), 89–112.

Cooley, K. A., Frame, P. S., and Eberly, S. W. (1999). After the grant runs out. Long-term provider health maintenance compliance using a computer-based tracking system. *Archives of Family Medicine, 8*(1), 13–17.

Coyne, J. C., Schwenk, T. L., and Smolinski, M. (1991). Recognizing depression: A comparison of family physician ratings, self-report, and interview measures. *Journal of the American Board of Family Practice, 4*(4), 207–215.

Crane, L. A., Leakey, T. A., Rimer, B. K., Wolfe, P., Woodworth, M. A., and Warnecke, R. B. (1998). Effectiveness of a telephone outcall intervention to promote screening mammography among low-income women. *Preventative Medicine, 27*(5 Pt 2), S39–49.

Cullinane, P., Hyppolite, K., Zastawney, A., and Friedman, R. (1994). Telephone linked communication-activity counseling and tracking for older patients. *Journal of General Internal Medicine (Suppl), 9*(86A).

Cummings, K. (1999). Community-wide interventions for tobacco control. *Nicotine and Tobacco Research, 1*, S113–S116.

Curry, S., McBride, C., Grothaus, L., Louie, D., and Wagner, E. (1995). A randomized trial of self-help materials personalized feedback and telephone counseling with nonvolunteer smokers. *Journal of Consulting and Clinical Psychology, 63*(6), 1005–1014.

Curry, S. J. (1993). Self-help interventions for smoking cessation. *Journal of Consulting and Clinical Psychology, 61*(5), 790–803.

Davis, D. T., Bustamante, A., Brown, C. P., Wolde-Tsadik, G., Savage, E. W., Cheng, X., and Howland, L. (1994). The urban church and cancer control: A source of social influence in minority communities. *Public Health Report, 109*(4), 500–506.

DePue, J. D., Wells, B. L., Lasater, T. M., and Carleton, R. A. (1990). Volunteers as providers of heart health programs in churches: A report on implementation. *American Journal of Health Promotion, 4*(5), 361–366.

Devesa, S., and Diamond, E. (1980). Association of breast cancer and cervical cancer incidence with income and education among whites and blacks. *Journal of the National Cancer Institute, 65*, 515–528.

Devesa, S., and Diamond, E. (1983). Socioeconomic and racial differences in lung cancer incidence. *American Journal of Epidemiology, 118*, 818–831.

Dietrich, A. J., O'Connor, G. T., Keller, A. et al. (1992). Cancer: Improving early detection and prevention. A community practice randomized trial. *British Medical Journal, 304*, 687–691.

Dijkstra, A., De Vries, H., Roijackers, J., and van Breukelen, G. (1998). Tailored interventions to communicate stage-matched information to smokers in different motivational stages. *Journal of Consulting and Clinical Psychology, 66*(3), 549–557.

DiPietro, L., and Caspersen, C. (1991). National estimates of physical activity among white and black Americans. *Medicine, Science, Sports, and Exercise, 23*(Suppl), S105.

Dishman, R. K., Oldenburg, B., O'Neal, H., and Shephard, R. J. (1998). Worksite physical activity interventions. *American Journal of Preventative Medicine, 15*(4), 344–361.

Dutton, J., Posner, B., Smigelski, C., Noonan, J., and Friedman, R. (1995). Use of an automated telephone counselor to reduce serum lipids in hypercholesterolemia. *Clinical Research (Suppl), 10*(99A).

Easton, D., and Peto, J. (1990). The contribution of inherited predisposition to cancer incidence. *Cancer Surveys, 9*, 395–416.

Ebrahim, S., and Davey Smith, G. (1999). Multiple risk factor interventions for primary prevention of coronary heart disease. The Cochrane Library, Oxford: Update Software.

Elkin, I., Shea, M. T., Watkins, J. T., Imber, S. D., Sotsky, S. M., Collins, J. F., Glass, D. R., Pilkonis, P. A., Leber, W. R., Docherty, J. P., et al. (1989). National Institute of Mental Health treatment of depression collaborative research program. General effectiveness of treatments. *Archives of General Psychiatry, 46*(11), 971–982; discussion 983.

Ellenbecker, M. J. (1996). Engineering controls as an intervention to reduce worker exposure. *American Journal Industrial Medicine, 29*(4), 303–307.

Emmons, K. (2000). Health Behaviors in Social Context. In L. Berkman and I. Kawachi, Eds., *Social Epidemiology.* New York: Oxford Press.

Emmons, K., Atwood, K., Dart, H., Weinstein, N., and Colditz, G. (in press). The Harvard Cancer Risk Index: A interactive tool designed to increase understanding of risk for colorectal cancer. *Information Design Journal.*

Emmons, K., Marcus, B., Linnan, L., Rossi, J., and Abrams, D. (1994). Mechanisms in multiple risk factor interventions: Smoking, physical activity, and dietary fat intake among manufacturing workers. *Preventative Medicine, 23*, 481–489.

Emmons, K., and Rollnick, S. (in press). Motivational interviewing in public health settings: Opportunities and limitations. *American Journal of Preventative Medicine.*

Emmons, K., Shadel, W., Linnan, L., Marcus, B., and Abrams, D. (1999a). A prospective analysis of change in multiple risk factors for cancer. *Cancer Research Therapy and Control, 8*, 15–23.

Emmons, K. M., Kawachi, I., and Barclay, G. (1997) Tobacco control: A brief review of its history and prospects for the future. In: A. Elias, B. Barlogie (Eds.), *Multidisciplinary Care of Lung Cancer Patients, Part I: Multiple Myeloma, Part II: Hematology/Oncology Clinics of North America,* chapter 11: 177–196.

Emmons, K. M., Linnan, L. A., Shadel, W. G., Marcus, B., and Abrams, D. B. (1999b). The Working Healthy Project: A worksite health-promotion trial targeting physical activity, diet, and smoking. *Journal of Occupational and Environmental Medicine, 41*(7), 545–555.

Eng, E., Hatch, J., and Callan, A. (1985). Institutionalizing social support through the church and into the community. *Health Education Quarterly, 12*(1), 81–92.

Eng, E., Parker, E., and Harlan, C. (1997). Lay health advisor intervention strategies: A continuum from natural helping to paraprofessional helping. *Health Education and Behavior, 24*, 413–417.

Eng, E., and Smith, J. (1995). Natural helping functions of lay health advisors in breast cancer education. *Breast Cancer Research Treatment, 35*, 23–29.

Eng, E., and Young, R. (1992). Lay health advisors as community change agent. *Family and Community Health, 15*(1), 24–40.

Erfurt, J., Foote, A., Heirich, M., and Brock, B. (1991). *Worksite Wellness Programming: How to Do It Effectively.* Bethesda, MD: National Heart, Lung and Blood Institute.

Evans, R., Barer, M., and Marmor, T. (1994). *Why Are Some People Healthy and Others Not? The Determinants of Health of Populations.* New York: Aldine de Gruyter.

Farkas, A., Gilpin, E., Diatefan, J., and Pierce, J. (1999). The effects of household and workplace smoking restrictions on quitting behaviours. *Tobacco Control, 8*, 261–265.

Farquhar, J. W. (1978). The community-based model of life style intervention trials. *American Journal of Epidemiology, 108*(2), 103–111.

Farquhar, J. W., Fortmann, S. P., Flora, J. A., Taylor, B., Haskell, W. L., Williams, P. T., Maccoby, N., and Wood, P. D. (1990). Effects of communitywide education on cardiovascular disease risk factors. *Stanford Five-City Project, 264*(3), 359–365.

Farquhar, J. W., Fortmann, S. P., Maccoby, N., Haskell, W. L., Williams, P. T., Flora, J. A., Taylor, C. B., Brown Jr, B. W., Solomon, D. S., and Hulley, S. B. (1985). The Stanford five-city project: Design and methods. *American Journal of Epidemiology, 122*(2), 323–334.

Farquhar, J. W., Wood, P. D., Breitrose, H., Haskell, W. L., Meyer, A. J., Maccoby, N., Alexander, J. K., Brown Jr, B. W., McAlister, A. L., Nash, J. D., and Stern, M. P. (1977). Community education for cardiovascular health. *Lancet*, 1192–1195.

Farrelly, M., Evans, W., and Sfekas, A. (1999). The impact of workplace smoking bans: Results from a national survey. *Tobacco Control, 8*, 272–277.

Feinleib, M. (1996). Editorial: New directions for community intervention studies. *American Journal of Public Health, 86*(12), 1696–1697.

Ferguson, T. (1996). *Health Online*. Reading, MA: Addison-Wesley Publishing.

Fielding, J. (1984). Health promotion and disease prevention at the worksite. *Annual Review of Public Health, 5*, 237–265.

Fiore, M., Bailey, W., and Cohen, S. (1996). *Smoking cessation* (No. 96-0692). Rockville, MD: U.S. Department of Health and Human Services.

Fisher, E. B. J. (1995a). Editorial: The Results of the COMMIT Trial. *American Journal of Public Health, 85*(2), 159–160.

Fisher, E. B. J. (1995b). The results of the COMMIT Trial. *American Journal of Public Health, 85*, 159–161.

Fisher, E. B. J., Lichtenstein, E., Haire-Joshu, D., Morgan, G. D., and Rehberg, H. R. (1993). Methods, successes, and failures of smoking cessation programs. *Annual Review of Medicine, 44*, 481–513.

Flora, J., Lefebvre, R., Murray, D., et al. (1993). A community education monitoring system: Methods from the Stanford Five-City Project, the Minnesota Heart Health Program, and the Pawtaucket Heart Health Program. *Health Education and Research, 8*, 81–95.

Folsom, A. R., Caspersen, C. J., Taylor, H. L., Jacobs, D. R., Jr., Luepker, R. V., Gomez-Marin, O., Gillum, R. F., and Blackburn, H. (1985). Leisure time physical activity and its relationship to coronary risk factors in a population-based sample. The Minnesota Heart Survey. *American Journal of Epidemiology, 121*(4), 570–579.

Fortmann, S. P., Taylor, C. B., Flora, J. A., and Jatulis, D. E. (1993a). Changes in adult cigarette smoking prevalence after 5 years of community health education: The Stanford Five-City Project. *American Journal of Epidemiology, 137*(1), 82–96.

Fortmann, S. P., Taylor, C. B., Flora, J. A., and Winkleby, M. A. (1993b). Effect of community health education on plasma cholesterol levels and diet: The Standard Five City Project. *American Journal of Epidemiology, 137*, 1039–1055.

Fortmann, S. P., Winkleby, M. A., Flora, J. A., Haskell, W. L., and Taylor, C. B. (1990). Effect of long-term community health education on blood pressure and hypertension control. The Stanford Five-City Project. *American Journal of Epidemiology, 132*(4), 629–646.

Freed, L. H., Vernick, J. S., and Hargarten, S. W. (1998). Prevention of firearm-related injuries and deaths among youth. A product-oriented approach. *Pediatric Clinics of North America, 45*(2), 427–438.

Freemantle, N., Harvey, E., Wolf, F., Grimshaw, J., Grilli, R., and Bero, L. (1999). Printed educational materials: Effects on professional practice and health care outcomes. The Cochrane Library, Oxford: Update Software.

French, S. A., Hennrikus, D. J., and Jeffery, R. W. (1996). Smoking status, dietary intake, and physical activity in a sample of working adults. *Health Psychology, 15*(6), 448–454.

Friedman, C., Brownson, R. C., Peterson, D. E., and Wilkerson, J. C. (1994). Physician advice to reduce chronic disease risk factors. *American Journal of Preventative Medicine, 10*(6), 367–371.

Friedman, R. H. (1998). Automated telephone conversations to assess health behavior and deliver behavioral interventions. *Journal of Medical Systems, 22*(2), 95–102.

Friedman, R. H., Kazis, L. E., Jette, A., Smith, M. B., Stollerman, J., Torgerson, J., and Carey, K. (1996). A telecommunications system for monitoring and counseling patients with hypertension. Impact on medication adherence and blood pressure control. *American Journal of Hypertension, 9*(4 Pt 1), 285–292.

Friedman, S. R., Chapman, T. F., Perlis, T. E., Rockwell, R., Paone, D., Sotheran, J. L., and Des Jarlais, D. C. (1999). Similarities and differences by race/ethnicity in changes of HIV seroprevalence and related behaviors among drug injectors in New York City, 1991–1996. *Journal of Acquired Immune Deficiency Syndrome, 22*(1), 83–91.

Galuska, D. A., Will, J. C., Serdula, M. K., and Ford, E. S. (1999). Are health care professionals advising obese patients to lose weight? *Journal of American Medical Association, 282*(16), 1576–1578.

Glanz, K. (1997). Progress in dietary behavior change. *American Journal of Health Promotion, 14(2),* 112–117.

Glanz, K. (1997a). Behavioral research contributions and needs in cancer prevention and control: Dietary change. *Preventative Medicine, 26*(5Pt 2), S43–S55.

Glanz, K. (1997b). Dietary Change. *Cancer Causes and Control, 8* Suppl *1*, S13–16.

Glanz, K., Hewitt, A., and Rudd, J. (1992). Consumer behavior and nutrition education: An integrative review. *Journal of Nutrition Education, 24*(267–77).

Glanz, K., Lankenau, B., Foerster, S., Temple, S., Mullis, R., and Schmid, T. (1995). Environmental and policy approaches to cardiovascular disease prevention through nutrition: Opportunities for state and local action. *Health Education Quarterly, 22*(4), 512–527.

Glanz, K., Lewis, F., and Rimer, B. (1997). Linking Theory, Research, and Practice. In K. Glanz, F. Lewis, and B. Rimer (Eds.), *Health Behavior and Health Education: Theory, Research and Practice,* pp. 19–40. San Francisco: Jossey-Bass.

Glanz, K., Sorensen, G., and Farmer, A. (1996). The health impact of worksite nutrition and cholesterol intervention programs. *American Journal of Health Promotion, 10*(6), 453 470.

Glasgow, R., McKay, H., Piette, J., and Reynolds, K. (1999). The RE-AIM criteria for evaluating population-based interventions: What can they tell us about different chronic illness management strategies? *American Journal of Public Health, 89,* 1322–1327.

Glasgow, R., Vogt, T., and Bowles, S. (in press-a). Evaluating the public health impact of health promotion interventions: The RE-AIM framework. *American Journal of Public Health, 89(9),* 1322–1327.

Glasgow, R., Wagner, E., Kaplan, R., Vinicor, F., Smith, L., and Norman, J. (in press-b). If diabetes is a public health problem, why not treat it as one? A population-based approach to chronic illness. *Annals of Behavioral Medicine.*

Glasgow, R. E., Cummings, K. M., and Hyland, A. (1997a). Relationship of worksite smoking policy to changes in employee tobacco use: Findings from COMMIT. Community Intervention Trial for Smoking Cessation. *Tobacco Control, 6*(Suppl 2), S44–48.

Glasgow, R. E., Terborg, J. R., Hollis, J. F., Severson, H. H., and Boles, S. M. (1995). Take heart: Results from the initial phase of a work-site wellness program. *American Journal of Public Health, 85*(2), 209–216.

Glasgow, R. E., Terborg, J. R., Stycker, L. A., Boles, S. M., and Hollis, J. F. (1997b). Take Heart II: Replication of a Worksite Health Promotion Trial. *Journal of Behavioral Medicine, 20,* 143–161.

Golaszewski, T., Barr, D., and Cochran, S. (1998). An organization-based intervention to improve support for employee heart health. *American Journal of Health Promotion, 13*(1), 26–35.

Gomel, M. K., Oldenburg, B., Simpson, J. M., Chilvers, M., and Owen, N. (1997). Composite cardiovascular risk outcomes of a work-site intervention trial. *American Journal of Public Health, 87*(4), 673–676.

Goodman, R., and Steckler, A. (1989). A model for the institutionalization of health promotion programs. *Family and Community Health, 11,* 63–78.

Graham, H. (1994). *When Life's a Drag: Women, Smoking and Disadvantage.* London: University of Warwick, Department of Health.

Greenlund, K. J., Giles, W. H., Keenan, N. L., Croft, J. B., Casper, M. L., and Matson-Koffman, D. (1998). Prevalence of multiple cardiovascular disease risk factors among women in the United States, 1992 and 1995: The Behavioral Risk Factor Surveillance System. *Journal of Women's Health, 7*(9), 1125–1133.

Greenwald, P., Kramer, B., Weed, D., and eds. (1995). *Cancer Prevention and Control.* New York: Marcel Dekker.

Griffin, S., and Kinmonth, A. (1999). Diabetes care: The effectiveness of systems for routine surveillance for people with diabetes. *The Cochrane Library*(4), Oxford: Update Software.

Guthrie, J., Fox, J., Cleveland, L., and Welsh, S. (1995). Who uses nutrition labeling, and what effects does label use have on diet quality? *Journal of Nutrition and Education, 27,* 163–172.

Hall, H., May, D., Lew, R., Koh, H., and Nadel, M. (1997). Sun protection behaviors of the U.S. white populations. *Preventative Medicine, 26,* 401–407.

Hall, S. M., Tunstall, C. D., Vila, K. L., and Duffy, J. (1992). Weight gain prevention and smoking cessation: Cautionary findings. *American Journal of Public Health, 82*(6), 799–803.

Hancock, L., Sanson-Fisher, R., Redman, S., Burton, R., Burton, L., Butler, J., Girgis, A., Gibberd, R., Hensley, M., McClintock, A., Reid, A., Schofield, M., Tripodi, T., and

Walsh, R. (1997). Community action for health promotion: A review of methods and outcomes 1990–1995. *American Journal of Preventative Medicine, 13*(4), 229–239.

Hansen, W. B., and McNeal, J. R. B. (1996). The law of maximum expected potential effect: Constraints placed on program effectiveness by mediator relationships. *Health Education and Research Theory Practice, 11*, 501–507.

Harris, M. (1998). Diabetes in America: Epidemiology and scope of the problem. *Diabetes Care, 21*(Suppl 3), C11–C14.

Harvey, E., Glenny, A., Kirk, S., and Summerbell, C. (1999). Improving health professionals' management and organization of care for overweight and obese people. *The Cochrane Library*(4), Oxford: Update Software.

Hayaki, J., and Brownell, K. D. (1996). Behaviour change in practice: Group approaches. *International Journal of Obesity Related Metabolism Disorders, 20 Suppl 1*, S27–30.

He, J., and Whelton, P. (1997). Epidemiology and prevention of hypertension. *Medical Clinics North America, 81*(5), 1077–1097.

Heaney, C., and Goldenhar, L. (1996). Worksite health programs: Working together to advance employee health. *Health Education Quarterly, 23*(2), 133–136.

Heath, G. W., Temple, S. P., Fuchs, R., Wheeler, F. C., and Croft, J. B. (1995). Changes in blood cholesterol awareness: Final results from the South Carolina Cardiovascular Disease Prevention Project. *American Journal of Preventative Medicine, 11*(3), 190–196.

Heimendinger, J., Thompson, B., Ockene, L., Sorensen, G., Abrams, D. B., Emmons, K. M., Varnes, J. W., Eriksen, M. P., Probart, C., and Himmelstein, J. S. (1990). Reducing the risk of cancer through worksite intervention, *Occupational Medicine: State of the Art Reviews*, Vol. 7. Philadelphia: Henley and Belfus, Inc.

Heirich, M. A., Foote, A., Erfurt, J. C., and Konopka, B. (1993). Work-site physical fitness programs: Comparing the impact of different program designs on cardiovascular risks. *Journal of Occupational Medicine, 35*(5), 510–517.

Henderson, S., Duncan-Jones, P., Byrne, D., Scott, R., and Adcock, S. (1979). Psychiatric disorder in Canberra. *Acta Psychiatrica Scandinavica, 60*, 355–374.

Hennrikus, D. J., and Jeffery, R. W. (1996). Worksite intervention for weight control: A review of the literature. *American Journal of Health Promotion, 10*(6), 471–498.

Henry, M., Hollander, J., Alicandro, J., Cassara, G., O'Malley, S., and Thode, H. (1996). Prospective countrywide evaluation of the effects of motor vehicle safety device use on hospital resource use and injury severity. *Annals of Emergency Medicine, 28*, 627–634.

Hobfoll, S. E., Jackson, A. P., Lavin, J., Britton, P. J., and Shepherd, J. B. (1994). Reducing inner-city women's AIDS risk activities: A study of single, pregnant women. *Health Psychology 13*(5), 397–403.

Hodiamont, P., Peer, N., and Syben, N. (1987). Epidemiological aspects of psychiatric disorder in a Dutch health area. *Psychological Medicine, 17*, 495–505.

Holmberg, S. (1996). The estimated prevalence and incidence of HIV in 96 large US metropolitan areas. *American Journal of Public Health, 86*, 642–654.

Hunt, J. R., Kristal, A. R., and White, E. (1995). Physician recommendations for dietary change: Their prevalence and impact in a population-based sample. *American Journal of Public Health, 85*(5), 722–725.

Interagency Board for Nutrition Monitoring and Related Research. (1993). *Nutrition monitoring in the United States. Chartbook I: Selected findings from the national nutrition monitoring and related research program* . Hyattsville, MD: Public Health Service.

Israel, B. A., Cummings, K. M., Dignan, M. B., Heaney, C. A., Perales, D. P., Simons-Morton, B. G., and Zimmerman, M. A. (1995). Evaluation of health education programs: Current assessment and future directions. *Health Education Quarterly, 22*(3), 364–389.

Israel, B. A., Schultz, A. J., Parker, E. A., and Becker, A. B. (1998). Review of community based research: Assessing partnership approaches to improve public health. *Annual Review of Public Health, 19*, 173–202.

Jackson, C., Altman, D., Howard-Pitney, B., and Farquahar, J. (1989). Evaluating community level health promotion and disease prevention interventions. *New Directions for Program Evaluation, 43*, 19–32.

Jackson, C., Fortmann, S., Flora, J., Melton, R., Snider, J., and Littlefield, D. (1994). The capacity-building approach to intervention maintenance implemented by the Stanford Five-City Project. *Health Education and Research, 9*, 385–396.

Jeffrey, R. (1989). Risk behaviors and health: Contrasting individual and population perspectives. *American Psychologist, 44*, 194–202.

Jeffery, R., French, S., Raether, C., and Baxter, J. (1994). An environmental intervention to increase fruit and salad purchases in a cafeteria. *Preventative Medicine, 23*, 788–792.

Jeffery, R. W., Forster, J. L., Dunn, B. V., French, S. A., McGovern, P. G., and Lando, H. A. (1993). Effects of work-site health promotion on illness-related absenteeism. *Journal of Occupational Environmental Medicine, 35*(11), 1142–1146.

Johnson, S., and Walker, J. (1996). *The Crash Outcome Data Evaluation System (CODES)* (DOT HS 808 338). Springfield, VA: National Technical Information Service.

Kahn, C., Vicent, D., and Doria, A. (1996). Genetics of non-insulin dependent (type II) diabetes mellitus. *Annual Review of Medicine, 47*, 509–531.

Kalsbeek, W., Mauney, J., Brock, S., and Campbell, M. (under review). Assessing the bias effect of noncompliance in community intervention trials.

Kamb, M., and Wortley, P. (2000). Human immunodeficiency virus and AIDS in women. In M. Goldman and M. E. Hatch (Eds.), *Women and Health*, pp. 336–351. New York: Academic Press.

Kaplan, G. (1995). Where do shared pathways lead? Some reflections on a research agenda. *Psychosomatic Medicine, 57*, 208–212.

Kelly, J. A., Murphy, D. A., Washington, C. D., Wilson, T. S., Koob, J. J., Davis, D. R., Ledezma, G., and Davantes, B. (1994). The effects of HIV/AIDS intervention groups for high-risk women in urban clinics. *American Journal of Public Health, 84*(12), 1918–1922.

Kennedy, B. P., Kawachi, I., and Prothrow-Stith, D. (1996). Income distribution and mortality: Cross sectional ecological study of the Robin Hood index in the United States. *British Medical Journal, 312*(7037), 1004–1007.

Kessler, R. C., McGonagle, K. A., Zhao, S., Nelson, C. B., Hughes, M., Eshleman, S., Wittchen, H. U., and Kendler, K. S. (1994). Lifetime and 12-month prevalence of

DSM-III-R psychiatric disorders in the United States. Results from the National Comorbidity Survey. *Archives of General Psychiatry, 51*(1), 8–19.

King, A. C., Jeffery, R. W., Fridinger, F., Dusenbury, L., Provence, S., Hedlund, S. A., and Spangler, K. (1995). Environmental and policy approaches to cardiovascular disease prevention through physical activity: Issues and opportunities. *Health Education Quarterly, 22*(4), 499–511.

King, E., Rimer, B., Seay, J., Balshem, A., and Enstrom, P. (1994). Promoting mammography use through progressive interventions: Is it effective? *American Journal of Public Health, 84*(1), 104–106.

King, T. K., Marcus, B. H., Pinto, B. M., Emmons, K. M., and Abrams, D. B. (1996). Cognitive-behavioral mediators of changing multiple behaviors. *Preventative Medicine, 25*(6), 681–691.

Kintner, M., Boss, P., and Johnson, N. (1981). The relationship between dysfunctional family environments and family member food intake. *Journal of Marriage and the Family, 43*, 633–641.

Kirsch, I., Jungeblut, A., Jenkins, L., and Kolstad, A. (1993). *Adult Literacy in America: A First Look at the Results of the National Adult Literacy Survey.* Washington, DC: National Center for Education Statistics, Educational Testing Service.

Koffman, D. M., Lee, J. W., Hopp, J. W., and Emont, S. L. (1998). The impact of including incentives and competition in a workplace smoking cessation program on quit rates. *American Journal of Health Promotion, 13*(2), 105–111.

Kottke, T., Puska, P., Salonen, J., Tuomilehto, J., and Nissinen, A. (1985). Projected effects of high risk versus population based prevention strategies in coronary heart disease. *American Journal of Epidemiology, 121*, 697–704.

Kottke, T. E., Battista, R. N., and DeFriese, G. H. (1988). Attributes of successful smoking cessation interventions in medical practice. A meta-analysis of 39 controlled trials. *Journal of the American Medical Association, 259*, 2883–2889.

Krebs-Smith, S., Cook, A., Subar, A., Cleveland, L., and Friday, J. (1995). U.S. adults' fruit and vegetable intakes, 1989–1991: A revised baseline for the Healthy People 2000 objective. *American Journal of Public Health, 85*, 1623–1629.

Kreuter, M., and Brennan, L. (1997). Do nutrition label readers eat healthier diets? Behavioral correlates of adults use of food labels. *American Journal of Preventative Medicine, 13*, 277–283.

Kreuter, M. W., Bull, F. C., Clark, E. M., and Oswald, D. L. (1999). Understanding how people process health information: A comparison of tailored and nontailored weight-loss materials. *Health Psychology, 18*(5), 487–494.

Kreuter, M. W., and Strecher, V. J. (1996). Do tailored behavior change messages enhance the effectiveness of health risk appraisal? Results from a randomized trial. *Health Education Research, 11*(1), 97–105.

Krieger, N., Rowley, D. I., Herman, A. A., Avery, B., and Phillips, M. T. (1993). Racism, sexism, and social class: Implications for studies of health, disease, and well-being. *American Journal of Preventative Medicine, 9*(Suppl 6), 82–122.

Kumanyika, S., and Morssink, C. (1997). Cultural appropriateness of weight management programs. *Overweight and Weight Management.* Gaithersburg, MD: Aspen Publishers.

Kumanyika, S. K., and Charleston, J. B. (1992). Lose weight and win: A church-based weight loss program for blood pressure control among black women. *Patient Education Counsel, 19*, 19–32.

LaMontagne, A., and Christiani, D. (in press). Prevention of work-related cancers, *Cancer Causes, Cancer Prevention*, (Vol. 1). The Netherlands: Klewer Publishers.

LaMontagne, A., Kelsey, K., Ryan, C., and Christiani, D. (1992). A participatory workplace health and safety training program for ethylene oxide. *American Journal of Industrial Medicine, 22*(5), 651–664.

Lancaster, T., and Stead, L. (1999). Self-help interventions for smoking cessation. *The Cochrane Library*(4), Oxford: Updated software.

Lefebvre, R., and Flora, J. (1988). Social marketing and public health intervention. *Health Education Quarterly, 15*, 299–315.

Lehmann, E. D., and Deutsch, T. (1995). Application of computers in diabetes care—a review. II. Computers for decision support and education. *Medical Informatics, 20*(4), 303–329.

Leigh, J., Markowitz, S., Fahs, M., Shin, C., and Landrigan, P. (1997). Occupational injury and illness in the United States. Estimates of costs, morbidity, and mortality. *Archives of Internal Medicine, 157*, 1557–1568.

Lerman, C. (1997). Translational behavioral research in cancer genetics. *Preventative Medicine, 26*(5 Pt 2), S65–69.

Levin, J. (1984). The role of the black church in community medicine. *Journal of the American Medical Association, 76*, 477–483.

Levine, B. S., Wigren, M. M., Chapman, D. S., Kerner, J. F., Bergman, R. L., and Rivlin, R. S. (1993). A national survey of attitudes and practices of primary-care physicians relating to nutrition: Strategies for enhancing the use of clinical nutrition in medical practice. *American Journal of Clinical Nutrition, 57*, 115–119.

Levine, D. M. (1987). The physician's role in health-promotion and disease prevention. *Bulletin of the New York Academy of Medicine*, 950–956.

Levine, D. M., Becker, D. M., Bone, L. R., Hill, M. N., Tuggle, M. B., 2nd, and Zeger, S. L. (1994). Community-academic health center partnerships for underserved minority populations. One solution to a national crisis. *Journal of the American Medical Association, 272*(4), 309–311.

Levy, A., Matthews, O., Stephenson, M., Tenney, J., and Schucker, R. (1985). The impact of a nutrition information program on food purchases. *Journal of Public Policy Marketing, 4*(1), 1–13.

Lewis, C. E. (1988). Disease prevention and health promotion practices of primary care physicians in the United States. *American Journal of Preventative Medicine, 4*(suppl), 9–16.

Lichtenstein, E., Glasgow, R., Lando, H., Ossip Klein, D., and Boles, S. (1996). Telephone counseling for smoking cessation: Rationales and meta-analytic review of evidence. *Health Education and Research Theory Practice, 11*(2), 243–257.

Linenger, J. M., Chesson, C. V. d., and Nice, D. S. (1991). Physical fitness gains following simple environmental change. *American Journal of Preventative Medicine, 7*(5), 298–310.

Lipkus, I., Lyna, P., and Rimer, B. (in press). Using tailored interventions to enhance smoking cessation among African-Americans at a community health center. *Nicotine Tobacco Research, 1* 77–85.

Luepker, R. V., Murray, D. M., Jacobs, D. R. J., Mittlemark, M., and Bracht, N. (1994). Community education for cardiovascular disease prevention: Risk factor changes in the Minnesota Heart Health Program. *American Journal of Public Health, 84*, 1383–1389.

Lundberg, G. (1991). National health care reform: An aura of inevitability is upon us. *Journal of the American Medical Association, 265*, 2566–2567.

Lutz, S. F., Ammerman, A. S., Atwood, J. R., Campbell, M. K., DeVellis, R. F., and Rosamond, W. D. (1999). Innovative newsletter interventions improve fruit and vegetable consumption in healthy adults. *Journal of the American Dietetic Association, 99*(6), 705–709.

Mallonee, S., Istre, G. R., Rosenberg, M., Reddish-Douglas, M., Jordan, F., Silverstein, P., and Tunell, W. (1996). Surveillance and prevention of residential-fire injuries. *New England Journal of Medicine, 335*(1), 27–31.

Manley, M. W., Epps, R. P., and Glynn, T. J. (1992). The clinician's role in promoting smoking cessation among clinic patients. *Medical Clinics of North America, 76*(2), 477–494.

Marcus, B., Albrecht, A., Niaura, R., Taylor, E., Simkin, L., Feder, S., Abrams, D., and Thompson, P. (1995). Exercise enhances the maintenance of smoking cessation in women. *Addictive Behavior, 20*(1), 87–92.

Marcus, B. H., Albrecht, A. E., King, T. K., Parisi, A. F., Pinto, B. M., Roberts, M., Niaura, R. S., and Abrams, D. B. (1999). The efficacy of exercise as an aid for smoking cessation in women: A randomized controlled trial. *Archives of Internal Medicine, 159*(11), 1229–1234.

Marcus, B. H., Albrecht, A. E., Niaura, R. S., Abrams, D. B., and Thompson, P. D. (1991). Usefulness of physical exercise for maintaining smoking cessation in women. *American Journal of Cardiology, 68*(4), 406–407.

Marcus, B. H., Goldstein, M. G., Jette, A., Simkin-Silverman, L., Pinto, B. M., Milan, F., Washburn, R., Smith, K., Rakowski, W., and Dube, C. E. (1997). Training physicians to conduct physical activity counseling. *Preventive Medicine, 26*, 382–388.

Marian, A. (1998). Genetic risk factors for myocardial infarction. *Current Opinion in Cardiology, 13*, 171–178.

Marmot, M., Adelstein, A., Robinson, N., and Rose, G. (1978). The changing social class distribution of heart disease. *British Medical Journal, 2*, 1109–1112.

Marmot, M., Bobak, M., and Davey Smith, G. (1996). Explanations for social inequalities and health. In B. Amick, S. Levine, A. Tarlov, and D. Walsh (Eds.), *Society and Health*. London: Oxford University Press.

Marmot, M., and Davey Smith, G. (1997). Socioeconomic differentials in health: The contribution of the Whitehall studies. *Journal of Health Psychology, 2*(3), 283–296.

Marrero, D. (1993). Computers in the assessment of diabetes control: In C. Mogensen and E. Staid (Eds.), *Diabetes Forum Series, Volume IV: Concepts of the Ideal Diabetes Clinic* . Berlin/New York: Walter de Gruyter.

Mavreas, V., Beis, A., Mouyias, A., Rigoni, F., and Lyketsos, G. (1986). Prevalence of psychiatric disorders in Athens. *Social Psychiatry, 21*, 172–181.

McBeath, W. (1991). Health for all: A public health vision. *American Journal of Public Health, 81*, 1560–1565.

McConnaughy, J., Lader, W., Chin, R., and Everette, D. (1997). *Falling Through the Net II: New Data on the Digital Divide; National Telecommunications and Information*

Administration: Office of Policy Analysis and Development. Internet report: www. ntia.doc.gov.

McKinlay, J. (1995). The new public health approach to improving physical activity and autonomy in older populations. In E. Heikkinon (Ed.), *Preparation for Aging*. New York: Plenum Press.

McLeroy, K. R., Bibeau, D., Steckler, A., and Glanz, K. (1988). An ecological perspective on health promotion programs. *Health Education Quarterly, 15*(4), 351–377.

McWhorter, W., Schtzhin, A., Horm, J. et al. (1989). Contribution of socioeconomic status to black/white differences in cancer incidence. *Cancer, 63*, 982–987.

Meister, J. S., Warrick, L. H., Zapien, J. G., and Wood, A. H. (1992). Using lay health workers: Case study of a community-based prenatal intervention. *Journal of Community Health, 17*(1), 37–51.

Minkler, M., and Wallerstein, N. (1997). *Improving Health Through Community Organization and Community Building*, 2nd ed. San Francisco: Jossey-Bass.

MMWR. (1991). Child passenger restraint use and motor vehicle related fatalities among children—United States, 1982–90. *Morbidity and Mortality Weekly Review, 40*, 600–602.

MMWR. (1993). Mortality trends and leading causes of death among adolescents and young adults. *Morbidity and Mortality Weekly Review, 42*, 459–462.

MMWR. (1997). Trends in the prevalence and incidence of self-reported diabetes mellitus—United States, 1980–1994. *Morbidity and Mortality Weekly Review, 46*, 1014–1018.

MMWR. (1998). Self-reported frequent distress among adults—United States, 1993–1996. *Morbidity and Mortality Weekly Review, 279*, 1772–1773.

MMWR. (1999). State-specific prevalence of current cigarette and cigar smoking among adults—United States, 1998. *Morbidity and Mortality Weekly Review, 48*(45), 1034–1039.

Mokdad, A. H., Serdula, M. K., Dietz, W. H., Bowman, B. A., Marks, J. S., and Koplan, J. P. (1999). The spread of the obesity epidemic in the United States, 1991–1998. *Journal of the American Medical Association, 282*(16), 1519–1522.

Moorman, P., Hames, C., and Tyroler, H. (1991). Socioeconomic status and morbidity and mortality in hypertensive blacks. In E. Saunders (Ed.), *Cardiovascular Diseases in Blacks*, pp. 179–194. Philadelphia: FA Davis Co.

Morrow, G. R., and Bellg, A. J. (1994). Behavioral science in translational research and cancer control. *Cancer, 74*(4 Suppl), 1409–1417.

Morton, W., Baker, H., and Fletcher, W. (1983). Geographic pathology of uterine cancers in Oregon: Risks of double primaries and effects of socioeconomic status. *Gynecologic Oncology, 16*, 63–77.

Must, A., Spadano, J., Coakley, E. H., Field, A. E., Colditz, G., and Dietz, W. H. (1999). The disease burden associated with overweight and obesity. *Journal of the American Medical Association, 282*(16), 1523–1529.

National Cancer Institute. (1987). Working guidelines for early cancer detection: Rationale and supporting evidence to decrease mortality. Internet report: *National Cancer Institute*. www.NCI.gov.

National Cancer Institute. (1997). *Americans Closer to Eating "5-a-Day," Food Survey Finds*. Bethesda, MD: National Cancer Institute.

National Center for Health Statistics. (1996a). *Healthy People 2000 Progress Review: Diabetes and Chronic Disabling Conditions.* Hyattsville, MD: Department of Health and Human Services.

National Center for Health Statistics. (1996b). *Healthy People 2000 Review: 1995–1996* (DHHS Pub No. 96-1256). Hyattsville, MD: Public Health Service.

National Diabetes Information Clearinghouse. (1999). *Diabetes Statistics* (NIH Publication No. 99-3892). Bethesda, MD: National Institute of Health.

National Highway Traffic Safety Administration. (1996a). *Effectiveness of Occupant Protection Systems and Their Use: Third Report to Congress.* Washington, DC: NHTSA.

National Highway Traffic Safety Administration. (1996b). *Traffic Safety Facts 1995: A Compliance of Motor Vehicle Crash Data from the Fatal Accident Reporting System and the General Estimates System.* Washington, DC: NHTSA.

National Research Council. (1989). *A Common Destiny: Blacks and American Society.* Washington DC: National Academy of Sciences.

Neuhouser, M., Kristal, A., and Patterson, R. (1999). Use of food nutrition labels is associated with lower fat intake. *Journal of the American Dietetic Association, 99,* 45–50,53.

Neumark Sztainer, D., Story, M., French, S., Cassuto, N., Jacobs, D. R. J., and Resnick, M. D. (1996). Patterns of health-compromising behaviors among Minnesota adolescents: Sociodemographic variations. *American Journal of Public Health, 86*(11), 1599–1606.

NIOSH. (1996). *National Occupational Research Agenda* (Public Law 91-596, Section 5 (a1). Bethesda, MD: US Public Health Service, Centers for Disease Control, National Institute for Occupational Safety and Health.

Novotny, T., Warner, K., Kendrick, J., and Remington, P. (1988). Smoking by blacks and whites: Socioeconomic and demographic differences. *American Journal of Psychiatry, 78,* 1187–1189.

Novotny, T. E., and Healton, C. G. (1995). Research linkages between academia and public health practice. *American Journal of Preventative Medicine, 11*(supp), 1–61.

Ockene, I. S., Hebert, J. R., Ockene, J. K., Merriam, P. A., Hurley, T. G., and Saperia, G. M. (1996). Effect of training and a structured office practice on physician-delivered nutrition counseling: The Worcester-Area Trial for Counseling in Hyperlipidemia (WATCH). *American Journal of Preventative Medicine, 12*(4), 252–258.

Ockene, I. S., Hebert, J. R., Ockene, J. K., Saperia, G. M., Stanek, E., Nicolosi, R., Merriam, P. A., and Hurley, T. G. (1999). Effect of physician-delivered nutrition counseling training and an office-support program on saturated fat intake, weight, and serum lipid measurements in a hyperlipidemic population: Worcester Area Trial for Counseling in Hyperlipidemia (WATCH). *Archives of Internal Medicine, 159*(7), 725–731.

Ockene, J. K., Kristeller, J., and Goldberg, R. (1991). Increasing the efficacy of physician delivered smoking interventions: A randomized clinical trial. *Journal of General Internal Medicine, 6*(1), 1–8.

Ockene, J. K., Ockene, I. S., Quirk, M. E., Hebert, J. R., Saperia, G. M., Luippold, R. S., Merriam, P. A., and Ellis, S. (1995). Physician training for patient-centered nutrition counseling in a lipid intervention trial. *Preventative Medicine, 24,* 563–570.

Olds, D. L., Eckenrode, J., Henderson, C. R. J., Kitzman, H., Powers, J., Cole, R., Sidora, K., Morris, P., Pettott, L. M., and Luckey, D. (1997). Long-term effects of home visitation on maternal life course and child abuse and neglect. *Journal of the American Medical Association, 278*(8), 637–643.

Olds, D. L., Henderson, C. R. J., Tatelbaum, R., and Chamberlin, R. (1986). Improving the delivery of prenatal care and outcomes of pregnancy: A randomized trial of nurse home visitation. *Pediatrics, 77*(1), 16–28.

O'Malley, S. S., Jaffe, A. J., Chang, G., Schottenfeld, R. S., Meyer, R. E., and Rounsaville, B. (1992). Naltrexone and coping skills therapy for alcohol dependence. A controlled study. *Archives of General Psychiatry, 49*(11), 881–887.

Orleans, C., Gruman, J., Ulmer, C., Emont, S., and Hollendonner, J. (in press). Rating our progress in population health promotion: Report card on six behaviors. *American Journal of Health Promotion.*

Orleans, C. T., George, L. K., Houpt, J. L. et al. (1985). Health promotion in primary care: A survey of U.S. family practitioners. *Preventative Medicine, 14*, 636–647.

Panzarino, P., Jr. (1998). The costs of depression: Direct and indirect; treatment versus nontreatment. *Journal of Clinical Psychiatry, 59*, 11–14.

Parker, E. A., Schulz, A. J., Israel, B. A., and Hollis, R. (1998). Detroit's East Side Village health worker partnership: Community-based health advisor intervention in an urban area. *Health Education and Behavior, 25*(1), 24–45.

Pasick, R., D'Onofrio, C., and Otero Sabogal, R. (1996). Similarities and differences across cultures: Questions to inform a third generation for health promotion research. *Health Education Quarterly, 23*(Supplement), S142–S161.

Pate, R. R., Heath, G. W., Dowda, M., and Trost, S. G. (1996). Associations between physical activity and other health behaviors in a representative sample of U.S. adolescents. *American Journal of Public Health, 86*(11), 1577–1581.

Patterson, R. E., Kristal, A. R., Glanz, K., McLerran, D. F., Hebert, J. R., Heimendinger, J., Linnan, L., Probart, C., and Chamberlain, R. M. (1997). Components of the working well trial intervention associated with adoption of healthful diets. *American Journal of Preventative Medicine, 13*(4), 271–276.

Peterson, T. R., and Aldana, S. G. (1999). Improving exercise behavior: An application of the stages of change model in a worksite setting. *American Journal of Health Promotion, 13*(4), 229–232, iii.

Pierce, J. P., Fiore, M. C., Novotny, T. E., Hatziandreu, E. J., and Davis, R. M. (1989). Trends in cigarette smoking in the United States: Projections to the year 2000. *Journal of the American Medical Association, 26*(1), 61–65.

Pietinen, P., Vartianinen, E., Seppanen, R., Aro, A., and Puska, P. (1996). Changes in diet in Finland from 1972 to 1992: Impact on coronary heart disease risk. *Preventative Medicine, 25*, 243–250.

Puska, P., Salonen, J. T., Nissinen, A., Tuomilehto, J., Vartianinen, E., Korhonen, H., Tanskanen, A., Ronnqvist, P., Koskela, K., and Huttunen, J. (1983). Change in risk factors for coronary heart disease during 10 years of a community intervention programme (North Karelia project). *British Medical Journal, 287*, 1840–1844.

Rachuba, L., Stanton, B., and Howard, D. (1995). Violent crime in the United States. An epidemiologic profile. *Archives of Pediatric and Adolescent Medicine, 149*, 953–960.

Rakowski, W., Ehrich, B., Goldstein, M. G., Rimer, B. K., Pearlman, D. N., Clark, M. A., Velicer, W. F., and Woolverton, H., 3rd. (1998). Increasing mammography among women aged 40–74 by use of a stage-matched, tailored intervention. *Preventative Medicine, 27*(5 Pt 1), 748–756.

Ramelson, H. Z., Friedman, R. H., and Ockene, J. K. (1999). An automated telephone-based smoking cessation education and counseling system. *Patient Education Counseling, 36*(2), 131–144.

Rastenyte, D., Tuomilehto, J., and Sarti, C. (1998). Genetics of stroke—A review. *Journal of Neurologic Science, 153*, 132–145.

Regier, D. A., Farmer, M. E., Rae, D. S., Myers, J. K., Kramer, M., Robins, L. N., George, L. K., Karno, M., and Locke, B. Z. (1993a). One-month prevalence of mental disorders in the United States and sociodemographic characteristics: The Epidemiologic Catchment Area Study. *Acta Psychiatrica Scandinavica, 88*(1), 35–47.

Regier, D. A., Narrow, W. E., Rae, D. S., Manderscheid, R. W., Locke, B. Z., and Goodwin, F. K. (1993b). The de facto U.S. mental and addictive disorders service system. Epidemiologic catchment area prospective 1-year prevalence rates of disorders and services. *Archives of General Psychiatry, 50*(2), 85–94.

Resnicow, K., Baranowski, T., Ahluwalia, J. S., and Braithwaite, R. L. (1999). Cultural sensitivity in public health: Defined and demystified. *Ethnicity and Disease, 9*(1), 10–21.

Resnicow, K., Futterman, R., Weston, R., Royce, J., Parms, C., Freeman, H., and Orlandi, M. (1996). Harlem Hospital smoking prevalence. *Smoking Prevalence in Harlem, New York, 10*(5), 343–346.

Rimer, B., Conaway, M., Lyna, P., Glassman, B., Yarnell, K., Lipkus, I., and Barber, L. (1999). The impact of tailored interventions on a community health center population. *Patient Education Counseling, 37*(2), 125–140.

Rimer, B., and Glassman, B. (1997). Tailored communications for cancer prevention in managed care settings. *Outlook*, 4–5.

Rimer, B., and Glassman, B. (1999). Is there a use for tailored print communications (TPC's) in cancer risk communication (CRC)? 25, 140–148.

Rimer, B. K., Orleans, C. T., Fleisher, L., Cristinzio, S., Resch, N., Telepchak, J., and Keintz, M. K. (1994). Does tailoring matter? The impact of a tailored guide on ratings and short-term smoking-related outcomes for older smokers. *Health Education and Research, 9*(1), 69–84.

Rivara, F., Grossman, D., and Cummings, P. (1997). Injury Prevention (2 part review article). *New England Journal of Medicine, 337*(8), 543–618; 613–618.

Robins, L., Helzer, J., Croughan, J., Williams, J., and Spitzer, R. (1981). *Diagnostic Interview schedule: Version III.* Rockville, MD: NIMH.

Rogers, E. M. (1983). *Diffusion of Innovations,* 3rd ed. New York: The Free Press.

Roman, P., and Blum, T. (1996). Alcohol: A review of the impact of worksite interventions on health and behavioral outcomes. *American Journal of Health Promotion, 11*(2), 136–149.

Rose, G. (1982). Strategy of prevention: Lessons from cardiovascular disease. *British Medical Journal, 282*, 1847–1851.

Rose, G. (1985). Sick individuals and sick populations. *International Journal of Epidemiology, 14*(1), 32–38.

Rose, G. (1992). *The Strategy of Preventive Medicine.* New York, NY: Oxford University Press.

Rosenburg, M. (1995). An integrated approach to understanding and prevention. *Journal of Health Care for the Poor and Underserved, 6,* 102–110.

Rothman, J. (1970). Three models of community organization practice. In E. J. Cox , Rothman J., Tropman J.E. (Ed.), *Strategies of Community Organization,* pp. 86–162. Itasca, NJ: Peacock.

Salina, D., Jason, L. A., Hedeker, D., Kaufman, J., Lesondak, L., McMahon, S. D., Taylor, S., and Kimball, P. (1994). A follow-up of a media-based worksite smoking cessation program. *American Journal of Community Psychology, 22*(2), 257–271.

Sanders-Phillips, K. (1996). The ecology of urban violence: Its relationship to health promotion behaviors in low-income black and latino communities. *American Journal of Health Promotion, 10*(4), 308–317.

Schafer, R. (1978). Factors affecting food behavior and the quality of husbands' and wives' diets. *Journal of the American Dietetic Association, 72,* 138–143.

Schafer, R., and Keith, P. (1982). Social psychological factors in the dietary quality of married and single elderly. *Journal of the American Dietetic Association, 81,* 30–34.

Schensul, S. (1985). Science, theory and application in anthropology. *American Behavioral Scientist, 29,* 164–185.

Schulberg, H., Saul, M., McLelland, M., Ganguli, M., Christy, W., and Frank, R. (1985). Assessing depression in primary medical and psychiatric practices. *Archives of General Psychiatry, 44,* 152–156.

Schultz, A., Israel, B., Becker, A., and Hollis, R. (1997). "It's a 24-hour thing A living for each other concept": Identity, networks, and community in an urban village health worker project. *Health Education and Behavior, 24*(4), 465–480.

Sebastian, J. L., McKinney, W. P., and Young, M. J. (1989). Epidemiology and interaction of risk factors in cardiovascular disease. *Primary Care, 16*(1), 31–47.

Seetharam, S. (1999). *Selecting a Process for Identifying Tobacco Reduction Best Practices: A preview of the issues.* Ottawa, Canada: Office of Tobacco Reduction Programs.

Shepard, R. (1996). Worksite fitness and exercise programs: A review of methodology and health impact. *American Journal of Health Promotion, 10*(6), 436–452.

Shiffman, S. (1993). Smoking cessation treatment. *Journal of Consulting and Community Psychology, 61*(5), 718–722.

Siegal, P., Fraizer, E., and Mariolis, P. (1993). Behavioral Risk Factor Surveillance, 1991: Monitoring Progress Toward the Nation's Year 2000 Health Objectives. *Morbidity and Mortality Weekly Report, 42*(SS-4), 1–30.

Skinner, C., Campbell, M., Rimer, B., Curry, S., and Prochaska, J. (1999). How effective is tailored print communication? *Annals of Behavioral Medicine, 21*(4), 290–298.

Skinner, C. S., Siegfried, J. C., Kegler, M. C., and Strecher, V. J. (1993). The potential of computers in patient education. *Patient Education and Counseling, 22*(1), 27–34.

Snow, L. F. (1974). Folk medical beliefs and their implications for care of patients. A review bases on studies among black Americans. *Annals of Internal Medicine, 81*(1), 82–96.

Sobell, L. C., Sobell, M. B., Kozlowski, L. T., and Toneatto, T. (1990). Alcohol or tobacco research versus alcohol and tobacco research. *British Journal of Addiction, 85*(2), 263–269.

Sorensen, G., Emmons, K., Hunt, M., Eisenberg, M., and Johnston, D. (in press). Public Health Interventions Targeting Health Behaviors: Building on Research to Date. Washington, DC: Institute of Medicine.

Sorensen, G., Emmons, K., Hunt, M., and Johnston, D. (1998a). Implications of the results of community intervention trials. *Annual Review of Public Health, 19*, 379–416.

Sorensen, G., Himmelstein, J., Hunt, M., Youngstrom, R., Hebert, J., Hammond, S. et al. (1995). A model for worksite cancer prevention: Integration of health protection and health promotion in the Wellworks Project. *American Journal of Health Promotion, 10*(1), 55–62.

Sorensen, G., Hunt, M., Cohen, N., Stoddard, A., Stein, E., Phillips, J., Baker, F., Combe, C., Hebert, J., and Palombo, R. (1998b). Worksite and family education for dietary change: The Treatwell 5-a-Day Program. *Health Education and Research, 13*(4), 577–591.

Sorensen, G., Lando, H., and Pechacek, T. F. (1993). Promoting smoking cessation at the workplace: Results of a randomized controlled intervention study. *Journal of Medicine, 35*(2), 121–126.

Sorensen, G., Morris, D., Hunt, M., Hebert, J., Harris, D., Stoddard, A., and Ockene, J. (1992). Work-site nutrition intervention and employees' dietary habits: The Treatwell program. *American Journal of Public Health, 82*(6), 877–880.

Sorensen, G., Stoddard, A., and Hunt, M. (1998c). Behavior change in a worksite cancer prevention intervention: The WellWorks Study. *American Journal of Public Health, 88*, 1685–1690.

Sorensen, G., Stoddard, A., Peterson, K., Cohen, N., Hunt, M., Stein, E., Palumbo, R., and Lederman, R. (1999). Increasing fruit and vegetable consumption through worksites and families in the Treatwell 5-a-Day Study. *American Journal of Public Health, 89*(1), 54–60.

Sorensen, G., Thompson, B., Basen-Enquist, K., Abrams, D., Kuniyuki, A., DiClemente, C., and Biener, L. (1998d). Durability, dissemination, and institutionalization of worksite tobacco control programs: Results from the Working Well Trial. *International Journal of Behavioral Medicine, 5*(4), 335–351.

Sorensen, G., Thompson, B., Glanz, K., Feng, Z., Kinne, S., DiClemente, C., Emmons, K., Heimendinger, J., Probart, C., and Lichtenstein, E. (1996a). Work site-based cancer prevention: Primary results from the Working Well Trials. *American Journal of Public Health, 86*(7), 939–947.

Sorensen, G., Thompson, B., Glanz, K., Feng, Z., Kinne, S., DiClemente, C., Emmons, K., Heinmendinger, J., Probart, C., and Lichtenstein, E. (1996b). Work site-based cancer prevention: Primary results from the Working Well Trial. *American Journal of Public Health, 86*(7), 939–947.

Sorensen, G., Thompson, B., Glanz, K., Feng, Z., Kinne, S., DiClemente, C., Emmons, K. M., Heimendinger, J., Probart, C., and Lichtenstein, E. (1996c). Working Well: Results from a worksite based cancer prevention trial. *American Journal of Public Health, 86*, 939–947.

Stead, L., and Lancaster, T. (1999). Group behaviour therapy programmes for smoking cessation. *The Cochrane Library*(4), Oxford: Updated software.

Stokols, P., Allen, J., and Bellingham, R. L. (1996b). The social ecology of health promotion: Implications for research and practice. *American Journal of Health Promotion, 10*, 247–251.

Stokols, D., Pelletier, K. R., and Fielding, J. E. (1996a). The ecology of work and health: Research and policy directions for the promotion of employee health. *Health Education Quarterly, 23*(2), 137–158.

Strecher, V. J., Kreuter, M., Den Boer, D. J., Kobrin, S., Hospers, H. J., and Skinner, C. S. (1994). The effects of computer-tailored smoking cessation messages in family practice settings. *Journal of Family Practice, 39*(3), 262–270.

Street, R., Jr., Gold, W., and Manning, T. (1997). *Health Promotion and Interactive Technology: Theoretical Applications and Future Directions.* London: Lawrence Erlbaum Associates.

Subar, A. S., Heimdinger, J., Krebs-Smith, S. M., Patterson, B. H., Kessler, R., and Pivonka, E. (1995). Fruit and vegetable intake in the United States: The baseline survey of the Five a Day for Better Health Program. *American Journal of Health Promotion, 9*(5), 352–360.

Sundstrom, E. (1986). *Workplaces: The Psychology of the Physical Environment in Offices and Factories.* New York: Cambridge University Press.

Surtees, P., Dean, C., Ingham, J., Kreitman, N., Miller, P., and Sashidharan, S. (1983). Psychiatric disorder in women from an Edinburgh community: Associations with demographic factors. *British Journal of Psychiatry, 142*, 238–246.

Susser, M. (1985). Editorial: The tribulations of trials-Intervention in communities. *American Journal of Public Health, 85*(2), 156–158.

Syme, S. (1997). Individual vs. community interventions in public health practice: Some thoughts about a new approach. *Vic Health*(2).

Tarr, K., Highstein, G., Sykes, R., Musick, J., Strunk, R., and Fisher, E. (2000). *Asthma Coaches Reach Underserved Medicaid Enrolled Through Nondirective Support and Proactive Strategies.* Paper presented at the SBM Annual Meeting. Nashville, TN.

Taylor, V., Robson, J., and Evans, S. (1992). Risk factors for coronary heart disease: A study in inner London. *British Journal of General Practice, 42*(362), 377–380.

Thomas, S. B., Quinn, S. C., Billingsley, A., and Caldwell, C. (1994). The characteristics of northern black churches with community health outreach programs. *American Journal of Public Health, 84*(4), 575–579.

Thorndike, A., Rigotti, N., Stafford, R., and Singer, D. (1998). National patterns in the treatment of smokers by physicians. *Journal of the American Medical Association, 279*(8), 604–608.

Tilley, B. C., Glanz, K., Kristal, A. R., Hirst, K., Li, S., Vernon, S. W., and Myers, R. (1999a). Nutrition intervention for high-risk auto workers: Results of the next step trial. *Preventative Medicine, 28*, 276–283.

Tilley, B. C., Vernon, S. W., Myers, R., Glanz, K., Lu, M., Hirst, K., and Kristal, A. R. (1999b). The Next Step Trial: Impact of a worksite colorectal cancer screening promotion program. *Preventative Medicine, 28*(3), 276–283.

Tomatis, L. (1992). Poverty and cancer. *Cancer Epidemiology, Biomarkers, and Prevention, 1*, 167–175.

Tosteson, A. N., Weinstein, M. C., Hunink, M. G., Mittleman, M. A., Williams, L. W., Goldman, P. A., and Goldman, L. (1997). Cost-effectiveness of populationwide educational approaches to reduce serum cholesterol levels. *Circulation, 95*(1), 24–30.

Troutt, D. (1993). *The Thin Red Line: How the Poor Still Pay More.* San Francisco: Consumers Union of the United States.

Unger, J. (1996). Stages of change of smoking cessation: Relationships with other health behaviors. *American Journal of Preventative Medicine, 12,* 134–138.

U.S. Department of Agriculture. (1991). *USDA Continuing Survey of Food Intakes by Individuals, 1989–1991.* Washington, DC: ARS, Beltsville Hum. Nutr. Res. Cent. Food Surv. Res Group.

U.S. Preventative Services Task Force. (1996). *Guide to Clinical Preventative Services.* Baltimore: Williams & Wilkins.

USDHHS. (1991). *Healthy People 2000: National Health Promotion and Disease Prevention.* Bethesda, MD: Public Health Service.

USDHHS. (1994). *A Report on Research, Training, Career Development, Education, and Other Activities Related to Nutrition, Fiscal Year 1994.* Washington, DC: U.S. Department of Health and Human Services, National Institutes of Health, National Heart Lung and Blood Institute Programs in Nutrition.

USDHHS. (1996a). *Healthy People 2000 Progress Review: Diabetes and Chronic Disabling conditions.* Hyattsville, MD: National Institute of Health.

USDHHS. (1996b). *Physical Activity and Health: A Report of the Surgeon General.* Atlanta: Center for Disease Control and Prevention; National Center for Chronic Disease Prevention and Health Promotion.

USDHHS. (1996c). *Vital Statistics of the U.S., 1992, vol. 2, Mortality Part A* (Pub No. 96-1101). Hyattsville, MD: National Center for Health Statistics.

USDHHS. (1998). *Socioeconomic Status and Health Chartbook.* Washington, DC: Department of Health and Human Services.

USDHHS. (1999). *Healthy People 2000, Progress Review: Heart Disease and Stroke.* Bethesda, MD: Department of Health and Human Services.

Vazquez-Barquero, J., Diez-Manrique, J., Pena, C. et al. (1987). A community mental health survey in Cantabria: A general description of morbidity. *Psychological Medicine, 17,* 227 241.

Velasquez, M., Hecht, J., Quinn, V., Emmons, K., DiClemente, C., and Mullen, P. (in press). The application of motivational interviewing to prenatal smoking cessation: Training and implementation issues. *Tobacco Control.*

Velicer, W. F., Prochaska, J. O., Bellis, J. M., DiClemente, C. C., Rossi, J. S., Fava, J. L., and Steiger, J. H. (1993). An expert system intervention for smoking cessation. *Addictive Behavior, 18,* 269–290.

Velicer, W. F., Prochaska, J. O., Fava, J. L., Laforge, R. G., and Rossi, J. S. (1999). Interactive versus noninteractive interventions and dose-response relationships for stage-matched smoking cessation programs in a managed care setting. *Health Psychology, 18*(1), 21–28.

Vogt, T., Hollis, J., Lichtenstein, E., Stevens, V., Glasgow, R., and Whitlock, E. (1998). The medical care system and prevention: The need for a new paradigm. *HMO Practice, 12,* 6–14.

Voorhees, C. C., Stillman, F. A., Swank, R. T., Heagerty, P. J., Levine, D. M., and Becker, D. M. (1996). Heart, body, and soul: Impact of church-based smoking cessation interventions on readiness to quit. *Preventative Medicine, 25,* 277–285.

Wallack, L., and Winkleby, M. (1986). Primary prevention: A new look at basic concepts. *Social Science and Medicine, 25*, 923–930.

Wang, J., Carson, E., Lapane, K., Eaton, C., Gans, K., and Lasater, T. (1999). The effect of physician office visits on CHD risk factor modification as part of a worksite cholesterol screening program. *Preventative Medicine, 28*, 221–228.

Warner, K. E., Slade, J., and Sweanor, D. T. (1997). The emerging market for long-term nicotine maintenance. *Journal of the American Medical Association, 278*(13), 1087–1092.

Webber, D., Balsam, A., and Oehlke, B. (1995). The Massachusett's farmer's market coupon program for low-income elders. *American Journal of Health Promotion, 9*(4), 251–253.

Wegman, D., and Levy, B. (1995). Preventing occupational disease. In D. Wegman and B. Levy (Eds.), *Occupational Health: Recognizing and Preventing Work-Related Disease*, pp. 83–101. Boston: Little, Brown, and Company.

Weinstein, N. (1988). The precaution adoption process. *Health Psychology, 7*, 355–386.

Weiss, B. D., Hart, G., McGee, D. L., and D'Estelle, S. (1992). Health status of illiterate adults: Relation between literacy and health status among persons with low literacy skills. *Journal of the American Board of Family Practice, 5*, 257–264.

Wells, K., Lewis, C., Leake, B., Schleiter, M., and Brook, R. (1986). The practice of general and subspecialty internists in counseling about smoking and exercise. *American Journal of Public Health, 76*, 1009–1013.

Wells, K., Stewart, A., Hays, R. et al. (1989a). The functioning and well-being of depressed patients. *Journal of the American Medical Association, 262*, 914–919.

Wells, K. B., Hays, R. D., Burnam, M. A., Rogers, W., Greenfield, S., and Ware, J. E., Jr. (1989b). Detection of depressive disorder for patients receiving prepaid or fee-for-service care. Results from the Medical Outcomes Study. *Journal of the American Medical Association, 262*(23), 3298–3302.

Wells, K. B., and Lewis, B. (1984). Do physicians practice what they preach? *Journal of the American Medical Association, 252*, 2846–2848.

Wiist, W. H., and Flack, J. M. (1990). A church-based cholesterol education program. *Public Health Reports, 105*(4), 381–388.

Wilkinson, R. G. (1992). Income distribution and life expectancy. *British Medical Journal, 304*(6820), 165–168.

Willemsen, M. C., de Vries, H., van Breukelen, G., and Genders, R. (1998). Long-term effectiveness of two Dutch work site smoking cessation programs. *Health Education and Behavior, 25*(4), 418–435.

Willett, W., Colditz, G., and Mueller, N. (1996). Strategies for minimizing cancer risk. *Scientific American, 275*(3), 58.

Williams, A. (1982). Passive and active measures for controlling disease and injury: The role of health psychologists. *Health Psychology, 1*, 399–409.

Williams, M. V., Parker, R. M., Baker, D. W., Parikh, N. S., Pitkin, K., Coates, W. C., and Nurss, J. R. (1995). Inadequate functional health literacy among patients at two public hospitals. *Journal of the American Medical Association, 274*(21), 1677–1682.

Williams, R., and Horm, J. (1977). Association of cancer sites with tobacco and alcohol consumption and socioeconomic status of patients: Interview study from the Third National Cancer Study. *Journal of the National Cancer Institute, 58*, 525–547.

Wilson, D. M., Taylor, D. W., Gilbert, J. R., Best, J. A., Lindsay, E. A., Willms, D. G., and Singer, J. (1988). A randomized trial of a family physician intervention for smoking cessation. *Journal of the American Medical Association, 260*(11), 1570–1574.

Wilson, M. G., Holman, P. B., and Hammock, A. (1996a). A comprehensive review of the effects of worksite health promotion on health-related outcomes. *American Journal of Health Promotion, 10*(6), 429–435.

Wilson, M. G., Jorgensen, C., and Cole, G. (1996b). The health effects of worksite HIV/AIDS interventions: A review of the research literature. *American Journal of Health Promotion, 11*(2), 150–157.

Wilson, P. W., and Culleton, B. F. (1998). Epidemiology of cardiovascular disease in the United States. *American Journal of Kidney Disease, 32*(5 Suppl 3), S56–65.

Winett, R., King, A., and Altman, D. (1989). *Health Psychology and Public Health: An integrative approach.* New York: Pergamon Press.

Winkleby, M. (1994). The future of community-based cardiovascular disease intervention studies. *American Journal of Public Health, 84*(9), 1369–1371.

Winkleby, M. A., Feldman, H. A., and Murray, D. M. (1997). Joint analysis of three U.S. community intervention trials for reduction of cardiovascular disease risk. *American Journal of Public Health, 87*.

Winkleby, M. A., Taylor, B., Jatulis, D., and Fortmann, S. P. (1996). The long-term effects of a cardiovascular disease prevention trial: The Stanford five-city project. *American Journal of Public Health, 86*(12), 1773–1779.

Womble, K. (1988). *The Impact of Minimum Drinking Age Laws on Fatal Crash Involvements: An Update of the NHTSA Analysis.* Washington, DC: National Highway Traffic Safety Administration.

The Behavioral and Social Dynamics of Aging Well

George L. Maddox, Ph.D.

In the last half of the twentieth century the United States discovered the implications of an aging population for both social institutions and individuals. In the context of public health, aging populations were of interest because they were large and observed to be growing rapidly at mid century. At the end of the century, 13% of the population of the United States was 65 years of age or older and an estimated 4%, 80 or older. In Europe, aging populations are already much larger, rising to 20% in Germany, for example. Public health interest is also sustained by evidence that older adults have high rates of chronic conditions accompanied by functional disability, consume health and social services at a high rate, and illustrate so consistently the negative consequences for health of lower socioeconomic status (SES). The bad news from research has been that individuals could be expected to live longer but they could not depend on dying conveniently with functional capacity and financial resources intact. The social institutions through which a society does its essential business of transportation, housing, retirement at the end of a work career, personal income maintenance, and providing essential health and social care for elderly citizens have been seriously challenged. The good new from behavioral and social research on aging, however, has delivered increasingly positive evidence that aging well is possible

Dr. Maddox is professor emeritus, Center for Studies of Aging and Human Development, at Duke University. This paper was prepared for the symposium "Capitalizing on Social Science and Behavioral Research to Improve the Public's Health," the Institute of Medicine and the Commission on Behavioral and Social Sciences and Education of the National Research Council, Atlanta, Georgia, February 2–3, 2000.

for the substantial majority of older adults. And the prospects of beneficial behavioral and social interventions to enhance well-being in later life continue to improve. The mind set of contemporary gerontology is increasingly interventionist and optimistic about change.

The challenges of individual and population aging are real and should not be underestimated. Demographers have documented, and often viewed with alarm, the increase in dependency ratios (the number of nonworking individuals versus those actively in the workforce) and the age gradient of risk of dependency, and have forecast problems for pension, income maintenance, and health care financing. Epidemiologists have documented both the significance and the persistent age gradient of morbidity and comorbidity and, with behavioral and social scientists, have also documented notable variation in life expectancy and risk of functional disability associated with socioeconomic status, ethnicity, and gender. The documented diversity of older populations has been a significant factor in the growing awareness of gerontologists that chronological age per se is a relatively weak explanatory variable in assessing the prospects of continuing to age well in later life, which is the experience of a substantial majority of older adults (Campbell et al., 1976; Maddox and Glass, 1999).

The established behavioral and social diversity of older adults has had important practical and theoretical consequences in gerontological research. Practically, sampling older populations for research and for generalizing about older adults, who constitute about 13% of the U.S. population currently, typically requires oversampling to insure inclusion of minorities and the very old. Theoretically, repeatedly observed diversity within age cohorts suggests both that behavioral and social factors are involved in aging processes and that such factors are potentially modifiable. The intellectual shot that was heard around the world in gerontology was fired by Stanford's James Fries (1980) in a seminal article on "the compression of morbidity." Fries argued that even if the life span is typically limited (he optimistically and incorrectly concluded that the limit is 85 years), the risk of morbidity and related functional disability can be delayed through interventions designed to improve physical activity, social integration, and cognitive performance. Critics initially scoffed and dismissed such optimism, but not for long. The evidence supporting the modifiability of functional disability in later life has continued to accumulate and has laid the foundation for the increasing interest of gerontologists in purposive behavioral and social interventions to improve the well-being of older adults (e.g., Rowe and Kahn, 1987; Berkman, 1988; Manton, 1988; Fries, 1995).

Unlike their clinical colleagues who view interventions at the personal level to be a natural extension of practical knowledge, behavioral and social scientists have moved cautiously in developing enthusiasm for psychosocial interventions. And they have remained particularly cautious about macrosocial legislated interventions such as Social Security and Medicare or Medicaid, both of which are viewed as important and beneficial natural experiments but outside the competence of most behavioral and social scientists to initiate and evaluate as political interventions (see, e.g., Marmor and Okma, 1998). An important turning point in interest in psychosocial interventions in research on aging on a modest scale occurred, however, when the Institute of Medicine, responding to a request of the National Institute on Aging to propose a research agenda for the future, recommended increased emphasis on psychosocial interventions and field trials (Lonergan, 1991). Interest in psychosocial interventions in later life has increased markedly in the past decade.

What follows in this paper are three sections, beginning with an overview of what is known about aging individuals and populations. Evidence from epidemiology and medical demography provides a clear characterization of the health and well-being of older adults and populations. While the evidence is primarily from the United States, the characteristics of aging populations in other industrial societies are similar. A second section presents brief accounts of four quite varied psychosocial interventions that range from emphasis on health promotion and disease prevention through physical activity for well elderly persons through rehabilitation regimes for persons with diagnosed disease to enhancement of autonomy among institutionalized elderly. A concluding section illustrates how the convergence of theory and research on the social structuring of living and work environments, and on the reconceptualization of dependency in later life as a modifiable interpersonal strategy, suggests a distinctive psychosocial intervention for frail, nursing home-eligible older adults living in the community. The intervention is a distinctive new type of housing with services known as "assisted living."

HEALTH AND WELL-BEING IN LATER LIFE: KNOWING THE TERRITORY OF AGING

The basic evidence for characterizing the health and well-being of older populations is now well established (Berkman, 1988; Manton, 1988; Manton et al., 1997; Maddox and Glass, 1999):

• The distinctive age gradients of morbidity, disability, and mortality vary significantly by gender, ethnicity, and socioeconomic status, although the gradients are attenuated in very late life as a result of selective survival.

• The top four conditions in the National Health Interview Survey's league table of chronic conditions in the mid-1990s for women were arthritis, hypertension, hearing loss, and chronic heart disease; for men the predominant conditions were arthritis, hearing loss, hypertension, and ischemic heart disease (Verbrugge, 1995).

• The expected age gradient in medical care utilization occurs, but the utilization patterns of men and women vary significantly; higher total utilization by women reflects the fact that older women are more likely to be functionally disabled than men, and they live longer.

• Comorbidity is a condition well known to geriatricians; the average older adult has two chronic conditions at any time of observation.

Older populations are typically characterized in terms of functional status in addition to health status. The usual designations of functioning are Activities of Daily Living (ADLs) and Instrumental Activities of Daily Living (IADLs). The former reference self-care activities such as bathing, toileting, and eating; the latter, activities such as ambulation, cooking, and money management. These designations have stood up well in both research and practice for use in characterizing types and levels of need in populations and as triggers for authorizing services for individuals. Manton (1988), for many years the data manager of the Health Care Financing Administration's longitudinal National Long Term Care Survey (NLTCS), observes that functional status complements medical diagnoses in a useful way: functional assessment suggests the range of services likely to be required in care management while diagnosis suggests the possible length of time services may be required. Functional status has also been a key construct in the Medical Outcome Study of patients being seen in primary care settings (Stewart et al., 1989) as an outcome measure; and the concept has been broadened to include the capacity to perform social roles.

In reviewing the evidence on the prevalence and distribution of functional disability in later life, one finds many expectations fulfilled, but also a few surprises:

- The most significant surprise is that 8 or 10 older adults report no functional disability at all and 95% live in the community.
- A persistent 5% of older adults reside in nursing homes at any observation, and the lifetime risk of any individual for at least some exposure to a nursing home is an estimated 20%. An additional estimated 5% of older adults in the community have functional disabilities that make them "nursing home eligible."
- For both men and women, arthritis and circulatory problems are the most totally disabling conditions. Total disablement is the experience of 30% of older adults with circulatory problems and 26% of those with arthritis. For both conditions, women are more likely than men to be totally disabled.
- Senility, an outmoded term that persists to indicate cognitive deficit in late life, ranks fourth (15%) in the NLTCS league table of chronic conditions producing total disability.
- Depression, a common mental health problem in adulthood, has not been found to be consistently elevated in older populations. However, when present, both depression and cognitive impairment increase the risk of functional impairment from chronic conditions, complicate the management of chronic conditions, and increase the risk of extraordinary outcomes such as suicide among older males (Stewart et al., 1988; Roberts et al., 1997; Reynolds et al., 1998).
- The consequences of the socioeconomic gradient of chronic conditions (see, e.g., Evans et al., 1994) is dramatically underscored by the distribution of active life expectancy in later life (Guralnick et al., 1993). Active life expectancy designates disability-free years of living post-age 65. Higher educational attainment, for example, predicts for men an 18% increase in disability-free

years and for women, 25%. The SES gradient of health and illness is observed worldwide, although the gradient can be affected by sociocultural factors.

• Ethnicity as well as socioeconomic status affects functioning and well-being in later life (Clark et al., 1993; Markides and Wallace, 1996). These effects are observed in distinctive patterns of disability and dependency, need for long-term care services, and cultural expectations about responsibility for providing care for family members.

• Longitudinal trajectories of disability over a 4-year period in the NLTCS document stability of functional status for a substantial majority (80%), and for those whose functional status changes, the change is positive for 30%.

• Healthy life-styles are observed as frequently among older adults as among adults generally and have the expected positive effects (see, e.g., Berkman and Breslow, 1983; Rowe and Kahn, 1997). But commitment to healthy life-styles among adults in the United States remains suboptimal.

In sum, the demography and epidemiology of later life have reinforced some of the basic maxims of contemporary gerontology: Older populations are and remain substantially diverse; the gradients of chronic conditions and related functional disability vary significantly by gender, ethnicity, and socioeconomic status; and the mutability of functional status and well-being in later life is well established. In my 40 years in gerontology, probably the most significant event has been increasing evidence-based interest in psychosocial interventions. Gerontology has rediscovered the venerable maxim of clinical and scientific research: *If you want to understand something (aging), try to change it.* This maxim has increasingly dominated my own thinking about the feasibility of beneficial psychosocial interventions (Maddox, 1987) and my research (Maddox and Clark, 1992; Maddox et al., 1994). The Social Security Administration's Longitudinal Retirement History Survey, which was designed to explore retirement as a social process for a large population (11,000) over the period of a decade, sensitized me to the SES and gender gradients in disability among older adults. What we found in my research was the following:

• The expected age gradient of functional disability was confirmed for both men and women in the observed trajectories of functional impairment over the period of a decade; women were and remained consistently more impaired than men; and the expected socioeconomic gradient of disability was found.

• But two significant surprises were revealed in the analysis. (1) At the upper ranges of age, the trajectories of disability converged for men and women, a finding anticipated from research on African Americans that indicated a convergence and reversal of disability rates at upper age ranges, probably reflecting selective survival. (2) The more important surprise was that when socioeconomic status was controlled, the initially observed gender difference disappeared.

With such information one does not leap to the conclusion that gender does not have a biological component. But the evidence clearly suggests that gender differences in functional status and well-being have psychosocial components, particularly income and education, known to be modifiable. As noted earlier, the most obvious political interventions at the societal level focused on access to education and higher income have obvious merit but are beyond the scope of this paper. There is merit, however, in keeping in mind that the modest psychosocial interventions we typically choose to consider do not exhaust the possibilities. As noted above, the enactment of Social Security in 1933 and of Medicare and Medicaid in 1965 has had far-reaching benefits for the welfare of older adults in the United States. Similarly, a brief note about the Black report (Townsend and Davidson, 1982) will remind us just how much we prefer modest nonpolitical interventions in the interest of improving the public's health and well-being.

In Great Britain at the end of 25 years of the National Health Services, a Labour government asked a commission to review how well this free at the point of access health care system had done in improving the health of the British people. Not enough, came the answer from Sir Douglas Black and his colleagues; pronounced social class differences in health persist. What should be done to improve this discrepancy? Do not increase the number of physicians and hospital beds came the answer. Instead, came an answer that might have been and quite possibly was copied from an epidemiology textbook: Concentrate public policy initiatives on redistributing income and increasing access of the young to education. This interesting advice, as luck would have it, had to be offered to the Conservative government of Mrs. Thatcher who came into power in 1980, and it was promptly shelved. Mrs. Thatcher had a different view of the role of government in beneficial interventions that concentrated on private-sector initiatives.

A SAMPLER OF PSYCHOSOCIAL INTERVENTIONS IN LATER LIFE

Evidence of the modifiability of aging processes and the experience of aging has stimulated an increasing number of psychosocial interventions in later life. Strategies for design and implementation of such interventions and the variety of their objectives are conveniently summarized in a recent volume edited by Schulz et al. (1998). The substance of the interventions summarized ranges broadly over topics that include uses of pharmacologic agents in combination with psychosocial therapy in control of depression; physical activity regimes to improve physical health and psychological functioning; improvement of memory; home modification to improve ambulation; incontinence control; improving motivation in nursing homes; and a comparative review of what one learns from societal policy initiatives about the modifiability of aging processes. In each instance, extensive bibliographies permit a review of a broad range of research on each topic.

The sampler of psychosocial interventions in later life presented here features four illustrative initiatives beginning with a macroanalysis of a very large number of activity regimes designed to improve physical health and sense of well-being. Two illustrations follow that address interventions to improve management of patients diagnosed with chronic conditions, specifically, osteoporosis and diabetes. One of these interventions addresses the issue of psychosocial interventions with minority and low-income patients. The fourth illustration is from a comparative study of interventions to reduce excessive dependency among very frail nursing home residents. Although these four interventions were chosen to illustrate variety in objectives and strategies, their findings proved to have two dominant themes in common: (1) emphasis on the benefits of social support groups and social network integration for health and well-being; and (2) self-efficacy as a key predictor variable in successful intervention outcomes.

The importance of social support groups and social integration in a variety of natural settings has been a major theme in most psychosocial research on aging in recent decades. In particular, Berkman (1988) and colleagues (Berkman and Syme, 1979; Berkman and Breslow, 1983; see also House et al., 1988) have consistently documented the positive relationships between social integration and support and favorable morbidity and mortality outcomes. Such a transactional view of the person as an active agent negotiating within a structured social context continues to be a central theme in a social ecological view of development over the life course. Further, a social learning perspective on development in later life that stresses the importance of self-efficacy is a central theme in a wide range of health intervention research in the last decade.

Activity Interventions in Later Life

• *Objective*—McAuley and Katula (1998) provide a meta-analysis of 1,300 studies of "physical activities interventions" in later life intended to improve physical health and cognitive or emotional functioning (mood, morbidity, and sense of well-being). The straightforward hypothesis typically advanced is that activity is beneficial.

• *Design Issues*—Overall the studies reviewed are given low marks regarding their weak conceptualization of causation, inadequate measurement of key variables, and poor sample maintenance and motivation.

• *Findings and Conclusions*—Consistent evidence of a direct causal link between physical activity and beneficial outcomes across the various intervention studies reviewed was "surprisingly weak and equivocal." The evidence was particularly unclear that physical activity per se, as distinct from social activity, generally was the primary causal factor in outcomes (see, e.g., Glass et al., 1999). Further, in many studies, favorable outcomes appeared to require a sense of social efficacy and a favorable outcome expectancy as intervening variables (see Bandura, 1997; also Antonovsky, 1987, for a discussion of the meaning of activities as a component of motivation).

An Educational Intervention with Osteoporotic Patients

• *Objective*—Osteoporosis, a common chronic condition among women, results in considerable pain and the possibility of significant skeletal deformity that often produces negative emotional outcomes such as depression, hostility, stress, and reduced self-esteem. To explore effective ways to counter these negative outcomes a multidisciplinary team of clinicians in a specialty clinic at Duke Medical Center created a controlled trial of education and exercise to reduce these unwanted outcomes (Gold et al., 1993).

• *Design*—Subjects in their mid-60s, primarily women, were recruited from surrounding life care communities and offered individual evaluations by a physician; personal tutoring regarding best ways to achieve pain reduction; and group exercise regimens in structured support groups. Subjects were interviewed 6 months later and compared with controls from the same clinic.

• *Findings and Conclusion*—While the intervention had no significant effect on pain reduction, psychiatric symptoms such as depression and stress were significantly reduced as were obsessive-compulsive behavior and anxiety. In subsequent research, investigators followed up what appeared to be higher levels of anxiety about self-image resulting from deformity than clinical assessment would suggest. This anticipatory anxiety appeared to be reduced by participation in a structured group-supported exercise regime that participants described as offering an "element of hope" and a feeling of being better in control of their lives even in the absence of pain reduction. This finding is reminiscent of many intervention studies indicating that structured social support groups are a key variable in achieving beneficial effects from activity and that a sense of self-efficacy is a critical component of this effectiveness.

Exercise Interventions with Poor and Minority Populations

• *Objective*—While the intervention was initially prompted by interest in the benefits of exercise in management of diabetes in older adults, a greater interest was found in exploring how poor and minority populations can be attracted and motivated to continue in such structured activities (Clark, 1997; Clark and Nothwehr, 1999).

• *Design*—A large population of inner-city residents in a metropolitan area was invited to participate in a straightforward exposure to exercise as a component in managing diabetes. From a review of literature on successful exercise interventions, investigators concentrated on the more basic question of motivating patients to participate at all. Motivation to participate was found to be affected substantially by a sense of self-efficacy and outcome expectancy. These were the key intervening variables in achieving beneficial outcomes.

• *Findings and Conclusions*—The expectation that sense of efficacy and outcome expectance would be the key modifiable variables in whether patients made themselves available to beneficial exercise interventions was confirmed.

Further, the importance of involving local neighborhood institutions such as churches in interventions in the community was also confirmed.

Reducing Excessive Behavioral Dependency in Nursing Homes

• *Objective*—Using social-ecological theory to understand how various forms of dependency are created in later life, Margaret Baltes (1996; see also Baltes and Baltes, 1990) explored the dynamic transaction between frail older adults and those who care for them in nursing homes, primarily in Germany but also in the United States. She asked four questions: (1) Is behavioral dependency modifiable? (2) What kinds of social environments foster dependence? (3) Why do caregivers foster dependency? (4) Can dependency-creating environments be modified?

• *Design*—An important conceptual distinction was made at the outset between "learned helplessness," in which any sense of self-efficacy and favorable outcome expectancy is abandoned, and dependency as an interpersonal strategy that a nursing home resident can use to receive attention and parlay a social exchange advantageously. Seven observational studies provided evidence to document how "scripts" in different care settings typically promote dependency if not helplessness, particularly in the more individualistically oriented United States.

• *Findings and Conclusions*—Evidence answered the four questions asked. The promotion of dependency is reinforced by a stereotypic association by caregivers of dependency in later life with incompetence. Through training, frail individuals could selectively increase their capacity for self-care and institutional caregivers could be trained to change their "script" so that they could attribute competence to frail residents and promote greater autonomy of action. As in the other interventions illustrated above, Bandura's concepts of "sense of efficacy" and outcome expectancy are central. Also, dependency was found to have "many faces," including being a device for increasing the sense of social contact and control on the part of a frail resident living in an environment scripted to assume incompetence. The behavior of both residents and caregivers in institutional settings, being learned, can be modified. Baltes' emphasis on the consequences of organizational structuring of the everyday contexts of living parallels Kohn's (1995) extensive research on the behavioral effects of work environments. Varied, challenging environments, Kohn found, promote satisfaction, a sense of efficacy, and the willingness and ability to respond to subsequent environmental change. And Bandura's complementary concept of self-efficacy and its key role in a theory of social learning appear with notable frequency in literature searches for reports of beneficial psychosocial interventions across the life course. Self-efficacy is a likely product of exposure to a supportive, socially integrated environment.

ASSISTED LIVING HOUSING: A PARADIGM FOR ENHANCING BEHAVIORAL INDEPENDENCE IN LATE LIFE

Evidence has established that the debilitating behavioral dependence of a substantial minority of older adults can be countered beneficially with appropriate psychosocial interventions. Some beneficial interventions directed primarily toward individuals, small groups of older adults, or those with identified clinical conditions have been illustrated. Major federal interventions at the societal level benefiting the functioning and well-being of older adults, such as Social Security and Medicare, have been noted but only briefly because the conceptualization and implementation of such interventions are essentially complex political undertakings beyond the scope of this paper. The final section of this paper, however, discusses a timely and potentially consequential intervention that shifts from interventions primarily with individuals or small groups to an intervention focused on the structural, policy, and program enhancements of a type of organization of increasing importance to frail older adults in the United States. The particular type of organization of interest is *assisted living housing.*

Assisted living housing is of interest as a strategic intervention site in aging for both theoretical and practical reasons. Kohn (1995), in an overview of his research on the effect of work environments on personality and behavior, has documented that the complexity of work environments and opportunities for personal involvement and mastery not only tends to produce a sense of well-being but also enhances the prospects for subsequent personal initiative and the willingness to take on and master the challenges of environmental change with confidence. Further, Moos and Lemke (1994) have documented that group living environments that maximize policies emphasizing personal control and involvement of residents in group decision making tend to enhance the sense of well-being of residents and reduce their inappropriate use of facility care services. From the perspective of Bandura's theory of social cognition, care environments can be designed to maximize social support resources that, rather than encouraging behavioral dependence, produce a sense of self-efficacy and outcome expectancy of independent living among frail older adults at both the personal and the group levels. Environments designed to maximize appropriate behavioral independence are not a recommendation of rugged individualism and the denial of appropriate care but a recognition that Baltes and Baltes (1990; see also Baltes, 1996) are on strong theoretical ground in describing the process of successful aging as "selective optimization with compensation." That is, realistically, while later life is a season of increased risk of chronic conditions and functional disability, functional competence is not lost at the same rate in all areas of functioning; as the risks of disability increase, successful agers are observed to strive to do a smaller number of things but to do them well and seek environments in which compensatory help can be found in areas of decline.

Assisted living housing has emerged as a naturally occurring strategic site in which housing becomes the reasonable counterpart of a work site whose structure is consequential for the competence and well-being of its participants. And for a subset of assisted living housing facilities in the United States, an emergent philosophy is identifiable that stresses the intention to maximize the residential quality of assisted living environments and at the same time enhance the sense of self and group efficacy among residents (Kane and Wilson, 1993; Wilson, 1996). Regnier et al., (1995) noted four basic concepts of a distinctive assisted living philosophy: (1) creating a place of one's own; (2) matching services to individual need; (3) sharing responsibility among caretakers, family, and resident; and (4) providing residents with choice and control of their lives.

Good theory has converged with some practical considerations to highlight assisted living housing as a strategic site for psychosocial intervention on a relatively large scale. Historically, housing, much less housing with services, has not been considered an integral component of health and health care policy or provision in the United States. Without much enthusiasm, nursing homes may call their inhabitants residents, but they are really patients in what operates very much like a hospital. Federal housing policy until recently has forced a separation between housing and service provision in minimally regulated and supervised settings variously known as old-age, retirement, or board-and-care homes. For an aging population in this country that clearly has expressed its preference to age at home if possible, the prospect of a purpose-built facility that invites residents at an affordable price to buy housing and at the same time purchase levels of service appropriate to their assessed needs has been just what they wanted. Private-sector developers got the picture quickly, and by 1998 there were 28,000 assisted living housing facilities in the United States with provision for more than 612,000 residents, and the level of investment in this market continues to be high. Twenty-five percent of the available places for residents are in California, Florida, and Pennsylvania alone (Mollica, 1998).

The potential size of this obviously attractive market is not known. Some portion of persons currently served in nursing homes, say at least 10%, might be accommodated more appropriately and economically in assisted living facilities. The size of the community-dwelling population that is assessed as having functional disability at a level qualifying individuals as "nursing home equivalent" is at least as large, possible larger, than the 5% already in nursing homes. A population of more than 1.5 million persons could easily constitute the market for assisted living housing as an effective way to deal with chronic health problems and functional disability. For the evidence that underlies such an estimate, see the population projections, including demographic characteristics of income, disability, and living arrangements, in *Health, United States, 1999* (U.S.DHHS, 1999), and the multivariate analyses of how demographic and health characteristics of older adults relate to both institutionalization and management of disability in the community (Manton, 1988; see also Wiener et al., 1990). While special housing with services is neither a desirable nor a realistic option for all disabled older adults, it is an attractive option for many.

The research of Moos and Lemke (1994) has applied a carefully evaluated methodology (the Multiphasic Environmental Assessment Procedure [MEAP])

for characterizing the structural and resident characteristics of group living facilities and generated normative data on how these characteristics relate to outcomes. This methodology is just what is needed to ask two really important
questions about assisted living housing: (1) When a philosophy of housing is
implemented to maximize autonomy, self-efficacy, social support, and participation in decisions about community, does assisted living housing achieve
promised outcomes of quality residential care with economy? (2) Can this philosophy be implemented more widely through feasible interventions?

Bandura (1997) has extended the personal variable *self-efficacy* to suggest a
social and organizational variable *collective efficacy* in a way that is particularly
relevant for understanding the potential of assisted living housing. Individuals
can and do experience collectively in particular settings a shared sense of mission, cooperative behavior, and resilience in the face of challenge to one's
group. The empowerment or enablement implied in one's sense of self-efficacy
is not bestowed by edict but is an observed outcome based on experience that
conjoint behavior can be organized and implemented to attain group objectives.
The concept of collective efficacy has been used in a variety of community research settings to explore how a neighborhood, for example, can develop a sense
of social cohesion and unity of purpose that promotes not only networks of social support but also willingness to intervene in behalf of attaining some shared
social good (see, e.g., Sampson et al., 1997). The concept clearly has relevance
to explore how, in an assisted living setting, a sense of collective efficacy in
support of compensatory care role modeling could arise and be sustained.

A feasible intervention cannot be spelled out in detail here, but what is suggested meets the essential tests this observer learned to apply over a quarter
century of "study sectioning" to ask about proposals under review at the National Institutes of Health. Is the theory behind a proposal sound and will theory
be advanced? Is methodology available that will make what is proposed feasible? And is the proposal significant, certainly in the sense of being compatible
with the priorities of the research community and, if possible, also recognizable
within the priorities of the policy and attractive to programming persons responsible for advancing the public's health.

On all of these counts the recommended intervention would receive high
marks. The theoretical background is very strong. The experience of Moos and
Lemke has obvious applicability to assisted living housing as a tested systems
analytic strategy for identifying the structuring of organizations likely to improve the functionality, sense of well-being, and adaptability of frail older
adults. The population likely to benefit is large, as large—probably larger—than
the current nursing home population. And one final note: An intervention intended to benefit assisted living housing residents would necessarily deal with a
key issue in the implementation of information from the initiative proposed—the
intersection of public and private interests. In the best of all possible worlds in
the United States, the aging care business will discover that "good care is good
business." It is just such a discovery that is most likely to promote the public's
health in an aging society and generate a political will reinforced by private eco-

nomic incentives to promote careful study of assisted living as one promising feasible option for dealing with older adults at risk for a level of dependency requiring some level of compensatory care.

The Moos and Lemke research that lays the groundwork for the recommended intervention has included more than 300 group residences—congregate, residential, sheltered environments, and nursing homes. But regardless of the type of shelter, the MEAP strategy has proved to be applicable in characterizing (1) resident and staff; (2) physical and architectural features; (3) the basic objectives of institutional policy and programs; and (4) the social climate of the housing community.

In the initial research, structural features such as ownership, size, and level of care required were found to be important. But more important was the factor of social climate, particularly a climate in which autonomy and choice are legitimate and promoted; residents are involved in decisions about their community; and staff are committed to a climate in which privacy, choice, and resident involvement are encouraged.

Initial research has already provided the preliminary documentation that a pro-choice, pro-involvement social climate promotes well-being, better adaptation to change, and reduction of inappropriate use of facility care resources. These are all evidence of positive outcomes for frail older adults that theory would predict.

In their final chapter, Moos and Lemke themselves point to the next task: Now that we have identified the favorable outcomes deliverable in assisted living housing dedicated to enhancing a pro-choice and pro-involvement social climate, we should demonstrate how to promote such a social climate in assisted living facilities more widely. This is a challenge of one significant and promising intervention in the interest of the public's health in later life likely to enhance the functioning and well-being of a large number of frail older adults while reducing unnecessary use of care resources. Assisted living housing is not the only feasible intervention to improve the public's health in our aging society. But it is an opportunity with the possibility of significant positive effect.

REFERENCES

Antonovosky, A. (1987). *Unraveling the Mysteries of Health: How People Manage Stress and Stay Well*. San Francisco: Jossey Bass.

Baltes, M. (1996). *The Many Faces of Dependency in Old Age*. Cambridge, UK: Cambridge University Press.

Baltes, P., and Baltes, M. (1990). Psychological perspectives on successful aging: The model of selective optimization with compensation. In P. Baltes and M. Baltes (eds), *Successful Aging: Perspectives from Behavioral Sciences*. Cambridge, UK: Cambridge University Press.

Bandura, A. (1997). *Self-Efficacy: The Exercise of Control*. New York: Freeman.

Berkman, L. (1988). The changing and heterogeneous nature of aging and longevity: A social and biomedical perspective. In G. Maddox and P. Lawton (Eds.). *Varieties of*

Aging. Annual Review of Gerontology and Geriatrics, Volume 8, pp. 37–67. New York: Springer Publishing Company.

Berkman, L., and Breslow, S. (1983). *Health and Ways of Living: The Alameda County Study*. New York: Oxford University Press.

Berkman, L., and Syme, L.S. (1979). Social networks, host resistance and mortality: A nine year follow-up of Alameda County residents. *American Journal of Epidemiology, 109*, 684–694.

Campbell, A., Converse, P., and Rogers, W. (1976). *The Quality of American Life*. New York: Russell Sage Foundation.

Clark, D., (1997). Physical activity efficacy and its correlates among socioeconomically Disadvantaged older adults. *Diabetes Care, 20*(7), 1176–1182.

Clark, D., Maddox, G., and Steinhauser, K. (1993). Race, aging, and functional health. *Journal of Aging and Health, 5*(4), 536–553.

Clark, D., and Nothwehr, F. (1999). Exercise self-efficacy and its correlates among socioeconomically disadvantaged older adults. *Health Education and Behavior, 26*(4), 535–546.

Evans, R., Barer, M., and Marmor, T. (1994) *Why Are Some People Healthy and Others Not? The Detrements of Health Populations*. New York: Aldine de Gruyter.

Fries, J. (1980). Aging, natural death and the compression of morbidity. *New England Journal of Medicine, 303*, 130–36.

Fries, J. (1995). Compression of morbidity/disease postponement. In G. Maddox (Ed.), The Encyclopedia of Aging, 2nd edition, pp. 213–216. New York: Springer Publishing Company.

Glass, T., Menzes de Leon, C., and Berkman, L. (1999). Population based study of productive activities as predictors of survival among elderly Americans. *British Medical Journal, 319*, 478–482.

Gold, D., Stegmaier, K., Bales, C., et al. (1993). Psychosocial functioning and osteoporosis in late life: Results from a multidisciplinary intervention. *Journal of Women's Health, 2*(2), 149–155.

Guralnik, J., Land, K., Blazer, D., et al. (1993). Educational status and active life expectancy in older blacks and whites. *New England Journal of Medicine, 329*,110–116.

House, J., Landis, K., and Umberson, D. (1988). Social relationships and health. *Science, 241*, 540–545.

Kane, R., and Wilson, K. (1993). Assisted Living in the United States: *A New Paradigm for Residential Care for Frail Older Persons?* Washington, DC: American Association of Retired Persons.

Kohn, M. (1995). Social structure and personality through time and space. In: P. Moen, G. Elder, and K. Luscher (Eds.). *Lives in Context: Perspectives on the Ecology of Human Development*, pp. 141–169. Washington, DC: American Psychological Association.

Lonergan, E., (Ed.). (1991) *Extending Life, Enhancing Life: A National Research Agenda*. Washington, DC: Institute of Medicine, National Academy of Sciences.

Maddox, G. (1987). Aging differently. *The Gerontologist, 27*(5), 557–564.

Maddox, G., and Clark, D. (1992). Trajectories of functional impairment in later life. *Journal of Health and Social Behavior, 33*(2), 114–125.

Maddox, G., Clark, D., and Steinhauser. K. (1994). Dynamics of functional impairment in late adulthood. *Social Science and Medicine, 38*(7), 925–936.

Maddox, G., and Glass, T. (1999). Sociology of aging. In W. Hazzard et al., (Eds.). *Principles of Geriatric Medicine and Gerontology*, pp. 191– 202. New York: McGraw Hill.

Manton, K. (1988). Planning long term care for heterogeneous older populations. In G. Maddox and P. Lawton (Eds.), *Varieties of Aging. Annual Review of Gerontology and Geriatrics, Volume 8*. New York: Springer Publishing Company.

Manton, K., Corder, L., and Stollard, E. (1997). Chronic disability trends in the U.S. elderly population 1982 to 1984. *Proceedings of the National Academy of Sciences, 94*:2593–2598.

Markides, K., and Wallace, S. (1996). Health and long-term care needs of minority elderly. In J. Romeis, R. Coe, and J. Morley (Eds.). *Applying Health Services Research to Long-Term Care*. New York: Springer Publishing Company.

Marmor, T., and Okma, G. (1998). Societal intervention affecting elderly citizens: A comparative approach. In R. Schulz, G. Maddox, and P. Lawton (Eds.), Interventions Research with Older Adults. *Annual Review of Gerontology and Geriatrics, Volume 18*,pp. 321–338. New York: Springer Publishing Company.

McAuley, J., and Katula, J. (1998). Physical activity interventions in the elderly: Influence on physical health and psychological function. In R. Schulz, G. Maddox, and P. Lawton (Eds.). *Interventions Research with Older Adults. Annual Review of Gerontology and Geriatrics, Volume 18*, pp. 111–155. New York: Springer Publishing Company.

Mollica, R. (1998) *State Assisted Living Policy: 1998*. Portland, ME: National Academy of State Health Policy.

Moos, R., and Lemke, S. (1994). *Group Residences for Older Adults: Physical Features, Policies, and Social Climate*. New York: Oxford University Press.

Regnier, V., Hamilton, J., and Yatabe, S. (1995). *Assisted Living for the Aged: Innovations in Design, Management, and Financing*. New York: Columbia University Press.

Reynolds, C., et al. (1998). Behavioral and pharmacologic interventions for depression in later life. In R. Schulz, G. Maddox and P. Lawton (Eds.). *Focus on Interventions Research with Older Adults. Annual Review of Gerontology and Geriatrics, Volume 18*, pp. 48–73. New York: Springer Publishing Company.

Roberts, E., Kaplan, G. et al. (1997). Does growing old increase the risk for depression? *American Journal of Psychiatry, 154*(10), 1384–1390.

Rowe, J., and Kahn, R. (1987). *Human aging: Usual and successful. Science, 237*, 143–149.

Sampson, R., Rudenbush, S., and Earls, F. (1997). Neighborhoods and violent crime: A multilevel study of collective efficacy. *Science 27*, 918–925.

Schulz, R., Maddox, G., and Lawton, P. (1998). *Interventions Research with Older Adults. Annual Review of Gerontology and Geriatrics, Volume 18*. New York: Springer Publishing Company.

Stewart, A., et al. (1989). Functional status and well-being of patients with chronic conditions. *Journal of the American Medical Association, 262*(7), 907–913.

Townsend, P., and Davidson, N. (1982). *Inequalities in Health: The Black Report*. London: Penguin.

U.S.Department of Health and Human Services. (1999). *Health, United States, 1999: Health and Aging Chartbook*. Washington, DC: DHHS.

Verbrugge, L. (1995). Sex differences in health. In G. Maddox (Ed.), *Encyclopedia of Aging*, 2nd edition , pp. 850–854. New York: Springer Publishing Company.

Wells, K., et al. (1987). The functioning and well-being of depressed patients: Results from the MOS study. *Journal of the American Medical Association, 261*(7), 914–919.

Wiener, J., et al. (1990). Measuring the activities of daily living across national surveys. *Journal of Gerontology: Social Sciences, 45*(6), 229–237.

Wilson, K. (1996). *Assisted Living*. Washington, DC: AARP.

The Role of Mass Media in Creating Social Capital: A New Direction for Public Health

Lawrence Wallack, Dr.P.H.[1,2]

INTRODUCTION

In the summer of 1999 the East Coast was suffering through a terrible heat wave and deaths were mounting (Barstow, 1999). New York City sagged under the oppressive weight of the heat and city officials were struggling to address the crisis. The apparent cause of death for those who died was the physical effects of the heat. However, the underlying cause simply may have been fear and isolation, in part the consequence of not being connected to a broader community. One news report related the observation of emergency workers who said "an alarming number of city residents without air-conditioning keep their windows shut because they fear becoming victims of crime, and instead became

[1]Dr. Wallack is professor and director, School of Community Health, College of Urban and Public Affairs, Portland State University. This paper was prepared for the symposium "Capitalizing on Social Science and Behavioral Research to Improve the Public's Health," the Institute of Medicine and the Commission on Behavioral and Social Sciences and Education of the National Research Council, Atlanta, Georgia, February 2–3, 2000.

[2]I want to express my special gratitude to Ray Catalano, Lori Dorfman, Arthur Kellermann, Linda Nettekoven, Esther Thorson, and Katie Woodruff whose comments helped shape this work. In addition, Tony Chen, Rachel Dresbeck, Michael Antecol, and Raquel Bournhonesque provided editing, referencing, and other assistance. I also want to express my appreciation to the Institute of Medicine, Committee on Capitalizing on Social Science and Behavioral Research to Improve the Public's Health, for commissioning me to write this paper. Finally, I would like to especially acknowledge Professor S. Leonard Syme, Committee Chair. I learned much from him as his student and continue to benefit from his wisdom as his colleague.

patients" (*New York Times*, 1999, p. 1). An earlier heat wave killed more than 700 in Chicago (Semenza et al., 1996). Of course these deaths were not random occurrences; those most likely to die were isolated, disconnected, and likely to live in high homicide areas (Shen et al., 1995). A lower risk of death was associated with "anything that facilitated social contact, even membership in a social club" (Semenza et al., 1996, p. 90).

Heat waves provide a useful reference for thinking about the role of media in public health. It is a seemingly simple matter to reduce personal risk by opening a window or going out to a cooling station. Yet, people's behavior is strongly influenced by the social, economic, and political context of the larger community. Failure to account for the influence of community forces on behavioral choices will lead to narrowly focused media approaches that perilously ignore significant determinants of health.

The media matter in public health. But just how they matter is often a contentious issue. The way media matter is based on how we conceptualize the nature of public health issues and hence their solutions—and this is often controversial. If public health problems are viewed as largely rooted in personal behaviors resulting from a lack of knowledge, then media matter because they can be a delivery mechanism for getting the right information to the right people in the right way at the right time to promote personal change. If, on the other hand, public health problems are viewed as largely rooted in social inequality resulting from the way we use politics and policy to organize our society, then media matter because they can be a vehicle for increasing participation in civic and political life and social capital to promote social change. Of course, media matter in both these ways and other ways as well.

The central argument of this paper is that mass media approaches to improving the public's health need to be rethought in light of recent developments in social epidemiology, political science, sociology, and mass communication. Of particular importance is how these findings relate to social capital and population health. Traditional behavioral-oriented media campaigns, while useful, have been limited in creating significant behavior change and improvements in health status (e.g., McGuire, 1986). While there are many reasons for these modest results, this may be due in part to the failure of these campaigns to adequately integrate fundamental public health values related to social justice, participation, and social change—values made more important by the increasing research on the relationship between social inequality and health inequality.

There is an expanding science base for understanding public health as a product of social and political arrangements rather than of primarily personal behaviors. This is not to say that individual actions and personal responsibility are not important, but only to emphasize that behavior is inextricably linked to a larger social, political, and economic environment. Attempting to address public health problems without attending to the context in which they exist inevitably produces, at best, limited solutions. An important part of that context may be the range of opportunities for people to participate in the life of the community. The importance of involvement in civic life may well be a fundamental characteristic of socially and economically healthy communities (e.g., Sampson et al., 1997; Gittell and Vidal, 1998). Thus, future media approaches must focus on skill development for participation in the social change process rather than primarily on information for personal change. Civic or public journalism, media advocacy, and photovoice are particularly well suited to this task and are explored in this paper.

This paper provides a framework for understanding the role of media in advancing public health and social goals. It briefly reviews the implications of recent social epidemiological and political science research for developing mass media interventions, the limits of previous public health efforts to use mass communication strategies, and prospects for a new public health media of engagement and participation.

SOCIAL INEQUALITY AND HEALTH

There is a long history establishing the role of social status, measured in various ways, as a strong determinant of health (Haan et al., 1989a,b; Adler et al., 1993; Adler et al., 1994; Marmot and Mustard, 1994; Anderson and Armstead, 1995; Blane, 1995; Kaplan, 1995; Lantz et al., 1998). This extensive body of research indicates that social class differences exist for virtually every type of adverse health outcome and for treatable as well as nontreatable diseases. Rather than this being a rich–poor dichotomy or a factor just of poverty, the distribution of disease follows a gradient. This means that even among those in the upper quadrant of income or education levels in the society, those lower in the quadrant have poorer health. These findings are robust and appear consistent over time and across western industrialized countries. The health differences cannot be explained by traditional risk factors or access to health care. So access to health care is not the defining factor for population health status. The explanation for the social gradient is unclear. A wide range of material (physical resources) and nonmaterial (psychosocial) factors has been suggested.

More recently, this line of research has focused on the specific issue of income inequality as a property of the larger social system. This research suggests that it is not the individual's absolute level of resources that matters as much as one's position relative to everyone else (Smith and Egger, 1992; Wilkinson, 1992, 1996; Duleep, 1995; Kaplan et al., 1996; Kennedy et al., 1996; Navarro, 1997). The central concept is that up to a point the level of absolute income or resources in a society contributes to increasing health status. After that point, however, the way that the resources are distributed has the greatest impact on health: "In the developed world, it is not the richest countries which have the best health, but the most egalitarian" (Wilkinson, 1996, p. 3).

WHAT IS SOCIAL CAPITAL?

Social capital appears to be an umbrella concept that includes anything that helps to remove the barriers to collective action in communities. The general concept is certainly not foreign to the social and community emphasis of public health and is related to various concepts such as collective efficacy, psychological sense of community, neighborhood cohesion, and community competence (Lochner et al., 1999). Specifically, Gittell and Vidal (1997) define social capital as "the resources embedded in social relations among persons and organizations that facilitate cooperation and collaboration in communities" (p. 16). Social capital seems rather like a glue made from various ingredients that holds communities together and allows them to work better together to achieve common goals. It is a component of social cohesion that includes social trust and civic participation (Putnam, 1993). Coleman (1990, p. 302) explains that social capital is defined by its function—what it does rather than what it is:

> It is not a single entity, but a variety of different entities having two characteristics in common: They all consist of some aspect of a social structure, and they facilitate certain actions of individuals who are within the structure. Unlike other forms of capital, social capital inheres in the structure of relations between and among persons.

However, there are specific things that appear to be markers for higher levels of social capital. These include increased social trust, generalized norms of reciprocity, group membership, interdependence, and networks or social organizations through which the cooperation of individuals can be facilitated toward action (Coleman, 1990; Putnam, 1993, 1995a,b). In addition, there is an important prescriptive norm associated with social capital that calls on people to "forego self interests to act in the interests of the collectivity" (Coleman, 1990, p. 311). In sum, social capital is marked by norms, skills, or other individual characteristics, and structures that facilitate groups of people working toward the collective or community good. Civic engagement, when combined with social trust and facilitated by social connectedness, creates social capital (Putnam, 1995b).

Social capital, then, generates new opportunities for communities to participate in civic life. It allows groups to work together toward shared goals that create mutual benefits, and it smoothes the process because high levels of trust and connectedness help to overcome the traditional obstacles to collective action (Putnam 1993, 1995b)—social capital allows groups to achieve ends that otherwise would be beyond their capacity (Coleman, 1990). Importantly, social capital is cumulative and generalizable. It can be created for one purpose and used for other purposes. For example, a group working to increase the responsiveness of a local school board to community concerns might also be effective in mobilizing people to change the way police interact with the neighborhood.

Another important aspect of social capital is that it is not "owned" by any individual. A community with higher levels of social capital creates benefits for all of those in the community whether they helped create the social capital or not. Consider the East Coast heat wave: if communities had stronger social cohesion—marked, perhaps, by neighborhood watch groups—then individuals might be more likely to open their windows or go to a cooling station regardless of whether they participated personally in a neighborhood watch group.

Social capital, of course, can also be used for ends that many might not view as socially desirable. For example, youth gangs might be seen as reservoirs of social capital for young people in certain communities, and hate groups might flourish because of the social capital generated by the trust, norms, and dense quality of group membership. Thus, from a public health perspective, social capital should have a social justice criteria—does it contribute to a fairer, more equitable, and just society (Beauchamp, 1976)?

SOCIAL CAPITAL: A SIGNIFICANT PATHWAY

Drawing on research from political science and sociology (Coleman, 1990; Putnam, 1993, 1995a,b), public health research has now moved beyond identifying the relationship between social inequality and health inequality. It has begun to identify potential explanations for the relationship and implications for the design of public health interventions. The work of Kawachi and colleagues (Kawachi and Kennedy, 1997; Kawachi et al., 1997a,b; Kennedy et al., 1998) and others (Wilkinson, 1996; Lynch and Kaplan, 1997) is especially important in that it has identified lower levels of social capital as a pathway that may channel income inequality into increased mortality. For example, higher overall mortality and rates for most major causes of death were associated with lower measures of social capital as measured by group membership, voting levels, and social trust across 39 states in the United States (Kawachi and Berkman, 1998). Kennedy et al. (1998) reported that the depletion of social capital was strongly associated with homicide and violent crime, even when controlling for poverty and access to firearms. Also, self-reported health status, a strong indicator of actual health (Idler and Benyamini, 1997), is significantly related to the amount of social capital at the state level (Kawachi and Berkman, 1998).

There are various ways that social capital might influence population health. For example, areas with higher levels of social inequality may "systematically underinvest in human, physical, health and social infrastructure" (Lynch and Kaplan, 1997, p. 306). Also, lack of social capital might inhibit the flow of health information through populations, could make it less likely that communities band together for collective action to insure basic health and social services, and might influence psychosocial processes that increase the sense of isolation and low sense of self-efficacy of those living in less cohesive communities (Kawachi and Berkman, 1998).

Social capital appears to be an "elastic" commodity in the economic sense. That is, small increases in various components of this public good can result in significant benefits. For example, a 10% increase in the level of social trust, a marker of social capital, could result in an 8% reduction in overall mortality (Kawachi et al., 1997). Addressing a related concept, Sampson and his colleagues (1997) found that a 2-standard deviation increase in collective efficacy—a community's willingness to intervene in community life that is linked to social trust and solidarity—was associated with an almost 40% reduction in the expected homicide rate.

PUBLIC HEALTH, MASS MEDIA, AND
SOCIAL CAPITAL

The mass media are a significant part of the environment in which the pursuit of public health goals occurs. The mass media facilitate the pursuit of public health goals in some ways and obstruct it in other ways. On the one hand, large-scale, mass-mediated educational programs to inform the public about health threats have long been a staple of public health practice (Wallack, 1981). Over the years, these campaigns have become increasingly sophisticated with new standards set for the integration of research, theory, planning, and evaluation by the Stanford Heart Disease Prevention Program in the 1970s (Farquhar et al., 1984, 1990; Flora et al., 1989; Fortmann et al., 1990). Current programs involve much greater levels of resources and a strong focus on high-impact advertising. Nonetheless, current efforts, like previous efforts, have generally been limited in achieving the goals for which they were designed.

On the other hand, the public health community has long been concerned about the mass media as a source of problems. Various types of advertising and the portrayal of health-compromising behaviors and products in the media have been identified as promoting disease rather than health. The potential influence of movies, advertising media, and television programming has been considered in regard to alcohol, tobacco, and other drug use; violence; nutritional behavior; sexual behavior; traffic safety; and various other public health threats (e.g., Gerbner, 1990; Centerwall, 1992; Strasburger and Comstock, 1993; Strasburger, 1995; Singorielli and Staples, 1997; Kilbourne, 1999; Kunkel et al., 1999). Over the years, various interventions have been developed to influence the producers, directors, and writers of television series to change or include specific information on various health topics such as alcohol, tobacco, immunization, drunk driving, emergency contraception, and other topics (e.g., Breed and DeFoe, 1982; Montgomery, 1989; DeJong and Wallack, 1992; Glik et al., 1997; Langlieb, Cooper, and Gielen, 1999).

The research on social capital has significant implications for developing media strategies in public health. It expands our attention to whether the very nature of the structure and organization of the media might build or destroy social capital, might add to or detract from public health. It suggests that broader issues must be addressed—*the nature of commercialism rather than advertising about a specific product, the impact of television on social relations rather than on specific behaviors*—but public health has not raised these issues in a substantive way. The introduction of social capital as a concept that cuts across many categories of public health threats demands consideration of the broader effect of media on our social fabric rather than just on our specific behaviors.

The rugged individualism inherent in American society is one of the major barriers to collective action and a cornerstone of a market system that generates excess public health casualties (Beauchamp, 1976, 1981, 1988; Bellah et al., 1986). Technological trends will likely increase individualism and further undercut the foundation for the type of social cohesion necessary for a civil society

(Putnam, 1995a; McChesney, 1999). Hypercommercialism, the commodification and marketing of virtually everything, cuts across all media and into all aspects of everyday living. Hypercommercialism may well increase a sense of hyperindividualism and contribute to a focus on increasing personal accumulation rather than enhancing social participation. This has serious implications for social capital and creates urgency for innovative media approaches to build social capital.

There are various ways that mass media may inhibit the formation of, or reduce, the stock of social capital in the society. If the concept of social capital and civic engagement is broadened to political participation, its potential effects can expand considerably. From a public health perspective, increasing engagement in community health issues is likely to lead to increased participation in the political process. Those working to prevent alcohol problems, limit availability of handguns, prevent tobacco use, improve nutrition in schools, or prevent unsafe sexual activity quickly find themselves moving from simply working with others to confronting political institutions and interest groups on policy issues.

Undermining Social Capital: The Role of the Media

If social capital is the glue that helps communities work effectively on collective issues, then it is important that the media do not dissolve the bonding capacity of the glue. Unfortunately, television, and mass media in general, may function to reduce rather than reinforce or nurture social capital. Putnam (1995a) asserts that there has been a significant decline of social capital in the United States and attributes a substantial part of the blame to television. Both of these claims have been disputed, with Ladd (1999) arguing that social capital, far from declining, is being generated at levels beyond anything in the past, and others questioning the focus on television as a significant variable (Schudson, 1996). However, for purposes of this paper, my concern is whether social capital is related to indicators of public health and whether mass media might influence the level of civic participation from a public health perspective.

Television viewing contributes to lower levels of group membership and civic trust—two key components of social capital (Putnam, 1995a). This occurs because the time spent watching television displaces time that might be allocated to other activities related to civic life. Further, increased television viewing may lead to higher levels of pessimism and cynicism about the world.

George Gerbner and his colleagues (1994a) have argued that television cultivates a very distorted perception of the world in heavier viewers. For example, these heavy viewers score low on social trust and are less accepting of norms of reciprocity. When compared with lighter viewers, heavier viewers are more likely to believe that most people "cannot be trusted" and are "just looking out for themselves" (p. 30). Further, compared with lighter viewers, they are more likely to overestimate their chances of being victimized by crime or violence, believe that their neighborhood is unsafe, and assume crime is rising regardless of the actual facts. Television "facts" become the basis for making judgments about the real world. Not surprisingly, heavier viewers are more likely to express "gloom and alienation. . . . [and] express a heightened sense of living in a mean world of danger, mistrust, and alienation" (Gerbner et al., 1994b, p.9). So, not only do people have less time to participate in civic activities, but their level of fear, mistrust, and alienation would hardly make such participation inviting.

Another issue raised by Putnam is that of the passivity-inducing role of television. Indeed, Postman (1985) argues that television, and the media in general, provide an information glut that trivializes public discourse, distracts people from substantive issues, and renders the population passive. The issue of passivity draws us to the broader issue of the structure and function of the mass media. Writing before the diffusion of television, Lazarsfeld and Merton (1948) worried that the mass media inhibited social change and suggested that they might contribute to a population that was "politically apathetic and inert" (p. 501). Similar to Postman who followed, they were concerned that the flood of information from a mass media motivated primarily by profit rather than public interest would "narcotize rather than energize the average reader or listener" (p. 502). Schiller (1973) picks up this theme and argues that it is, in fact, the aim of the mass media to lessen rather than raise concern about social issues.

The primary source of news for people is local television, though newspaper reading is more strongly associated with voting (Stempel and Hargrove, 1996). Journalism, in general, has been severely criticized for its contribution to the trivialization of public discourse and the alienation of the public from the political process (e.g., Fallows, 1997; McChesney, 1999). Part of the reason for this is the way that the news fragments issues and thus obscures the connections among them (Schiller, 1973). Iyengar (1991) argues that television news overwhelmingly frames social issues episodically in concrete, individual, personal stories that communicate personal responsibility rather than social accountability. The result is that viewers are more likely to "blame the victim" for the cause and solution of the problem rather than hold public officials or institutions accountable. He explains, "Because television news generally fails to activate (and may indeed depress) societal attributions of responsibility, . . . it tends to obscure the connections between social problems and the actions or inactions of political leaders. By attenuating these connections, episodic framing impedes electoral accountability" (Iyengar, 1991, pp. 141–142).

Most recently, McChesney (1997, 1999) has argued that the very nature of the media system in the United States "undermines all three of the meaningful criteria for self-government" (1997, p. 7). These criteria are lack of significant disparities in wealth, a sense of community and acceptance of the idea that one's well-being is linked to the larger well-being, and an effective system of political communication that engages citizens. He argues that the mass media through corporate concentration, conglomeration, and hypercommercialism create a depoliticized, passive citizenry who are largely cynical and apathetic.

In sum, the mass media may adversely affect the development or maintenance of social capital in the United States. A fundamental question is whether the media relate to people as consumers or citizens (Burns, 1989). If they are valued only as demographics that are more or less likely to consume various types of products, then media will offer little to efforts to build social capital. If, on the other hand, the media relate to people as citizens who are valued for their potential participation, then media may well offer much support for building social capital. An equally important issue is how people relate to the media.

Public Health Mass Media Campaigns: Building Human Capital

If you ask a group of public health practitioners whether improvements in health status will come about *primarily* as a result of people getting more information about their personal health habits or of people getting more power to change the social and environmental conditions in which they live, they will inevitably voice the latter belief. Because many people enter the public health profession motivated by the opportunity for contributing to social change, and because practitioners are closely connected to people with the problems, they either bring or quickly develop an understanding of social causation of disease. However, when asked where most of their work effort is focused, they explain that they spend most of their time trying to change personal health behaviors, not social factors.[3] The practice of public health, and certainly conventional health education, has, to a great extent, been the practice of building human capital—providing people with the tools for good health, in this case health information.

James Coleman (1990) distinguishes between human and social capital, a distinction that is fundamental to understanding the role of public health media campaigns to improve health. He explains, ". . . [H]uman capital is created by changing persons so as to give them skills and capabilities that make them able to act in new ways. Social capital, in turn, is created when the relations among persons change in ways that facilitate action" (p. 304). The history of media campaigns shows that they try to increase human capital, not promote collective action. These campaigns provide individuals with knowledge about risks such as alcohol, tobacco, sedentary life-styles, diet, unsafe sex, and the like in the hope that they will change the way they act. Sometimes such campaigns might attempt to link people, such as the recent $2 billion antidrug campaign that tries to get parents to talk to their children about drugs, but for the most part they simply provide people with health information (DeJong and Wallack, 1999). *These campaigns are governed by the idea that people need more and better personal information to navigate a hazardous health environment rather than that people need skills to better participate in the public policy process to make the environment less hazardous.*

---

[3]I have asked this question at many professional meetings over the years and the response is very consistent. Usually, at least 90% of the audience believes that social conditions are the major determinants of health but less that 10% ever say their work focuses on the social-structural aspects of public health.

Mass-mediated health communication efforts generally flow from a pragmatic logic that assumes an information gap in individuals—if people just knew and understood that certain behaviors were bad for them and others good, then these people would change to the behaviors that benefited their health. Filling the information gap becomes the purpose of the campaign; if enough people changed their behavior, then this would lead to a healthier society. The problem is operationally defined as people just not knowing any better. The goal, then, is to warn and inform people so they can change. In order to make this happen, campaigns focus on developing the right message to deliver to the largest number of people through the mass media. Finding the right message is central to the campaign and extremely important. The message, however, is always about personal change rather than social change or collective action.

Better health communication campaigns are characterized by at least three important factors. First, these campaigns are more likely to use mass communication and behavior change theory as a basis for campaign design. This means using a variety of mass communication channels, making sure the audience is exposed to the message, and providing a clear and specific action for the individual to take. Second, they are more likely to use formative research such as focus groups in order to develop messages and inform campaign strategy. Many better-designed interventions also include various social marketing strategies such as market segmentation, channel analysis, and message pretesting (Lefebvre and Flora, 1988). Third, they are more likely to link media strategies with community programs, thus reinforcing the media message and providing local support for desired behavior changes (Wallack and DeJong, 1995).

While there are many ways that a well-designed campaign can increase the potential for success, meaningful success itself has been elusive. In a comprehensive review of communication campaigns Rogers and Storey (1987) noted, "The literature of campaign research is filled with failures, along with qualified successes—evidence that campaigns *can* be effective under certain conditions" (italics in original, p. 817). This review, more optimistic than some and slightly more pessimistic than others, generally echoed previous reviews (Wallack, 1981, 1984; Alcalay, 1983; Atkin, 1983; McGuire, 1986) and anticipated later reviews (Salmon, 1989; Brown and Walsh-Childers, 1994; Wallack and DeJong, 1995; DeJong and Winsten, 1998).

Overreliance on public education campaigns constitutes a barrier to the accomplishment of public health goals. First, such an emphasis conflicts with the social justice ethic of public health, which calls for a fair sharing of the burden for prevention (Beauchamp, 1976). At worst, such campaigns may contribute to the problem they seek to address. This happens when the narrow behavioral focus of the campaign deflects our attention away from social and structural determinants of health by focusing exclusively on the behavior of individuals—in effect blaming the victim for the problem and placing the sole burden for change on him or her (Ryan, 1976; Wallack, 1989, 1990; Dorfman and Wallack, 1993).

Second, participation in civic life is generally not advanced by most of these campaigns since they tend to focus on personal behaviors that individuals can take on their own behalf in order to improve their health. Public policy or social action is seldom, if ever, a focus of public health media campaigns because these campaigns are usually supported with public money that makes advocacy for specific policies problematic. Also, many media outlets will not accept public service announcements or even paid advertisements that are considered controversial—and policy issues that inevitably confront corporate interests are inherently controversial.

Third, such actions may be necessary or desirable but do not appear to be sufficient for improving the health of populations. Lomas (1998) argues that individual risk factor modification, an approach at the core of most mass media campaigns, has been "spectacularly unsuccessful" (p. 1183).

Finally, it is not possible to define a problem at the community or societal level and then focus primarily on solutions at the personal or individual level. There are many definitions of public health but one clear thread running through these is the fundamental idea that the primary focus must be on the health and well-being of communities or populations, not individuals (Rose, 1985, 1992; Mann, 1997). It does not follow then that applying primarily individual-level solutions can effectively address public health problems.

MEDIA STRATEGIES THAT BUILD
SOCIAL CAPITAL

The Institute of Medicine suggests a broad vision of the mission of public health, explaining that it requires creating the conditions in which people can be healthy. It goes on to say, "Clearly, public health is 'public' because it involves organized community effort" (Institute of Medicine, 1988, p. 39). Social capital is a fundamental fuel for generating the kind of collective action that is required for public health to adequately pursues its mission. The crucial issue, then, is what kinds of media approaches can increase the capacity of groups, and broader communities, to act on matters related to public health that potentially benefit the entire society.

Developing media strategies to build social capital has two significant public health implications. First, in general, by increasing the level of social capital in the community, there may be benefits to the public's health in the form of lower overall mortality rates. Second, by increasing the level of social capital, groups may become more effective in advancing policies that may help to build a more egalitarian society and protect health (e.g., early childhood education). In addition, the skills and social structures associated with social capital can be put to use for other issues that might appear less central to health but nonetheless are still central to strong communities.

There are at least three promising media approaches that have the potential to build social capital and thus contribute to public health. These approaches are civic or public journalism, media advocacy, and photovoice.

Civic Journalism

Public health and journalism at their best hold an important value in common: attention to and concern for the well-being of the public. The former seeks to create the conditions in which people can be healthy (Institute of Medicine, 1988), and the latter seeks to create the conditions in which people can be good citizens (Merritt, 1995). It is now clear that these "conditions" are inextricably linked through the concept of social capital.

In the late 1980s and early 1990s, journalism was in crisis. There was great concern about the loss of public civility and the decline of public life. The 1988 presidential campaign had the lowest voter turnout since 1924 and journalism was being blamed for citizen apathy and cynicism. In 1994, a Times Mirror Poll reported that 71% of national respondents agreed that "the news media gets in the way of society solving its problems" (Merritt, 1995). The public was alienated from the political process; there was a sense that public life, politics, and journalism all seemed to be caught in a downward spiral (Clark, 1993; Merritt, 1995; Fallows, 1997).

Journalism in general, and newspapers in particular, began a process of soul searching about whether they might do a better job in serving the democratic process. What evolved in the early 1990s was the controversial concept of public journalism (Rosen, 1991, 1993; Merritt, 1995), and soon the term "civic journalism" was being used interchangeably (Rosen, 1994).[4] It was not long before interesting collaborations among local newspapers, television stations, and radio stations were developing around the country.

Civic journalism projects seek to engage the community in the process of civic life by providing information and other forms of support to increase community debate and public participation in problem solving. Jay Rosen, an academic, and Davis Merritt, a long-time print journalist, are among the best-known architects of civic journalism. They argue that civic journalism represents a fundamental shift in thinking by the journalist. This shift requires the journalist to be attached to community life rather than maintain the traditional pose of detachment (Rosen, 1994). They argue that journalists have a greater responsibility than just reporting the news. They have a responsibility to help the community work better. The purpose of civic journalism is to create a process by which citi-

---

[4]The concept is controversial because many journalists feel it changes the traditional role of the journalist from reporting the news to participating in the news. Some were concerned that it was simply a marketing tool to stem the decline in readership. Others felt it trampled on the core journalistic value of objectivity by associating journalists with various solutions to community problems. Still others felt that it gave away the power and responsibility of journalists to community people who lacked any special training or insight, particularly as it related to covering political campaigns. Many simply dismissed the more innovative examples of civic or public journalism as good journalism that they were already doing or that they would do if sufficient resources were available. See Black (1997) for an extensive review of this debate.

zens can participate in the life of the community through public discussion, deliberation, collective problem solving, and ongoing involvement. By the end of the century, there were approximately 300 civic journalism projects in cities of varying sizes around the country (Friedland et al., 1998). These projects have addressed a diverse set of issues, including race relations, crime and violence, juvenile delinquency, alcohol, land use planning, domestic violence, economic development, community leadership, and voting participation.

Civic journalism projects are themselves quite diverse, employing a wide range of approaches. Generally, these projects are initiated by newspapers and involve television and radio stations as partners. They generally are based on three broad activities undertaken by civic journalists:

1. There is an extensive information development and data-gathering process. This can take the form of in-depth coverage of an issue where teams of reporters rather than just one or two are put on the story. In addition, in an effort to develop more insight into the community, special polls, focus groups, interviews, and other techniques are used (Wiley, 1998). Reports for various neighborhoods might be produced based on polling data, follow-up interviews by journalists with poll respondents, dialogues at town meetings, and detailed analysis of crime data.

2. There is far more extensive news coverage of the issue than is commonly seen, and the coverage is coordinated with other media outlets. This serves to increase the visibility, legitimacy, and urgency of the issue and set the public and policy agenda.

3. There are structures developed to insure that information and community concern are translated into action. Substantial efforts are often made to insure community participation and are facilitated through various means. In some cases a person is hired by the newspaper to coordinate the process. The Poverty Among Us project in St. Paul, Minnesota, provided money for child care and translators to remove barriers to participation in community discussions.

Civic journalism is still at an early stage, and the evaluation of projects is moving from case studies to more sophisticated survey research and statistical modeling analyses. Case studies provide an impressionistic view of problems, processes, challenges, and successes. For the most part the news is encouraging (Pew Center for Civic Journalism, 1997; Ford, 1998). High levels of media coverage of significant *local* problems are being generated, and participation in the projects seems extensive. In Charlotte, the *Observer* ran a front-page story on crime and violence that was augmented with four inside pages. The following month, the *Observer* provided almost seven pages to exploring life in the community. A local television station and two radio stations followed up with roundtables and call-in shows focused on solutions to the crime and violence problem (Taking Back Our Neighborhoods, 1995). Subsequently, more than 700 groups and individuals volunteered to work on various community needs. The city responded by razing dilapidated buildings, clearing overgrown lots, and opening parks and recreation facilities. Local law firms got involved by providing pro bono services to close crack houses.

In Peoria, Illinois ("Leadership Challenge"), several hundred people met to develop a citywide action plan. New leaders emerged and the shape of city government changed when a person who had been influenced by the project ran for mayor and won. In Springfield, Missouri, the *News-Leader's* "Good Community" program focused on juvenile crime. One event attracted 700 people who pledged 13,000 hours to community service. After three years the project is continuing and "crime is down in Springfield and public involvement is up" (Ford, 1998, p. 15).

In Binghamton, New York, the *Press and Sun Bulletin* ("Facing Our Future") convened a town meeting and devised 10 action teams on topics important for economic development. In addition to hiring a former city official to find discussion leaders for the teams, the newspaper provided special group process training for the team leaders. More than 100 meetings were held and more than 300 people participated in the team meetings. The media partners in the project covered recommendations of the teams. In this particular project, "Facing Our Future" continued on to become "Building Our Future" (Ford, 1998). More rigorous evidence is now available to support these anecdotal claims of effectiveness.

The most extensive evaluations of civic journalism have examined five projects in four cites. The first project, "Taking Back Our Neighborhoods," addressed crime and violence in parts of Charlotte, North Carolina. The second and third projects, "We the People," focused on land use issues and juvenile delinquency in Madison, Wisconsin. The fourth project, "Voice of the Voter," tried to increase the vote among low-turnout groups in a mayoral election in San Francisco, California, and the final project, "Facing Our Future," in Binghamton, New York, sought to stimulate citizen involvement in finding solutions to economic decline.

A series of evaluation studies provides encouraging findings on the effects of the civic journalism efforts (Chaffee et al., 1997; Ognianova et al., 1997; Thorson et al., 1997; Denton and Thorson, 1998). In general, the survey evaluations focused on outcomes as well as theoretical pathways and found promising results for the hypothesis that the news media can enhance the democratic process by increasing involvement (Denton and Thorson, 1998). It was fairly clear that interest in and discussion of civic issues could be attributed to the civic journalism projects (Madison). More importantly, the projects were associated with increased participation in neighborhood problem solving (Charlotte, Madison, San Francisco) and increased voting in groups with usually low turnout (San Francisco) (Chaffee et al., 1997). Chaffee and his colleagues were encouraged by their findings and concluded that "[civic journalism] programs appear from our evidence to be effective" (p. 26).

While finding evidence of success, Chaffee and his colleagues were concerned that selective exposure might explain their findings. This would mean that people already interested in the issues and perhaps predisposed to civic participation sought the programs rather than being stimulated by the programs. In a related study that also included the Binghamton site, Ognianova and her colleagues (1997) tested whether the civic journalism project leads to increased concern about issues and civic involvement (media stimulation of involvement) or whether existing involvement leads people to be aware of the civic journalism project (selective exposure). Their conclusion was that awareness of the project led to concern, knowledge, and subsequent involvement: "Analyses of the two alternative models with data from four different cities in the United States showed clear and consistent support for the media stimulation model" (Ognianova et al., 1997, p. 21). Other work on all four cities (Thorson et al., 1997) explored the potential of a two-step model of civic journalism where awareness of projects helps to shift attitudes and leads to subsequent increases in civic involvement. This research concluded that indeed civic journalism was an effective means for reconnecting citizens to public life.

Media Advocacy

Media advocacy is the strategic use of mass media in combination with community organizing to advance healthy public policies. The primary focus is on the role of news media, with secondary attention to the use of paid advertising (USDHHS, 1988; Wallack and Sciandra, 1990–1991; Wallack, et al., 1993, 1999; Wallack, 1994; Wallack and Dorfman, 1996; Winett and Wallack, 1996). Media advocacy seeks to raise the volume of voices for social change and shape the sound so that it resonates with the social justice values that are the presumed basis of public health (Beauchamp, 1976; Mann, 1997). It has been used by a wide range of grass roots community groups, public health leadership groups, public health and social advocates, and public health researchers (Wallack et al., 1993, 1999).

The practical origins of media advocacy can be traced to the late 1980s. It grew from a collaboration of public health groups working on tobacco and alcohol issues with public interest and consumer groups also working on these or similar issues. The public interest and consumer groups brought a new array of strategies and tactics that were more familiar to a political campaign than a public health effort. The public health people provided a clearer understanding of the substantive scientific issues and the importance of theory in creating change. The result has been an approach that blends science, politics, and advocacy to advance public health goals.

From a theoretical perspective, media advocacy borrows from mass communication, political science, sociology, and political psychology to develop strategy. Central to media advocacy are the concepts of agenda setting (McCombs and Shaw, 1972; Deering and Rogers, 1997) and framing (Gamson, 1989; Iyengar, 1991; Ryan, 1991). From a practical perspective, media advocacy borrows from community organizing, key elements of formative research (i.e., focus groups and polling), and political campaign strategy (e.g., application of selective pressure on key groups or individuals) (Wallack et al., 1993). Blending theory with practice provides an overall framework for advocacy and social change.

Media advocacy differs in many ways from traditional public health campaigns. It is most marked by an *emphasis* on:

- linking public health and social problems to inequities in social arrangements rather than to flaws in the individual;
- changing public policy rather than personal health behavior;
- focusing primarily on reaching opinion leaders and policy makers rather than on those who have the problem (the traditional audience of public health communication campaigns);
- working with groups to increase participation and amplify their voices rather than providing health behavior change messages; and
- having a primary goal of reducing the power gap rather than just filling the information gap.

Media advocacy is generally seen as a part of a broader strategy rather than as a strategy per se. One of the fundamental rules of media advocacy is that it is not possible to have a media strategy without an overall strategy. Media advocacy is part of the overall plan, but is not the plan, for achieving policy change. For example, a group in Oakland, California, effectively used media advocacy to advance a city ordinance to place a tax on liquor stores and institute a moratorium on new licenses in the city (Seevak, 1997). The effort took 4 years to implement, starting at the local zoning commission and ending up in the California State Supreme Court. Over that period, the group used media advocacy to provide legitimacy to the issue, to increase the credibility of its position and add urgency to the problem, and to let politicians know that the community was very involved in the issue and would be following all votes. To achieve this, the group used a variety of tactics to generate news coverage and discussion on the editorial pages. This increased the effectiveness of the grass roots coalition advancing the policy but would have made little difference if the coalition did not have strong community support (resulting in large turnouts at key meetings and hearings, and visits and calls to politicians), a clear and reasonable policy, and research to back up its claims. The group might have failed, lacking any one of the ingredients for change: a reasonable policy goal that could make a difference, an issue that the community supported and was willing to work for, and a media strategy to advance the policy and support community organizing.

Media advocacy focuses on four primary activities in support of community organizing, policy development, and advancing policy:

1. Overall Strategy Development: Media advocacy uses critical thinking to understand and respond to problems as social issues rather than personal problems. Following problem definition, the focus is on elaborating policy options; identifying the person, group, or organization that has the power to create the

necessary change; and identifying organizations that can apply pressure to advance the policy and create change (for example, in the Oakland illustration above, various elements of the community were organized to apply pressure on the zoning commission, mayor's office, city council, and state legislature, which were all targets at various points in the campaign). Finally, various messages for the different targets of the campaign are developed.

2. Setting the Agenda: Getting an issue in the media can help set the agenda and provide legitimacy and credibility to the issue and group. Media advocacy involves understanding how journalism works in order to increase access to the news media. This includes maintaining a media list, monitoring the news media, understanding the elements of newsworthiness, pitching stories, holding news events, and developing editorial page strategies for reaching key opinion leaders.

3. Shaping the Debate: The news media generally focus on the plight of the victim, while policy advocates emphasize social conditions that create victims. Media advocates frame policy issues using public health values that resonate with broad audiences. Some of the steps include "translat[ing] personal problems into public issues" (Mills, 1959); emphasizing social accountability as well as personal responsibility; identifying individuals and organizations who must assume a greater burden for addressing the problem; presenting a clear and concise policy solution; and packaging the story by combining key elements such as visuals, expert voices, authentic voices (those with experience of the problem), media bites, social math (creating a context for large numbers that is interesting to the press and understandable to the public), research summaries, fact sheets, policy papers, and so forth.

4. Advancing the Policy: Policy battles are often long and contentious, and it is important to make effective use of the media to keep the issue on the media agenda. The Oakland effort took 4 years and now must focus media attention to ensure that the policy is implemented properly. Thus, it is important to develop strategies to maintain the media spotlight on the policy issue on a continuing basis. This means identifying opportunities to reintroduce the issue to the media, such as key anniversaries of relevant dates, publication of new reports, significant meetings or hearings, and linking the policy solution to breaking news.

Media advocacy has been applied to a number of public health and social issues including affirmative action, child care, alcohol, tobacco, childhood lead poisoning, health promotion, violence, handgun control, and suicide prevention, as well as others. To date, most evaluations of media advocacy have been case studies (Wallack et al., 1993, 1999; DeJong, 1996; Jernigan and Wright, 1996; Wallack and Dorfman, 1996; Woodruff, 1996). These case studies have shown that community groups trained in media advocacy can effectively gain access to the news media and enhance their participation in the process of public policy making. In California, for example, media advocacy training, follow-up, and support were provided to hundreds of community activists, researchers, service providers, and others working on violence prevention. These skills were used in the process of passing substantial numbers of local ordinances limiting the availability of firearms and ultimately passing statewide legislation banning the manufacture and sale of Saturday night specials or junk guns (Wallack, 1997, 1999). Nonetheless, media advocacy can be controversial, and there are risks to the organizations that use it as part of their strategy (DeJong, 1996).

In a more systematic evaluation of the role of media advocacy in a controlled study designed to advance community policies to reduce drinking and driving, Holder and Treno (1997) concluded that media advocacy was effective in several areas and "an important tool for community prevention" (p. S198). For example, local people trained in media advocacy were able to increase local news coverage in television and newspapers and presumably frame it around policy issues. They suggest that results of the media advocacy component of the intervention "can focus public and leader attention on specific issues and approaches to local policies of relevance to reducing alcohol-involved injuries" (p. S198). Another evaluation looked at the effects of media advocacy in the Stanford Five City Heart Disease Prevention Project (Schooler et al., 1996). Dependent variables included coverage of the issue, prominence of the article, framing of the article (e.g., prevention versus treatment), and impact on the media agenda (i.e., ratio of locally generated articles on heart disease to those on other health issues). The study concluded that "media advocacy efforts can be successful" (p. 361) but found that maintenance of the effects was weak. In both of these evaluation studies (particularly Schooler et al., 1996) it was unclear whether there was a focus on advancing public policies or whether, like many media efforts, the focus was more related to increasing awareness. Also, it was unclear whether a comprehensive media advocacy approach was implemented as was found in the case studies on limiting alcohol outlets in Oakland or banning junk guns in California.

Photovoice

Photovoice, a relatively new concept, is the use of photography for social change by marginalized and traditionally powerless groups. It has deep roots in documentary photography, feminist theory, empowerment theory, and participatory research (Wang and Burris, 1994, 1997; Wang et al., 1996a, 1996b, 1998, 1999; Wang and Pies, 1999). Photovoice is "designed to enable people to create and discuss photographs as a means of catalyzing personal and community change" (Wang et al., 1999, p. 4). Much health education and health promotion have at their core a great passion for community participation and social change (e.g., Minkler, 1997), and photovoice is a media approach designed to increase the likelihood of this occurring by "engaging the community to act on its own behalf" (Wang and Burris, 1994, p. 182).

Photovoice focuses on grass roots involvement and attempts to increase the participation of marginalized groups in the policy process. Various projects have been implemented with women in rural China (Wang and Burris, 1994; Wang, et al., 1996a,b, 1998; Wang and Burris, 1997), homeless men and women in

Ann Arbor, Michigan (Wang et al., 1999), and people recruited from public health and social service sites in Contra Costa County, California (Wang and Pies, 1999). The goals of these projects are quite similar and clearly reflect the theory and values of the approach:

1. To understand local issues and concerns through the perspective of specific groups of people. This means seeing health, work, and community issues through the eyes of the participants and those most affected by the problems rather than just the usual experts.

2. To promote knowledge and critical discussion about significant community issues. This involves group discussion among participants regarding their photographs.

3. To reach policy makers and others who can be mobilized to create change. This means finding ways to translate and make visible the "data" in the photographs so that others can be enlisted in the social change process.

The photovoice process has been documented in a series of articles by Wang and her colleagues. Once a project is defined, a target audience of policy makers or community leaders is identified and participates in the planning process. Its primary role is to serve as a group with the political will to put participants' ideas and recommendations into practice (Wang et al., 1999). At the same time, facilitators are trained. This involves grounding in the process of photovoice, including ethical issues such as privacy and power, which might arise in the process of taking pictures. Technical knowledge about cameras and photography is provided as are basic group process skills for leading discussion.

Trainers or facilitators then recruit participants through a variety of means depending on the project. (For example, in the "Language of Light," homeless project participants were recruited through shelters and provided with cameras and small stipends.) Participants, in turn, attend a series of workshops to learn about the methods of photovoice, the technical aspects of using and caring for a camera, and the safety and privacy issues that might arise from using a camera in public or social service settings. After the first workshop, the meetings are used for group discussion and feedback on the pictures. Participants who wish to write about their photographs may follow a series of "root-cause questions" similar to those used in discussion.

In the final stage of the project, facilitators and participants select pictures to share with journalists and policy makers in order to move the documentation process to the action process. Each of the projects achieved some success in reaching broader audiences and policy makers. In China, project facilitators organized a slide show that attracted some of the most powerful policy makers in the province. Three policy decisions regarding day care for toddlers, training programs for midwives, and educational scholarships for girls were enacted as a result of facilitators' and participants' advocacy using the photovoice process. The participating Chinese village women highlighted each of these issues through their photographs and stories (Wang et al., 1996a).

In Ann Arbor, the "Language of Light" project provided pictures and captions for a series of articles in local newspapers, a gallery exhibition, and a major public forum. These activities communicated concerns of the homeless to a broader population and also put a human face on the issue. The public forum was attended by several hundred people and allowed the project to provide input to policy makers on a proposal to build a new homeless shelter that would have resulted in major disadvantages to the homeless population (Wang et al., 1999).

The "Picture This" project in Contra Costa County held exhibitions of its pictures at the County Office of Maternal and Child Health and the state capitol during a statewide meeting. In addition, more than a full page in the local newspaper was provided to show pictures and report on the project. Several stories of change came out of the project, including one resulting from a picture of a closed hospital with a caption complaining about inadequate health services for low-income people: "The picture and other complaints prompted the county to improve care at its Pittsburgh [California] clinic" (Spears, 1999).

Photovoice, though a new concept that has not been subject to rigorous evaluation, appears to have promise for increasing community involvement. The use of pictures in addition to words may well increase the power of local groups to effectively press their case for social change. Perhaps most important is that this approach may be a particularly useful tool for those who find the usual means of participation in community discussion to be a foreign and unfriendly process that seems to uphold the views of those who already make the decisions.

A NOTE ON THE INTERNET

The Internet promises to provide people with unprecedented access to information about the kinds of factors that affect their health and affords health educators the opportunity to use this medium to design interventions to change health behavior (e.g., Cassell et al., 1998). An estimated 33.5 million adults seek out medical information on the Internet (Davis and Miller, 1999), and many others use the Internet to find social support (Bly, 1999) Also, Cart (1997) has discussed the potential of the Internet for local communities to organize, gain immediate access to critical facts, and increase their power as citizens to effectively participate in policy debates. She also suggests that on-line networks "[have] the potential to bring back 'communities that disappeared with front porches' " (Cart, 1997, p. 328).

The Internet has the potential to supplement and possibly increase the value of any media approach used. Mass media campaigns that can direct people to the Internet for more detailed and personalized information, as well as social support, will no doubt increase their potential to help people. Civic journalism projects that use the Internet will make it easier for people to participate in a more informed way. For the media advocate, the Internet allows fast and easy access to policy information that was simply unavailable in the past as well as specialized information and strategic help from colleagues on the other side of the world as easily as from those down the street. This will help increase the potential contribution of media advocacy and other activist approaches because it will build social capital by providing one of the basic elements for effective collective action—easy, fast, and direct communication.

McChesney (1999), however, raises an important question about the Internet: "In fact, cannot the ability of people to create their own 'community' in cyberspace have the effect of terminating a community in the general sense?" (p. 146). Just as the Internet will speed many desirable aspects of our society along, so will it likely accelerate the path to hyperindividualism and hypercommercialism that McChesney warns about. From a social capital perspective this would not be a welcome direction because of the potential adverse effects of the corporate dominance of media technologies on citizen activism (McChesney, 1997, 1999).

Another important Internet issue is the amount and quality of information. While more people have access to unprecedented amounts of information, the quality of such information is uneven. Those seeking cancer information, for example, could easily end up in sites that might offer information that was potentially damaging to one's health. The flood of health and medical advice without some added ability to critically assess accuracy could have significant unintended consequences for consumers of health information.

Finally, access to the Internet is very much influenced by economic status. Efforts to promote universal access have largely faltered, raising the possibility of the information "haves" and "have nots" and further increasing the effects of income inequality.

DISCUSSION

Recent research points to the urgency of rethinking the role of mass media to advance the public's health. Research strongly suggests that media approaches should focus on increasing the reservoir of social capital by engaging people and increasing their involvement and participation in community life. This, per se, may have a positive generalized effect on the population's health. In addition, because public health seeks to "create the conditions in which people can be healthy" (Institute of Medicine, 1988), mass media strategies should also provide citizens with the skills to better participate in the policy process to create these conditions. Furthermore, it is crucial that social capital be seen not as a substitute for the kinds of policies that are important to reduce social inequality but as a foundation that makes policy change possible. Social capital then is a prerequisite for policy change and a consequence of the process of generating that change (Putnam, 1993).

In the new century, sophisticated versions of the classic mass-mediated public health campaigns will play a role in increasing awareness, providing knowledge, and shifting attitudes. However, these campaigns have not had a significant impact on the health of populations and should be a relatively small part of a comprehensive strategy. Public health should not be seduced by a primarily information-based approach that focuses on the individual and ignores more potentially effective, but controversial, approaches emphasizing policy or political participation.

Civic journalism, media advocacy, and photovoice have been presented as promising approaches, but this is not the same as suggesting that these are successful approaches. Early evaluations are indeed promising, but more important is the set of values underlying these approaches. The goal of these approaches is to engage people in the process of improving their communities through deliberation about problems, discussions about solutions, and participation in the processes that lead to social or political change. They seek to give people a voice rather than leave them with a message, and they point people to solutions that benefit the entire community, not just the individual. Their goal is nothing short of making democracy work better and by doing so affecting the public's health on the most global level.

As a society, we exalt the person that can "beat the odds" and succeed against adversity (Schorr, 1988). This "triumphant individual" story is, in fact, one of the dominant parables that guide political thought, rhetoric, and policy development in our society (Reich, 1988). Public health is a profession that should work to reduce the odds so that more people can succeed, not a profession that simply provides information, services, and encouragement to people so they might be among the few lucky ones to beat the odds (Beauchamp, 1981).

In considering media approaches we must select the kinds of strategies that have the long-range potential to change the odds. The income gap between the rich and the poor has more than doubled in the past 20 years. Currently, 20% of the population earns more than one-half of all the income in America. The 20% with the lowest income earns only 4.2% of all the income (Johnston, 1999). This inequality gap is bad for society overall, not just those on the bottom rungs, and the public health body count will be one tragic indicator of this. Building social capital is not a panacea, but it can make an important contribution to changing the odds.

Developing media approaches that can enhance social capital and level the playing field is important for the future of public health. There are a number of questions that must be addressed in considering the selection of media strategies:

1. Does the approach increase the capacity of individuals or small groups to participate in collective action by

- providing participatory skills, and
- creating a structure or network through which individuals, groups, and organizations can act?

2. Does the approach connect the problems or issues to broader social forces?

3. Does the approach increase the community's capacity to collaborate and cooperate by strengthening existing groups (create bonding capital) and connecting various groups (create bridging capital)?

4. Does the approach reflect a social justice orientation—the idea that "each member of the community owes something to all the rest, and the community owes something to each of its members" (Etzioni, 1993, p. 263)?

The greater the degree to which a media approach can respond affirmatively to these questions, the more likely it is to build social capital. The public health profession should support such approaches even though in some cases the link to public health might seem tenuous.

The research on the effects of these approaches on public health outcomes is limited, and more comprehensive and systematic evaluations are necessary. One of the problems in determining effects is that these approaches must be seen as supporting and advancing larger interventions for policy change. Civic journalism, media advocacy, and photovoice are likely means to increase social capital and enhance the capacity of communities to act. This should, if the social epidemiological research is on the right track, lead to improved health across a number of areas. Isolating and linking the contribution of specific media approaches to this kind of social and policy change will be very difficult. Nonetheless, increased participation at the local school board may well result in less activity at the local hospital.

Public health is, at its core, a political process, and one of our best strategies is to use the democratic process to advance public health goals and objectives. Social and political participation is important, and it is necessary that we develop media strategies that foster community participation rather than just inform personal behavior. The safe and familiar path of mass media campaigns has not been sufficient for change. It is time to travel a new path—even if its terrain is not well mapped and its specific direction must still be clearly marked.

REFERENCES

Adler N, Boyce T, Chesney M, Folkman S, Syme SL. Socioeconomic Inequalities in Health. *Journal of the American Medical Association*. 1993;269(24):3140–3145.

Adler NE, Boyce T, Chesney MA, Cohen S, Folkman S, Kahn RL, Syme SL. Socioeconomic Status and Health. *American Psychologist*. 1994;49(1):15–24.

Alcalay R. The Impact of Mass Communication Campaigns in the Health Field. *Social Science Medicine*. 1983;17:87–94.

Anderson NB, Armstead CA. Toward Understanding the Association of Socioeconomic Status and Health. *Psychosomatic Medicine*. 1995;57:213–225.

Atkin CK. Mass Media Information Campaign Effectiveness. In Rice R, Paisley W, eds. *Public Communications Campaigns*. 1983:265–279.

Bal DG, Kizer KW, Felten PG, Mozar HN, Niemeyer D. Reducing Tobacco Consumption in California. *Journal of the American Medical Association*. 1990;264(12):1570–1574.

Barstow D. A Heat Wave Sizzles. *The New York Times*. July 7, 1999:A1.

Beauchamp D. Public Health as Social Justice. *Inquiry*.1976;8:3–14.

Beauchamp D. Lottery Justice. *Journal of Public Health Policy*. 1981;2(3):201–205.

Beauchamp D. *The Health of the Republic*. Philadelphia: Temple University Press; 1988.

Bellah R, Masden R, Sullivan W, Swindler A, Tipton S. *Habits of the Heart: Individualism and Commitment in American Life*. New York: Harper & Row; 1986.

Black, J., ed. *Mixed News*. Mahwah, NJ: Lawrence Erlbaum Associates, 1997.

Blane D. Social Determinants of Health. *American Journal of Public Health*. 1995;85(7): 903–906.

Bly, L. A Network of Support. *USA TODAY*. July 14, 1999:D1,D2.

Breed W, DeFoe JR. Effecting Media Change: The Role of Cooperative Consultation on Alcohol Topics. *Journal of Communication*. 1982;32(2):88–99.

Brown JB, Walsh-Childers K. Effects of Media on Personal and Public Health. In Bryant J, Zillmann D. eds. *Media Effects: Advances in Theory and Research*. Hillsdale, NJ: Lawrence Erlbaum Associates; 1994.

Burns K. Moyers: A Second Look—More than Meets the Eye. *New York Times*. May 14, 1989.

Cart CU. Online Computer Networks. In Minkler M, ed. *Community Organizing and Community Building for Health*. New Brunswick, NJ: Rutgers University Press; 1997:325–338.

Cassell MM, Jackson C, Cheuvront B. Health Communication on the Internet: An Effective Channel for Behavior Change? *Journal of Health Communication*. 1998;3(1): 71–79.

Centerwall BS. Television and Violence. *Journal of the American Medical Association*. 1992;267(22):3059–3063.

Chaffee S, McDevitt M, Thorson E. Citizen Response to Civic Journalism. Paper presented at the annual meeting of the Association for Education in Journalism and Mass Communication; Chicago; August 1997.

Clark RP. Foreword. In Rosen J. *Community Connectedness Passwords for Public Journalism*. St. Petersburg, FL: The Poynter Institute for Media Studies, 1993.

Coleman J. *Foundations of Social Theory*. Cambridge, MA: The Belknap Press of Harvard University Press;1990.

Davis R, Miller L. Millions Scour the Web to get Medical Information *USA Today*. July 14, 1999:A1,A2.

Deering JW, Rogers EM. *Agenda-Setting*. Thousand Oaks, CA: Sage Publications;1997.

DeJong W. MADD Massachusetts Versus Senator Burke: A Media Advocacy Case Study. *Health Education Quarterly*. 1996;23(3):318–329.

DeJong W, Wallack, L. The Role of Designated Driver Programs in the Prevention of Alcohol-Impaired Driving: A Critical Reassessment. *Health Education Quarterly*. 1992;19:429–442.

DeJong W, Wallack L. A Critical Perspective on the Drug Czar's Antidrug Media Campaign. *Journal of Health Communication*. 1999;5:155–160.

DeJong W, Winsten JA. *The Media and the Message*. Washington, DC: The National Campaign to Prevent Teen Pregnancy; 1998.

Denton F, Thorson E. Effects of a Multimedia Public Journalism Project on Political Knowledge and Attitudes. In Lambeth EB, Meyer PE, Thorson E, eds. *Assessing Public Journalism*. Columbia: University of Missouri Press; 1998:143–178.

Dorfman L, Wallack L. Advertising Health: The Case for Counter-Ads. *Public Health Reports*. 1993; 108(6):716–726.

Duleep HO. Mortality and Income Inequality Among Economically Developed Countries. *Social Security Bulletin*. 1995; 58(2):34–50.

Etzioni, A. *The Spirit of Community*. New York: Simon & Schuster; 1993.

Fallows J. *Breaking the News*. New York. Vintage Books; 1997.

Farquhar J, Maccoby N, Solomon D. Community Applications of Behavioral Medicine. In Gentry W, ed. *Handbook of Behavioral Medicine*. New York: Guilford Press; 1984.

Farquhar, J, Fortmann SP, Flora J. Effects of Communitywide Education on Cardiovascular Disease Risk Factors: The Stanford Five-City Project. *Journal of the American Medical Association*. 1990;264:359–365.

Flora JA, Maccoby N, Farquhar JW. Communication Campaigns to Prevent Cardiovascular Disease. In Rice RE, Atkin CK, eds. *Public Communication Campaigns*. Newbury Park, CA: Sage Publications; 1989:233–252.

Ford P. *Don't Stop There!* Washington, DC: The Pew Center for Civic Journalism; 1998.

Fortmann S, Winkleby M, Flora J, Haskell W, Taylor C. Effect of Long-Term Community Health Education on Blood Pressure and Hypertension Control. *American Journal of Epidemiology*. 1990;132(4):629–646.

Friedland L, Sotirovic M, Daily K. Public Journalism and Social Capital. In Lambeth EB, Meyer PE, Thorson E, eds. *Assessing Public Journalism*. Columbia: University of Missouri Press; 1998:191–220.

Gamson WA. News as Framing: Comments on Graber. *American Behavioral Scientist*. 1989;33(2):157–162.

Gerbner G. Stories That Hurt: Tobacco, Alcohol, and Other Drugs in the Mass Media. In U.S. Department of Health and Human Services, *Youth and Drugs: Society's Mixed Messages*. Rockville, MD; 1990:53–127.

Gerbner G, Gross L, Morgan M, Signorielli N. Growing Up with Television: The Cultivation Perspective. In Bryant J, Zillmann D, eds. *Media Effects: Advances in Theory and Research*. Hillsdale, NJ: Lawrence Erlbaum Associates; 1994a:17–42.

Gerbner G, Morgan M, Signorielli. Television Violence Profile No. 16: The Turning Point Journal. January 1994b.

Gittell R, Vidal A. *Community Organizing*. Thousand Oaks, CA: Sage Publications; 1998.

Glik D, Berkanovic E, Stone K, et al. Health Education Goes Hollywood: Working with Prime-Time and Daytime Entertainment Television for Immunization Promotion. *Journal of Health Communication*. 1997;3(3):263–282.

Goldman LK, Glantz S. Evaluation of Antismoking Advertising Campaigns. *Journal of the American Medical Association* 1998;279(10):772–777.

Haan MN, Kaplan GA, Syme SL. Socioeconomic Status and Health: Old Observations and New Thoughts. In Bunker JP, Gomby DS, Kehrer BH, eds. *Pathways to Health: The Role of Social Factors*. Menlo Park, CA: Henry J. Kaiser Family Foundation; 1989a:76–135.

Haan MN, Kaplan GA, Syme SL, O'Neil A. Recent Publications on Socioeconomic Status and Health. In Bunker JP, Gomby DS, Kehrer BH, eds. *Pathways to Health: The Role of Social Factors*. Menlo Park, CA: Henry J. Kaiser Family Foundation; 1989b:319–420.

Holder HD, Treno AJ. Media Advocacy in Community Prevention: News as a Means to Advance Policy Change. *Addiction*. 1997;92(suppl 2):S189–S199.

Idler EL, Benyamini Y. Self-Rated Health and Mortality: A Review of Twenty-Seven Community Studies. *Journal of Health and Social Behavior*. 1997;38:21–37.

Institute of Medicine. *The Future of Public Health*. Washington, DC: National Academy Press; 1988.

Iyengar S. *Is Anyone Responsible?* Chicago: University of Chicago Press; 1991

Jernigan DH, Wright PA. Media Advocacy: Lessons from Community Experiences. *Journal of Public Health Policy*. 1996;17(3):306–330.

Johnston D. Gap Between Rich and Poor Substantially Wider. *New York Times*. September 5, 1999.

Kaplan GA. Where Do Shared Pathways Lead? Some Reflections on a Research Agenda. *Psychosomatic Medicine*. 1995;57:208–212.

Kaplan GA, Pamuk ER, Lynch JW, Cohen RD, Balfour JL. Inequality in Income and Mortality in the United States. *British Medial Journal*. 1996;312:999–1003.

Kawachi I, Berkman LF. Social Cohesion, Social Capital, and Health. In Berkman LF, Kawachi I. eds. *Social Epidemiology*. New York: Oxford University Press; 1998.

Kawachi I, Kennedy BP. Socioeconomic Determinants of Health. *British Medical Journal*. 1997;314:1037.

Kawachi I, Kennedy BP, Lochner K. Long Live Community. *The American Prospect*. November–December 1997a:56–59.

Kawachi I, Kennedy BP, Lochner K, Prothrow-Stith D. Social Capital, Income Inequality, and Mortality. *American Journal of Public Health*. 1997b;87:1491–1498.

Kennedy BP, Kawachi I, Prothrow-Stith D. Income Distribution and Mortality. *British Medical Journal*. 1996;312:1004.

Kennedy BK, Kawachi I, Prothrow-Stith D, Lochner K, Gupta V. Social Capital, Income Inequality, and Firearm Violent Crime. *Social Science Medicine*. 1998;47:7–17.

Kilbourne J. *Deadly Persuasion: Why Women and Girls Must Fight the Addictive Power of Advertising*. New York: Free Press; 1999.

Kunkel D, Cope KM, Farinola WJM, Biely E, Rollin E, Donnerstien E. Sex on TV. *A Biennial Report to the Kaiser Family Foundation;* 1999.

Ladd EC. *The Ladd Report*. New York: The Free Press; 1999.

Langlieb AM, Cooper CP, Gielen A. Linking Health Promotion with Entertainment Television. *American Journal of Public Health*. 1999;89(7):1116–1117.

Lantz PM, House JS, Lepkowski JM, Williams DR, Mero RP, Chen J. Socioeconomic Factors, Health Behaviors, and Mortality. *Journal of the American Medical Association* 1998;279:1703–1708.

Lazarsfeld P, Merton R. Mass Communication, Popular Taste and Organized Social Action. In Schramm W, ed. *Mass Communications*. Urbana: University of Illinois Press; 1975. (Original work published in 1984.)

Lefebvre C, Flora J. Social Marketing and Public Health Intervention. *Health Education Quarterly*. 1988;15(3):299–315.

Lochner K, Kawachi I, Kennedy BP. Concepts of Social Capital: Approaches to Measurement. *Health and Place*. 1999.

Lomas J. Social Capital and Health: Implications for Public Health and Epidemiology. *Social Science Medicine*. 1998;47(9):1181–1188.

Lynch JW, Kaplan GA. Understanding How Inequality in the Distribution of Income Affects Health. *Journal of Psychology*. 1997;2:297–314.

Mann JM. Medicine and Public Health, Ethics and Human Rights. *Hastings Center Report*. 1997;27(3):6–13.

Marmot MG, Mustard JF. Coronary Heart Disease from a Population Perspective. In Evan RG, Barer ML, Marmor TR. *Why Are Some People Healthy and Others Not?* New York: Aldine De Gruyter; 1994:1–25.

McChesney R. *Corporate Media and the Threat to Democracy*. New York: Seven Stories Press; 1997.

McChesney R. *Rich Media, Poor Democracy*. Urbana and Chicago: University of Illinois Press; 1999.

McCombs M, Shaw D. The Agenda Setting Function of Mass Media. *Public Opinion Quarterly.* 1972;36:176–187.

McGuire, W. Myth of Massive Media Impact: Savagings and Salvagings. In Comstock G., ed. *Public Communication and Behavior.* Orlando, FL: Academic Press Inc; 1986;173–257.

Merritt D. *Public Journalism and Public Life.* Hillsdale, NJ: Lawrence Erlbaum Associates; 1995.

Mills C. *The Sociological Imagination.* New York: Oxford University Press; 1959.

Minkler M. *Community Organizing and Community Building for Health.* New Brunswick, NJ: Rutgers University Press; 1997.

Montgomery K. *Target: Prime Time.* New York: Oxford University Press; 1989.

Navarro V. Topics for Our Times: The "Black Report" of Spain—The Commission on Social Inequalities in Health. *American Journal of Public Health.* 1997;87(3):334–335.

New York Times. Stifling Heat Retains Grip on East Coast. July 6, 1999: A1, A19.

Ognianova E, Thorson E, Mendelson A. What Makes an Active Citizen? Do the Media Play a Role? Paper presented at Communication Theory and Methodology Division of the Association for Education in Journalism and Mass Communication; August 1997.

Pew Center for Civic Journalism. *Civic Lessons: Report on Four Civic Journalism Projects.* Philadelphia: The Pew Charitable Trusts; 1997.

Postman N. *Amusing Ourselves to Death.* New York: Viking Penguin; 1985.

Putnam RD. The Prosperous Community. *The American Prospect.* Spring 1993(13):35–42.

Putnam RD. Tuning In, Tuning Out: The Strange Disappearance of Social Capital in America. *PS: Political Science and Politics.* 1995a;664–683.

Putnam RD. Bowling Alone: America's Declining Social Capital. *Journal of Democracy.* 1995b;6:65–78.

Reich RB. *Tales of a New America: The Anxious Liberal's Guide to the Future.* New York: Vintage; 1988.

Rogers EM, Storey JD. Communication Campaigns. In Berger CR, Chaffee SH., eds. *Handbook of Science Communication.* Newbury Park, CA: Sage Publications; 1987, 817.

Rose G. Sick Individuals and Sick Populations. *International Journal of Epidemiology.* 1985;14(1):32–38.

Rose G. *The Strategy of Preventive Medicine.* New York: Oxford University Press; 1992.

Rosen J. Making Journalism More Public. *Communication.* 1991;12:267–284.

Rosen J. *Community Connectedness Passwords for Public Journalism.* St. Petersburg, FL: The Poynter Institute for Media Studies; 1993.

Rosen J. Making Things More Public: On the Political Responsibility of the Media Intellectual. *Critical Studies in Mass Communication.* December 1994;363–388.

Ryan C. *Blaming the Victim.* New York: Vintage; 1976.

Ryan C. *Prime Time Activism.* Boston: South End Press; 1991.

Salmon C. *Information Campaigns: Balancing Social Values and Social Change.* Newbury Park, CA: Sage Publications; 1989.

Sampson RJ, Raudenbush SW, Earls F. Neighborhoods and Violent Crime: A Multilevel Study of Collective Efficacy. *Science.* 1997;277:918–924.

Schiller H. *The Mind Managers.* Boston: Beacon Press; 1973.

Schooler C, Sundar SS, Flora J. Effects of Stanford Five-City Project Media Advocacy Program. *Health Education Quarterly.* 1996;23(3):346–364.

Schorr L. *Within Our Reach.* New York: Anchor/Doubleday; 1988.

Schudson M. What if Civic Life Didn't Die? *The American Prospect.* March–April 1996; 25:17–20.

Seevak A. Oakland Shows the Way: The Coalition on Alcohol Outlet Issues and Media Advocacy as a Tool for Policy Change. *Berkeley Media Studies Group.* Issue #3; December 1997.

Semenza JC, Rubin CH, Falter KH, Selanikio JD, Flanders WD, Howe HL, Wilhelm JL. Heat Related Deaths During the July 1995 Heat Wave in Chicago. *New England Journal of Medicine.* 1996;335:84–90.

Shen T, Howe HL, Tobias RA, Roy C. Community Characteristics Correlated with Heat-Related Mortality. Springfield, IL: Illinois Department of Public Health, Division of Epidemiological Studies.

Siegel M. Mass Media Antismoking Campaigns: A Powerful Tool for Health Promotion. *Annals of Internal Medicine.* 1998;129(2):128–132

Signorielli N, Staples J. Television and Children's Conceptions of Nutrition. *Health Communication.* 1997;9(4):289–301.

Smith GD, Egger M. Socioeconomic Differences in Mortality in Britain and the United States. *American Journal of Public Health.* 1992;82(8):1079.

Spears L. Picturing Concerns. *Contra Costa Times.* April 11, 1999;A1, A32.

Stempel GH, Hargrove T. Mass Media Audiences in a Changing Media Environment. *Journalism & Mass Communication Quarterly.* 1996;73(3):549–559.

Strasburger VC. *Adolescents and the Media.* Thousand Oaks, CA: Sage Publications; 1995.

Strasburger VC, Comstock GA. *Adolescent Medicine: State of the Art Reviews.* Philadelphia: Hanley and Belfus; 1993.

Taking Back Our Neighborhoods. *A Joint Report by the Pew Center for Civic Journalism and the Poynter Institute for Media Studies.* Philadelphia: Pew Center for Civic Journalism; 1995.

Thorson E, Mendelson A, Ognianova. Affective and Behavioral Impact of Civic Journalism. Paper submitted to Mass Communication and Society Division of the Association for Education in Journalism and Mass Communication; April 1, 1997.

U.S. Department of Health and Human Services. *Media Strategies for Smoking Control.* January 1988.

Wallack L. Mass Media Campaigns: The Odds Against Finding Behavior Change. *Health Education Quarterly.* 1981; 8(3):209–260.

Wallack L. Mass Media Campaigns in a Hostile Environment: Advertising as Anti-Health Education. *Journal of Alcohol and Drug Education.* 1983;28(2):51–63.

Wallack L. Drinking and Driving: Toward a Broader Understanding of the Role of Mass Media. *Journal of Public Health Policy.* 1984;5(4):471–498.

Wallack L. Mass Communication and Health Promotion: A Critical Perspective. In Rice R, Atkin C., eds. *Public Communication Campaigns.* Newbury Park, CA: Sage Publications; 1989.

Wallack, L. Improving Health Promotion: Media Advocacy and Social Marketing Approaches. In Atkin C, Wallack L, eds. *Mass Communication and Public Health: Complexities and Conflicts.* Newbury Park, CA: Sage Publications; 1990.

Wallack L. Media Advocacy: A Strategy for Empowering People and Communities. *Journal of Public Health Policy.* 1994;15(4):420–436.

Wallack L. Strategies for Reducing Youth Violence: Media, Community and Policy. In University of California/the California Wellness Foundation, *1997 Wellness Lectures.* Berkeley, CA: The Regents of the University of California; 1997:37–69.

Wallack L. The California Violence Prevention Initiative: Advancing Policy to Ban Saturday Night Specials. *Health Education and Behavior.* 1999;26(6):841–857.

Wallack L, DeJong W. Mass Media and Public Health. In U.S. Department of Health and Human Services, ed. *The Effects of Mass Media on the Use and Abuse of Alcohol.* Bethesda, MD: National Institutes of Health; 1995:253–268.

Wallack L, Dorfman L. Media Advocacy: A Strategy for Advancing Policy and Promoting Health. *Health Education Quarterly.* 1996;23(3):293–317.

Wallack L, Sciandra R. Media Advocacy and Public Education in the Community Trial to Reduce Heavy Smoking. *International Quarterly of Community Health Education.* 1990–1991;11:205–222.

Wallack L, Dorfman L, Jernigan D, Themba M. *Media Advocacy and Public Health: Power for Prevention.* Newbury Park, CA: Sage Publications; 1993.

Wallack L, Woodruff K, Dorfman L, Diaz I. *News for a Change. An Advocates Guide to Working with the Media.* Newbury Park, CA: Sage Publications; 1999.

Wang CC, Burris MA. Empowerment Through Photo Novella: Portraits of Participation. *Health Education Quarterly.* 1994;21(2):171–186.

Wang CC, Burris MA. Photovoice: Concept, Methodology, and Use for Participatory Needs Assessment. *Health Education Quarterly.* 1997;24(3):369–387.

Wang CC, Pies CA. Family, Maternal, and Child Health Through Photovoice. Submitted to *Maternal and Child Health Journal.* October 1999.

Wang CC, Burris MA, Xiang PY. Chinese Village Women as Visual Anthropologists. *Social Science Medicine.* 1996a; 42(10):1391–1400.

Wang CC, Yuan YL, Feng ML. Photovoice as a Tool for Participatory Evaluation. *Journal of Contemporary Health.* 1996b;4:47–49.

Wang CC, Cash JL, Powers LS. Who Knows the Streets as Well as the Homeless? Revised for *Health Promotion Practice* (HPP99-002). April 1999.

Wang CC, Wu YK, Zhan TW, Carovano K. Photovoice as a Participatory Health Promotion Strategy. *Health Promotion International.* 1998;13(1):75–86.

Wiley S. Civic Journalism in Practice. *Newspaper Research Journal.* 1998;19:16–29.

Wilkinson RG. National Mortality Rates: The Impact of Inequality? *American Journal of Public Health.* 1992;82:1082–1084.

Wilkinson RG. *Unhealthy Societies: The Afflictions of Inequality.* London: Routledge; 1996.

Winett L, Wallack L. Advancing Public Health Goals Through the Mass Media. *Journal of Health Communication.* 1996:173–196.

Woodruff K. Alcohol Advertising and Violence Against Women: A Media Advocacy Case Study. *Health Education Quarterly.* 1996;23(3):330–345.

Public Health and Safety in Context: Lessons from Community-Level Theory on Social Capital[*]

Robert J. Sampson, Ph.D., and Jeffrey D. Morenoff, Ph.D.[1,2]

A long-standing body of research has underscored the association of multiple health-related outcomes with the social and economic characteristics of community contexts. As reviewed below, for example, child and adolescent outcomes correlated with the ecological concentration of poverty include infant mortality, low birthweight, child maltreatment, and adolescent violence; health risks for adults include depression, homicide victimization, cardiovascular disease, and all-cause mortality. At the other end of the spectrum, communities with high socio-economic status appear to promote the health of children and adults.

Why are so many health-related outcomes concentrated ecologically? A new generation of neighborhood-level research has emerged in recent years to tackle this question. This research has extended across the disciplines of sociology, public health, psychology, economics, and political science. A visible example is provided by the recent publication of two research volumes supported by the Social Science Research Council on "neighborhood effects" (Brooks-Gunn et al., 1997a,b). In public health, renewed interest in neighborhood envi-

[1]Dr. Sampson is Lucy Flower Professor of Sociology at the University of Chicago and Dr. Morenoff is assistant professor of sociology and faculty associate at the Population Studies Center at the University of Michigan. This paper was prepared for the symposium "Capitalizing on Social Science and Behavioral Research to Improve the Public's Health," the Institute of Medicine and the Commission on Behavioral and Social Sciences and Education of the National Research Council, Atlanta, Georgia, February 2–3, 2000.

[2]We thank the Institute of Medicine panel along with discussants at the Atlanta symposium for helpful comments. Portions of this paper draw from Sampson et al. (1999) and Sampson (1999a,b,c).

ronments has resulted in the publication of two recent review articles (Roberts, 1999; Yen and Syme, 1999) and a collection of classic and contemporary works on neighborhoods and health (Kawachi et al., 2000).

The goal of this paper is to make sense of current knowledge on health and public safety in local communities. We do so by drawing on the concept of "social capital" to unpack what it is about neighborhoods, above and beyond the status and attributes of the individuals who live there, that might lead to various health outcomes. Indeed, despite the wide range of evidence documenting relationships between community socioeconomic status and health, we still know very little about what these associations mean. As we shall elaborate, the basic idea of social capital provides a possible clue. According to James Coleman, social capital is a resource stemming from the structure of social relationships, which in turn facilitates the achievement of specific goals (Coleman 1990:300). Such resources, be they actual or potential, are often linked to durable social networks (Bourdieu 1986: 249). Putnam defines social capital more expansively to include not only the networks themselves, but also shared norms and mutual trust, which "facilitate coordination and cooperation for mutual benefit" (1993: 36).

In short, social capital is a resource that is realized through relationships (Coleman 1990:304), as compared to physical capital, which takes observable material form, and human capital, which rests in the skills and knowledge acquired by an individual. Whatever the specific formulation, social capital is not an attribute of individuals but rather a property of a social structure, such as an organization, an extended family, or a community (Coleman 1990; Bourdieu 1986). This paper employs the concept of social capital as a mode of inquiry into why community environments may be consequential for health. We review theoretical formulations on what social capital means at the community level, criticisms and weaknesses of the concept, and recent theoretical innovations. We also highlight research frontiers and promising community-level strategies that put social capital to work in promoting health. Before articulating social capital in more detail, we first note the regularities in prior empirical research that motivate its consideration.

A BRIEF HISTORY OF COMMUNITY HEALTH RESEARCH

The study of community environments and health-related outcomes actually has a long lineage in both sociology and public health. In sociology, the urban ecological approach of the "Chicago School" brought neighborhood-centered research to the fore of the discipline during the early 20th Century.[3] One influen-

---

[3]We set aside a detailed discussion of equally longstanding debates on how to define "neighborhood." The traditional definition of neighborhood, as proposed by Robert Park, referred to an ecological subsection of a larger community—a collection of both people and institutions occupying a spatially defined area that is conditioned by a set of ecological, cultural, and political forces (Park, 1916: 147–154). Neighborhoods are ecological

tial framework in this tradition was Shaw and McKay's (1942) theory of neighborhood social disorganization. Although focusing on delinquency, Shaw and McKay constructed a general framework for understanding how community processes relate to a wide range of outcomes, including health. Community social disorganization was conceptualized as the inability of a community structure to realize the common values of its residents and maintain effective social controls. Social control refers to the capacity of a social unit to regulate itself according to desired principles—to realize *collective,* as opposed to forced, goals (Janowitz 1975: 82, 87). Common ends include the desire of residents to live in neighborhoods characterized by economic sufficiency, good schools, adequate housing, freedom from predatory crime, and a generally healthy environment. The capacity to achieve such goals is linked to both formal, purposive efforts to achieve social regulation through institutional means, and to informal role relationships established for other purposes (Kornhauser 1978).

Shaw and McKay argued that delinquency was not an isolated phenomenon, and showed in their research the association between communities and health. In particular, Chicago neighborhoods characterized by poverty, residential instability, and dilapidated housing were found to suffer disproportionately high rates of infant mortality, delinquency, crime, low birth weight, tuberculosis, physical abuse, and other factors detrimental to health (1969: 106). In another seminal study, Faris and Dunham (1965, 1939) applied the idea of social disorganization to mental health, arguing that more disorganized areas had higher rates of hospitalization for mental disorders. Interestingly, both Shaw and McKay and Faris and Dunham observed that high rates of adverse outcomes tended to persist in the same communities over time, despite the movement of different population

---

units nested within successively larger communities (1916: 114). That is, there is no one neighborhood, but many neighborhoods that vary in size and complexity depending on the social phenomenon of interest and the ecological structure of the larger community. In most cities there exist local community or city planning areas that, although relatively large, usually have well-known names and borders such as freeways, parks, and major streets. For example, Chicago has 77 local community areas averaging about 40,000 persons that were designed to correspond to socially meaningful and natural geographic boundaries. Some boundaries have undergone change over time, but these areas are widely recognized by administrative agencies and local institutions. Census tracts refer to smaller and more socially homogeneous areas of roughly 3,000–5,000 residents on average; their boundaries are usually, but not always, drawn to take into account major streets, parks, and other geographical features. A third and even smaller area more likely to approximate common notions of a "neighborhood" is the block group—a set of blocks averaging approximately 1,000 residents. Although widely used in empirical research, the fact remains that community or planning areas, census tracts, and block groups all offer flawed operational definitions of neighborhood. In addition, social networks are potentially boundless in physical space.

groups through them.[4] From these findings, the Chicago School sociologists concluded that neighborhoods possess relatively enduring features that transcend the idiosyncratic characteristics of particular ethnic groups that inhabit them—so-called "emergent properties." In any event, what makes the Chicago-School framework relevant to present concerns is its theoretical emphasis on the characteristics of *places* rather than *people*.

Community environments were a focus of early epidemiological research as well. An exemplar in this tradition is the research of Goldberger and his colleagues on pellagra in Southern villages. In a classic study of family income and the incidence of pellagra, Goldberger et al. (1916) found that the probability of contracting pellagra was related not only to individual-level socioeconomic status but also to the availability of nutritional foods in villages. They amassed an impressive array of both individual- and village-level data relating to food supply and malnutrition that included village-level measures of the prevalence of retail grocery establishments and home-provided foods, and contrasts in the type of agriculture in farm areas surrounding the villages. Their study also provided some of the earliest evidence of an interaction between individual- and community-level health risks: in villages with fewer supplies of nutritious food, family income was "less efficient as a protective factor than in other similar localities with better conditions of food availability" (Goldberger et al., 1916: 2707).

Although Goldberger may have been "rowing against the epidemiologic current" with his focus on the social context of individual risk factors (Schwartz et al., 1999: 19), his work was nonetheless widely influential and illustrative of a much broader tradition of epidemiological research on the ecological context of health that dates back to the early 19th Century. As Susser (1998: 609) argues, "Epidemiology, a population science, is in its essence ecological in the original biological sense of organisms in a multilevel interactive environment."

Recent Evidence

The importance of an ecological perspective has, in our opinion, increased in recent years. Social characteristics continue to vary systematically across communities along dimensions of socioeconomic status (e.g., poverty, wealth, occupational attainment), family structure and life cycle (e.g., female-headed households, child density), residential stability (e.g., home ownership and tenure), and racial/ethnic composition (e.g., racial segregation). In fact, there is evidence that the concentration of poverty and inequality has increased in the 1980s and 1990s (Wilson 1996; Massey and Denton 1993). A prominent explanation for the clustering of multiple forms of social and economic disadvantage

---

[4]The assumption of ecological stability has been called into question in recent decades. Ironically, many social scientists have returned to basic Chicago School principles to explain ecological transformations such as those brought on by white flight in the 1950s and the increasing concentration of poverty in the 1970s and 1980s (see Morenoff and Sampson, 1997).

is Wilson's (1987) theory of *concentration effects* arising from living in an impoverished neighborhood. Wilson argues that the social transformation of inner-city areas in recent decades (due primarily to out-migration of the middle class and industrial restructuring that depleted the demand for unskilled labor) has increased the concentration of the most disadvantaged segments of the population—especially black, poor, female-headed families with children. Massey and Denton (1993) describe how the interaction between rising economic dislocation and persistent racial residential segregation created a set of structural circumstances that reinforce the effects of economic deprivation. Massey (1996) notes also the growing geographic concentration of *affluence*, suggesting an increasingly bifurcated society by wealth.

There is an unfortunate parallel in health regarding ecological concentration; the "co-morbidity" or spatial clustering of homicide, infant mortality, low birth weight, accidental injury, and suicide continues to the present day (e.g., Wallace and Wallace 1990; Almgren et al., 1998). In the period 1995–1996, for example, data from the city of Chicago reveal that census tracts with high homicide rates tend to be spatially contiguous to other tracts high in homicide. Perhaps more interesting, more than 75% of such tracts also contain a high level of clustering for low birth weight and infant mortality, and more than half for accidental injuries (Sampson 1999a). Suicide is more distinct although even here the spatial clustering is significant. The ecological concentration of homicide, low birth weight, infant mortality, and injury indicates that there may be geographic "hot spots" for a number of unhealthy outcomes. The range of child and adolescent outcomes correlated with multiple forms of concentrated disadvantage is quite wide, and includes infant mortality, low birth weight, teenage childbearing, low academic achievement and educational failure, child maltreatment, and delinquency (see Brooks-Gunn et al., 1997a,b).

A growing body of research has also examined community characteristics and *individual-level* health. Although the evidence is mixed and the magnitudes often small, a number of studies have linked health outcomes to neighborhood context even when individual attributes and behaviors are taken into account (Robert 1999), including coronary risk factors and heart disease mortality (Diez-Roux et al., 1997; LeClere et al., 1997), low birth weight (Roberts 1997; O'Campo et al., 1997; Gorman 1999), smoking (Duncan et al., 1999; Diehr et al., 1993), morbidity (Robert 1998), all-cause mortality (Haan et al., 1987; Anderson et al., 1997), and self-reported health (Jones and Duncan 1995; Sooman and Macintyre 1995). Recent analyses of the longitudinal Alameda County Health study in Northern California, for example, revealed that self-reported fair/poor health was 70 percent higher for residents of concentrated poverty areas than for residents of nonpoverty areas, independent of age, sex, income, education, smoking status, body mass index, and alcohol consumption (Yen and Kaplan 1999a). In a related study, age and sex-adjusted odds for mortality were more than 50% higher (odds ratio = 1.58) for residents in areas characterized by poverty and deteriorated housing, after adjusting for income, race/ethnicity, smoking, body mass index, alcohol consumption, and perceived health status

(Yen and Kaplan 1999b). Such patterns are not limited to the United States. A multilevel study in Sweden found a similar elevated risk of poor health for residents of lower socioeconomic-status communities, controlling for age, sex, education, body mass index, smoking, and physical activity (Malmstrom et al., 1999).

Experiments

Correlational and observational studies suffer well-known weaknesses with respect to making causal inferences. Much research on communities and health implicitly assumes that the social characteristics of neighborhood environments cannot be reduced to the compositional characteristics of individual residents, just as the liquidity of water is a property that does not pertain to the individual molecules of hydrogen and oxygen (Schwartz et al., 1999: 26–27). Alternatively, however, it may be that individuals with poor health selectively migrate to, or are left behind in, poor neighborhoods. Under this interpretation, the observed correlations between community characteristics and health may simply be a reflection of the unmeasured processes through which individuals sort themselves into different neighborhoods (Manski 1995).

To address this "reflection problem," researchers have begun to explore community-level effects on health outcomes with experimental and quasi-experimental research designs. One such example is found in the "Moving to Opportunity" (MTO) program, a series of housing experiments in five cities that randomly assigned housing-project residents to one of three groups: an experimental group receiving housing subsidies to move into low-poverty neighborhoods, a group receiving conventional (Section 8) housing assistance, and a control group receiving no special assistance. A study from the Boston MTO site showed that children of mothers in the experimental group had significantly lower prevalence of injuries, asthma attacks, and personal victimization during follow-up. The move to low-poverty neighborhoods also resulted in significant improvements in the general health status and mental health of household heads (Katz et al., 1999). Because the experimental design was used to control individual-level risk factors, a reasonable inference from these studies is that an improvement in community socioeconomic environment leads to better health and behavioral outcomes.

In summary, research in the social and behavioral science has established a reasonably consistent set of findings relevant to the community context of health. Although causality and magnitude are still at issue, there seems to be broad agreement that (a) there is considerable inequality between neighborhoods and local communities along multiple dimensions of socioeconomic status, (b) a number of health problems tend to cluster together in geographically defined ecological units such as neighborhoods or local community areas, (c) these two phenomena are themselves related—community-level predictors common to many health-related outcomes include concentrated poverty and/or affluence, racial segregation, family disruption, residential instability, and poor quality housing, and (d) the relationship between community context and health out-comes—especially all-cause mortality, depression, and violence—appears to maintain when controls are introduced for individual-level risk factors. An asso-ciation between the social environment and individual-level health has emerged in experimental studies as well.

Despite this suggestive body of evidence on the association between com-munity social contexts and health, the question remains as to why. Until re-cently, answers from the dominant perspectives in social science and epidemio-logy were not forthcoming given their (ironically) individualistic bent in the modern era. In sociology, the Chicago School paradigm, with its emphasis on ecological and social systems, gave way in the 1950s and 1960s to a focus on estimating individual parameters in national surveys (Coleman 1994). Modern epidemiology became dominated by an analogous "risk factor paradigm" that elevated individual-level causes of disease and generally demoted more "up-stream" social and economic antecedents of health (Schwartz et al., 1999; Susser and Susser 1996a, b; Susser 1998; Diez-Roux 1998). The theoretical framework that underlies this paradigm has been described as "biomedical individualism" that "considers social determinants of disease to be at best secondary (if not ir-relevant), and views populations simply as the sum of individuals and popula-tion patterns of disease as simply reflective of individual cases" (Krieger 1994).

In the last several years, notable programmatic essays assailing the risk factor paradigm have appeared in major public health journals, with titles such as "Does Risk Factor Epidemiology Put Epidemiology at Risk?" (Susser 1998); "The Failure of Academic Epidemiology: Witness for the Prosecution" (Shy 1997); "Bringing Context Back into Epidemiology" (Diez-Roux 1998); "The Fallacy of the Ecological Fallacy" (Schwartz 1994); and "The Logic in Ecologi-cal" (Susser 1994a; b). One theme that runs throughout these articles is the need for more research on the social context of health risks. Some prominent epide-miologists—Krieger (1994) and Susser and Susser (1996a, b)—have called for a new paradigm centered around an ecological metaphor that would emphasize the broader context of individual risk factors, both at the macro level, with more attention to social environments, and at the micro level of molecular biology (Schwartz et al., 1999). Within sociology, Abbott (1997) makes a similar plea for a "contextualist" paradigm, premised on the idea that "no social fact makes any sense abstracted from its context in social (and often geographic) space and social time" (1152). The need for a contextualist paradigm in health is, we would argue, clear. We thus turn to such a paradigm, that of social capital.

SOCIAL CAPITAL THEORY AND BEYOND

The spatial patterning of crime and health provides a potentially important clue in thinking about why it is that communities and larger collectivities might matter for health. Namely, if multiple and seemingly disparate health outcomes are linked together empirically across communities and are predicted by similar structural characteristics, there may be common underlying causes or mediating mechanisms at the neighborhood level. For example, if "neighborhood effects" of concentrated poverty on health really exist, presumably they stem from social processes that involve collective aspects of neighborhood life (e.g., social cohesion, spatial diffusion, local support networks, informal social control). The theory of social capital addresses such social processes. (So too did the early Chicago School, if less rigorously. The connection between social disorganization and social capital is this: Communities high in social capital are better able to realize common values and maintain the social controls that foster public safety.)

Although he was not the originator of the idea, Coleman's writings on social capital elevated the concept to the forefront of social science research (1988, 1990).[5] He argued that social capital takes a variety of different forms, all of which involve relationships among persons that facilitate the realization of goals (Coleman 1990:300). One form of social capital relevant to health is *reciprocal obligations* among neighbors, which create a source of "credit" that individuals can draw upon when in need of a favor (Coleman 1990: 306–310). A second form of social capital occurs when social relations are used to *exchange information* (1990: 310). Neighbors sometimes provide each other with advice, tips, or other types of information that might be costly to acquire elsewhere. A third form is *intergenerational closure*. When parents know the parents of their children's friends, they have the potential to observe the child's actions in different circumstances, talk to each other about the child, compare notes, and establish rules (Coleman 1988). Such intergenerational closure of local networks provides the parents and children with social capital of a collective nature. Coleman also argued that *voluntary associations* can generate social capital either intentionally, by generating community action around a specific purpose, or unintentionally, by creating new ties between people that are then used to facilitate other types of action. For example, parents who join school-based organizations like the PTA or a local school council may form new ties with some of their neighbors and decide to employ those ties towards non-educational pursuits, such as establishing an informal system of childcare.

Since Coleman introduced the idea to a wider audience, there has been an explosion of interest in social capital. The concept is currently so popular that the World Bank maintains an entire web site dedicated to social capital (http://www.worldbank.org/poverty/scapital/index.htm). Unfortunately, the growing popularity of social capital has led to a proliferation of its meanings. Even some proponents of social capital theory (e.g., Portes 1998) worry that the concept has come to represent so many different things to different people that it is in danger of losing its distinctive social meaning. Part of this confusion stems

---

[5]Earlier essays exploring the meaning of social capital can be found in the works of Jane Jacobs, George Homans, Glen Loury, and Pierre Bourdieu. For a more extensive discussion of the theoretical origins and development of social capital, see Portes (1998), Sandefur and Laumann (1998), Woolcock (1998), Astone et al. (1999), and Kawachi and Berkman (2000).

from the way Coleman originally formulated the concept. Rather than undertaking a systematic analysis of how social capital is generated and what its consequences are, Coleman chose to illustrate its operation through vignettes. Recent work bearing on health has thus set out to clarify, extend, and operationalize the concept, a trend particularly evident in the fields of epidemiology, criminology, and urban sociology.

In epidemiology, the recent application of social capital to understanding variations in health has focused largely on norms that encourage cooperation and facilitate social cohesion. Drawing on Putnam (1993) perhaps more so than Coleman, Kawachi and Berkman (2000) argue that the core meaning of social capital is tied to the broader notion of *social cohesion*, which refers to the absence of social conflict, coupled with the presence of strong social bonds and mutual trust. There is a small but intriguing body of research linking cohesion to health-related outcomes, although usually at higher levels of aggregation than the neighborhood. For example, measures of social cohesion and trust have been found to predict mortality rates at the state level. Kawachi et al. (1997) reported that the level of distrust (the proportion of residents in each state agreeing that most people can't be trusted) was strongly correlated with the age-adjusted mortality rate ($r = .79$, $p < .001$). Lower levels of trust were associated with higher rates of most major causes of death, including coronary heart disease, unintentional injury, and cerebrovascular disease. A one standard deviation increase in trust was associated with about a 9% lower level of overall mortality. A negative association between levels of trust/cohesion and homicide rates was found at the state level as well (Kawachi et al., 1998). Kawachi et al. (1999) also found a relationship between state-level social capital and individual self-rated health. Controlling for individual risk factors (e.g., smoking, obesity, income, lack of access to health care), individuals living in states with low levels of social capital (low trust, reciprocity, and voluntary associations) exhibited a significantly greater risk of poor self-rated health.

A rich line of research on social networks in the fields of both health and urban sociology also shares a natural affinity with the surge of interest in neighborhood social capital. In particular, much evidence reveals that friendship ties and family social support networks promote individual health (see House et al., 1988; Berkman and Syme 1979). And contrary to the popular belief that metropolitan life has led inexorably to the decline of personal ties, sociological research has shown that while urbanites may be exposed to more unconventionality and diversity, they retain a set of personal support networks just like their suburban and rural counterparts (see e.g., Fischer 1982). The difference is that the social ties of city dwellers tend to be more dispersed spatially. In other words, social ties are alive and well in American cities, even if not concentrated geographically, and at the individual level they appear to be a protective factor in health.

At the same time, however, we would maintain that local social ties (whether urban or rural in nature) do not necessarily translate into high social capital at the neighborhood level. Wilson (1996), for example, argued that many poor neighborhoods with strong social ties do not produce collective resources such as the social control of disorderly behavior. His research suggests that disadvantaged urban neighborhoods are places where dense webs of social ties among neighbors actually impede social organization: "(I)t appears that what many impoverished and dangerous neighborhoods have in common is a relatively high degree of social integration (high levels of local neighboring while being relatively isolated from contacts in broader mainstream society) and low levels of informal social control (feelings that they have little control over their immediate environment, including the environment's negative influences on their children)" (Wilson 1996: 63–64). Although members of such communities share strong social linkages with one another, they remain socially isolated, in Wilson's terms, because their network ties do not extend beyond immediate social environs to include *non*-community members and institutions. The limits of tight-knit social bonds were recognized earlier in Granovetter's (1973) seminal essay on the strength of "weak ties" in obtaining job referrals. Whether or not weak ties promote health is unknown.

Collective Efficacy

We believe that the research on cohesion and social ties reveals somewhat of a paradox. Namely, many urbanites have an abundance of friends and social support networks that are no longer organized in a parochial, local fashion. Moreover, urbanites whose "strong ties" *are* tightly restricted geographically may actually produce an environment that discourages collective responses to local problems. To address this issue, Sampson et al. (1997, 1999) have proposed a focus on mechanisms that facilitate social control without requiring strong ties or associations. As Warren (1975) noted, the common belief that neighborhoods have declined in importance as social units "is predicated on the assumption that neighborhood is exclusively a primary group and therefore should possess the 'face-to-face,' intimate, affective relations which characterize all primary groups" (p. 50). Sampson et al. (1997) reject this outmoded assumption and highlight instead working trust and the shared willingness of local residents to intervene in support of public order. Personal ties notwithstanding, it is the linkage of mutual trust and shared expectations for intervening on behalf of the common good that defines the neighborhood context of what Sampson et al. (1997) term *collective efficacy*. Just as individuals vary in their capacity for efficacious action, they argue that so too do neighborhoods vary in their capacity to achieve common goals. Moreover, just as self-efficacy is situated rather than global (one has self-efficacy relative to a particular task or type of task), neighborhood efficacy exists relative to collective tasks such as maintaining public order.

Sampson et al. (1999) thus view social capital as referring to the resources or potential inherent in social networks, whereas collective efficacy is a task-specific construct that refers to shared expectations and mutual engagement by residents in local social control. Moving away from a focus on private ties, the term collective efficacy is meant to signify an emphasis on shared beliefs in a neighborhood's conjoint capability for action to achieve an intended effect, and hence an active sense of engagement on the part of residents. As Bandura (1997) argues, the meaning of efficacy is captured in expectations about the exercise of control, elevating the "agentic" aspect of social life over a perspective centered on the accumulation of "stocks" of social resources. This conception of collective efficacy is consistent with the redefinition of social capital by Portes and Sensenbrenner in terms of "expectations for action within a collectivity" (1993: 1323).

The theory of collective efficacy was tested in a survey of 8,782 residents of 343 Chicago neighborhoods in 1995. A five-item Likert-type scale measured shared expectations about "informal social control." Residents were asked about the likelihood that their neighbors could be counted on to take action if: (1) children were skipping school and hanging out on a street corner, (2) children were spray-painting graffiti on a local building, (3) children were showing disrespect to an adult, (4) a fight broke out in front of their house, and (5) the fire station closest to home was threatened with budget cuts. "Social cohesion/trust" was measured by asking respondents how strongly they agreed that "People around here are willing to help their neighbors"; "This is a close-knit neighborhood"; "People in this neighborhood can be trusted"; and (reverse coded): "People in this neighborhood generally don't get along with each other"; "People in this neighborhood do not share the same values." Social cohesion and informal social control were strongly related across neighborhoods ($r = .80$), and were combined into a summary measure of "collective efficacy."

Collective efficacy was associated with lower rates of violence, controlling for concentrated disadvantage, residential stability, immigrant concentration, and a set of individual-level characteristics (e.g., age, sex, SES, race/ ethnicity, home ownership). Whether measured by official homicide events or violent victimization as reported by residents, neighborhoods high in collective efficacy had significantly lower rates of violence. This finding held up controlling for prior neighborhood violence that may have depressed later collective efficacy (e.g., because of fear); a two standard-deviation elevation in collective efficacy was associated with a 26 percent reduction in the expected homicide rate (1997: 922). Concentrated disadvantage and residential instability were also linked to lower collective efficacy, and the association of disadvantage and stability with violence was significantly reduced when collective efficacy was controlled. In particular, collective efficacy appears to be undermined by the concentration of disadvantage, racial segregation, family disruption, and residential instability (Sampson et al., 1997, 1999). The cross sectional nature of the data and the likelihood of reciprocality (crime may reduce collective efficacy) means that causal effects could not be reliably determined. Nonetheless, these patterns are consistent with the inference that neighborhood characteristics influence violence in part through the construct of neighborhood collective efficacy (see also Elliott et al., 1996).

Institutions and Public Control

A theory of social capital and collective efficacy should not ignore institutions, or the wider political environment in which local communities are embedded. Communities can exhibit intense private ties (e.g., among friends, kin) and perhaps even shared expectations yet still lack the institutional capacity to achieve social control (Hunter 1985; Woolcock 1998). The institutional component of social capital is the resource stock of neighborhood organizations and their linkages with other organizations, both within *and* outside the community (Sampson 1999b). Kornhauser (1978: 79) argues that when the horizontal links among institutions within a community are weak, the capacity to defend local interests is weakened. Vertical integration is potentially more important. Similar to the idea of "bridging" social capital, Bursik and Grasmick (1993) highlight the importance of *public* control, defined as the capacity of local community organizations to obtain extralocal resources (e.g., police, fire protection; block grants; health services) that help sustain neighborhood stability and control. Hunter (1985) identifies the dilemma of public control in a civil society. The problem is that public control is provided mainly by institutions of the State, and we have seen a secular decline in public (citizenship) obligations in society accompanied by an increase in civil (individual) rights. This imbalance of collective obligations and individual rights undermines social control, and by implication, social capital. According to Hunter (1985), local communities must thus work together with forces of public control to achieve social order, principally through interdependence among private (family), parochial (neighborhood) and public (State) institutions such as the police and schools.

Caveat

Any discussion of social capital needs to acknowledge its potential downside. After all, social networks can be drawn upon for negative as well as positive goals—the same strong social ties that benefit members of one particular group can be used to exclude others outside the group from sharing in those resources (Portes 1998: 15). As but one example, racial exclusion is not desirable yet dense social networks have been used to facilitate it. As Sugrue's (1996) research on Detroit circa 1940–1970 revealed, strong neighborhood associations were exploited by whites to keep blacks from moving to white working-class areas.

Social capital (and by implication, collective efficacy) may thus be said to have a valence depending on the goal in question (Sandefur and Laumann 1998: 493). Recognizing the valence of social capital, Sampson et al. (1999) apply the nonexclusivity requirement of a social good (Coleman 1990: 315–316) to judge whether neighborhood structures serve the collective needs of residents. We believe that resources such as neighborhood safety and healthy environments produce positive externalities (see Coleman 1990: 250–251) that are consensually desired but problematically achieved, owing in large part to variabilities in structural constraints. Moreover, even if health and safety are consensually desired, there may be conflicts over the setting of priorities when resources are limited. One can imagine, for example, that in some contexts a disagreement over whether a violence reduction program or a toxic waste cleanup deserves priority would lead to paralysis and not collective action. As with the existence of strong ties, consensus on ultimate goals does not automatically lead to enhanced outcomes. Like Sampson et al. (1999), then, we view social capital and collective efficacy not as some all-purpose elixir but as normatively situated and endogenous to specific structural contexts (Portes 1998).[6]

RECENT DEVELOPMENTS IN NEIGHBORHOOD RESEARCH

Consideration of neighborhoods and health should not be confined strictly to social capital, of course. Two developments in particular bear noting—research on spatial inequality and routine activities. Although distinct conceptually from social capital, we believe there are sufficient grounds for integrating these developments to better understand the ecology of health.

Metropolitan-Wide and Spatial Inequality

Research on the political economy of American cities has shown that the stratification of places is shaped, both directly and indirectly, by the extralocal decisions of public officials and businesses. For example, the decline of many central-city neighborhoods has been facilitated not only by individual preferences, as manifested in voluntary migration patterns, but by government decisions on public housing that concentrate the poor, incentives for suburban sprawl in the form of tax breaks for developers and private mortgage assistance, highway construction, economic disinvestment in central cities, and haphazard zoning on land use (Logan and Molotch 1987).

The embeddedness of neighborhoods within the larger system of citywide spatial dynamics is equally relevant (Sampson et al., 1999). Recent research on population change shows that population abandonment is driven as much by spatial diffusion processes (e.g., changes in proximity to violent crime) as by the internal characteristics of neighborhoods (Morenoff and Sampson 1997). In particular, housing decisions are often made by assessing the quality of neighborhoods relative to what is happening in surrounding areas. Parents with young children appear quite sensitive to the relative location of neighborhoods and schools in addition to their internal characteristics. Spatial diffusion processes for dimensions of social capital are even more likely, mainly because social

---

[6]Although we are critical of the undisciplined appropriation of social capital rhetoric by many health researchers, the renewed attention to what are in fact old ideas about the social nature of life does have an upside. Namely, the excessively individualistic paradigm of "risk factors" has been challenged in an unprecedented way, opening a window of opportunity for consideration of macrolevel strategies for community intervention. We return to this issue in the final section of this paper.

networks and exchange processes unfold across the artificial boundaries of analytically defined neighborhoods. A neighborhood-level perspective on health cannot afford to ignore the relative geographic position of neighborhoods and how that bears on internal dimensions of social capital. The importance of spatial externalities is shown by the finding that ecological proximity to areas high in collective efficacy bestows an advantage above and beyond the structural characteristics of a given neighborhood (Sampson et al., 1999).

Routine Activities

A concern with ecology suggests another often-overlooked mechanism in discussions of neighborhood effects—how land use patterns and the ecological distributions of daily routine activities bear on well being. The location of schools, the mix of residential with commercial land use (e.g., strip malls, bars), public transportation nodes, and large flows of nighttime visitors, for example, are relevant to organizing how and when children come into contact with other peers, adults, and nonresident activity. The "routine activities" perspective in criminology provides the important insight that predatory violence requires the intersection in time and space of motivated offenders, suitable targets, and the absence of capable guardians (Cohen and Felson 1979). Rooted in social control theory, the routine activity approach assumes a steady supply of motivated "offenders," and focuses on how targets of opportunity and guardianship combine to explain criminal events. This strategy has appeal in thinking about a range of adolescent health behaviors, such as drinking, early sexual behavior, smoking, and "hanging out," that reflect natural desires yet can yield negative outcomes both personally and for others (e.g., teen childbearing, low birth weight, low achievement, poor health). For example, not only do mixed-use neighborhoods offer greater opportunities for expropriative crime, they offer increased opportunity for children to congregate outside the home in places conducive to peer-group influence (Sampson 1999a,b).

In short, because illegal and "deviant" activities feed on the spatial and temporal structure of routine legal activities (e.g., transportation, work, entertainment, and shopping), the differential land use of neighborhoods is a key to comprehending the ecological distribution of situations and opportunities conducive to a wide range of potentially adverse behaviors. In particular, the ecological placements of bars, liquor stores, strip-mall shopping outlets, subway stops, and unsupervised play spaces play a direct role in the distribution of high-risk situations. The ecology of routine activities is not usually thought of in the "neighborhood effects" literature, much less as a mechanism. We suggest, however, that it holds considerable promise as an explanatory factor, especially in combination with a theory of social capital. For instance, decisions to locate high-risk businesses are often targeted precisely to lower-income communities known to lack the organizational capacity to resist. Thus one arena where collective efficacy is likely to matter is in the differential ability of neighborhoods to organize against local threats such as disorderly bars, licensing of new liquor stores, and the mixing of strip malls with residences and schools.

METHODOLOGICAL CHALLENGES AND
RESEARCH FRONTIERS

Despite promising leads from existing research, several limitations must be addressed if scientific knowledge on social capital and health is to progress. First, aside from the experimental designs discussed above, neighborhood research has been largely silent on the issue of differential residential selection of individuals. This selection issue raises not only a methodological challenge to causal inference but also important substantive questions about how individuals sort themselves into neighborhoods. This sorting process surely has a bearing on how social capital gets produced. Closely related is the issue of "endogeneity" bias –does social capital affect health, or does health status determine the need and capacity for a neighborhood to produce social capital?

Second, health environments are not limited to geographical communities. Families, the workplace, religious institutions, and peer groups, to name just a few, generate their own collective properties that bear on health. As noted earlier, for example, friendship ties and family social support networks have been found to promote individual health (Berkman and Syme 1979). Nor are the relevant health environments limited to urban settings and areas of disadvantage. Most of the United States' population lives in suburban areas, and the relationship of socioeconomic status and health holds at the upper end of the socioeconomic distribution as well as the lower end (Robert 1999). Yet much of the extant research literature is limited to the study of poverty in inner-city communities, underscoring the need to assess suburban and rural contexts.

Third, there is a need to further develop multi-level methodologies for contextually based research. Health data collected at nested levels of aggregation (e.g., neighborhood, city, state) pose important challenges to the standard analytic procedures that are prevalent among health researchers. In particular, the use of multi-level models has yet to fully incorporate the analysis of spatial interdependence. If social capital is a public good then there is reason to believe that its benefits may diffuse over arbitrary neighborhood boundaries. Spatial processes may also influence some health-related behaviors, such as drug use and utilization of health services. A methodological challenge is thus to integrate multi-level methods with spatial dynamics.

A fourth research frontier is to build strategies for the direct measurement of social mechanisms and collective properties hypothesized to predict health (Mayer and Jencks 1989). Raudenbush and Sampson (1999) argue that while interest in the social sciences has turned to an integrated scientific approach that emphasizes individual factors in social context, a mismatch has arisen in the quality of measures. Decades of psychometric and biological research have produced individual-level measures that often have excellent statistical properties. By contrast, much less is known about measures of ecological settings. Neighborhood-level research is dominated by poverty and other demographic characteristics drawn from census data or other government statistics that do not provide information on the collective properties of administrative units.

A major research frontier is thus methodological —the science of ecological assessment ("ecometrics") of social environments relevant to health (Raudenbush and Sampson 1999). A major component of ecometrics is the development of systematic procedures for directly measuring community social processes, such as in population-based health surveys and systematic social observation of community environments. For example, the latter approach has used videotaping techniques to capture aspects of microcommunity environments (e.g., streetblocks) that bear on health risks (e.g., garbage in the streets, public intoxication, unsafe housing). Lochner et al. (1999) suggest other inventive measures of mutual trust and social cohesion that can be obtained through direct observation, such as the proportion of gas stations that require customers to pay before they pump their gas. Field-based experimental techniques, such as dropping stamped envelopes on the street and counting how many get returned, could also be used in communities to observe collective efficacy "in action."

IMPLICATIONS AND DIRECTIONS

Consideration of the collective properties of social environments promises a deeper understanding of the etiology of health outcomes and the development of community based prevention strategies. Indeed, the health sciences can "capitalize on social capital" by thinking creatively about the implications of extant research for community-based prevention strategies. Because community contexts are important units of analysis in their own right, we suggest the need for concrete "community-level" strategies that have been neglected in the health field. We thus turn to some possible directions for future research and community intervention efforts.

Data Collection and Methodology

An important "first step" in fostering intervention from a social capital perspective would be to support the systematic collection of benchmark data on social environments that can be compared across communities (see Sampson 1999c). The goal would be to develop a standardized approach to the collection and dissemination of data that individual communities could use to evaluate where they stand in regard to national and/or regional norms. Similar to school "report cards" that are used to track the progress of educational reform, a standardized approach to assessing collective properties would eventually allow cities and local communities to gauge how well or poorly they are doing on a variety of health-related dimensions.[7]

An exemplar that might be used as a framework on which to build is the "Sustainable Seattle" project, where some 40 indicators have been collected for use as a benchmark to gauge the progress of Seattle in meeting various goals of public and civic health (Sampson 1999c). An innovative combination of archival records, census data, and surveys have been used to compile sustainability trends across five basic areas—environment (e.g., air quality), population and resources (e.g., fuel consumption), economy (e.g., housing affordability, poverty), youth and education (e.g., high school graduation, literacy), and community health (e.g., low birth weight, neighborliness). The Leaders Roundtable in Portland, Oregon has undertaken a similarly ambitious initiative (The Caring Community) that has collected data on community health using a combination of focus groups, surveys, key stakeholder interviews, and document reviews. We also noted above some strategies for new data collection involving social observation and field experiments. If measurement standards and systematic procedures at the national level could be developed, communities could then use benchmark data to develop early warning signs with respect to changes in the quality of health environments.

Alongside such data collection, there is a need for strategic investment in methodologies that are central to building an infrastructure capable of supporting the assessment and analysis of community social capital on a systematic and flexible scale. In addition to multi-level spatial methods, a practical move is to invest in Geographical Information Systems (GIS) and support the geographical linkage of ongoing data collection efforts in the health sciences. For instance, data on health outcomes can now be linked virtually in real time to address-level data bases on employment, density of liquor stores, mixed land use, and building code violations. Such "geo-coding" would support the ability to use existing health records to construct community health profiles, thereby aiding in the development of benchmark standards. A principal advantage of GIS is community profiling and the ability to overlay multiple health-related phenomena (e.g., deaths, cancer clusters, and accident hot spots) in time and space (see also below).

"Natural" Experiments

Many urban communities across the U.S. are witnessing unprecedented changes in their social environments resulting from the devolution of public housing. Especially in large cities, families are being relocated and entire housing projects are being dispersed. The quasi-experimental nature of these changes provides opportunities to learn about the connection between health outcomes

---

[7]Robert Putnam has recently proposed launching just such a benchmark survey, both nationwide and in about 40 American communities, with the goal of assessing baseline levels of social capital. The possibilities for coordinating between his and other efforts seem rich with promise.

and environmental change. We noted some early evidence on the significance of such changes, and recommend that, wherever possible, health considerations be taken into account in ongoing and new evaluations. The experimental nature of many housing-related interventions provides strategic leverage in addressing individual selection bias, hence improving our understanding of the connection between communities and health in a way not possible with passive, observational designs. By integrating "ecometric" strategies for collecting theoretically relevant data on the collective properties of social environments with the random assignment of individuals to new social contexts, researchers are in a better position to sort out selection mechanisms and social causation mechanisms in health outcomes.

Intervention

Finally, our paper implies that it is possible to focus on designing prevention strategies from the lens of research on social capital and communities. Traditional thinking about disease has emphasized behavioral change among individuals as a means to reduce disease risk. For example, smoking interventions have targeted smokers and include hypnosis, smoking cessation programs, and nicotine patches. Environmental approaches look instead to macrolevel factors such as taxation policies, regulation of smoking in public places, and restriction of advertising in places frequented by adolescents (Yen and Syme 1999). Such approaches appear to have had notable successes in reducing the aggregate level of cigarette consumption. It follows that community-level prevention that attempts to change places and social environments rather than people may yield similar payoffs that complement traditional individual and disease-specific approaches. Although scant, there is some evidence that community-based interventions may be successful in promoting prenatal health care and children's health. An evaluation by the National Academy of Sciences (1981: 58) reported that community-based interventions were significantly associated with lower rates of infant mortality and premature birth. Similarly, Wallace and Wallace (1990: 417–418) argue that governmental community intervention helped to reduce the infant mortality rate in New York from 1966 to 1973. Hence there is reason to believe that connecting health initiatives for children with strategies for community social organization is promising (Sampson 1999a).

Drawing on social capital and routine activity theory as explicated in this paper, we would argue that advances in computer mapping technology be used to promote safety by exploiting information on ecological "hot spots." In Chicago, Block (1991) pioneered the use of what is termed an "early warning system" for gang homicides. By plotting each homicide incident and using mapping and statistical clustering procedures, the early warning system allows police to identify potential neighborhood crisis areas at high risk for suffering a "spurt" of gang violence. With rapid dissemination of information, police can intervene in hot spots to quell emerging trouble. Places may also be modified or put under periodic surveillance to reduce the opportunities for trouble to occur. Sherman and colleagues (Sherman 1994; Sherman et al., 1989: 48) have reviewed "hot-spot" neighborhood interventions such as differential patrol allocations by place, selective revocation of bar licenses, and swift removal of vacant "crack" houses. The idea of hot spots suggests a neighborhood-level response that may be more effective than policies that simply target individuals or families. By responding proactively to neighborhoods and places that disproportionately generate crimes and adverse health events (e.g., high incidence of heat related deaths, alcohol fatalities), intervention strategies can more efficiently stave off "epidemics" and their spatial diffusion. Also, neighborhood strategies to monitor the ecological placements of bars, liquor stores, strip-mall shopping outlets, subway stops, and unsupervised play spaces may play an important role in controlling the distribution of high-risk situations for crimes and accidents.

Another intervention strategy implied by this paper is to foster activities and policies that directly promote social capital by encouraging community social interaction, in the hopes that it will in turn lead to greater cohesion, shared expectations, and social control. Such initiatives include both "bottom-up" and "top-down" approaches (Kawachi and Berkman 2000). Community organizing through voluntary associations is a prime example of a bottom-up approach. In the field of crime prevention, these efforts often take the form of collective surveillance programs such as neighborhood watch and citizen patrols. Unfortunately, there is no convincing evidence that attempts at informal community surveillance can successfully "implant" social organization in neighborhoods where such processes are naturally lacking, but there have also been very few rigorous evaluations of such efforts (Rosenbaum et al., 1998: 51). Social capital theory suggests that the bottom up approach would be more viable if community organizations form partnerships with other organizations both inside and outside their community (Meares and Kahan 1998).

There is some encouraging news in this regard from the evaluation of community policing interventions designed to increase the involvement of local residents, especially in those communities that have called upon faith-based organizations to be partners in the co-creation of social order (Meares and Kahan 1998). One of the major goals of community policing is for the police to act as a catalyst in sparking among residents a sense of local ownership over public space and greater activation of informal social control. An organizational strategy designed to accomplish this outcome is the "beat meeting"—regularly scheduled meetings of the police with residents of their beats. Early evidence from the Chicago Alternative Policing Strategy (CAPS) suggests that beat meetings were one of the most visible and unique features of community policing. About 25 residents and five officers attended per meeting, with attendance highest in African-American and minority neighborhoods. Skogan and Hartnett's evaluation (1997: 160) estimated that residents turned up on almost 15,000 occasions to discuss local problems with the police. To be sure, the news is not all positive. Skogan and Hartnett (1997: 125, 130) found that the police took the lead in almost all beat meetings; despite much prodding, it was difficult to sustain resident input and to induce collective problem solving among residents.

Another model for encouraging grassroots participation in community initiatives is for public health researchers to collaborate with community members and organizational representatives in all aspects of the research process, in what has become known as "community-based research" (Minkler and Wallerstein 1998; Israel et al., 1998; Wallerstein 1999). One of the core ideas of this approach is that the research process can become a vehicle through which communities empower themselves (and thus become more collectively efficacious) by promoting "the reciprocal transfer of knowledge, skills, capacity, and power" (Israel et al., 1989: 179) and by facilitating the formation of linkages between local agencies and organizations. As is the case in the crime prevention literature, there has been a shortage of high-quality evaluations of such efforts, making their success difficult to gauge even though the idea of building upon existing community resources and encouraging linkages between institutions is theoretically compelling.

In sum, community-level interventions to increase neighborhood "social capital" are hard to implement and have achieved only limited success in the areas that need them the most—poor, unstable neighborhoods with high crime rates (Hope 1996; Skogan and Hartnett 1997). Short-run interventions that try to change isolated or specific behaviors without confronting their common antecedents are also susceptible to failure. The paradox is that self-help strategies to "build community" give priority to the very activities undermined by the social isolation and spatial vulnerability of unstable and economically deprived neighborhoods (Hope 1996: 24, 51). Neglecting the spatial dynamics of neighborhood social organization and the vertical connections (or lack thereof) that residents have to extracommunity resources obscures the structural backdrop to social capital (Sampson et al., 1999; Sampson 1999a). Overall, then, social capital is at once promising and yet no panacea, and accordingly should not be uncritically adopted as an isolated intervention strategy. "Top-down" or systemic policies, such as the promotion of housing-based neighborhood stabilization, the deconcentration of poverty, code enforcement, improvement of municipal health services, and fostering the community's organizational base, need to be creatively linked to "bottom-up" strategies that involve local residents and institutions in partnership.

REFERENCES

Almgrem, Gunnar, Avery Guest, George Imerwahr, and Michael Spittel. 1998. "Joblessness, Family Disruption, and Violent Death in Chicago, 1970–1990. *Social Forces* 76: 1465–1493.

Anderson, Roger T., Paul Sorlie, Eric Backlund, Norman Johnson, and George A. Kaplan. 1997. "Mortality Effects of Community Socioeconomic Status." *Epidemiology* 8:42–47.

Astone, Nan, C. Nathanson, Robert Schoen, and Young Kim. 1999. "Family Demography, Social Theory, and Investment in Social Capital." *Population Development and Review* 25:1–31.

Bandura, Albert. 1997. *Self Efficacy: The Exercise of Control*. New York: W. H. Freeman.

Berkman, Lisa and S. L. Syme. 1979. "Social Networks, Host Resistance, and Mortality: A Nine-Year Follow-Up Study of Alameda County Residents." *American Journal of Epidemiology* 109: 186–204.

Block, Carolyn.1991. "Early Warning System for Street Gang Violence Crisis Areas: Automated Hot Spot Identification in Law Enforcement." Chicago: Illinois Criminal Justice Information Authority.

Bourdieu, Pierre. 1986. "The Forms of Capital." Pp. 241–258 in *Handbook of Theory and Research for the Sociology of Education*, edited by J. Richardson. New York: Greenwood Press.

Brooks-Gunn, Jeanne, Greg J. Duncan, and Lawrence Aber (eds.). 1997a. *Consequences of Growing up Poor*. New York: Russell Sage Foundation.

—. 1997b. *Neighborhood Poverty: Policy Implications in Studying Neighborhoods*. New York: Russell Sage Foundation.

Bursik, Robert J. and Harold Grasmick. 1993. *Neighborhoods and Crime: The Dimensions of Effective Community Control*. New York: Lexington.

Cohen, Lawrence and Marcus Felson 1979. "Social Change and Crime Rate Trends: A Routine Activity Approach." *American Sociological Review* 44: 588–608.

Coleman, James S. 1988. "Social Capital in the Creation of Human Capital." *American Journal of Sociology* 94:S95–S120.

—. 1990. *Foundations of Social Theory*. Cambridge, MA: Harvard University Press.

—. 1994. "My Vision for Sociology." *Society*.

Diehr, Paula, Thomas Koepsell, Allen Cheadle, Bruce M. Pstay, Edward Wagner, and Susan Curry. 1993. "Do Communities Differ in Health Behaviors?" *Journal of Clinical Epidemiology* 46:1141–1149.

Diez-Roux, Ana V. 1998. "Bringing Context Back into Epidemiology: Variables and Fallacies in Multilevel Analysis." *American Journal of Public Health* 88:216–222.

Diez-Roux, Ana V., Javier Nieto, Carles Muntaner, Herman A. Tyroler, George W. Comstock, Eyal Shahar, Lawton S. Cooper, Robert L. Watson, and Moyses Szklo. 1997. "Neighborhood Environments and Coronary Heart Disease: A Multilevel Analysis." *American Journal of Epidemiology* 146:48–63.

Duncan, Craig, Kelvyn Jones, and Graham Moon. 1999. "Smoking and Deprivation: Are There Neighborhood Effects?" *Social Science and Medicine* 48:497–505.

Elliott, Delbert, William Julius Wilson, David Huizinga, Robert J. Sampson, Amanda Elliott and Bruce Rankin. 1996. "Effects of Neighborhood Disadvantage on Adolescent Development." *Journal of Research in Crime and Delinquency* 33:389–426.

Faris, Robert and Warren H. Dunham. 1939 (1965, 2nd edition). *Mental Disorders in Urban Areas: An Ecological Study of Schizophrenia and Other Psychoses*. Chicago: University of Chicago Press.

Fischer, Claude. 1982. *To Dwell Among Friends: Personal Networks in Town and City*. Chicago: University of Chicago Press.

Goldberger J, Wheeler GA, Sydenstrycker E. 1920. "A Study of the Relation of Family Income and Other Economic Factors to Pellagra Incidence in Seven Cotton Mill Villages of South Carolina in 1916." *Public Health Reports* 35:2673–2714.

Gorman, Bridget K. 1999. "Racial and Ethnic Variation in Low Birthweight in the United States: Individual and Contextual Determinants." *Health and Place* 5: 195–207.

Granovetter, Mark. 1973. "The Strength of Weak Ties." *American Journal of Sociology* 78: 360–380.

Haan, Mary, George A. Kaplan, and Terry Camacho. 1987. "Poverty and Health: Prospective Evidence from Alameda County Study." *American Journal of Epidemiology* 125(6): 989–998.

Hope, Tim. 1995. "Community Crime Prevention." Pp. 21–89 in *Building a Safer Society* edited by Michael Tonry and David Farrington. Chicago: University of Chicago Press.

House, James S., Debra Umberson, and Karl R. Landis. 1988. "Structures and Processes of Social Support." *Annual Review of Sociology* 14:293–318.

Hunter, Albert. 1985. "Private, Parochial and Public Social Orders: The Problem of Crime and Incivility in Urban Communities." In *The Challenge of Social Control*, edited by Gerald Suttles and Mayer Zald. Norwood, NJ: Ablex.

Israel, Barbara A., Amy J. Schulz, Edith A. Parker, and Adam B. Becker. 1998. "Review of Community-Based Research: Assessing Partnership Approaches to Improve Public Health." *Annual Review of Public Health 19*: 173–202.

Janowitz, Morris. 1975. "Sociological Theory and Social Control." *American Journal of Sociology* 81:82–108.

Jones, Kelvyn and Craig Duncan. 1995. "Individuals and Their Ecologies: Analysing the Geography of Chronic Illness within a Multilevel Modeling Framework." *Health and Place* 1(1):27–40.

Katz, Lawrence, Jeffrey Kling, and Jeffrey Liebman. 1999. "Moving to Opportunity in Boston: Early Impacts of a Housing Mobility Program." Paper presented at the conference, "Neighborhood Effects on Low Income Families," Joint Center for Poverty Research, Northwestern University/University of Chicago, Chicago, IL.

Kawachi, Ichiro and Lisa F. Berkman. 2000. "Social Cohesion, Social Capital, and Health." In *Social Epidemiology*, edited by Lisa F. Berkman and Ichiro Kawachi. New York: Oxford University Press.

Kawachi, Ichiro, Bruce P. Kennedy, and Roberta Glass. 1999. "Social Capital and Self-Rated Health: A Contextual Analysis" *American Journal of Public Health* 89:1187–1193.

Kawachi, Ichiro, Bruce Kennedy, Kimberly Lochner, and Deborah Prothrow-Stith. 1997. "Social Capital, Income Inequality, and Mortality." *American Journal of Public Health* 87:1491–1498.

Kawachi, Ichiro. Kennedy, Bruce P. Wilkinson, Richard G. 2000. *The Society and Population Health Reader: Income Inequality and Health*. New York: The New Press.

Krieger Nancy. 1994. "Epidemiology and the Web of Causation: Has Anyone Seen the Spider?" *Social Science and Medicine* 39:887–903.

Kornhauser, Ruth. 1978. *Social Sources of Delinquency*. Chicago: University of Chicago Press.

LeClere, Felicia B., Richard G. Rogers, and Kimberley Peters. 1998. "Neighborhood Social Context and Racial Differences in Women's Heart Disease Mortality." *Journal of Health and Social Behavior* 39: 91–107.

Lochner, Kimberly, Ichiro Kawachi, and Bruce P. Kennedy. 1999. "Social Capital: A Guide To Its Measurement." *Health and Place* 5: 259–270.

Logan, John and Harvey Molotch. 1987. *Urban Fortunes: The Political Economy of Place*. Berkeley, CA: University of California Press.

Malmstrom, Marianne, Jan Sundquist, and Sven-Erik Johansson. 1999. "Neighborhood Environment and Self-Reported Health Status." *American Journal of Public Health* 89:1181–1186.

Manski, Charles. 1995. *Identification Problems in the Social Sciences*. Cambridge, MA: Harvard University Press.

Massey, Douglas S. 1996. "The Age of Extremes: Concentrated Affluence and Poverty in the Twenty-First Century." *Demography* 33:395–412.

Massey, Douglas S. and Nancy Denton. 1993. *American Apartheid: Segregation and the Making of the Underclass.* Cambridge, MA: Harvard University Press.

Mayer, Susan E. and Christopher Jencks. 1989. "Growing up in Poor Neighborhoods: How Much Does it Matter? *Science* 243:1441–1445.

Meares, Tracey and Dan Kahan. 1998. "Law and (Norms of) Order in the Inner City." *Law and Society Review* 32: 805–838.

Minkler, Meredith and Nina Wallerstein. 1988. "Improving Health through Community Organization and Community Building: A Health Education Perspective." Pp. 30–54 in *Community Organization and Community Building for Health.* New Brunswick, NJ: Rutgers University Press.

Morenoff, Jeffrey and Robert J. Sampson. 1997. "Violent Crime and the Spatial Dynamics of Neighborhood Transition: Chicago, 1970–1990." *Social Forces*, 76:31–64.

National Academy of Sciences. 1981. *Toward a National Policy for Children and Families.* Washington, D.C.: United States Government Printing Office.

O'Campo, Patricia, Xiaonan Xue, Mei-Cheng Wang, and Margaret O'Brien Caughy. 1997. "Neighborhood Risk Factors for Low Birthweight in Baltimore: A Multilevel Analysis." *American Journal of Public Health* 87:1113–1118.

Park, Robert. 1916. "The City: Suggestions for the Investigations of Human Behavior in the Urban Environment." *American Journal of Sociology* 20: 577–612.

Portes, Alejandro.1998. "Social Capital: Its Origins and Applications in Modern Sociology."*Annual Review of Sociology* 24:1–24.

Portes, Alejandro and Julia Sensenbrenner. 1993. "Embeddedness and Immigration: Notes on the Social Determinants of Economic Action." *American Journal of Sociology* 98:1320–1350.

Putnam, Robert. 1993. "The Prosperous Community: Social Capital and Community Life." *The American Prospect* (35–42).

Raudenbush, Stephen and Robert J. Sampson. 1999b. " 'Ecometrics': Toward A Science of Assessing Ecological Settings, with Application to the Systematic Social Observation of Neighborhoods." *Sociological Methodology* 29:1–41.

Robert, Stephanie. 1998. "Community-Level Socioeconomic Status Effects on Adult Health." *Journal of Health and Social Behavior* 39:18–37.

——. 1999. "Socioeconomic Position and Health: The Independent Contribution of Community Socioeconomic Context." *Annual Review of Sociology* 25:489–516.

Rosenbaum, Dennis P., Arthur J. Lurigio, and Robert C. Davis. 1998. *The Prevention of Crime: Social and Situational Strategies.* Belmont, CA: Wadsworth.

Sampson, Robert J. 1999a. "How Do Communities Undergird or Undermine Human Development? Relevant Contexts and Social Mechanisms." In *Does It Take a Village? Community Effects on Children, Adolescents, and Families*, edited by Alan Booth and Nan Crouter. Mahwah, New Jersey: Lawrence Erlbaum. In press.

——. 1999b. "Crime and Public Safety: Insights from Community-Level Perspectives on Social Capital." Paper prepared for the Ford Foundation conference on "Social Capital and Poor Communities: Building and Using Social Capital to Combat Poverty," New York City, March 11–13th, 1999.

——. 1999c. "Collective Properties and Healthy Communities." Draft chapter for the National Academy of Sciences, Panel on "Future Directions of Social and Behavioral Sciences Research at the National Institutes of Health." Burton Singer, Chair. Washington, D.C.: National Academy of Sciences.

Sampson, Robert J., Stephen Raudenbush, and Felton Earls. 1997. "Neighborhoods and Violent Crime: A Multilevel Study of Collective Efficacy." *Science* 277:918–924.

Sampson Robert J. Jeffrey Morenoff, and Felton Earls. 1999. "Beyond Social Capital: Spatial Dynamics of Collective Efficacy for Children." *American Sociological Review* 64:633–660.

Sandefur, Rebecca and Edward O. Laumann. 1998. "A Paradigm for Social Capital." *Rationality and Society* 10:481–501.

Schwartz S. 1994. "The Fallacy of the Ecological Fallacy: The Potential Misuse of a Concept and the Consequences." *American Journal of Public Health* 84(5):819–824.

Schwartz, S., E. Susser, and M. Susser. 1999. "A Future for Epidemiology?" *Annual Review of Public Health* 20:15–33.

Shaw, Clifford, and Henry McKay. 1942. (2nd edition, 1969). *Juvenile Delinquency and Urban Areas*. Chicago: University of Chicago Press.

Sherman, Lawrence. 1995. "The Police." In *Crime,* edited by J. Q. Wilson and J. Petersilia. San Francisco, CA: ICS Press.

Sherman, Lawrence, Patrick Gartin, and M. Buerger. 1989. "Hot Spots of Predatory Crime: Routine Activities and the Criminology of Place." *Criminology* 27: 27–56.

Skogan, Wesley and Susan Hartnett. 1997. *Community Policing, Chicago Style*. New York: Oxford University Press.

Shy, C.M. 1997. "The Failure of Academic Epidemiology: Witness for the Prosecution." *American Journal of Epidemiology*. 145: 479–487.

Sooman, Anne and Sally Macintyre. 1995. "Health Perceptions of the Local Environment in Socially Contrasting Neighbourhoods in Glasgow.' " *Health and Place* 1(1):15–26.

Susser, Mervyn. 1994a. "The Logic in Ecological: I. The Logic of Analysis." *American Journal of Public Health* 84:825–829.

Susser, Mervyn. 1994b. "The Logic in Ecological: II. The Logic of Design." *American Journal of Public Health* 84:830–835.

Wallace, Rodrick and Deborah Wallace. 1990. "Origins of Public Health Collapse in New York City: The Dynamics of Planned Shrinkage, Contagious Urban Decay and Social Disintegration." *Bulletin of the New York Academy of Medicine* 66(5): 391–434

Wallerstein, Nina. 1999. "Power between Evaluator and Community: Research Relationships within New Mexico's Healthier Communities." *Social Science and Medicine* 49(1): 39–53.

Wilson, William Julius. 1987. *The Truly Disadvantaged: The Inner City, the Underclass, and Public Policy*. Chicago: University of Chicago Press.

—. 1996. *When Work Disappears*. New York: Knopf.

Woolcock, Michael. 1998. "Social Capital and Economic Development: Toward a Theoretical.Synthesis and Policy Framework." *Theory and Society* 27:151–208.

Yen, Irene H. and S.L. Syme. 1999. "The Social Environment and Health: A Discussion of the Epidemiologic Literature." *Annual Review of Public Health* 20: 287–308.

Yen, Irene H. and George Kaplan. 1999a. "Poverty Area Residence and Changes in Depression and Perceived Health Status: Evidence from the Alameda County Study." *International Journal of Epidemiology* 28: 90–94.

—. 1999b. "Neighborhood Social Environment and Risk of Death: Multilevel Evidence from the Alameda County Study." *International Journal of Epidemiology* 28: 90 94.

PAPER CONTRIBUTION J
Legal and Public Policy Interventions to Advance the Population's Health

Lawrence O. Gostin, J.D., LL.D (Hon.)[1]

Government has a number of "levers" at its disposal to try to prevent injury and disease and promote the population's health.[2] Laws and regulations, like other prevention strategies, can intervene at a variety of levels, each designed to secure safer behavior among the population—individual behavior, agents of behavior change, and the environment (Haddon et al., 1964; Institute of Medicine, 1999).

First, government interventions are aimed at *individual behavior*—through education, incentives, or deterrence. For example, health communications campaigns educate and persuade people to make healthier choices; taxing and spending powers discourage risk behaviors or encourage healthy activities; and police powers deter risk behaviors by imposing civil and criminal penalties. Second, the law regulates the *agents of behavior change* by requiring safer product design. For example, government regulates unsafe products directly by requiring safety features or indirectly through the tort system. Finally, the law

---

[1]Dr. Gostin is professor of law, Georgetown University; professor of public health, The Johns Hopkins University; and codirector, Georgetown/Johns Hopkins Program on Law and Public Health. This paper was prepared for the symposium "Capitalizing on Social Science and Behavioral Research to Improve the Public's Health," the Institute of Medicine, and the Commission on Behavioral and Social Sciences and Education of the National Research Council, Atlanta, Georgia, February 2–3, 2000.

[2]While the emphasis here will be on "public policy" interventions undertaken by government, the analogous role that can be served by other large institutions, such as employers and health care organizations, should not be overlooked.

alters the *informational, physical, social, or economic environment* to facilitate safer behavior. For example, government demands accurate labeling and instructions or restricts commercial advertising of hazardous products; enacts housing and building codes to prevent injury and disease; and regulates the environment in diverse ways.

Despite the importance of legislation and regulation to promote the public's health, the effectiveness of government interventions is poorly understood. In particular, policy makers often cannot answer important empirical questions—do legal interventions work and at what economic and social cost? Policy makers need to know if legal interventions achieve their intended goals (e.g., reducing risk behavior). If so, do legal interventions unintentionally increase other risks ("risk–risk" trade-offs)?[3] Similarly, cost is important because, if legal interventions are very expensive, they can reduce opportunities to spend those resources in more effective ways.

Policy makers need to understand not only the cost or effectiveness of an intervention, but also the burdens it imposes on individuals and groups. Public health regulations can intrude on personal interests, economic interests, and the rights of minorities. Some public health regulations affect personal interests in autonomy, privacy, expression, or liberty. Other regulations affect economic interests in property and, more generally, dampen economic development. Still other regulations are unjust because they disproportionately burden vulnerable groups such as the poor and racial minorities. The laws themselves may be unfair or they may be enforced selectively and in a discriminatory manner. These intrusive regulations should concern us not only because freedom has intrinsic value in our democracy, but because denial of human rights can undermine public health efforts (Mann et al., 1994). Even detriments to professional opportunities and economic prosperity can have health effects. Researchers, for example, have long understood the positive correlation between socioeconomic status and health (DHHS, 1991).

In this paper, I first examine legal interventions as a tool in achieving the public's health and safety. Here, I present five models of public health regulation: (1) economic incentives and disincentives (taxing and spending powers); (2) the informational environment (education, labeling, and commercial speech regulation); (3) direct regulation (penalties for engaging in risk behavior); (4) indirect regulation (the tort system); and (5) deregulation (dismantling legal barriers to desired public health behaviors). In relation to each of these five models, I explore the trade-offs entailed between advancing the population's health and invading private rights and interests. Second, I examine the empirical question, do legal interventions work? Here, I present data from two of the most studied areas of intervention—one involving disease control (cigarettes) and the other

---

[3]Consider one study reporting that helmet laws reduce the use of bicycles: The benefits of cycling, even without a helmet, have been estimated to outweigh the hazards by a factor of 20 to 1. Consequently, a helmet law, whose most notable effect was to reduce cycling, may have generated a net loss of health benefits to the nation." (Robinson, 1996).

injury control (automobile crashes). I also examine some of the methodological problems that thwart many evaluations of law reform, as well as the striking absence of systematic research evaluating the large majority of legal interventions. Finally, I draw some conclusions about the use of the law as a tool for achieving public health goals. How important is the law, what risks are entailed in legal strategies, and how can legal interventions best be used in combination with other public health strategies?

LAW AS A TOOL FOR ACHIEVING THE PUBLIC'S HEALTH AND SAFETY

Elsewhere, I define public health law as the study of the legal powers and duties of the state to assure the conditions for people to be healthy and the limits on that power to constrain the liberty or property of individuals for protection or promotion of community health (Gostin, 2000). Through this definition, I suggest five essential characteristics of public health law: (1) *government* has the responsibility to advance the public's health; (2) *populations* are the main focus of public health interventions; (3) *relationships* are primarily between the state and the population; (4) *services* meet the needs of populations and are grounded in scientific methodologies; and (5) *coercion* of individuals and businesses may be necessary for the protection of the community.

If government has an obligation to assure the conditions for the population's health, what tools are available to accomplish that task? Here, I present five regulatory models intended to demonstrate the breadth and importance of legal and public policy interventions to advance the public's health. Public health interventions, however, are not an inherent good. More often than not, when government acts to promote the population's health it undermines an important private right or interest. In this section, I also explore the trade-offs between the common good and private interests in liberty and property.

Model One: Economic Incentives and Disincentives— Taxing and Spending Powers

The government has a number of powers at its disposal to create potent incentives or disincentives for changing the behavior of individuals and businesses—the power to tax and spend. By Article I, Section 8 of the Constitution, "Congress shall have Power To lay and collect Taxes . . . and provide for the common Defence and general Welfare of the United States." State constitutions provide similar taxing and spending powers. On its face, the power to tax and spend has a single, overriding purpose—to raise revenue and allocate resources to provide for the good of the community. Absent the ability to generate sufficient revenue, the legislature could not provide services such as education, medical services to the poor, sanitation, and environmental protection.

The taxing power, while affording government the financial resources to provide public health services, has another, equally important, purpose. The power to tax is also the power to regulate risk behavior and influence health-promoting activities. Virtually all taxes achieve ancillary regulatory effects by imposing an economic burden on the taxed activity or providing economic relief for certain kinds of private spending. Consequently, the tax code provides incentives and disincentives to perform, or to refrain from performing, certain acts.

Through various forms of tax relief (e.g., excluding benefits from taxable income, deducting spending from gross income, and providing credits against tax owed), government provides incentives for private activities that it views as advantageous to community health. Employer-sponsored health plans, for example, receive generous tax incentives that "deeply [affect] how health care is provided in the United States, to whom it is provided, and who provides it." (Fox and Schaffer, 1987, p. 610). The tax code influences private health-related spending in many other ways: encouraging child care to enable parents to enter the work force; inducing investment in low-income housing; and stimulating charitable spending for research and care.

Public health taxation also regulates private behavior by economically penalizing risk-taking activities. Tax policy discourages a number of activities that government regards as unhealthy or dangerous. Consider excise or manufacturing taxes on tobacco and alcoholic beverages. Tax policy also influences individual and business decisions that adversely affect human health or the environment, such as taxes on gasoline or on ozone-depleting chemicals that contribute to environmental degradation. It is difficult to imagine a public health threat caused by human behavior or business activity that cannot be influenced by the taxing power.

While many Americans resent the use of government taxing power, they generally understand its importance in a good society. Still, high taxation of inherently dangerous products such as cigarettes and alcoholic beverages is not universally supported. On one level, businesses and consumers denounce increased taxation of hazardous products as they would any tax—liberal government overreaching and economically burdening the population. To some, excessive taxation of lawful conduct represents government intrusion into the private sphere, where individuals should be permitted to make free, autonomous choices. To others, the taxation itself appears regressive because the poorer and working classes disproportionately engage in the taxed behavior.

A high tax on cigarettes, for example, is widely supported by public health professionals because it provides a disincentive to smoking. Taxation may reduce smoking particularly among young people whose demand for the product is elastic. The cigarette tax, however, is burdensome. It may compel individuals to pay a "health tax" on a behavior that is addictive and, to a certain extent, beyond the person's control. More importantly, the tax is highly regressive because most adults who smoke are in lower socioeconomic classes.

The power to spend is closely aligned with the power to tax. Economists regard legislative decisions to provide tax relief for certain activities as indirect expenditures because government is, in fact, subsidizing the activity from the national treasury. Economists project, for example, that favorable tax treatment afforded to employer-sponsored health care plans will cost the federal government $438 billion between 1999 and 2003 (OMB, 1998).

The spending power does not simply grant legislatures the authority to allocate resources; it is also an indirect regulatory device. Congress may prescribe the terms upon which it disburses federal money to the states. The conditional spending power is akin to a contract: in return for federal funds, the states agree to comply with federally imposed conditions.[4] For example, in the mid-1980s, Congress appropriated highway funds on the condition that states adopt a 21-year-old minimum drinking age. Since a major purpose of highway funds is traffic safety, the Supreme Court upheld this public health measure.[5]

Congress' power to set the terms upon which state appropriations shall be distributed is an effective regulatory device. States and localities can seldom afford to decline public health grants. Congress and the federal agencies use conditional appropriations to induce states to conform to federal standards in numerous public health contexts. Federal funding programs for AIDS/HIV, for example, require involuntary postconviction testing of sex offenders, adoption of Centers for Disease Control and Prevention (CDC) guidelines for HIV counseling and testing of pregnant women, and compliance with specific community planning and program priorities. Conditional spending induces states to conform to federal regulatory requirements in other areas as well: eligibility and quality standards relating to Medicare and Medicaid, prohibition on recipients of family-planning funds from engaging in abortion counseling, and state and local planning for land use and solid waste management.

The federal government and the states also award grants and contracts to individuals and groups in the private and charitable sectors. These awards frequently contain conditions that require individuals to refrain from, or conform with, specific behavior. For example, the Supreme Court upheld a federal regulation that prohibited recipients of federal family-planning funds from providing abortion counseling or referrals.[6]

It is obvious that the power to tax and spend is not value neutral, but rather laden with political overtones. Collection of revenues and allocation of resources go to the very heart of the political process. Legislators, as influenced by the public and interest groups, purport to promote the public's health, safety, and security. Many of their economic decisions do promote the common welfare, such as taxes on cigarettes and expenditures for antismoking campaigns. But their vision is also influenced by moral, social, and cultural values so that government's economic power may be used to discourage fetal research, sex educa-

---

[4]*Pennhurst State School and Hospital* v. *Halderman,* 451 U.S. 1, 17 (1981).
[5]*South Dakota* v. *Dole,* 483 U.S. 203 (1987).
[6]*Rust* v. *Sullivan,* 500 U.S. 173 (1991).

tion, or needle exchange. The power to tax and spend, then, may be used to impede, as well as to promote, legitimate public health goals.

Model Two: Informational Environment—Education, Labeling, and Commercial Speech

The field of public health is deeply concerned with the communication of ideas. Human behavior is a powerful contributor to injury and disease, so government strives to influence behavioral choices. Public health authorities understand that many factors influence behavior, but information is a prerequisite for change. The population must at least be aware of the health consequences of risk behaviors to make informed decisions. The citizenry is bombarded with behavioral messages that affect its health—by the media and entertainment, trade associations and corporations, religious and civic organizations, and family and peers. Public health authorities strive to be heard above the din of conflicting and confusing communications. Consequently, the field of public health is a virtual battleground of ideas. Consider the controversy surrounding the Office of Drug Policy's approving scripts in lieu of public service announcements on prime-time programming. While many people would applaud the government's attempts to promote antidrug messages, they might object to the deceptive manner in which those messages are conveyed.

Public health agencies deliver messages to promote healthy behavior and restrict messages that encourage risktaking. Health authorities exert influence on behavior at various levels of intervention: at the individual level, they counsel individuals at risk for injury and disease (e.g., HIV prevention, genetic disease, or reproductive choice); at the group level, they inform and promote behavior change (e.g., hospital or health maintenance organizations [HMO] newsletters, support groups for stress reduction, or smoking cessation); at the population level, they educate the public and market healthy life-styles (e.g., health communication campaigns or school-based health education).

We like to think that public health's concern with "healthy messages" is an inherent good, and we are prepared to give government considerable leeway in constructing a "favorable" informational environment. But the concern of public health authorities with health, communication, and behavior conflicts with other important social values. When public health authorities counsel individuals or educate groups or populations about the government's view concerning unsafe sex, abortion, smoking, a high-fat diet, or a sedentary life-style, there is no formal coercion. Yet education conveys more than information; it is also a process of inculcation and acculturation intended to change behavior. Even though they are not always particularly adept or successful, public health authorities routinely construct social norms or meanings to achieve healthier populations. Not everyone believes that public funds should be expended, or the veneer of government legitimacy used, to prescribe particular social orthodoxies (Lessig, 1995).

No matter how much government educates the public, it is bound to have difficulty changing risk behaviors. The reason is that the private sector has a strong economic interest in influencing consumer preferences. Advertising commands ever-increasing resources and engenders ever more creative approaches to stimulate consumer demands. As a result, government regulation of commercial speech is an important strategy to safeguard consumer health and safety. First, government is concerned with advertising that increases use of hazardous products and services such as cigarettes, alcoholic beverages, firearms, and gambling. For example, advertisements extol the virtues of handguns for home defense and safety, despite scientific evidence of increased risk of suicide, domestic violence, and unintended death (Vernick et al., 1997). Second, government is concerned with marketing "age-restricted" products to children and adolescents. For example, the Distilled Spirits Council lifted its 48-year-old voluntary ban on liquor advertising on radio and television, prompting concern about the targeting of young people (Elliott, 1996). Third, government is concerned with industry health claims that mislead the public. For example, government actively reviews food and dietary supplement labels[7] and direct-to-consumer pharmaceutical marketing for unsubstantiated health claims. Regulation of commercial speech is becoming even more challenging as government monitors Internet marketing of the sale of hazardous products or the expression of deceptive health messages.

Government regulation of commercial speech raises profound social and constitutional questions. Substantial public health benefits can be achieved by reducing risk behavior, but regulation of communications can stifle freedom of expression. Nominally, the Supreme Court affords commercial speech "lower-value" constitutional protection than social or political discourse.[8] But in reality, the level of scrutiny for commercial speech has changed over the years and the modern Court steadfastly defends truthful, nonmisleading advertisements. Most public health advocates argue that advertisements that associate hazardous products with glamorous, adventuresome, sexy life-styles are, in fact, misleading. But the Court has not viewed mere "puffery" as inherently misleading and appears to prefer to have consumers make the decisions for themselves.

Perhaps more importantly, the Court is insisting that the government must demonstrate, most probably with credible evidence, that the regulation will, in fact, achieve the asserted public health goal and not be an "ineffective" or "remote" method.[9] This standard demands an empirical response. Absent careful research into the effectiveness of commercial speech regulation, this form of

---

[7]Compare *Nutritional Health Alliance* v. *Shalala,* 144 F.3d 220 (2d Cir.), *cert. denied,* 119 S. Ct. 589 (1998) (upholding Food and Drug Administration [FDA] requirement for prior approval of health claims on dietary supplement labels because of health and safety risk) with *Pearson* v. *Shalala,* 164 F.3d 650, denying petition for rehearing *en banc,* 172 F.3d 72 (D.C. Cir. 1999) (invalidating same regulation because FDA was required to consider whether inclusion of appropriate disclaimers would negate potentially misleading health claims).

[8]*Central Hudson Gas* v. *Public Service Commission,* 447 U.S. 557, 563 (1980).

[9]*44 Liquormart, Inc.* v. *Rhode Island,* 517 U.S. 484 (1996).

public health intervention may be found unconstitutional by the Supreme Court.[10]

Model Three: Direct Regulation—Penalties for Engaging in Risk Behavior

Public health authorities have the power to set health and safety standards as well as to monitor compliance and punish noncompliance. Monitoring activities include injury and disease surveillance, screening individuals for disease and reporting positive cases to health authorities, and inspecting commercial premises. Government can directly prohibit behavior (e.g., exceeding highway speed limits) or require individual behavior (e.g., wearing seatbelts); mandate businesses to alter product designs to promote safety (e.g., air bags in automobiles, trigger locks on firearms, safety caps on medicines); or modify sales practices (e.g., sale of cigarettes or alcoholic beverages to children). In the area of infectious diseases, government can compel vaccination, treatment, or isolation.

The state's authority to monitor, prohibit, or mandate behavior is derived from the "police power"—the most famous expression of the natural authority of sovereign governments. The police power is the state's inherent authority to regulate private interests to protect, preserve, and promote the health, safety, morals, and general welfare of the people. To achieve these communal benefits, the state retains the power to restrict—within federal and state constitutional limits—private interests.

In the foundational case of *Jacobson v. Massachusetts*, the Supreme Court explained its early twentieth century community-oriented philosophy: "There are manifold restraints to which every person is necessarily subject for the common good. On any other basis organized society could not exist with safety to its members... A fundamental principle of the social compact is that the people covenant that each citizen shall be governed by certain laws for the common good, and that government is instituted for the common good, for the protection, safety, prosperity and happiness of the people."[11]

Despite the undoubted police power authority of government to act for the welfare of society, there are constitutional limits beyond which it cannot go. Every measure that sets health and safety standards, monitors compliance and punishes noncompliance, creates individual burdens. Surveillance (i.e., government collection of personal health data) affects privacy; compulsory screening affects autonomy; mandatory treatment affects bodily integrity; isolation affects liberty. Commercial regulation also affects proprietary interests. Licenses affect professional opportunities, while inspections and nuisance abatements affect

---

[10]*Greater New Orleans Broadcasting Association* v. *United States,* 119 S. Ct. 1923 (1999).
[11]197 U.S. 11, 26–27 (1905).

property rights. These trade-offs "between public goods and private interests" are highly complex and politically contested in a constitutional democracy.

Perhaps the most controversial area of police power regulation is the control of so-called self-regarding behavior—that is, behavior that risks primarily the health or safety of the individual concerned. Classical regulation of self-regarding behavior includes mandatory motorcycle helmet and seatbelt use, as well as gambling prohibitions. From the public health perspective, these kinds of laws are justified because they reduce behavioral risks, thereby improving the population's health and longevity. At the same time, many argue that individuals should have the right to make their own decisions about behaviors that primarily affect themselves. After all, a person declines to wear a motorcycle helmet not because he or she is oblivious to the risk, but presumably because that person places one value (freedom) above another (physical security). There is a special resistance to regulation that involves government controlling how people behave when they pose little public risk.

Court decisions usually support regulation of self-regarding behavior, but often reduce the justification to a strained conception of social harms rather than recognizing certain public health interventions as justified paternalism. Consider one state court's justification for motorcycle helmet regulation: "From the moment of the [motorcycle] injury, society picks the person up off the highway, delivers him to a municipal hospital, and provides him with unemployment compensation . . . We do not understand a state of mind that permits plaintiff to think that only he himself is concerned."[12]

If public health authorities continue to press for regulation of self-regarding behavior, it will certainly be important to be able to point to empirical evidence of effectiveness in reducing harms within the population.

Model Four: Indirect Regulation—The Tort System

The foregoing methods of regulation are comprised principally of actions taken by legislatures and administrative agencies to prevent injury or disease or to promote public health. The creation of private rights of action in the courts can also be an effective means of public health regulation (Jacobson and Warner, 1999). Perhaps the most important form of civil litigation for public health purposes can be found in tort law to redress harms to people and the environment they inhabit.

A tort is a civil, noncontractual wrong for which an injured person or group of persons seeks a remedy in the form of monetary damages. Tort law, then, characteristically is a private, rather than a public, right of action, a civil rather than a criminal proceeding; it remedies a wrong by awarding monetary damages rather than an injunction or civil or criminal penalties. Tort law is comprised of

---

[12]*Simon* v. *Sargent,* 346 F.Supp. 277, 279 (D. Mass. 1972).

a series of related doctrines that impose civil liability upon persons or businesses whose (usually) substandard conduct causes injury or disease.

The functions, or goals, of tort law—although highly controversial and imperfectly achieved—are the (1) assignment of *responsibility* to individuals or businesses that impose unreasonable risks, causing injury or disease; (2) *compensation* of persons for loss caused by the conduct of individuals or businesses; (3) *deterrence* of unreasonably hazardous conduct; and (4) encouragement of *innovation* in product design, packaging, labeling, and advertising to reduce the risk of injury or disease. In thinking about tort law as a tool of public health, it is important to emphasize the role of litigation in preventing risk behavior and providing incentives for safer product design.

There exists a vast potential for using tort litigation as an effective tool to reduce the burden of injury and disease. Attorneys general, public health authorities, and private citizens resort to civil litigation to redress many different kinds of public health harms: environmental damage or exposure to toxic substances; unsafe pharmaceuticals or vaccines; and hazardous products such as tobacco, firearms, or alcoholic beverages.

Private citizens, as well as government officials, have adopted a civil litigation strategy in two highly publicized public health contexts—cigarettes and firearms. In the context of cigarettes, lawsuits have been filed by private litigants, populations of smokers (class actions), and government entities (medical reimbursement suits) (Gostin et al., 1991; Daynard and Kelder, 1998). For example, in November 1998, a Settlement Agreement between tobacco companies and 46 states required industry to compensate states in perpetuity, with payments totaling $206 billion through the year 2025. The agreement also restricted outdoor advertising, the use of cartoon characters, tobacco merchandising, and sponsorship of sporting events. In exchange, the industry received civil immunity for future state claims, but not for individual or class action lawsuits.[13]

Thus far, litigants have not been as successful in firearm litigation. Most firearm design defect cases fail because courts rule that consumers have a "reasonable expectation" that firearms will be dangerous.[14] Firearm risks, for the most part, are open and obvious, and consumers do not require expert knowledge to assess the risks.[15] Firearms, moreover, are in "common use." If they are functioning properly, they may be exempt from strict liability based on the the-

---

[13]Master Settlement Agreement, http://www.tobaccoresolution.com/msa.html.

[14]See, for example, *Richman* v. *Charter Arms Corp.,* 571 F. Supp. 192 (E.D.La. 1983) (criminal use of handgun was a "normal" use and marketing to the public was not an "unreasonably dangerous activity").

[15]See, for example, *Perkins* v. *F.I.E. Corp.,* 762 F.2d 1250 (5th Cir. 1985), *reh=g. denied en banc,* 768 F.2d 1350 (where guns functioned as designed and dangers were obvious and well known, strict liability was not an available remedy).

ory that they are "good" (well-made) guns.[16] Nevertheless, recent litigation has followed the model used against cigarette manufacturers. Many cities (e.g., New Orleans and Chicago) have filed, or intend to file, tort actions against the gun industry (Kairys, 1998). The city lawsuits proceed on different theories of recovery including product liability theory[17] and public nuisance theory claiming that industry marketing practices encourage movement of firearms into the possession of criminals.[18]

Tobacco and firearm litigation strategies are premised on the theory that these industries have made conscious choices that increase disease, injury, and death, particularly among children and adolescents. Tort litigation is seen as one strategy, among many, to encourage safer design, greater disclosure, and reduced consumption of potentially hazardous products. Whether tort law can achieve all of these public health goals is uncertain. Litigation is still languishing in the terrain of personal responsibility—the idea that it is not the manufacturer of the product that creates harm, but the user. It is in this regard that the emerging tort strategy of government lawsuits has advantages over individual tort actions. Governments have the resources to engage in mass litigation and seek damages incurred collectively by taxpayers. Furthermore, a manufacturer cannot attribute blame for harm to government entities the way it can on those who purchase and use hazardous products. Finally, discovery powers in civil litigation may provide needed evidence about the industries' intentions in design, promotion, and sale.

Like other forms of regulation, the tort system does not achieve only socially desirable results. Tort costs (liability and litigation expenses) have potentially detrimental effects that warrant consideration. Tort costs are absorbed by the enterprise, which will often pass the costs onto its employees or consumers through loss of employment (or benefits of employment such as wages or health insurance) and/or higher prices. Since socioeconomic status has important health effects, lower employment or wages and higher consumer prices are important from a public health perspective. Tort costs may be, or may be perceived to be, so high that businesses leave the market or curtail research and development. Society, it may be argued, would not be any the poorer if tort costs made it difficult for dangerous enterprises (e.g., tobacco and firearms) to operate within the market. Tort costs, however, appear to be just as high for socially advantageous goods and services such as drugs, vaccines, and medical devices. While it is in

---

[16]See, for example, *Moore* v. *R.G. Indus., Inc.*, 789 F.2d 1326 (9th Cir. 1986) (strict liability not imposed on manufacturer of .25 caliber automatic handgun for injuries to woman shot by her husband since product "performed as intended").

[17]*Morial* v. *Smith and Wesson, et al.*, Civ. Action No. 98-18578 (Civ. Dist. Parish of New Orleans, filed October 30, 1998).

[18]*Chicago* v. *Beretta U.S.A. Corp., et al.*, No. 98 CH 15596 (Cook County Cir. Ct., Ill., filed November 12, 1998).

society's interest to encourage safety in the production of health-related products and services, overdeterrence may deter investment and innovation.

Model Five: Deregulation—Provide the Means for Behavior Change

Statutes and regulations may actually impede the achievement of public health objectives, and the necessary social response is to deregulate. Sometimes policy makers enact laws that criminalize or otherwise penalize provision of, or access to, the means for achieving behavior change. Consider government regulation designed to impede access to sterile syringes and needles even though public health authorities recommend their use to reduce transmission of blood-borne diseases such as HIV and HBV (hepatitis B virus). At least three kinds of statutes and regulations impede access to sterile drug injection equipment (Gostin and Lazzarini, 1997; Gostin, 1998).

Virtually all states have *drug paraphernalia statutes* that ban the manufacture, sale, distribution, possession, or advertisement of a wide range of devices, including syringes, if it is known that they may be used to introduce illicit substances into the body. It is not an offense under these statutes to sell or distribute syringes without knowledge that they will be used to inject illicit drugs. Thus, a pharmacist who sells syringes over the counter, believing they will be used for a lawful purpose such as to treat diabetes with insulin, commits no offense under drug paraphernalia laws. Most state statutes are based on the Model Drug Paraphernalia Act (DEA, 1991); the federal government also has enacted the Federal Mail Order Drug Paraphernalia Control Act that prohibits the sale and transportation of drug paraphernalia, including syringes, in interstate commerce.[19]

A minority of states (mostly in the Northeast corridor) have *syringe prescription statutes* that prohibit the dispensing or possession of syringes without a valid medical prescription. Prescription statutes differ from drug paraphernalia laws in that criminal intent is not required for a violation. The pharmacist dispensing a syringe without a prescription in a jurisdiction with a prescription law does not have to be aware that the buyer intends to use it to administer illegal drugs; the act of selling or dispensing the syringe without a prescription is itself a violation. In this sense, prescription laws have the potential to encompass many more transactions than paraphernalia laws.

The government also uses its spending powers to restrict access to sterile injection equipment. Since 1988, Congress has enacted statutes that contain provisions prohibiting or restricting the use of federal funds for syringe exchange programs (SEPs). The U.S. General Accounting Office concluded that the Department of Health and Human Services (DHSS) is authorized to conduct demonstration and research projects involving the provision of syringes, but is prohibited from using certain funds to support SEPs directly, which may prevent

---

[19]21 USC §857, reenacted 21 USC §863 (1990).

DHSS from funding ancillary support services provided by SEPs. Accordingly, SEPs must rely on state, local, or philanthropic funds for their operational activities, which is problematic given their uncertain legal status (GAO, 1993).

Under current law, before the federal government can fund SEPs, the Secretary of Health and Human Services must find that the programs effectively prevent the spread of HIV and do not encourage the use of illegal drugs. The National Research Council (1995) recommended that the Surgeon General make such a determination, and a National Institutes of Health (1997) consensus panel concurred. Nevertheless, the Secretary, while acknowledging that SEPs are effective, did not permit the use of federal funding.

Taken together, these laws and funding restrictions, make it difficult (but not impossible) for public health agencies and community groups to operate needle exchange programs in many states (Burris et al., 1996; Paone et al., 1999). They also make it difficult for injection drug users to reliably purchase sterile equipment in pharmacies (Case et al., 1998). There have been numerous research studies evaluating the effectiveness of deregulation of drug injection equipment. While the evidence for reduction of hepatitis B and hepatitis—is mixed (Hagan et al., 1999), most studies show that SEPs (Heimer, 1998; Heimer et al., 1998; Vlahov and Junge, 1998) and pharmacy access to syringes (Singer et al., 1998) reduce the incidence of HIV. In October 1999, the American Medical Association and many other national public health organizations sent a joint letter to the states urging the removal of legal penalties for possession of syringes that discourage injection drug users from carrying syringes and contribute to increased risk behaviors (AMA et al., 1999).

It is important to emphasize that the position of elected officials in these areas is not irrational. Rather, these officials, sensitive to the desires of many constituents, prefer one value (discouraging drug use) over another value (public health). Empirical evidence may help inform public policy in this controversy as well. It ought to be a "testable" proposition to inquire whether support for SEPs actually facilitates drug use. Most public health authorities believe that there is no relationship between access to syringes and greater drug use (AMA et al., 1999).

Empirical Evaluations of Public Health Regulation: Do Legal Interventions Work?

The five models of public health regulation just described are all highly complex, involving trade-offs between competing public goods as well as conflicting public and private interests. As the experience with drug injection equipment shows, politicians do not uniformly follow evidence of effectiveness because there exist many different values involved in policy making. Nevertheless, policy makers cannot even begin to assess the importance of public health regulation unless they have the benefit of impartial and rigorous research assessments. If policy makers are to support regulation they need to justify that decision by the probable achievement of an important public health objective.

Despite its importance, legal interventions often are not subjected to rigorous research evaluation. Part of the reason for the absence of systematic evaluative research is that universities do not always train investigators to evaluate legal interventions. Further, research in this area is not adequately funded. Finally, policy makers do not always understand the need for research. Many regulatory approaches have been in place for so long that they are simply presumed to be effective.

Just as important is the fact that evaluations of legal interventions face daunting methodological challenges. There exist so many variables that can affect behaviors (e.g., changes in the informational, physical, social, and cultural environment) that it can be extraordinarily difficult to demonstrate scientifically a causal relationship between the intervention and the perceived health effect (Flay and Cook, 1990). Consider the methodological constraints in identifying the causal effects of specific laws designed to reduce driving while under the influence of alcoholic beverages. Several different kinds of laws may be enacted within a short period of time, making it hard to isolate the effect of each law; publicity about the problem and the legal response may cross state borders, making state comparisons more difficult; people who drive under the influence may also engage in other risky driving behaviors (e.g., speeding, failing to wear safety belts, and running red lights), so that researchers need to control for changes in other highway safety laws and traffic law enforcement; and treatment and control communities may differ in unanticipated ways (Hingson, 1996; DeJong and Hingson, 1998).

Despite these challenges (relating to training, funding, and methodology), social science researchers have studied a number of discrete legal interventions, often with encouraging results. The following review of the social and behavioral science literature is not intended to be systematic, but does illustrate two important points. Firstly, legal interventions can be an essential part of a comprehensive strategy to influence behaviors desirable for the public health; and secondly, social and behavioral science research is pivotally important in evaluating the effectiveness and costs of legal interventions.

Of course, not only is research important in evaluating existing legislation; it is also important in helping policy makers to decide whether to enact legislation. Without adequate data, policy makers cannot make informed judgments about the need for, or importance of, legislation. For example, surveillance data demonstrated that increasing the minimum age for alcohol purchases from 18 to 21 resulted in fewer teenage traffic fatalities (Cook and Tauchen, 1984; GAO, 1987). These research findings were instrumental in influencing the Congress to enact legislation requiring states to adopt a 21-year-old drinking age as a condition for the receipt of federal highway funds (Wagenaar, 1993). All states currently have a 21-year-old drinking age, which is credited with saving many lives (NHTSA, 1996).

The social science, medical, and behavioral literature contains evaluations of interventions in a number of subject areas, particularly in relation to injury prevention (Rivara, 1997a,b; IOM, 1999). For example, studies have evaluated the effectiveness of regulation to prevent head injuries (bicycle helmets: Lund et al., 1991; Dannenberg et al., 1993; Kraus et al., 1994; Thompson et al., 1996a,b; Ni et al., 1997; Rivara et al., 1998), choking and suffocation (refrigerator disposal and warning labels on thin plastic bags: Kraus, 1985), child poisoning (childproof packaging: Rogers, 1996), and burns (tap water: Erdmann et al., 1991). The regulatory measures that have received a great deal of attention include reduction in cigarettes and motor vehicle crashes. Funding agencies and researchers should give much greater attention to systematic evaluation in other areas of governmental intervention that have not been subjected to systematic evaluation.

Anti-Tobacco Regulation: Evaluative Studies

Since tobacco is the primary preventable cause of morbidity and mortality, government has adopted multiple strategies to reduce smoking, particularly among children and adolescents. These interventions are directed mostly toward individual-level behavioral changes: education (e.g., antismoking campaigns), deterrence (e.g., bans on retail sales to minors), and disincentives (e.g., tobacco taxes). Government has also directed interventions at the level of the manufacturer (e.g., varied tobacco litigation strategies) and at the level of the informational (e.g., advertising restrictions) and physical environment (e.g., bans on smoking in the workplace and other public places). While there has been no systematic evaluation of all of these interventions, researchers have sought to analyze several governmental antitobacco strategies.

Perhaps the most encompassing studies have evaluated broad, multidimensional antitobacco campaigns that have been initiated in several states. While these state antitobacco initiatives differ in certain respects, they all involve taxation of cigarettes and use of the revenues for a multipronged approach to reducing smoking. In California, for example, the state mandated funding for health education campaigns, local health agencies to provide technical support and monitor adherence to antismoking laws, community-based interventions, and enhancement of school-based prevention programs (Bal et al., 1990). Evaluation studies in Massachusetts (Abt, 1997), California (Pierce et al., 1998), and Oregon (CDC, 1999a) all reported per capita reductions in cigarette consumption. An Institute of Medicine (IOM) analysis of these and other studies concluded that a regulatory approach toward cigarette use can be effective. The IOM found that states with "intense" tobacco control initiatives (as measured by laws, law enforcement, and funding) showed greater decreases in tobacco use than comparable states (IOM, 2000).

Despite the promising results of these studies, there are certain limitations—both empirical and methodological. The California study reported a sharp decline in smoking directly following the intervention, but the effect dissipated over time and, ultimately, failed to significantly affect smoking behavior (Pierce et al., 1998). There are several possible explanations for the fact that the program's initial effects did not persist. One possible reason is that the effect demonstrated was due as much to the political and social environment as it was to the interventions themselves. Undoubtedly, changes in the law, which are often associated with political debate and media coverage, have a "declarative effect" that influences behavior indirectly by changing attitudes; legal norms reinforce, stimulate, accelerate, or symbolize changes in public attitudes about socially desirable behaviors (Bonnie, 1986). Other possible explanations are temporary reductions in state funding for antitobacco programs, political interference with antitobacco messages, and industry advertising and pricing policy.

These studies also face difficult methodological challenges. Most importantly, public or private funding for evaluation research, including population surveys of smoking behavior, becomes available only after the intervention has occurred. Research funding after the fact thwarts a comparison of specific behaviors before and after the intervention. Even if this important methodological problem could be overcome, however, these studies will find it hard to identify precisely the intervention that is having the desired effect. The Massachusetts, California, and Oregon studies, by definition, examined multiple interventions without an ability to separate the effect of each element of the intervention.

The most distressing finding is that in spite of all the efforts, tobacco use among adolescents has recently increased. The data show, moreover, that current cigarette smoking prevalence among African Americans is similar to rates among whites and Hispanics (CDC, 2000).

There are, of course, numerous studies of discrete tobacco regulation strategies. Two of the major interventions that have been studied are programs to prevent youth access to cigarettes and bans on smoking in the workplace and other public places. In the absence of enforcement, banning cigarette sales to minors does not significantly reduce teenage tobacco use. Compliance with the law by retailers is low; youth access studies have demonstrated that the majority of retailers sell to children. The Tobacco Institute's own "It's the Law" campaign, perhaps predictably, has not been effective (DiFranza and Brown, 1992). Efforts to educate retailers to reduce cigarette sales to minors have shown an effect, but a small one (Wildey et al., 1995). The most successful legal strategy to reduce youth access imposes civil penalties against the store owner (not just the clerk), has progressive increases in fees culminating in suspension or revocation of the tobacco retailer's license and has regular enforcement using minors in unannounced purchase attempts to monitor compliance. This strategy, implemented by legislation in Woodbridge, Illinois, has been demonstrated to be successful over time (Jason et al., 1999). Other states, such as Minnesota, have also demonstrated the effectiveness of well-enforced antitobacco ordinances restricting youth access to tobacco (Forster et al., 1998). Additionally, locking devices on cigarette vending machines do not appear to be as effective as an outright ban on these machines (Forster et al., 1992). Finally, some states have reported modest success with antitobacco education campaigns directed toward youth (Noland et al., 1998).

Legal restrictions on smoking in the workplace and other public places have demonstrated high conformance with the rule and some reduction in cigarette use. A study of compliance with a clear indoor air act in Brookline, Massachusetts, showed that the law was popular and the incidence of smoking restrictions was high (Rigotti et al., 1992). Further, a summary of 19 studies that evaluated the effects of smoke-free workplaces on smoking habits showed that both smoking rates (cigarettes consumed in a 24-hour period) and smoking prevalence (proportion of workers who smoke) decreased as a result of the indoor smoking bans. The authors estimate an annual reduction of 9.7 billion cigarettes (2%) in the United States as a result of smoke-free workplaces (Chapman et al., 1999).

What is notably absent from the evaluative research are rigorous studies of the effects of tobacco and other forms of litigation. Although tort strategies are much used and publicized by private parties, classes, and national and state governments themselves, there remains considerable debate about the effects. Public health advocates strongly favor this approach, while some law and economic scholars are skeptical about the tort system as a useful and cost-effective intervention (Rose-Ackerman, 1991; Vicusi, 1992).

The experience with government strategies to reduce cigarette smoking shows that both the intervention and the behavior are highly complex. Many interventions have not been carefully evaluated and methodological difficulties have thwarted some of the studies that have been undertaken. A comprehensive, multipronged approach to cigarette reduction appears to work best, but problems still exist in the long term. This may suggest that government interventions may also have to restrict manufacturers, particularly in their advertisements and promotions. This, of course, is the current strategy of the federal Food and Drug Administration, but its proposed regulations are being challenged by the industry on jurisdictional grounds; the case is being heard in the Supreme Court's 1999–2000 term. At the same time, there are substantial societal issues surrounding the First Amendment protection to be afforded to commercial speech (Gostin et al., 1997). Once these legal issues are resolved, of course, it will be essential to study the effects of stricter regulation of the tobacco industry.

Unlike the case of tobacco, government has had relatively little difficulty regulating the automobile industry. Indeed, government regulation of motor vehicles has received such popular support and has been so successful that the CDC (1999b) called motor vehicle safety one of the 10 great public health achievements of the twentieth century.

Motor Vehicle Safety Regulation (including driving while under the influence of alcoholic beverages): Evaluation Studies

The twentieth century may be known more for the proliferation of automobiles and other motorized vehicles than for any other technological change. Six times as many people drive today as in 1925, and the number of motor vehicles has increased elevenfold since then to approximately 215 million. The number of miles traveled is also 10 times higher than in the mid-1920s (CDC, 1999b).

Systematic safety efforts began during the mid-1960s when 41% of the nearly 94,000 unintentional injury deaths were caused by motor vehicle crashes. In 1966, the Highway Safety Act and the National Traffic and Motor Vehicle Safety Act authorized the federal government to set and monitor standards for motor vehicles and highways. The Highway Safety Act also created the National Highway Safety Bureau, which later became the National Highway Traffic Safety Administration (NHTSA).

The pervasive regulation of motor vehicle safety over the last three decades resulted in a steep decline in the mileage-based motor vehicle death rate (Fingerhut and Warner, 1997). A broad and creative array of regulatory strategies have been used to reduce the vast toll of motor vehicle injuries and deaths. As the IOM Committee on Injury Prevention and Control observed: "Dramatic progress has been made in reducing motor vehicle injuries by understanding the factors that increase the risk of injury, designing interventions to reduce these risks, implementing and evaluating a wide array of interventions and assessing their benefits and costs, and providing a scientific foundation for individual and business choices and public policy judgments" (IOM, 1999, p. 115). In short, government has been successful largely because it has adopted a sophisticated and comprehensive approach that addresses safety issues for the host (driver and passenger), agent (vehicle), and physical environment (highway system) (Haddon, 1972, 1980).

Individual-level interventions have been carefully studied, including general and specific deterrence, alcohol control policies, mass communications campaigns (including advertising restrictions), and community traffic safety programs (DeJong and Hingson, 1998). Two of the most important individual-level interventions are legislative policies to prevent alcohol-impaired driving and to increase the use of seatbelts and child restraints.

Alcohol-Impaired Drivers

In 1996, 38.6% of fatal traffic crashes involved a driver or pedestrian who had been drinking (CDC, 1998; NHTSA, 1998a). Still, fatalities involving alcoholic beverages have decreased 39% since 1982 (CDC, 1999b). Government has sought to reduce drinking-impaired driving by aiming its interventions at those who have been convicted for driving under the influence (DUI) of alcoholic beverages (specific deterrence) and at the general driving population (general deterrence). A great deal of evaluative research has studied the differential impact of various rehabilitation and punishment schemes for those convicted of driving while under the influence of alcoholic beverages (Jacobs, 1989; Ross, 1993). One meta-analysis found that rehabilitation reduced alcohol-related driving recidivism and crashes by 7–9% when averaged across all kinds of offenders and rehabilitation techniques. Strategies that combined punishments with treatment were more effective than either strategy alone. Treatment did not substitute for sanctions, and sanctions did not substitute for treatment (Wells-Parker et al., 1995).

Various punishment strategies have been tried, with mixed results (Hingson, 1996): (1) *mandatory license suspension*, which has been found to be effective in reducing crashes and violations (e.g., administrative "per se" laws that automatically suspend driver's licenses as a penalty for driving under the influence of alcohol; McArthur and Kraus, 1999); (2) *jail terms*, which generally have not been found to effect postincarceration deterrence; (3) *probation*, which has a slight deterrent effect on drivers at low risk for DUI recidivism, but has no effect on those at high risk; (4) *lower blood alcohol concentration (BAC) limits* to 0.04% for previously convicted drivers, which resulted in a 38% decline in fatal nighttime crashes compared with a 50% increase in a neighboring state with no such law; and (5) *license plate impoundment*, which was effective when managed administratively, but not when managed through the courts.

The enactment of laws to impose firm and consistent punishment against convicted drunk drivers, with the hope of decreasing repeat offenses, worked only to a limited extent. Policy makers began to realize that successful prevention would require more than punishing the relatively small number of drunk drivers who are arrested and convicted each year. There emerged a policy of general deterrence targeted at the general population. DeJong and Hingson (1998) reviewed the extant research of various general deterrence policies: (1) *administrative license revocation* (where police remove driver's licenses if they exceed the legal BAC limit) probably reduces alcohol-related traffic fatalities, but studies have had difficulty isolating the effect from other policies (Hingson, 1996); (2) *sobriety checkpoints* (where police roadblocks check for drivers who have been drinking) resulted in reductions in alcohol-related fatalities compared with contiguous states; (3) *criminal per se laws* (which lower BAC limits from 0.10 to 0.08%) reduce fatalities (Hingson et al., 1996); (4) *reduced availability of alcoholic beverages* had positive effects if servers were trained (DeJong and Hingson, 1998), but not with respect to other server interventions (McKnight, 1996); and (5) *increased alcohol excise taxes*, which reduced fatality rates in the 15- to 24-year-old age group.

General deterrence strategies have particularly targeted young drivers who tend to take greater risks. Researchers have identified three successful strategies to reduce injuries and deaths among young drivers. One successful strategy has been to increase the minimum legal drinking age from 18 to 21 years of age. This strategy reduced traffic fatalities in the target ages, compared with states that did not adopt such laws (Hingson et al., 1983; Cook and Tauchen, 1984; GAO, 1987; Decker et al., 1988; O'Malley and Wagenaar, 1991; Jones et al., 1992; Hingson, 1996). A second strategy, which has been enacted in 49 states, is to establish lower legal blood alcohol limits for younger drivers than for adult drivers. Researchers in six studies reported that this approach reduced injuries: "Despite the methodologic difficulties of ecologic studies, the six studies reviewed represent accumulating evidence in support of the effectiveness of these laws" (Zwerling and Jones, 1999). A third strategy aimed at young persons is to place restrictions on the licenses of beginning drivers, such as proscribing nighttime driving or prohibiting beginning drivers from having other young passengers in the vehicle

(Foss and Evenson, 1999). Nighttime driving restrictions, for example, have been shown to reduce injuries and deaths (Williams and Preusser, 1997).

During the years 1985 to 1995, drivers younger than 21 years experienced nearly a 50% drop in fatal crashes involving alcoholic beverages (NHTSA, 1997). While much of this effect can probably be attributed to the declarative and actual effects of regulation, the reasons for the decrease remain unclear. For example, a recent study demonstrated that while drivers below the age of 21 were still drinking heavily, a smaller percentage of younger drivers than of older drivers had BACs of 0.01 or higher. The study concluded that younger drivers are more likely than drivers older than 21 years to separate drinking from driving (Roeper and Voas, 1999).

Seat Belts and Child Restraints

Another strategy aimed at individual-level interventions involves laws mandating child restraint and safety belt use (Graham, 1993). Since 1979, all states have had legislation requiring infants and young children to be restrained when traveling in passenger cars. While differences in penalties, enforcement, and public education make it difficult to compare states, the extant data show that these laws significantly reduced child injuries and deaths (Guerin and MacKinnon, 1985; Muller, 1986; Margolis et al., 1988; Goldstein and Spurlock, 1998). For example, following an Orange County statute that mandated restraints for children under 4, restraint use doubled, there were fewer injuries overall, and fewer head injuries, yet emergency room utilization did not decrease (Agran et al., 1987).

Child restraint laws, however, appear to have an insignificant effect on reducing the high-risk behavior of children traveling in the front seat of a car. Interventions aimed at promoting the use of rear seats by children traveling in motor vehicles continue to be very important (Segui-Gomez, 1998).

Since New York became the first state to enact a mandatory seat belt law in December 1984 (Preusser et al., 1988), studies have consistently demonstrated the beneficial safety effects of such laws (Thyer and Landis, 1988; Bernstein et al., 1989; Williams et al., 1996). After the enactment of seat belt laws, there are fewer crashes, the crashes are less severe, and the occupants require less medical treatment for head and face injuries (Lestina et al., 1991).

In 1993, California became the first state to modify existing safety belt laws from a secondary to a primary enforcement provision (Ulmer et al., 1994). A primary law gives police the authority to stop a vehicle solely on the basis of their observation of noncompliance with the safety belt law; a secondary law permits police officers to cite unbelted occupants only when the vehicle is stopped for another violation. After enactment of California's primary law, rates of safety belt use rose from 73 to 95.6% (Lange and Voas, 1998). Rivara and colleagues (1999) reviewed 48 studies of primary and secondary enforcement of seat belt laws, finding that primary enforcement laws are likely to be more effective. Nevertheless, these researchers observed that few studies are of good quality, and quantitative estimates of the relative effect of primary compared with secondary laws are limited.

Individual-level approaches, while often effective, do raise important constitutional and ethical issues in a constitutional democracy. As explained above, compulsory seat belt and motorcycle helmet laws have been attacked as unwarranted paternalism and challenged on the basis of personal freedom (Cole, 1995). Yet courts and philosophers have justified these minimally coercive measures on consequentialist grounds because they save lives.[20] Commentators also draw attention to the social and economic burdens caused by vehicular injuries and deaths (Dworkin, 1986). Various restrictions on drivers' freedoms are criticized because they reduce mobility, which is seen by the public as an important value. Indeed, mobility interests have prevailed over safety interests as speed limits have been increased in many states. As a result, vehicular fatalities have correspondingly increased (Farmer et al., 1997; NHTSA,1998b). Concerns about freedom and mobility have also been expressed about other effective strategies such as license restrictions on young persons (e.g., nighttime driving restrictions). Finally, and importantly, some personal-level interventions raise issues of fundamental fairness. For example, minority communities point to selective and discriminatory enforcement of primary enforcement laws. The communities' concerns are that police will use these laws to intrude on civil liberties, particularly of young persons and minorities.

Regulatory strategies have gone well beyond individual-level interventions. Legislation enacted in 1966 enabled the federal government to set safety standards for new vehicles[21] and to develop a coordinated national highway safety program.[22] The Highway Safety Act of 1970 charged NHTSA with the responsibility of reducing deaths, injuries, and economic losses resulting from motor vehicle crashes. At the state level, government has established programs for motor vehicle inspections, speed limits, road design, and highway maintenance. Federal and state agencies, moreover, fund research, which has demonstrated the effectiveness of multiple interventions on the vehicular and environmental level—for example, center high-mounted rear brake lights, improved tire and brake performance, breakaway sign and light poles, and protective guardrails (TRB, 1990; IOM, 1999).

CONCLUSION

Legal and regulatory interventions represent critically important components of societal strategies to prevent injury and disease and promote the public's health. Yet, regulation remains substantially underevaluated. There are many reasons for the absence of systematic evaluation, including lack of training

---

[20]See, for example, *Simon* v. *Sargent,* 346 F.Supp. 277, 279 (D. Mass. 1972).
[21]National Highway Traffic and Motor Vehicle Safety Act of 1966.
[22]Highway Safety Act of 1966.

and funding, difficulty in timing research strategies, and most importantly, the many methodological difficulties and confounding variables that are inherent in such research. Despite the challenges, rigorous research evaluations are critically important. Since society spends so much of its resources on regulation, policy makers need to better understand what works and at what cost. Arguably, the increasingly close working relationship among policy makers, industry, and researchers to improve traffic safety is a good model to emulate. Traffic safety interventions, despite concerns about mobility and civil liberties, have been broadly supported by consumers and the public. Careful and systematic research, moreover, has bolstered political and public support.

There have been many areas affecting the public health that have not had the same research base, industry cooperation, and public and political support. Many public health experts believe that regulation should be included within a broad, multidimensional strategy to reduce injuries and diseases. Yet we live in a society that is apathetic, and sometimes hostile, to government regulation. In order to assure political and public acceptance of regulation in America's future, interventions should be carefully and systematically evaluated; and the results should be made widely available to policy makers and the public. The best antidote to lack of political support for government regulation is to show that it works, at a reasonable cost, and with socially and constitutionally acceptable burdens on liberty and property.

REFERENCES

Abt. 1997. *Independent Evaluation of the Massachusetts Tobacco Control Program.* Cambridge, MA: Abt Associates.

Agran P.F., Dunkle D.E., Winn D.G. 1987. Effects of legislation on motor vehicle injuries to children. *American Journal of Diseases of Children* 141:959–964.

AMA (American Medical Association), American Pharmaceutical Association, National Alliance of State and Territorial AIDS Directors, et al. 1999. *HIV Prevention and Access to Sterile Syringes.* Chicago. AMA.

Bal D.G., Kizer KW, Felton PG, et al. 1990. Reducing tobacco consumption in California: Development of a statewide antitobacco use campaign. *Journal of the American Medical Association* 264:1570–1574.

Bernstein E., Pathak D, Rutledge L, Demarest G. 1989. New Mexico safety restraint law: Changing patterns of motor vehicle injury, severity, and cost. *American Journal of Emergency Medicine* 7(3):271–277.

Bonnie R.. 1986. The efficacy of law as a paternalistic instrument. In: Melton G, ed. Nebraska Symposium on Human Motivation, 1985: *The Law as a Behavioral Instrument.* Lincoln, NE: University of Nebraska Press. Pp. 131–211.

Burris S. et al. 1996. The legal strategies used in operating syringe exchange programs in the United States. *American Journal of Public Health* 86:1161–1165.

Case P., Meehan T, Jones TS. 1998. Arrests and incarceration of injection drug users for syringe possession in Massachusetts: Implications for HIV prevention. *Journal of Acquired Immune Deficiency Syndromes and Retrovirology* 18(Suppl. 1):S71–S75.

CDC (Centers for Disease Control and Prevention). 1998. Alcohol involvement in fatal motor-vehicle crashes—United States, 1996–1997. *Morbidity and Mortality Weekly Report* 47:1055–1056, 1063.

CDC (Centers for Disease Control and Prevention). 1999a. Decline in cigarette consumption following implementation of a comprehensive tobacco prevention and education program—Oregon, 1996–1998. *Morbidity and Mortality Weekly Report* 48:140–143.

CDC (Centers for Disease Control and Prevention). 1999b. Motor vehicle safety: A 20th century public health achievement. *Morbidity and Mortality Weekly Report* 48(18): 369–374.

CDC (Centers for Disease Control and Prevention). 2000. Tobacco use among middle and high school students—United States, 1999. *Morbidity and Mortality Weekly Report* 49:49–53.

Chapman S, Borland R, Scollo M, et al. 1999. The impact of smoke-free workplaces on declining cigarette consumption in Australia and the United States. *American Journal of Public Health* 89(7):1018–1023.

Cole P. 1995. The moral bases for public health interventions. *Epidemiology* 6(1):78–83.

Cook P.J., Tauchen G. 1984. The effect of minimum drinking age legislation on youthful auto fatalities. *Journal of Legal Studies* 13:169–190.

Dannenberg A.L., Gielen AC, Beilenson PL, et al. 1993. Bicycle helmet laws and educational campaigns: An evaluation of strategies to increase children's helmet use. *American Journal of Public Health* 83(5):667–674.

Daynard R., Kelder G., Jr., 1998. The many virtues of tobacco litigation. *Trial* 34:36–48.

DEA (U.S. Department of Justice, Drug Enforcement Administration). 1991. Controlled Substances Act: As Amended to July 1, 1991. Washington DC: Department of Justice.

Decker, M.D., Graitcer P.L., Schaffner W. 1988. Reduction in motor vehicle fatalities associated with an increase in the minimum drinking age. *Journal of the American Medical Association* 260(24):3604–3610.

DeJong W, Hingson R. 1998. Strategies to reduce driving under the influence of alcohol. *Annual Review of Public Health* 19:359–378.

DHHS (Department of Health and Human Services), 1991. *Health Status of Minorities and Low Income Groups*. Washington DC: U.S. Government Printing Office.

DiFranza J.R., Brown L.J. 1992. The Tobacco Institute's "It's the Law" campaign: Has it halted illegal sales of tobacco to children? *American Journal of Public Health* 82(9): 1271–1273.

Dworkin G. 1986. Paternalism. In: Feinberg J, Gross H, eds. *Philosophy of Law*. Belmont, CA: Wadsworth Publishing Co., 3rd edition.

Elliott S. 1996. *Liquor industry ends its ad ban in broadcasting*. N.Y. Times, November 8, A1.

Erdmann T.C., Feldman KW, Rivara FP, et al. 1991. Tap water burn prevention: The effect of legislation. *Pediatrics* 88(3):572–577.

Farmer C.M., Rettig R.A., Lund A.K. 1997. *Effect of 1996 Speed Limit Changes on Motor Vehicle Occupant Fatalities*. Arlington, VA: Insurance Institute for Highway Safety.

Fingerhut L.A., Warner M. 1997. *Injury Chartbook. Health, United States, 1996–97*. Hyattsville, MD: National Center for Health Statistics.

Flay B.R., Cook T..D. 1990. Evaluation of mass media prevention campaigns. In: Rice R.E., Atkin C.K., Eds. *Public Communication Campaigns*. Newbury park, CA: Sage Publications.

Forster J.L., Hourigan M.E., Kelder S. 1992. Locking devices on cigarette vending machines: Evaluation of a city ordinance. *American Journal of Public Health* 82(9): 1217–1219.

Forster J.L., Murray D.M., Wolfson M. 1998. The effects of community policies to reduce youth access to tobacco. *American Journal of Public Health* 88(8):1193–1198.

Foss R,D, Evenson K.R. 1999. Effectiveness of graduated driver licensing in reducing motor vehicle crashes. *American Journal of Preventive Medicine* 16 (1 Suppl.):47–56.

Fox D.M., Schaffer D.C. 1987. Tax policy as social policy: Cafeteria plans, 1978A–1985. *Journal of Health Politics Policy and Law* 12:609–621.

GAO (General Accounting Office). 1987. *Drinking-Age Laws: An Evaluation Synthesis of Their Impact on Highway Safety*. Washington, DC:GAO.PEMD-87-10.

GAO (General Accounting Office). 1993. *Needle Exchange Programs: Research Suggests Promise as an AIDS Prevention Strategy*. Washington, DC:GAO/HRD-93-60.

Goldstein LA, Spurlock CW. 1998. Kentucky's child restraint law has saved lives: A 20-year review of fatalities among children (aged 0–4) as motor vehicle occupants. *Kentucky Medical Journal* 96:97–100.

Gostin L.O. 1998. The legal environment impeding access to sterile syringes and needles: The conflict between law enforcement and public health. *Journal of Acquired Immune Deficiency Syndromes and Human Retrovirology* 18 (Suppl. 1):S60–S70.

Gostin L.O. 2000. *Public Health Law: Power, Duty, Restraint,*. Berkeley, CA: University of California Press.

Gostin L.O., Lazzarini Z. 1997. Prevention of HIV/AIDS among injection drug users: The theory and science of public health and criminal justice approaches to disease prevention. *Emory Law Journal* 46:587–696.

Gostin L.O., Arno P.S., Brandt A.M. 1997. FDA regulation of tobacco advertising and youth smoking: Historical, social, and constitutional perspectives. *Journal of the American Medical Association* 277(5):410–418.

Gostin L.O., Brant A.M., Cleary P.D.. 1991. Tobacco liability and public health policy. *Journal of the American Medical Association* 266:3178–3183.

Graham J.D., 1993. Injuries from traffic crashes: Meeting the challenge. *Annual Review of Public Health* 14:515–543.

Guerin D., MacKinnon D.P. 1985. An assessment of the California child passenger restraint requirement. *American Journal of Public Health* 75:142–144.

Haddon W. Jr. 1972. A logical framework for categorizing highway safety phenomena and activity. *Journal of Trauma* 12(3):193–207.

Haddon W. Jr. 1980. Options for the prevention of motor vehicle crash injury. *Israel Journal of Medical Science* 16(1):45–65.

Haddon W. Jr., Sussman EA, Klein D. 1964. *Accident Research: Methods and Approaches*. New York: Harper and Row.

Hagan H, McGough J.P. Thiede H. et al. 1999. Syringe exchange and risk of infection with hepatitis B and viruses. *American Journal of Epidemiology* 149(3):203–213.

Heimer R. 1998. Syringe exchange programs: Lowering the transmission of syringe-borne diseases and beyond. *Public Health Reports* 113(Suppl. 1):67–74.

Heimer R, Khoshnood K, Bigg D. 1998. Syringe use and reuse: Effects of syringe exchange programs in four cities. *Journal of Acquired Immune Deficiency Syndrome and Human Retroviruses* 18(Suppl. 1):S37–S44.

Hingson R. 1996. Prevention of drinking and driving. *Alcohol Health and Research World* 20(4):219–226.

Hingson R, Scotch N, Mangione T, et al. 1983. Impact of legislation raising the legal drinking age in Massachusetts from 18 to 20. *American Journal of Public Health* 73(2):163–170.

Hingson R, Heeren T, Winter M. 1996. Lowering state legal blood alcohol limits to 0.09%: The effect on fatal motor vehicle crashes. *American Journal of Public Health* 86(9):1297–1299.

IOM (Institute of Medicine). 1988. *The Future of Public Health.* Washington DC: National Academy Press.

IOM (Institute of Medicine). 1999. *Reducing the Burden of Injury: Advancing Prevention and Treatment.* Washington DC: National Academy Press.

IOM (Institute of Medicine). 2000. *State Programs Can Reduce Tobacco Use.* Washington DC: National Academy Press.

Jacobs J.B.. 1989. *Drunk Driving: An American Dilemma.* Chicago: University of Chicago Press.

Jacobson P, Warner K.E.. 1999. Litigation and public health policy making: The case of tobacco control. *Journal of Health Politics, Policy and Law.* 24:769–802.

Jason L.A.,, Berk M., Schnopp-Wyatt, Talbot B. 1999. Effects of enforcement of youth access laws on smoking prevalence. *American Journal of Community Psychology* 21(2):143–160.

Jones N.E., Pieper C.F., Robertson L.S. 1992. The effect of legal drinking age on fatal injuries of adolescents and young adults. *American Journal of Public Health* 82(1): 112–115.

Kairys D. 1998. Legal claims of cities against the manufacturers of handguns. *Temple Law Review* 71:1–32.

Kraus J.F., Peek C., McArthur D.L., Williams A. 1994. The effect of the 1992 California motorcycle helmet use law on motorcycle crash fatalities and injuries. *Journal of the American Medical Association* 272(19):1506–1511.

Kraus J.F. 1985. Effectiveness of measures to prevent unintentional deaths of infants and children from suffocation and strangulation. *Public Health Report* 100(2):231–240.

Lange J.E., Voas R.B. 1998. Nighttime observations of safety belt use: An evaluation of California's primary law. *American Journal of Public Health* 88(11):1718–1720.

Lessig L. 1995. The regulation of social meaning. *Columbia Law Review* 92:943B–1045.

Lestina D.C., Williams A.F., Lund A.K. et al. 1991. Motor vehicle crash injury patterns and the Virginia seat belt law. *Journal of the American Medical Association* 265(11):1409–1413.

Lund A.K., Williams A.F., Womack K.N. 1991. Motorcycle helmet use in Texas. *Public Health Reports* 106(5):576–578.

Mann J., Gostin L.O., Gruskin S. et al. 1994. Health and Human Rights, 1. *Journal of Health and Human Rights* 1:6–22.

Margolis L.H., Wagenaar A.C., Liu W. 1988. The effects of a mandatory child restraint law on injuries requiring hospitalization. *American Journal of Diseases of Children* 142:1099–1103.

McArthur D.L., Kraus J.F. 1999. The specific deterrence of administrative per se laws in reducing drunk driving recidivism. *American Journal of Preventive Medicine* 16(1S):68–75.

McKnight A.J. 1996. Server intervention to reduce alcohol-involved traffic crashes. *Alcohol Health and Research World* 20(4):227–229.

Muller A. 1986. Is the Oklahoma child restraint law effective? [Letter]. *American Journal of Public Health* 76(10):1251–1252.

National Institutes of Health. 1997. *Consensus Development Statement. Interventions to Prevent HIV Risk Behaviors*. February 11–13. http://odp.od.nih.gov/consensus.

National Research Council. 1995. *Preventing HIV Transmission: The Role of Sterile Needles and Bleach*. Normand J, Vlahov D, Moses LE, eds. Washington DC: National Academy Press.

NHTSA (National Highway Traffic Safety Administration). 1996. *Traffic Safety Facts, 1996*. Alcohol. Washington, DC: NHTSA.

NHTSA (National Highway Traffic Safety Administration). 1998a. *Traffic Safety Facts, 1997*. Washington, DC: NHTSA.

NHTSA (National Highway Traffic Safety Administration). 1998b. *The Effect of Increased Speed Limits in the Post-NMSL Era*. Report to Congress. Washington, DC: NHTSA.

NHTSA (National Highway Traffic Safety Administration). 1999. 1995 *Youth Fatal Crash and Alcohol Facts*. Washington, DC: NHTSA.

Ni H., Sacks J.J., Curtis L., Cieslak P.R., Hedberg K. 1997. Evaluation of a statewide bicycle helmet law via multiple measures of helmet use. *Archives of Pediatric and Adolescent Medicine* 151:59–65.

Noland M.P., Kryscio R.J., Riggs R.S. et al. 1998. The effectiveness of a tobacco prevention program with adolescents living in a tobacco-producing region. *American Journal of Public Health* 88(12):1862–1865.

O'Malley P.M., Wagenaar A.C. 1991. Effects of minimum drinking laws on alcohol use, related behaviors, and traffic crash involvement among American youth: 1976–1987. *Journal of the Study of Alcohol* 52:278–491.

OMB (Office of Management and Budget). 1998. *The Budget of the United States Government: Fiscal Year 1999*, p. 218. Washington, DC: OMB.

Paone D., Clark J., Shi Q. et al. 1999. Syringe exchange in the United States, 1996: A national profile. *American Journal of Public Health* 89(1):43–46.

Pierce J.P., Gilpin E.A., Emery S.L. 1998. Has the California tobacco control program reduced smoking? *Journal of the American Medical Association* 280(1):893–899.

Preusser D.F., Lund A.K., Williams A.F. et al. 1988. Belt use by high-risk drivers before and after New York's seat belt use law. *Accident Analysis and Prevention* 20(4): 245–250.

Rigotti N.A., Bourne D., Rosen A. et al. 1992. Workplace compliance with a no-smoking law: A randomized community intervention trial. *American Journal of Public Health* 82(2):229–235.

Rivara F.P., Grossman D.C., Cummings P. 1997a. Injury prevention. First of two parts. *New England Journal of Medicine* 337(8):543–548.

Rivara F.P., Grossman D.C., Cummings P. 1997b. Injury prevention. Second of two parts. *New England Journal of Medicine* 337(9):613–618.

Rivara F.P., Thompson D.C., Cummings P. Effectiveness of primary and secondary enforced seat belt laws. 1999. *American Journal of Preventive Medicine* 16(1 Suppl.): 30–39.

Rivara F.P., Thompson D.C., Patterson M.Q. Thompson R.S. 1998. Prevention of bicycle-related injuries: Helmets, education, and legislation. *Annual Review of Public Health* 19:293–318.

Rogers G.B. 1996. The safety effects of child-resistant packaging for oral prescription drugs. Two decades of experience. *Journal of the American Medical Association* 275(21):1661–1665.

Robinson D.L. 1996. Head injuries and bicycle helmet laws. *Accidental Analysis and Prevention* 28(4):463–475.

Roeper P.J. Voas. 1999. Underage drivers are separating drinking from driving. *American Journal of Public Health* 89(5):755–757.

Rose-Ackerman S. 1991. Tort law in the regulatory state. In: Schuck, ed. *Tort Law and the Public Interest*. New York: Norton. Pp. 105–126.

Ross H.L. 1993. Punishment as a factor is preventing alcohol-related accidents. *Addiction* 88:997–1002.Segui-Gomez M. 1998. Evaluating interventions that promote the use of rear seats for children. *American Journal of Preventive Medicine* 16(1S):23–29.

Singer M., Baer H.A., Scott G. et al.1998. Pharmacy access to syringes among injecting drug users: Follow-up findings from Hartford, Connecticut. *Public Health Reports* 113(Suppl. 1):81–89.

Thompson D.C., Nunn M.E., Thompson R.S., Rivara F.P.,1996a. Effectiveness of bicycle safety helmets in preventing serious facial injury. *Journal of the American Medical Association* 276(24):1974–1975.Thompson D.C., Rivara F.P., Thompson R.S. 1996b. Effectiveness of bicycle safety helmets in preventing head injuries: A case-control study. *Journal of the American Medical Association* 276(24):1968–1973.Thyer BA, Landis J. 1988. Is the Florida safety belt law effective? [letter]. *American Journal of Public Health* 78(3):323.

TRB (Transportation Research Board, National Research Council) 1990. *Safety Research for a Changing Highway Environment*. Washington, DC:TRB.

Ulmer R., Preusser C., Preusser D.F. 1994. Final Report (December 1992–December 1993): *Evaluation of California's Safety Belt Law Change to Primary Enforcement*. Washington, DC: NHTSA.

Vernick J.S., Teret S.P., Webster D.W. 1997. Regulating firearm advertisements that promise home protection. *Journal of the American Medical Association* 277:1391–1396.

Vicusi W.K. 1992. *Fatal Tradeoffs*. New York: Oxford University Press.

Vlahov D., Junge B. 1998. The role of needle exchange programs in HIV prevention. *Public Health Reports* 113(Suppl. 1):75–80.

Wagenaar A.C. 1993. Research affects public policy: The case of legal drinking age in the United States. *Addiction* 88(Suppl.):758–818.

Wells-Parker E., Bangert-Drowns R., McMillen R., Williams M. 1995. Final results from a meta-analysis of remedial interventions with drink/drive offenders. *Addiction* 90:907–926.

Wildey M.B., Woodruff S.I., Agro A. 1995. Sustained effects of educating retailers to reduce cigarette sales to minors. *Public Health Reports* 110:625–629.

Williams A.F., Preusser DF. 1997. Night driving restrictions for youthful drivers: A literature review and commentary. *Journal of Public Health Policy* 18(3):334–345.

Williams A.F., Reinfurt D. Wells J.K. 1996. Increasing seat belt use in North Carolina. *Journal of Safety Research* 27(1):33–41.

Zwerling C., Jones M.P. 1999. Evaluation of the effectiveness of low blood alcohol concentration laws for younger drivers. *American Journal of Preventive Medicine* 16(1S):76–80.

The Need for, and Value of, a Multi-Level Approach to Disease Prevention: The Case of Tobacco Control

Kenneth E. Warner[1]

NATURE AND MAGNITUDE OF THE HEALTH CONSEQUENCES OF TOBACCO CONSUMPTION[2]

In a prominent article published in 1993, McGinnis and Foege (1993) compared the leading disease causes of death with "the actual causes of death." Accounting for 1.1 million annual deaths among Americans, half of all mortality, these "actual causes"—unhealthy behaviors and environmental exposures—represent the principal challenge to public health in this new century. Topping the list was tobacco consumption, the source of nearly a fifth of all deaths among Americans.

Almost single-handedly, smoking has transformed lung cancer from a virtually unknown disease at the turn of the twentieth century to the leading cause of

---

[1]Dr. Warner is Richard D. Remington Collegiate Professor of Public Health and director, University of Michigan Tobacco Research Network, Department of Health Management and Policy, School of Public Health, University of Michigan. This paper was prepared for the symposium "Capitalizing on Social Science and Behavioral Research to Improve the Public's Health," the Institute of Medicine and the Commission on Behavioral and Social Sciences and Education of the National Research Council, Atlanta, Georgia, February 2–3, 2000.

[2]Throughout this paper, phrases such as "cigarette smoking" and "tobacco consumption" are used reasonably interchangeably. Unless the context dictates otherwise, the reader should interpret references to smoking as applying generally to other forms of tobacco consumption as well. (An example of a context that precludes generalization is the discussion of laws that prohibit smoking in public places. Clearly this would not apply to use of smokeless tobacco as well.) Cigarette smoking is referred to specifically in many instances primarily because it is far and away the most important source of tobacco-produced disease.

cancer death at its conclusion. Including mortality associated with environmental tobacco smoke and with interactions with other exposures (especially radon), smoking is responsible for more than 90% of the lung cancer deaths that fell Americans each year. Smoking is also the leading cause of chronic obstructive pulmonary disease mortality, accounting for at least 85% of deaths attributable to emphysema and chronic bronchitis. Although smoking accounts for only 17 to 30% of cardiovascular disease deaths, the dominance of heart disease as the leading disease cause of death accords this illness its dubious status as a contender, with lung cancer, as the chief tobacco-produced source of mortality. In addition to the "big three," smoking contributes to a host of less common causes of death, and it creates an enormous burden of preventable morbidity and disability as well (U.S. DHHS, 1989; Napier, 1996).

The enormity of the toll of smoking is due to a combination of the widespread prevalence of this behavior (more than 45 million Americans smoke), its intensity (smokers take 10–12 puffs per cigarette on an average of more than 25 cigarettes per day), and the chemical composition of the smoke inhaled (more than 4,000 chemicals, including tobacco-specific nitrosamines, ammonia, formaldehyde, naphthalene, carbon monoxide, hydrogen cyanide, arsenic, benzo[a]-pyrene, and polonium-210; 43 of the chemicals are known human carcinogens (U.S. DHHS, 1989). Over a typical smoking "career" of 50 years, a lifelong smoker inhales these 4,000 chemicals 4 million to 5 million times. Given such exposure, it is perhaps nothing short of remarkable that an estimated one-half of lifelong smokers do *not* die as a consequence of the behavior. Indeed, there may be no more impressive testimony to the strength of the human organism.

The fact remains, however, that reflecting its burden on the other half of the smoking population, this chemical onslaught takes a toll unparalleled in the course of human history. In the United States, the toll will subside over time, a reflection of a gradual and continuing decline in smoking rates dating from the 1960s. The prevalence of smoking has dropped from approximately 45% in 1963, the year prior to publication of the first Surgeon General's report on smoking and health (U.S. DHEW, 1964), to 25% in 1997 (CDC, 1999b). Among men, prevalence has halved. Despite a rising population, total cigarette consumption in the United States has fallen from 633 billion cigarettes in 1981 to 479 billion in 1997. Adult per capita cigarette consumption—a common measure of consumption that adjusts for population growth—has fallen almost annually since 1973 (Tobacco Institute, 1998). Based on projections of the demographics of smoking, even in the absence of stronger tobacco control education and policy than exist at present, and assuming no change in youth initiation of smoking, prevalence should continue to fall in the United States over the next two decades or so, "bottoming out" at around 18% of adults (Mendez and Warner, 1998).

Even at these diminished levels of smoking, however, the toll of smoking will remain substantial throughout at least the first half of the new century. Still, the achievements of America's "antismoking campaign," dating from publication of the Surgeon General's report, rank tobacco control among, and perhaps at the top of, the major public health success stories of the second half of the twentieth century (CDC, 1999a).[3] The consumption declines described above suggest the magnitude of the shift in smoking behavior since the early 1960s, but in fact they considerably understate the extent of the accomplishments. In the absence of the then-new knowledge about the dangers of smoking, and the publicizing of this knowledge that constituted the heart of the early antismoking campaign, smoking prevalence almost certainly would have continued to climb, reflecting the rapid rise of smoking rates among women. It is certainly plausible, even probable, that total smoking prevalence would have exceeded 50% by the end of the 1960s or early 1970s. Adult per capita cigarette consumption would have exceeded 6,000 per year, compared to 4,345 in 1963—the highest level ever attained in the United States—and 2,333, today's figure. According to one analysis, the first two decades of the antismoking campaign should be credited with avoiding nearly 3 million premature deaths through the year 2000 (Warner, 1989).

Reflecting on America's tobacco control victories, juxtaposed against the enormity of the continuing problem, one can consider America's situation as either a cup half full or a cup half empty. The picture for the rest of the world is far bleaker. The World Health Organization predicts that today's global smoking population of 1.1 billion will mushroom to 1.6 billion by the year 2030. By then, tobacco will have become the leading cause of death in developing countries as it is today in developed countries. Currently the cause of 4 million deaths worldwide, tobacco will kill 10 million of the globe's citizens annually beginning near the end of the third decade of the twenty-first century (World Bank, 1999). No other behavioral, environmental, or biological cause of death will come close (Murray and Lopez, 1996).

The magnitude of America's continuing tobacco-produced death toll, combined with the success of the nation's multifaceted smoking control endeavors, make tobacco control an excellent candidate for examining why a multilevel approach to disease intervention is essential. Lessons from the tobacco story certainly have relevance to other health behavior dilemmas within the United States, and they generalize to other countries' efforts to come to grips with their own emerging and existing epidemics of tobacco-produced disease.

DEVELOPMENT OF SMOKING AS A NORMATIVE BEHAVIOR

While American public health leaders like to fantasize about a "tobacco-free" country, the prospects for eliminating tobacco from the McGinnis-Foege list in the foreseeable future verge on the nonexistent. The fascinating history of tobacco use, eloquently related by Goodman (1994) and others (Wagner, 1971; U.S. DHHS, 1992), demonstrates the vise-like grip that tobacco, and its principal dependency-forming constituent, nicotine, have long held on the members of

---

[3]The nature of the campaign is discussed later in this paper.

all societies exposed to "the golden leaf." The earliest recorded evidence of tobacco use in the Americas dates from the ninth century, and in the intervening 1,000-plus years, people have developed an extraordinary array of methods of consuming tobacco, including as a suppository for medicinal purposes. In India at present, tobacco is consumed in about a dozen distinct forms by millions of people (Bhonsle et al., 1992). Although the principal early purposes of tobacco use were medicinal and religious, history reveals evidence of social use, multiple times per day, in several North American tribes in the early years of the second millennium.

Tobacco use spread rapidly throughout Europe and Asia beginning in the sixteenth century, when explorers of "the New World" first brought it back. So potent was the hold of nicotine that smokers defied official prohibitions of its use. Most notably, in the late sixteenth century, Sultan Murad IV of Turkey declared smoking punishable by beheading or being drawn and quartered; yet thousands of Turks persisted in inhaling the intoxicating fumes and, in many cases, suffering the consequences. This experience serves not merely as an interesting historical footnote. It demonstrates that official tobacco control policies have existed for centuries and that tobacco smoking has persisted in the face of far more draconian penalties than any contemplated today.[4]

Suspicions about the dangers of smoking have existed for at least four centuries. In 1604, writing in a document entitled *Counterblaste to Tobacco*, King James I of England called smoking "a custom loathsome to the eye, hateful to the nose, harmful to the brain, dangerous to the lungs and in the black stinking fume thereof, nearest resembling the horrible Stygian smoke of the pit that is bottomless" (as quoted in Wagner, 1971, p. 11).

Despite this early insight, true scientific understanding of the hazards is a strictly twentieth century phenomenon, dating primarily from the second half of the century (U.S. DHHS, 1989). In large part, this reflects the fact that smoking became a widespread threat to health beginning only in the second decade of the twentieth century, with the refinement of the easy-to-inhale cigarette. Prior to 1913, the harsh tobaccos used in cigarettes made cigarette smoking a minor form of tobacco consumption. Cigars, pipes, snuff, and chewing tobacco dominated the tobacco market. Rarely inhaled deeply and frequently, these forms of tobacco consumption, although hazardous to health, posed only a minor risk compared to that which would become associated with cigarette smoking.

In 1913, Camel cigarettes introduced the "American blend" of tobaccos, a combination of flavorful tobaccos imported from Turkey and Egypt with milder American tobaccos that permitted deep inhalation for the first time. Camels also introduced what is widely regarded as the first modern advertising campaign. The pairing of flavor and ease of inhalation with creative advertising has been credited with inaugurating the modern era of the cigarette (Tilley, 1985). Other

---

[4]One might credit Murad IV not only as the first government official to develop a tobacco control policy, but also, through its enforcement, as the first person to prove that smoking was hazardous to health!

factors contributed to the rapid emergence of cigarette smoking as well, however. They included the relatively low cost of the new cigarettes, the addictiveness of easily inhaled nicotine, and the convenience of packaged cigarettes: in an increasingly harried daily life, tobacco users appreciated the ease and brevity of the cigarette smoking experience. The latter constituted a principal reason that cigarettes were included in soldiers' rations in World War I and in every war thereafter until the Gulf War.

Previously considered effeminate, cigarette smoking was converted into a normative behavior among males by the return to America of tens of thousands of newly addicted soldiers. Through effective marketing, the cigarette manufacturers managed to associate smoking with athleticism and romance. A veritable who's who of baseball stars, such as Lou Gehrig and Joe DiMaggio, advertised cigarettes widely. And smoking became *de rigeur* in seduction scenes in the movies, epitomized by the cigarette dangling from Humphrey Bogart's lips whenever he was sweet-talking an attractive lady in one of his films. In the 1950s, America's most respected man, Edward R. Murrow, chain-smoked his way through his television news and commentary broadcasts[5]. When the cohort of men born in the 1911–1920 decade reached their age of peak smoking prevalence—their late 20s to mid-30s—fully 70% smoked cigarettes. As recently as the early 1960s, more than half of adult males smoked (Warner, 1986).

In contrast, at no time did a majority of women smoke. Smoking by women was considered completely socially unacceptable during the first two to three decades of the century, and "daring" thereafter until World War II opened the "man's world" to women (e.g., with so many men overseas fighting, women began working in factories in large numbers). The cigarette industry exploited the image of smoking as risqué in multiple ways. In early cigarette ads, women urged their male companions who were smoking to "blow some my way." In a precursor to the "liberated woman" advertising campaign for Virginia Slims in the late 1960s, ad agencies staged marches through downtown New York with defiant women smoking. Through such techniques, the agencies tried to link smoking by women to the suffragette movement.

By the 1940s, women were beginning to smoke in large numbers. Indeed, it is striking to note that four 10-year birth cohorts of women, those born from 1901 to 1940, all reached their rates of peak smoking prevalence within the single five-year period 1958–1963. For the oldest of the four cohorts, born during the century's first decade, this meant that they peaked at an average age of 52.5 (Warner, 1986). (By comparison, women born from 1951 to 1960 achieved their peak prevalence in 1976, at an average age of 20.5.) From the 1930s through the early 1960s, the diffusion of smoking among women was paralleling that experienced among men approximately three decades earlier. Unlike men, however,

---

[5]As a sad footnote, both Bogart and Murrow died of lung cancer in their 50s, along with a plethora of other prominent smokers from the era.

TABLE 1. Smoking Prevalence (%) by Gender and Racial or
Ethnic Group

Race or Ethnicity	Male	Female	Total
White, non-Hispanic	27.4	23.3	25.3
Black, non-Hispanic	32.1	22.4	26.7
Hispanic	26.2	14.3	20.4
American Indian or Alaska Native	37.9	31.3	34.1
Asian or Pacific Islander	21.6	12.4	16.9
TOTAL	27.6	22.1	24.7

SOURCE: CDC, 1999b.

women's smoking prevalence peaked at about a third. The growth of smoking
among women was interrupted by the advent of the national antismoking campaign, inaugurated in January 1964 with publication of the first Surgeon General's report (Warner and Murt, 1982).

The antismoking campaign has never been a single "campaign" in the conventional sense. Rather, it has consisted of an unorchestrated mix of varied private and public sector efforts, first to educate the public about the hazards of
smoking and, subsequently, to protect nonsmokers from exposure to environmental tobacco smoke. The major component parts of the campaign, and their
effects, constitute the focal point of this paper. As such, discussion of them is
deferred to the last section. However, as one indication of the overall impact of
the campaign, consider the subtle shift in the norms surrounding the act of
smoking. In the middle of the century it was considered impolite to light a cigarette without offering one to one's companions. Beginning in the 1970s, however, the question asked by a smoker contemplating lighting up switched from,
Would you like a cigarette? To do you mind if I smoke? By the 1990s, in many
social circles, the latter question had been mooted by the expectation that the
answer would be yes. Today, many smokers generally ask nothing and refrain
from smoking in the presence of nonsmokers.

WHO SMOKES AND WHY

Of adult Americans, 24.7% were smokers in 1997 (CDC, 1999b). Although
a greater percentage of men smoke than do women (27.6% and 22.1%, respectively), the gap between the two genders has declined gradually over time. Racial and ethnic differences in smoking prevalence are substantial, ranging from
16.9% for Asians and Pacific Islanders to twice as much, 34.1%, for American
Indians and Alaskan Natives. Race or ethnicity and gender differences in smoking prevalence are presented in Table 1.

Race or ethnicity prevalence differences mask other differences in smoking
behaviors that affect disease outcomes. For example, although more African-

American males smoke than do white males, African Americans smoke fewer cigarettes per day. Possibly mitigating the potential health advantage of lower daily consumption is African Americans' preference for mentholated cigarettes, believed to have an anesthetizing effect on the throat that may lead to deeper inhalation. Menthol may also contribute to a higher rate of addiction (Ramirez and Gallion, 1993).

Smoking rates vary substantially by age, with prevalence declining in the fourth and subsequent decades of life. In the older ages, differential death rates for smokers and nonsmokers account for a significant fraction of the prominent decrease in smoking prevalence (Harris, 1983). Smoking cessation, the principal determinant of the decline in prevalence with age, rises significantly with age. Cessation rates appear to have leveled off during the 1980s and early 1990s, with concern that they may actually have fallen in the late 1990s.

A real challenge to students of the demographics of smoking is assessing smoking initiation, a phenomenon that occurs almost exclusively during childhood. Much concern has been expressed about the documented increase in 30-day smoking prevalence among eighth, tenth, and twelfth graders during the first half of the 1990s, a trend that has, fortunately, reversed in the most recent years. In the 1999 Monitoring the Future Survey, 34.6% of high school seniors had smoked within the past 30 days. The comparable figures for tenth and eighth graders are 25.7 and 17.5% (Monitoring the Future, 1999). Troubling, however, is the question of how one should assess "smoking" by children, for while 30-day prevalence rates were rising during the 1990s, measures of regular and heavy smoking (e.g., half a pack or more per day) were not.

Data on youth smoking also raise perplexing questions about racial and ethnic differences. Most notably, the rates of smoking for African-American students were dramatically lower than those for whites, although the gap has narrowed in recent years. Yet smoking rates among young adult African Americans often exceed those of comparably aged whites. The difference is explained, in part, by lower quit rates among African Americans.

A large majority of children experiment with smoking, yet fewer than half go on to become regular smokers. Sociologists attribute much of the propensity to experiment with tobacco, as well as the propensity to become a regular smoker, to the influence of peer and parental behavior. It is widely believed, for example, that the children of smokers are twice as likely to smoke as the children of nonsmokers (although the data from multiple studies are not uniformly consistent in finding a significant association [U.S. DHHS, 1994]). There are important socioeconomic and educational links as well: in the United States, as in most developed nations today, smoking is increasingly becoming a marker for lower socioeconomic status (U.S. DHHS, 1989).

Clearly, the preeminent determinant of smoking dependency in a given individual is addiction to nicotine. A wealth of evidence from biology, brain chemistry, and sociology indicts nicotine as a classic addictive substance (U.S. DHHS, 1988; Henningfield et al., 1993). Ironically, when in 1988 the Surgeon General observed that nicotine was as addictive as heroin and cocaine, he may have been understating the case in one important respect: of all the dependency-forming substances of abuse, nicotine likely addicts the greatest proportion of its users. But the question remains as to why some people can take it or leave it, while others find themselves incapable of renouncing its use. Intriguing clues are emerging from the rapidly developing field of genetic science. Recent research offers provocative evidence of a genetic explanation for as much as half of the propensity to become a smoker and half of the apparent inability of some smokers to quit (Pomerleau, 1995).

That the social context in which smoking occurs affects the amount and nature of smoking is evident in the literature on children's role modeling (Lynch and Bonnie, 1994; U.S. DHHS, 1994). Intriguing new evidence on contemporary patterns of adult smoking illustrates just how influential societal norms can be. A recent (1992) change in the questions asked by the National Health Interview Survey (NHIS) to determine smoking status permitted analysts to assess how many people smoke cigarettes on a nondaily basis. The conventional wisdom among experts on smoking had always been that only 5% or so of smokers were "chippers"—recreational smokers who could smoke only a few cigarettes per day or even smoke on a nondaily basis. The NHIS data indicate that close to a fifth of all smokers do not smoke every day. Although multiple possible explanations come to mind, there is widespread agreement that the "clean indoor air" movement, prohibiting smoking in many public places and workplaces, likely has redefined smoking for a subset of smokers. These smokers have learned how to "survive" in a smoking-hostile environment by restricting their smoking to locations, and days, in which it is acceptable.

This shift in the social environment in which smoking takes place is but one example of the determinants of smoking that lend themselves to purposeful collective intervention. Another, of great concern within the tobacco control community, relates to the marketing of cigarettes and other tobacco products. It is an article of faith within the tobacco control community that advertising and, increasingly, other forms of marketing (ranging from sports sponsorship to distribution of cigarette brand-related paraphernalia) seduce youngsters into experimenting with cigarettes and keep adults hooked who otherwise would quit. Although the weight of the evidence supports this view, there is no "smoking gun" that demonstrates it conclusively (U.S. DHHS, 1989). The empirical evidence on the issue is mixed (Chaloupka and Warner, in press).

Nevertheless, it is clear that the marketing of tobacco products is a major front in the war on smoking, and notable tobacco control victories have been realized within the past few years, most recently the result of the multistate settlement concluded between the state attorneys general and the tobacco industry (National Association of Attorneys General, 2000). As a consequence of that settlement, tobacco billboards have disappeared and human subjects and cartoon characters will no longer grace the pages of cigarette ads. Product sampling is banned, as is product placement in movies and other media. Brand names are prohibited on merchandise (e.g., clothing and caps). Team sports sponsorship is prohibited and brand-name sponsorship is limited to one per year. In addition, the settlement provided for the establishment of a foundation (the American Legacy Foundation) that will devote substantial resources to marketing a strong antitobacco message to youth. Combined, the restrictions on tobacco marketing and the introduction of a well-funded counteradvertising campaign may have a significant influence on youth smoking by altering the social environment in which it has been glamorized so effectively for decades.

THE OBJECTIVES OF TOBACCO CONTROL AND BROAD STRATEGIES TO ATTAIN THEM

Tobacco control has three principal objectives, all directed toward avoiding the enormous burden of disease wrought by tobacco use. Although the three objectives are distinct in concept, realization of any one of them (partial or complete) will often affect one or both of the other objectives, as considered in the next section. The three objectives are the following:

1. preventing the initiation of tobacco use by young people,
2. helping adult smokers to quit (or at least to reduce their risk), and
3. protecting nonsmokers from the annoyance and risk posed by environmental tobacco smoke.

In principle, proponents of tobacco control should and do support all three objectives. In practice, however, a vigorous national debate has emerged, pitting advocates for a youth prevention focus (the first objective) against those who insist upon a more comprehensive strategy, one devoted more centrally to preservation of clean indoor air (the third objective) and more explicitly to helping adult smokers to quit (the second objective).

The youth prevention orientation has evolved in large part as a political strategy: preventing smoking by kids is a nearly universally lauded objective; even the tobacco industry pays lip service to this goal (Brown and Williamson, 2000; Philip Morris, 2000; R.J. Reynolds, 2000). This recognition drove the Food and Drug Administration (FDA) to adopt an exclusively youth-oriented set of policies when it courageously ventured into the realm of nicotine and tobacco product regulation (FDA, 1996). Similarly, state Medicaid lawsuits against the industry emphasized the prevention of youth smoking (Jacobson and Warner, 1999), and the multistate settlement's public health provisions all concentrated on that same goal (National Association of Attorneys General, 2000). In a congressional debate on policy measures designed to reduce smoking by kids, no representative or senator could afford to be depicted as opposing the legislation's purpose (although they could oppose its approaches, in part because they might impinge on the liberties of responsible adults).

Given these apple pie and motherhood characteristics, the youth prevention orientation pays homage to the art of the possible. In addition, from the perspective of many tobacco control advocates it permits a foot in the legislative door to achieve broader objectives by dressing them in prevention clothing. For example, the call for a large tax increase to discourage youth smoking would, if adopted, also decrease smoking by adults. A media antismoking campaign would reach adults both directly and indirectly, the latter by adults' awareness of the changing attitudes and behaviors of young people with regard to smoking. It is certainly reasonable to call for smoke-free indoor environments in locations frequented by young people, such as schools, malls, and sporting events. Adults work and play in those settings as well. Banning tobacco billboards has an effect on its ostensible target, youth, and on adults too.

Proponents of a more comprehensive strategy perceive the youth prevention approach as devious and, ultimately, counterproductive. They are not so sanguine about the ability to achieve broader tobacco control objectives when policies and programs are constrained to explicitly target youth. Even if this would work at least partially, in their judgment it would necessarily represent an inefficient attack on issues such as adult quitting and protection of nonsmokers' rights to clean air. Confronted with the massive war chests of the tobacco industry, their top-quality legal and public relations talent, and the inherent allure of nicotine, tobacco control can ill afford less than the best-possible approaches to achieving the three objectives. Further, many proponents of a frankly adult-oriented comprehensive strategy believe that any campaign explicitly focused on discouraging children from smoking will have exactly the opposite effect: rebellious kids often take their cues as to what to do based on what the adult world tells them not to do (Glantz, 1996).

Proponents of the comprehensive strategy, which targets smoking by adults quite explicitly, risk the charge that their objective smacks of paternalism. Lacking the easy political constituency of the youth orientation, the comprehensive tobacco control strategy creates an instant opposition in the form of the individual liberty and responsibility lobby. This is especially troublesome at the level of federal policy, which the comprehensive approach tacticians denounce as hopeless. At the national level the tobacco industry has repeatedly demonstrated its unrivaled strength to mobilize the troops to fight adult-affecting policy measures in Congress. Federal cigarette excise tax increase proposals are labeled, successfully, as ruinous and unfair "tax-and-spend" government "business as usual." Restrictions on cigarette advertising are an affront to First Amendment protections of commercial speech. Clean indoor air laws assault Americans' basic liberty rights, and the right and obligation to give "common courtesy" a chance to work first (Advocacy Institute, 1998).

Given the history of very timid tobacco control legislation in Congress, and the related ability of the tobacco industry to marshal its forces in successful opposition, the comprehensive tobacco control school emphasizes grass roots action, attacking tobacco at the local level (e.g., municipalities) and, when necessary, at the state level as well. A divide-and-conquer strategy—spreading the resources of the tobacco industry thinly across hundreds of local jurisdictions—has produced some impressive tobacco control victories, particularly in the domain of clean indoor air ordinances (Samuels and Glantz, 1991).

The division of the tobacco control forces into the two strategic camps reflects their terrain: the leadership of the youth prevention strategy comes from "establishment" national organizations, including the American Cancer Society, the American Heart Association, the American Medical Association, the National Center for Tobacco-Free Kids, and the new American Legacy Foundation. Savvy in the ways of Washington, replete with financial resources and congressional lobbying experience, these organizations believe that the greatest bang-for-the-buck ultimately must be achieved with a national strategy; for the reasons given, they believe that that strategy must necessarily be youth oriented.

In contrast, and not surprisingly, the comprehensive tobacco control school derives its support from state and local organizations, including local chapters of the major health voluntaries, tobacco control divisions of state and local units of government, and tobacco control grass roots organizations. The leadership of this school consists of individuals who have fought the tobacco wars in the trenches of state and local politics, directing state ballot initiatives to raise cigarette excise taxes and dedicate revenues to tobacco control, and heading campaigns to ban smoking in restaurants and other public places within cities and counties.

While the battle between the two schools of thought rages on, it is imperative to emphasize that virtually all tobacco control proponents concur that all three of the major objectives of tobacco control—youth smoking prevention, adult cessation, and protection of nonsmokers—are meritorious. The issues that divide the two camps are principally strategic, essentially pragmatic in nature. In truth, of course, as is invariably the case, they also reflect concerns about "turf" (Advocacy Institute, 1999).

Yet another strategic division appears poised on the horizon to dominate many coming debates about tobacco control, centered in, but certain to erupt outside, the community of smoking cessation experts. These experts are pondering the possibility of finding effective harm reduction strategies that fall short of smokers' completely renouncing their dependence on nicotine. The interest in harm reduction derives from frustration with the slow pace of smoking cessation—only 3% of smokers quit each year—and the emergence of a plethora of new nicotine delivery technologies, produced by both the tobacco and the pharmaceutical industries. The notion is that many smokers who find themselves unable (or unwilling) to give up nicotine might find lower-risk nicotine delivery devices acceptable substitutes for conventional cigarettes (Warner et al., 1997; Warner, in press).

Fraught with perils, the harm reduction concept faces considerable opposition among public health professionals, many of whom adhere strictly to a just-say-no philosophy. To many experts, however, harm reduction is the crucial new frontier in America's ongoing battle against tobacco-produced disease. This complicated and fascinating debate is certain to capture the attention of much of the tobacco control community as technology evolves and appropriate policy responses are contemplated. It explains why the second general objective of tobacco control—helping adult smokers to quit—was modified by "or at least to reduce their risk." For the purposes of the present paper, however, with few interventions having been studied to date, harm reduction will not be considered further. Interested readers should consult the provocative literature emerging on the subject (Tobacco Dependence, 1998; Ferrence et al., in press).[6]

APPROACHES TO TOBACCO CONTROL: WHAT ARE THEY AND HOW WELL DO THEY WORK?[7]

One of the defining characteristics of tobacco control—regardless of whether or not one adopts a youth-oriented focus—is recognition that a successful assault on the disease burden created by smoking necessarily must be multidimensional (CDC, 2000; National Cancer Policy Board, 2000). Individual interventions do work on their own. For example, smoking cessation treatments do help a subset of smokers to quit. Tax increases clearly discourage children from smoking and reduce smoking by adults as well. Prohibitions on smoking in public places clean the air for nonsmokers, decrease smoking prevalence and daily consumption among ongoing smokers, and help to establish and reinforce a non-smoking social norm. Yet, alone, each of these interventions succeeds by tinkering on the fringe. Collectively, these and other interventions may exhibit powerful synergism. The smoker committed to participating in a cessation treatment, for example, stands a better chance of quitting if the external environment discourages smoking, as it does when smoking is prohibited in public places. That same smoker is more likely to succeed in quitting if the price of cigarettes rises due to a tax increase.

In the remainder of this paper, attention focuses on understanding the varied dimensions of tobacco control intervention, briefly describing knowledge of their impacts and how they interact. First, however, a digression concerning the title and purpose of the paper seems warranted to set the stage for this section's discussion. The purpose is to examine a "multilevel" approach to improving the public's health, in this case by decreasing the use of tobacco products. The term "multilevel" is ambiguous, yet usefully so. One can envision a sizable number of alternative constructions of "level," each of which would permit the development of a different set of insights about public health intervention. By way of summary, Box 1 lists several obvious candidates for the meaning of "level."

---

[6]As this paper is being written, an Institute of Medicine committee is embarking on a study of the science base for evaluating the harm reduction potential of new nicotine delivery technologies.

[7]Given the brevity of this paper, this section can merely summarize important findings pertaining to this large subject. The most comprehensive review of tobacco control interventions, although now dated, is found in Chapters 6 and 7 of the 1989 Surgeon General's report (U.S. DHHS, 1989; see also U.S. DHHS, 1991). More recent references, discussing specific interventions, are cited in the text.

**BOX 1. Alternative Constructions of "Level" in
"Multilevel Approaches to Public Health"**

1. Size of the unit of interest (from the individual person to specific organizations to narrowly defined communities to the society as a whole).
2. Type of organization delivering an intervention (from governments to voluntary societies to businesses).
3. Level within a broad category of organization (e.g., local, state, and federal levels of government; local, national, and international levels of "society").
4. Intervention channels (e.g., the media, medical professional societies, workplaces, schools).
5. Sociodemographic and/or socioeconomic characteristics (age, gender, race or ethnicity, education, occupation, income or wealth).
6. Level of prevention (primary, secondary, tertiary).
7. Objectives (as in the three major objectives of tobacco control).
8. Discipline (e.g., social scientist, biological scientist, medical professional, lawyer, policy analyst, and ethicist, also specific disciplines within a category, such as—within social science—psychologist, sociologist, economist, political scientist).
9. Intervention function (education, incentives, regulation).

For the purposes of this paper, attention focuses on the last conception of level in Box 1—the intervention function. The section opens with a brief discussion of an intervention function typology that is applied in subsequent subsections. The section then turns to the application of this typology to each of the three major objectives of tobacco control.

A Typology of Intervention Functions

All tobacco control (and indeed other public health) interventions can be classified as one of three broad categorical types of interventions, here organized in increasing order of coerciveness (i.e., the degree to which they force behavior change): education and information interventions, incentives, and laws and regulations. The first of these encompasses all activities designed to inform the public about hazards or benefits to health and/or to persuade people to take health-enhancing behavioral action. In the case of tobacco control, dissemination of the findings published in the Surgeon General's reports on smoking and health serves to educate the public about the dangers of smoking (and of passive smoking) or the health benefits of quitting. Media "counteradvertising" campaigns attempt to persuade young people or adults to avoid tobacco use. Warning labels on cigarette packs and ads are intended to inform about dangers and, implicitly, to discourage use.

The second category, incentives, refers primarily to economic inducements to avoid tobacco. The most obvious and important example is an increase in a cigarette excise tax, driving up the price of cigarettes and thereby discouraging cigarette purchases by individuals who "feel the bite" of the higher price in their wallets. Other examples include differential life insurance rates (you pay more for given coverage if you smoke than if you do not) and explicit smoking cessation incentives, such as employers' rewarding workers who do not smoke with pay bonuses (Warner and Murt, 1984; U.S. DHHS, 1989).

The final category, laws and regulations, refers to explicit, legally binding requirements to do, or not do, something pertaining to tobacco consumption. Most notable here are clean indoor air laws, prohibiting smoking in public places, and minimum age of purchase laws that forbid vendors from selling cigarettes to minors and minors from buying them.

Walsh and Gordon (1986) described this method of classifying tobacco control interventions in an article written for the *Annual Review of Public Health*. Warner et al. (1990) developed a more general drug policy typology that elaborates on this classification, distinguishing the intervention type by point of intervention and end user. They observe that an intervention can represent a legal requirement of one party that serves to educate another. For example, cigarette and smokeless tobacco manufacturers are required to place warning labels on all packs of cigarettes and ads. This legal obligation of a member of the production and supply chain is intended to educate the end user, the purchaser of the tobacco product.

For the remainder of this section, intervention types will be judged by their relationship to the end user, the smoker or potential smoker. It is useful to recognize, nevertheless, that most education and incentive interventions, as viewed by consumers, represent legal or regulatory obligations imposed on either members of the production and supply chain or other "intermediaries" (e.g., schools required to present tobacco and health education to their students).

Preventing Initiation of Smoking[8]

Each of the major tobacco control objectives draws on interventions in all three categories of intervention types. Only in the case of preventing youth initiation of tobacco use, however, do interventions in all three categories receive roughly comparable emphasis. Education of children about the dangers of tobacco products, intended to discourage their use, was the hallmark of early youth prevention efforts (U.S. DHHS, 1994). This included both formal in-school education and media counteradvertising campaigns oriented toward children. Education and persuasion remain a core approach in youth prevention, as reflected in the new multimillion-dollar media campaign launched by the American Legacy Foundation in January 2000. Raising cigarette excise taxes,

---

[8]Good general references on this subject are the IOM report *Growing Up Tobacco Free* (Lynch and Bonnie, 1994) and Lantz et al. (in press).

the principal intervention from the incentive category, has become a central feature of nearly all comprehensive efforts to discourage youth smoking (Grossman and Chaloupka, 1997; National Cancer Policy Board, 2000). Recently, a great deal of emphasis has been placed on a legal strategy: strictly enforcing laws prohibiting sales of tobacco products to minors, generally defined as under age 18 (Forster and Wolfson, 1998; DiFranza, 1999). Indeed, strict enforcement is one of the main provisions of the Food and Drug Administration's 1996 regulatory policy designed to reduce youth smoking (FDA, 1996).

Preventing youth initiation of tobacco use logically appears to be critical to the overriding objective of breaking the seemingly endless cycle of youthful experimentation, addiction, subsequent long-term use, disease, and death. It is therefore exceedingly frustrating for the tobacco control community, and for public health more generally, that so little is understood about how to intervene effectively to reduce youth tobacco use. As it is implemented in practice, school health education, the quintessential ingredient of youth tobacco control, has contributed little to discouraging future experimentation or addiction. There is evidence that state-of-the-art education programs can reduce tobacco use (U.S. DHHS, 1994). But the reality, thus far, is that school systems lack the resources and the will to implement state-of-the-art programs effectively and on a sustained basis.

More encouraging, at least in the short run, have been media counteradvertising campaigns. In California, Massachusetts, Arizona, and Florida, well-funded media campaigns have caught the attention of young people and been followed by youth smoking rates that either declined or failed to rise at the rate experienced nationally through much of the 1990s (Popham et al., 1994; Florida Dept. of Health, 1999; Gregory Connolly, Massachusetts Dept. of Health, personal communication, 1999). In particular, advocates of media campaigns cite the apparent recent success of the Florida campaign, funded by resources from that state's settlement of its Medicaid lawsuit with the tobacco industry. Thirty-day smoking prevalence among teens fell from 23.3% to 20.9% from 1998 to 1999.

How long a media campaign can produce sustained decreases in youth tobacco use is unknown. Both logic and experience with cigarette advertising and counteradvertising suggest that as the novelty of an advertising or counteradvertising campaign recedes, so too will its effectiveness (Saffer and Chaloupka, 1999). Their novelty was likely one of the principal reasons that the broadcast media Fairness Doctrine antismoking ads of the late 1960s were so effective in discouraging smoking in the face of broadcast cigarette ads that outnumbered them by from 3:1 to 12:1 (Warner, 1979). Nevertheless, the apparent success of the state-funded campaigns has encouraged the American Legacy Foundation to devote a substantial proportion of its nearly $200 million in annual expenditures to a professionally designed media campaign.

The effect of price increases on discouraging youth smoking is clearly one of the best-documented and most encouraging stories in all of tobacco control. Although the evidence is not unequivocal, there is a consensus among economists who have studied the relationship that higher prices do decrease smoking by young people (National Cancer Institute, 1993; Warner et al., 1995; Chaloupka and Warner, in press). While the overall, primarily adult demand for cigarettes is only modestly responsive to price changes—a 10% increase in price decreases cigarettes demanded by approximately 4%—analysts believe that smoking by kids is roughly twice as price responsive as that of adults. As such, since tax constitutes only a fraction of total cigarette price, even a modest increase in a tax rate can reduce youth smoking significantly. To achieve maximal impact, however, such tax increases have to be sustained in real value over time. Since most taxes are set in nominal amounts, inflation gradually erodes their consumption-discouraging impact, unless further tax increases keep pace with inflation (Grossman and Chaloupka, 1997).

In contrast with most of the literature, a few studies by economists have not identified greater price responsiveness among children than among adults (Chaloupka, 1991; Wasserman et al., 1991). And a recent debate, inaugurated by conflicting interpretations of the same empirical data set (DeCicca et al., 1998; Dee and Evans, 1998), has broken out among health economists as to whether higher prices discourage youth smoking *initiation* per se. Despite these uncertainties, the overall strength of the evidence supporting the proposition that higher prices reduce youth smoking led a group of economists who had substantial experience working on tobacco economic issues to call for increased cigarette taxation primarily to reduce youth smoking (Warner et al., 1995).[9]

Interest in taxation as a means of combating youth tobacco use followed the early emphasis on education. The latest addition to the youth prevention armamentarium is policy oriented toward reducing youth access to tobacco products at retail outlets. A series of studies over several years established that minimum-age-of-purchase laws were enforced rarely; in monitored experiments, teenagers found it easy to buy cigarettes from stores in multiple states (Rigotti et al., 1997; Forster and Wolfson, 1998; Lancaster and Stead, 1999). Offended by vendors' utter disregard for the law and hopeful that enforcement might stem the tide of smoking by young people, a number of advocates pushed for legislative action. Federal and state laws were tightened, and most recently, the FDA's regulations required vendors to request photo identification from anyone appearing to be less than 27 years old (FDA, 1996). As a consequence, in some jurisdictions,

---

[9]Recent work by economists has found variations in the responsiveness of youth and young adults to price changes associated with race, gender, and socioeconomic status (Centers for Disease Control and Prevention, 1998; Chaloupka and Pacula, 1999). This new work introduces as many questions as it answers, since it does not explain why these differences exist. Still, the attempt to differentiate the effectiveness of policy interventions by race or ethnicity and gender, as well as age and income, seems an important step in refining policy approaches to tobacco control. To date, the literature on sociodemographic differences in smoking is related primarily to smoking prevalence, rather than to responses to educational and policy interventions (U.S. DHHS, 1998), although there are important exceptions (Townsend et al., 1994). Clearly, more work is needed on the latter.

compliance with the law has increased considerably, although not all states are in conformance with federal mandates (DiFranza, 1999).

Whether stricter enforcement of youth access laws will make a substantial difference in youth tobacco use remains to be seen. A study of what is likely the gold standard of enforcement, in Woodbridge, Illinois, produced very encouraging results: merchant sales to minors fell from 70% to 5% over one and a half years of compliance checks, following implementation of a youth access ordinance, and experimentation with and regular use of cigarettes by adolescents fell by more than 50% (Jason et al., 1991). In another study, however, while retail outlets reduced their cigarette sales to minors significantly (compliance with the law in three intervention communities rose to 82%, compared to 45% in three control communities), analysts found no evidence of a decline in smoking by youth (Rigotti et al., 1997). A recent analysis demonstrates convincingly why anything short of near-complete decreases in illegal retail sales is unlikely to substantially impact youth smoking. Young people will learn where cigarettes can be purchased and they have multiple other means of acquiring cigarettes as well (e.g., older siblings, friends, and black markets on school grounds) (Levy et al., 1998).

A more novel approach to youth smoking consists of directly penalizing youth caught smoking (or in possession of cigarettes). Approaches vary across the states, including requiring offenders to attend youth "tobacco courts," restricting law violators' driving privileges, and fining offenders. These demand-oriented approaches have drawn criticism from some members of the tobacco control community, who prefer to emphasize legal penalties against adult suppliers of cigarettes. To date, there is little evidence on the effectiveness of any of these new strategies (Lantz et al., 2000).

Analyses of the effects of comprehensive youth prevention programs are few in number and thin on empirical evidence. The state programs in California and Massachusetts consisted primarily of a tax increase and a tax revenue-funded media counteradvertising campaign. (Both states put additional resources into other activities, but these have received only modest funding and little if any analytical attention.) It is clear that these states' programs have reduced tobacco use by youth (as well as adults, as discussed in the following section) (National Cancer Policy Board, 2000). Given the paucity of evidence on the effects of media campaigns by themselves, however, it is impossible as yet to determine whether the tax increase and the media campaign together have decreased youth smoking by more than one might expect by adding the independent effects.

In concluding this examination of youth prevention efforts, and as a natural segue into the next section's discussion of adult smoking cessation, it is important to recognize a new frontier in tobacco control, one so new that there is insufficient literature to review: youth smoking cessation. Traditionally, youth and adult smoking concerns have been neatly distinguished as prevention and cessation, respectively (excluding, of course, exposure to environmental tobacco smoke—an issue for all age groups). Recently, however, recognition has dawned that there are likely hundreds of thousands of young people who, by virtue of early experimentation, are beyond the prevention stage; they, like most adult smokers, are addicted. Providing cessation assistance for youth raises a series of different issues than those confronted by professionals attempting to help adults to quit. For example, given strict prohibitions against being a young smoker in many families and some schools, many addicted children are unwilling to reveal their smoking status to professionals. Also, adults can walk into a pharmacy and buy nicotine replacement products over the counter. Underage minors cannot. Clearly, this is a problem crying out for attention.

Adult Smoking Cessation

If preventing youth smoking is necessary to breaking the generational transmission of nicotine addiction, speeding up the pace of adult smoking cessation is vital to reducing the disease toll of smoking in the foreseeable future. Even if prevention of youth smoking succeeded completely, in all countries of the world, starting today—that is, not another child ever started to smoke—the tragic milestone of 10 million annual global tobacco-produced deaths three decades from now will still be realized. Reflecting the long lag between initiation of smoking and its disease sequelae, those deaths will occur in people smoking today, young to early middle-age adults.

As with youth prevention, early efforts to foster adult smoking cessation all centered on education and related activities. When the first Surgeon General's report was released on January 11, 1964 (U.S. DHEW, 1964), the optimistic expectation among government public health officials was that it would lead to widespread quitting. (The report ranked as one of the major news stories of the year [U.S. DHHS, 1989].) Certainly the early response was encouraging: during the first three months of 1964, cigarette sales fell by 15%. By the end of the year, however, they were off by just 5%. Nicotine (and smoking) addiction was offering early evidence of its tenacity in the face of overwhelming evidence of its cost.

The Fairness Doctrine antismoking messages on the broadcast media from 1967 to1970 produced the first four-year decline in per capita cigarette smoking in the century (Warner, 1979). More recent evidence from California and Massachusetts indicates that those states' media campaigns have worked to decrease adult smoking as well (Harris et al., 1996; Goldman and Glantz, 1998). Since very few people start to smoke as adults, virtually all declines in adult smoking prevalence reflect quitting.

If antismoking media campaigns affect smoking by adults, less clear is the impact of restrictions on cigarette advertising. As industry critics have observed, with an annual budget of $6 billion devoted to advertising and other methods of promoting cigarettes in the United States, the tobacco companies are the nation's principal source of tobacco and health "education." The collective resources of all the health voluntary organizations devoted to antismoking education, combined with governmental monies dedicated to the same purpose, fall well short of a tenth of the industry's effort.

The tobacco control community believes fervently that cigarette advertising and marketing increase smoking, not only among children, who may be enticed to experiment by the seductive marketing campaigns, but also among adults. For adults, the effects of advertising are more subtle. Advertising works on adult smoking by creating an environment in which constant cues to smoke likely prompt subconscious desires to light up. Smokers contemplating quitting may find it harder to do so in such an environment, and recent quitters may find it more difficult to sustain their commitment (Warner, 1986). The ubiquity of advertising also sends a message that smoking cannnot really be as hazardous as "they" say it is; otherwise the government would not permit its presence everywhere (Marsh and Matheson, 1983). Finally, the media's dependence on cigarette ad revenues may restrict free and open discussion of the dangers of smoking. More than one empirical study has demonstrated that dependence on cigarette advertising reduces magazines' coverage of the hazards (Whelan et al., 1981; Warner et al., 1992).

Finding the "smoking gun" that demonstrates that cigarette advertising and promotion increase adult smoking has proven to be an elusive challenge. A decade ago, the Surgeon General concluded that the collective evidence supported the conclusion that advertising does increase smoking (U.S. DHHS, 1989). However, findings in the empirical literature have been mixed (Chaloupka and Warner, in press). A thorough new review of both theory and the empirical evidence presents a persuasive case that cigarette marketing does increase smoking and that comprehensive bans would decrease it (Saffer and Chaloupka, 1999). To date in the United States, however, restrictions on advertising and promotion have been partial. In 1971, cigarette ads went off the broadcast airways. In 1999, tobacco billboards came down and sports sponsorship by tobacco companies was limited (NAAG, 2000). The impacts of the latest restrictions on adult smoking, if any, remain to be established.

The other major government-produced education/information effort—placing warning labels on cigarettes and cigarette ads—has never been demonstrated to have had a significant impact on smoking. In part, this likely reflects the modest size and "drab" character of the warnings (U.S. DHHS, 1989). Dramatically larger labels, with graphic evidence of the harms caused by smoking, might be expected to command the attention of anyone who sees them (Lynch and Bonnie, 1994). That is the hope and expectation of Canadian tobacco control activists who have worked long and hard for plain packaging and large warning labels (Kennedy, 2000).

Judging intervention effectiveness by the percentage of those exposed who succeed in quitting, one must rank many formal smoking cessation programs, including medically directed treatments, as among the most effective weapons in the cessation arsenal (U.S. DHHS, 1996). Cessation programs are placed under the "education/information" category for lack of a better option. Not generally a policy measure (although there are exceptions, especially if one considers private business policies), participation in smoking cessation programs represents an individual smoker's choice, one adopted with the expectation that the smoker will learn methods to quit (hence the categorization as education/information).

While quit rates vary dramatically across participant and program types, formal programs commonly succeed in helping 15–25% of participants to quit (U.S. DHHS, 1996; Warner, in press). This is a dramatically higher figure than those associated with virtually all other tobacco control interventions. Nevertheless, one must acknowledge the high level of motivation of participants and the very modest reach of such programs. Relatively few smokers participate in them, and it remains true that the vast majority of smokers who quit do so without the aid of a formal program. Indeed, despite their high rate of effectiveness, individual cessation treatments have been criticized by Chapman (1985) as being socially undesirable. Given their low reach and high cost per participant, they are less cost-effective than a comparable level of resources devoted to a less effective, but high-reach, intervention such as a media quit campaign. This perspective has been challenged as being too narrow: specific individuals may need the individual attention accorded program participants; for them, formal programs may be the only effective option. And even if cessation programs cost more per quitter than public health interventions, as Chapman observed, they remain a highly cost-effective health care intervention (Warner, 1997).

Smoking cessation rates respond to interventions from the incentive and regulation categories, as well as education/information. Unlike the case for youth prevention, however, for which all categories of interventions are intended to reduce youth smoking, neither of the principal incentive and regulation interventions is explicitly intended to affect smoking rates among adults. Or at least proponents of these measures do not explicitly acknowledge reduction in adult smoking as their objective, although one suspects that many proponents harbor the hope and expectation that smoking prevalence will fall when the interventions are adopted.

As with youth smoking, the main incentive intervention is taxation. Although the impact of rising prices on adult smoking falls short of that for kids, adult smoking does respond to price. The empirical evidence suggests that the degree of price responsiveness is inversely related to age (Chaloupka and Warner, in press). That is, young adults are more price responsive than middle-aged adults, who in turn respond more to price than older smokers. Research also indicates that price responsiveness is inversely related to socioeconomic status (SES). Analysis of data in the United Kingdom demonstrates that in the highest social class, smoking is virtually unrelated to price changes. In striking contrast, in the lowest social class, the price elasticity of demand (the economist's measure of price responsiveness) is close to −1.0, meaning that a given percentage increase in price will reduce low-income smokers' demand for cigarettes by a comparable percentage (Townsend et al., 1994). In the United States, Farrelly and colleagues recently found that lower-income persons had a price responsiveness 70% greater than those with higher incomes (Farrelly et al., 1998).

Chaloupka (1991) earlier had found a qualitatively similar pattern comparing price responsiveness and education, which is highly correlated with income.

Collectively, as noted above, the adult price elasticity of demand is on the order of –0.4, meaning that a 10% increase in price will reduce the quantity of cigarettes demanded by 4%. As such, the tobacco control community recognizes that, translated into a price increase, a sizable tax increase can have a significant impact on adult smoking rates. In particular, it will reduce smoking more among young and poorer adults. The latter is particularly important since smoking and its disease sequelae are most common in groups of lower socioeconomic status.

From a political point of view, a cigarette tax increase has the added virtue that it will increase total tax revenues at the same time that consumption falls, simply because the tax rate rises much more than consumption declines. However, to avoid charges of social engineering, health professionals rarely advocate tax increases with the explicit objective of decreasing smoking by adults. Rather, they appeal to the impact of taxes on smoking by youth.

In a similar vein, the principal regulatory intervention that affects smoking by adults—prohibition against smoking in public places—is never advocated for that purpose. Rather, it is sought with the third major tobacco control objective in mind: protecting nonsmokers from the dangers posed by environmental tobacco smoke (ETS). In truth, clean indoor air laws were originally, and remain, motivated by the desire to protect nonsmokers. But as the research literature demonstrates, clean indoor air laws do decrease smoking in the aggregate, increasing the cessation rate modestly and causing continuing smokers to reduce their daily consumption (Evans et al., 1996; Brownson et al., 1997; Ohsfeldt et al., 1998). In addition, they help to establish and reinforce a nonsmoking social norm, which may help to discourage youth initiation (Lynch and Bonnie, 1994).

Evidence on the impacts of comprehensive tobacco control interventions on adult smoking prevalence is modest in quantity. Again, a major source of insight is provided by analyses of the experiences in California and Massachusetts, each of which has documented significant declines in smoking prevalence attributable to these states' campaigns (Harris et al., 1996; Goldman and Glantz, 1998). One major experimental effort to establish the effect of a multichannel community-based intervention, the COMMIT program, failed in its designated objective of reducing smoking among heavy smokers. However, researchers did find a statistically significant decline in smoking by light smokers (COMMIT Research Group, 1995).

The paucity of this empirical evidence notwithstanding, there is substantial reason to believe that multiple interventions produce at least an additive impact on smoking, and possibly a whole that is greater than the sum of its parts. The federal Office on Smoking and Health argues that comprehensive programs are vital to realizing substantial tobacco control success (CDC, 2000), and the Institute of Medicine has recently concurred (National Cancer Policy Board, 2000). What is unequivocally clear is that the modest resources devoted to all tobacco control programs to date require only modest success in controlling tobacco use to justify their existence. The prospect that they may yield more than modest success makes them a very attractive investment of public health resources.

In concluding consideration of the objective of adult smoking cessation, it seems critical to comment on the evidence on the changing demographic patterns of smoking since the inception of the antismoking campaign in 1964, because the numbers tell a compelling tale. Most notable is the change in smoking prevalence by education class. In 1965, the year following the first Surgeon General's report, less than 3 percentage points separated the prevalence of smoking among college graduates (33.7%) from that of Americans who did not graduate from high school (36.5%) (U.S. DHHS, 1989). By 1997, prevalence among college graduates had fallen by nearly two-thirds, to 11.6%. Among people without a high school diploma, in contrast, prevalence had fallen by only one-sixth (to 30.4%) (CDC, 1999b). The gap had grown to almost 19 points.

These numbers mirror others relating to income and occupation, which, of course, are closely related to education. Perhaps most striking is evidence that smoking prevalence among American physicians—among the nation's most highly educated persons—may now be less than 4% (Nelson et al., 1994; Frank et al., 1998), while it remains around 40% for certain blue-collar occupations. In short, smoking has moved from an "egalitarian" burden in the mid-1960s to a heavy weight today on those of low socioeconomic status.

Particularly given that high-income and highly educated smokers are less responsive to price increases than are low-income and education smokers (Chaloupka, 1991; Townsend et al., 1994; Farrelly et al., 1998), the socioeconomic evidence strongly suggests that the educational component of the antismoking campaign has had a far more substantial impact on high-income and education groups than on those less fortunate. To be sure, the dramatic changes in smoking prevalence among the more fortunate members of society likely reflect the interaction of effective information dissemination and social pressure. That is, as a portion of high-SES smokers quit in response to the newly emerging evidence on the dangers of smoking, smoking lost its social cache in this class quickly; indeed, it became socially less acceptable, and eventually unacceptable. But the conclusion that the lower-SES groups did not respond comparably to information dissemination and likely did not experience the same social disapprobation of their smoking, seems inescapable.

There are numerous possible explanations for the divergence in smoking trends by SES. One is that health educators communicated effectively with people like themselves—highly educated persons—and failed to deliver the tobacco-and-health message to less educated people in a manner they would comprehend and find compelling. Recent state-based campaigns devote specific resources to developing culturally and educationally relevant health education messages. Another possible explanation is that the affluent, well-educated population finds the future, especially the prospect of retirement, far more attractive than the lower-SES population for whom the future bodes only continuing economic worries. As a consequence, the low-SES population heavily discounts the future promised by not smoking.

Whatever the reason, the widening gap between high- and low-SES smoking suggests a dimension of tobacco control that, to date, has received very limited attention and clearly deserves more.

Protecting Nonsmokers from Environmental Tobacco Smoke

In many ways, the third major objective—protecting nonsmokers from environmental tobacco smoke—has proved to be the domain of the most interesting and politically contentious tobacco control activity. More than two decades ago, the tobacco industry was warned by its polling consultant, the Roper organization, that the issue of ETS, and the nonsmokers' rights movement it had spawned, posed the single greatest threat to the economic vitality of the industry (Roper, 1978). In subsequent years, grassroots activists succeeded in getting numerous and increasingly strong clean indoor air policies adopted, initially at the state level and then, increasingly, at the level of local government. The latter occurred first (and thus far most) in California, the clear leader in tobacco control policy innovation.

Californians' success in adopting scores of local ordinances demonstrated that even the financially muscular tobacco industry could be tackled with a divide-and-conquer strategy. Arguably, the industry has controlled the U.S. Congress for years (Taylor, 1984; Advocacy Institute, 1998). It has also carried enormous weight in the deliberations of state legislatures; the industry has impressive lobbying resources in all 50 states and it makes effective use of campaign contributions at the state level, as it long has at the federal level (Advocacy Institute, 1998; Monardi and Glantz, 1998). But its ability to curry favor with literally thousands of city council members is clearly limited. As one consequence, the industry adopted a strategy of working behind the scenes at the state level to promote weak state clean indoor air laws that preempted stronger local action. Initially, by carefully garbing such laws in seemingly attractive public health language, the industry often succeeded in garnering the support of local antitobacco advocates. Once it became clear, however, that the purpose of such laws was to preempt stronger measures, the tobacco control community became increasingly informed and vigilant (Siegel et al., 1997).

As with youth prevention and adult cessation, tobacco control efforts to protect the health of nonsmokers began with an educational effort to inform the public about the dangers of ETS. However, with the issue of tobacco control further along by the time ETS became a source of public concern (roughly the late 1970s), the public education effort had a more explicit policy orientation to it: the "educators" were attempting to mold public opinion, not merely inform it, with the objective of promoting legislated restrictions on smoking in public places. That this strategy has succeeded beyond their fondest hopes is demonstrated by the rapid diffusion of clean indoor air laws through the states (U.S. DHHS, 1989); the adoption of municipal ordinances in the heart of tobacco country, such as Winston-Salem, North Carolina; the fast transformation of the American workplace into a largely smoke-free environment; and the banning of smoking not only in restaurants but also in bars in California. Bars and gambling establishments have long been viewed as the last bastions of unrestricted smoking. Until California proved them wrong, most tobacco control advocates likely believed that prohibiting smoking in bars verged on the impossible. The early evidence indicates that in large part, the ban is working (Glantz and Smith, 1997).

The objective of protecting nonsmokers from ETS has been pursued by this highly effective combination of education and regulation strategies. Economic incentives have proven far less important to this objective than to either of the other two. They are not nonexistent, however. Although clean indoor air laws are largely self-enforcing, fines have been levied in a few instances of flagrant violations. Clearly, economic incentives have been significant motivators for businesses to adopt smoke-free policies on their own (many having done so prior to state mandates requiring smoke-free work environments): the absence of smoking in the workplace reduces a series of business costs, including cleaning and equipment maintenance, fire insurance, and the risk of liability lawsuits from employees allegedly injured by ETS in the workplace.

Lessons from the Experience with Tobacco Control

If one wishes to learn by example how a society can address a complicated and tenacious behavior-related public health problem—and to what effect—tobacco control is an excellent choice of subject matter. Tobacco is unrivaled as a source of avoidable premature mortality; as such, it clearly ranks among the nation's, and indeed world's, most important public health problems. In the complex web of its causes, ranging from nicotine addiction to a rich and influential industrial disease vector, tobacco illustrates the full spectrum of challenges to effective public health intervention. Tobacco demonstrates vividly how health professionals, motivated by the purest of causes, must learn to wrestle with unseemly politics driven by anything but pure motives. With 35 years of history under its belt, tobacco control offers a treasure trove of the dos and donts of intervention. Tobacco control is at once a model for public health optimism and a sobering reminder of the limits of intervention success.

Likely the most important lessons deriving from the tobacco control experience are all the obvious ones. A first lesson is that whenever possible, behavioral interventions should be grounded in solid science, here the evaluation research and policy analysis that have informed tobacco control for more than two decades. As one notable example, research on the effects of cigarette taxation has quite literally transformed the practice of public health policy in the domain of tobacco control and affected thinking about policy across a wide range of public health problems, including alcohol abuse (raising beer taxes to reduce underage drinking and driving (Grossman et al., 1994), unhealthy diets (California's snack tax), and even control of gun violence (taxing guns and bullets, as proposed by Senator Moynihan [Tax Treatment, 1994]). Research on the effects of clean indoor air laws, smoking cessation interventions, and other measures has increased their utilization and enhanced the efficiency of investments in tobacco control.

The qualification to the idea of grounding behavioral interventions in solid science—"whenever possible"—is itself important. When confronting large and urgent public health problems, the lack of definitive science should never paralyze action. As discussed throughout this paper, the evidence on the impacts of many individual tobacco control interventions and on comprehensive programs as well falls short of the kinds of definitive insights that constitute the lifeblood of science. But although the findings are imprecise, the evidence is good enough to warrant substantial investment in all but a handful of such interventions. Refinements in knowledge through further research promise the attainment of greater efficiency in mounting interventions in the future.

A leading lesson from tobacco control is a self-evident but important reminder: when one enters the fray, one should be prepared to stay for the long haul. After 35 years, tobacco control has achieved a great deal, enough that it is justifiably ranked among the great public health triumphs of the past 50 years (U.S. DHHS, 1989; CDC, 1999a). Yet despite this success, the toll of tobacco remains almost inconceivably high—higher in body count in the United States than the sum total of all other drugs, licit and illicit, all injuries, intentional and otherwise, and all the major infectious diseases, including AIDS. This is hardly the time to declare victory and go home, and few tobacco control advocates have done so.

Battles have been won, often small battles, and they should be savored. But they are never an excuse to lose sight of the bigger picture. Further, the small victories should never be considered immutable: just as the smoker who quits faces months and even years of risk of relapse, tobacco control successes are not necessarily ultimate victories. Witness, for example, how the industry converted federally mandated warning labels, which have never been demonstrated to discourage smoking, into successful product liability defenses and protection (preemption) against scores of more draconian and expensive state-based warning systems. Tobacco control—and, by extension, other behavioral health intervention issues—demands constant vigilance, evaluation and reevaluation, and creativity in looking forward to the next stages of intervention.

Yet another lesson is that innovation may prove crucial in finding new ways to attack old problems. Although not discussed much in this paper, the attorneys general's Medicaid tobacco lawsuits not only have broken new tobacco control ground with novel legal theories, but have made the judicial system an active participant in the crafting of public health policy on tobacco. Comparable creativity at the political level might redirect tobacco control policy making to the legislative and regulatory institutions designed for that purpose (Jacobson and Warner, 1999).

Certainly a major lesson, if also obvious, is that a multidimensional problem demands a multilevel intervention. The greatest U.S. success stories in tobacco control during the past decade reflect multipronged strategies, most notably the cigarette tax-financed state programs in California and Massachusetts. The notion that tobacco control programs must be comprehensive (be they youth oriented or not) is by now shared virtually universally within the tobacco control community (CDC, 2000; National Cancer Policy Board, 2000).

In fairness, as noted above, if one scrutinizes the evidence for this proposition in the harsh light of day, unassailable empirical support for the proposition is lacking. But this reflects the absence of experimental opportunities to evaluate the proposition, rather than any inherent weakness in the idea itself. The vast majority of multiply pronged tobacco control interventions are "natural experiments" lacking controls. Their successes have, in general, exceeded those that analysis permits us to attribute to one or more of their individual components; often prior research does not permit assessment of the likely effects of each component individually. For example, as noted above, the California and Massachusetts programs have decreased smoking by more than their associated tax increases, acting alone, would have. But lacking a sound body of evidence producing a consensus estimate of the impact of media campaigns, we cannot know how much credit to accord the media campaigns alone (although valiant attempts to do so have been made (Harris et al., 1996; Goldman and Glantz, 1998). Nor can we determine whether or not interaction of the component parts produced a synergistic effect. The absence of a more complete science of tobacco control precludes determination as to whether the sum is greater than, less than, or equal to its parts. A source of frustration to contemporary analysts, this situation also poses wonderful opportunities for future research, including integrative multidisciplinary research (Chaloupka, in press).

The dearth of empirical evidence notwithstanding, specific examples present a compelling case for multilevel interventions. To take but one, adult smoking cessation has resulted from dissemination of information about the dangers of smoking; from increased excise taxes; from responses to media antismoking campaigns; and from participation in formal smoking cessation programs. Two important observations verge on truisms. First, no one of these interventions could have successfully prompted all of the quitting that has occurred. The diversity of interventions was essential to bring us to the point that half of all Americans who ever smoked have quit. In the absence of any one of these interventions, a significant number of now former smokers might have remained smokers and perished prematurely as a result. That we cannot attribute a specific fraction of the quitting to information dissemination and another to media campaigns does not diminish the validity or importance of this observation. (It does, however, mean that until the evaluation science improves, we must live with the possibility that one or more of the interventions has had little impact or perhaps a cost-ineffective impact.[10])

----

[10]With one notable exception—cessation—the literature on the cost-effectiveness of tobacco control interventions is sparse to nonexistent. Cessation lends itself readily to cost-effectiveness analysis (CEA) and has been the subject of many CEAs (Cromwell et al., 1997; Warner, 1997). Other types of intervention, such as youth access law enforcement, should lend themselves nicely to CEA, and a few analysts are attempting to per-

Second, the interventions almost certainly reinforce each other. To contemplate how, consider further the example of smoking cessation raised at the beginning of this section. Information dissemination on the hazards of smoking may move smokers from the precontemplation stage to contemplation of quitting (Prochaska et al., 1993). A media campaign mocking smoking may move the now-ambivalent smoker toward action. A cigarette tax increase may push the smoker "over the top" toward successful quitting. And the elimination of tobacco billboards in 1999 may aid that former smoker's resolve to stay "quit." More generally, through specific interventions (such as clean indoor air laws) and the norms they help to create (a nonsmoking ethos), the social environment becomes increasingly conducive to quitting and to staying quit.

Throughout this paper, "multilevel" has referred to intervention functions. As observed in Box 1, however, other constructions of "multilevel" are equally valid. Although not discussed in this paper, a clear lesson of tobacco control is that any effective, comprehensive assault on a major behavior-related public health problem must avail itself of multiple "levels" along other dimensions. In tobacco control, for example, success has depended on the concerted efforts, sometimes coordinated, usually not, of professionals and volunteers from the full range of organizations within our society—government agencies, voluntary health societies, and private businesses (item 2 in Box 1). The need to rely on multiple intervention channels—the media, medical and public health societies, workplaces, schools, churches—verges on the self-evident (item 4).

Application of the lessons of tobacco control to other behavioral public health problems should proceed with caution. Some of the lessons will transfer quite directly; others likely will prove inappropriate in other substantive domains. The temptation is to think that problems most like tobacco will benefit most directly from the case study. Gun control and reduction of alcohol abuse come initially to mind as concerns that have borrowed intervention lessons directly from tobacco control (and vice versa; for example, the current youth access movement in tobacco control is modeled quite consciously on the experience with alcohol control). But the differences between any two behavior-related problems are invariably as profound as the similarities. Guns and alcohol

---

form such analysis at the time of this writing. Nevertheless, this intervention's susceptibility to useful CEA is limited by incomplete understanding of the effectiveness of the intervention (Forster and Wolfson, 1998; Lancaster and Stead, 1999). By definition, cost-effectiveness analysis presupposes the existence of good effectiveness knowledge. This problem plagues many areas of tobacco control, helping to explain why few CEAs have been completed outside the area of cessation. There is yet another important reason that many central tobacco control interventions have not been subjected to CEA: they represent the type of intervention for which costs are so hard to quantify that CEA may be meaningless, or at least controversial. For example, although taxation is documented to be a highly effective intervention, how does one value the cost of violating the economic neutrality of the fiscal system? How does one measure the cost of possible inequities associated with the burdens placed on poor smokers by tax increases?

each produce health consequences with an immediacy not experienced in tobacco; guns and alcohol kill children as well as adults. Tobacco is dangerous when used as intended. Consumed in moderation, alcohol benefits health.[11]

While applications of lessons from tobacco control to other problems (and vice versa) should proceed with caution, they definitely should proceed. To date, although a few adventurous scholars and activists have crossed the boundaries of individual public health problems, their numbers are almost shockingly low. It is nothing short of remarkable, for example, how little interaction one observes between the tobacco and alcohol control communities. The two major licit drugs—the two leading sources of death and disability in our society—have much in common. Yet consider the warning label on alcoholic beverages, "won" after a bitter political struggle. In its wordiness, diminutive size, and obscure placement, it goes virtually unnoticed. One day it may protect the alcohol producers in court. The lessons of tobacco labeling—far bolder than the labels themselves—have been available, and understood, for at least two decades.

If translation of the lessons from tobacco control to other behavioral health problems has proved limited to date, it is at least encouraging to recognize and celebrate the sharing of tobacco control lessons across nations. Thanks in part to a sophisticated Internet operation known as GlobaLink, some 1,000 tobacco control activists from scores of countries are in daily communication. Lessons about the effectiveness of taxation in discouraging youth smoking, the potential of state-based lawsuits to generate tobacco control action, and the need for comprehensive multilevel tobacco control programs are shared, learned, and put into play with increasing regularity. The challenges posed by tobacco worldwide are immense and urgent. The resources available to the public health community to address them pale in comparison with those the tobacco industry devotes to increasing them. Still, the sharing of knowledge, and the sophistication with which it is utilized, offer hope that the tobacco beast will eventually be contained. At the beginning of a new century, it may not be unrealistic to envision the elusive tobacco-free world before the next century dawns.

REFERENCES

Advocacy Institute. *Smoke and Mirrors: How the Tobacco Industry Buys and Lies Its Way to Power and Profits*. Washington, DC: Advocacy Institute, August 1998.

Advocacy Institute. *A Movement Rising: a Strategic Analysis of U.S. Tobacco Control Advocacy*. Washington, DC: Advocacy Institute, March 1999.

Bhonsle RB, Murti RP, Gupta PC. Tobacco habits in India. In: Gupta PC, Hamner JE III, Muri PR, eds. *Control of Tobacco-Related Cancers and Other Diseases*. Bombay: Oxford University Press, 1992.

Brown & Williamson, Inc. http://brownandwilliamson.com/8_yspc.html. 2000.

---

[11]This is a source of consternation to many public health educators who struggle with how one can convey the health message about moderate alcohol consumption without encouraging deadly abuse among the most vulnerable members of society.

Brownson RC, Eriksen MP, Davis RM, et al. Environmental tobacco smoke: Health effects and policies to reduce exposures. *Annual Review of Public Health* 1997;18: 163–185.

Centers for Disease Control and Prevention. Response to increases in cigarette prices by race/ethnicity, income, and age groups—United States, 1976–1993. *Morbidity and Mortality Weekly Report* 1998;47:605–609.

Centers for Disease Control and Prevention. Achievements in public health, 1900–1999: tobacco use—United States, 1900–1999. *Morbidity and Mortality Weekly Report* 1999a;48:986–993.

Centers for Disease Control and Prevention. Cigarette smoking among adults—United States, 1997. *Morbidity and Mortality Weekly Report* 1999b;48:993–996.

Centers for Disease Control and Prevention, National Center for Health Promotion and Chronic Disease Prevention, Office on Smoking and Health. *Best Practices for Comprehensive Tobacco Control Programs.* http://www.cdc.gov/tobacco/bestprac. htm. 2000.

Chaloupka FJ. Rational addictive behavior and cigarette smoking. *Journal of Political Economy,* 1991;99:722–742.

Chaloupka FJ. *Macro-social influences: the effects of prices and tobacco control policies on the demand for tobacco products.* Nicotine and Tobacco Research. In press.

Chaloupka FJ, Pacula RL. Sex and race differences in young people's responsiveness to price and tobacco control policies. *Tobacco Control* 1999;8:373–377.

Chaloupka FJ, Warner KE. Economics of smoking. In: Culyer AJ, Newhouse JP, eds. *Handbook of Health Economics.* Amsterdam: Elsevier, in press.

Chapman S. Stop smoking clinics: a case for their abandonment. *Lancet* 1985;1:918–920.

COMMIT Research Group. Community intervention trial for smoking cessation (COMMIT): I. Cohort results from a four-year intervention. *American Journal of Public Health* 1995;85:183–192.

Cromwell J, Bartosch WJ, Fiore MC, et al. Cost-effectiveness of the clinical practice recommendations in the AHCPR guideline for smoking cessation. Agency for Health Care Policy and Research. *Journal of the American Medical Association* 1997;278:1759–1766.

DeCicca P, Kenkel D, Mathios A. *Putting out the fires: will higher cigarette taxes reduce youth smoking?* Presented at the Annual Meetings of the American Economic Association, 1998.

Dee TS, Evans WN. *A comment on DeCicca, Kenkel, and Mathios.* Working Paper. School of Economics, Georgia Institute of Technology, 1998.

DiFranza JR. Are the federal and state governments complying with the Synar amendment? *Archives of Pediatrics and Adolescent Medicine* 1999;153:1089–1097.

Evans WN, Farrelly MC, Montgomery E. Do workplace smoking bans reduce smoking? Cambridge, MA: *National Bureau of Economic Research Working Paper No. 5567,* 1996.

Farrelly MC, Bray JW, Office on Smoking and Health. Response to increases in cigarette prices by race/ethnicity, income, and age groups—United States, 1976–1993. *Morbidity and Mortality Weekly Report* 1998;47:605–609.

Ferrence R, Slade J, Room R, Pope M, eds. *Nicotine and Public Health.* Washington, DC: American Public Health Association, in press.

Florida Department of Health, Office of Tobacco Control. *Report Regarding the Progress of the Tobacco Pilot Program,* March 17, 1999.

Food and Drug Administration. Regulations restricting the sale and distribution of cigarettes and smokeless tobacco to protect children and adolescents; final rule. *Federal Register* 1996 (August 28);61(168):44396–45318.

Forster JL, Wolfson DM. Youth access to tobacco: policies and politics. *Annual Review of Public Health* 1998;19:203–235.

Frank E, Brogan DJ, Mokdad AH, et al. Health-related behaviors of women physicians vs. other women in the United States. *Archives of Internal Medicine* 1998;158:342–348.

Glantz SA. Editorial: preventing tobacco use—the youth access trap. *American Journal of Public Health* 1996;86:156–158.

Glantz SA, Smith LR. The effect of ordinances requiring smoke-free restaurants and bars on revenues: a follow-up. *American Journal of Public Health* 1997;87:1687–1693.

Goldman LK. Glantz SA. Evaluation of antismoking advertising campaigns. *Journal of the American Medical Association* 1998;279:772–777.

Goodman J. *Tobacco in History: The Cultures of Dependence.* New York: Routledge, 1994.

Grossman M, Chaloupka FJ. Cigarette taxes: the straw to break the camel's back. *Public Health Reports* 1997;112:290–297.

Grossman M, Chaloupka FJ, Saffer H, et al. Alcohol price policy and youths: a summary of economic research. *Journal of Research on Adolescence* 1994;4:347–364.

Harris JE. Cigarette smoking among successive birth cohorts of men and women in the United States during 1900–80. *Journal of the National Cancer Institute* 1983;71:473–479.

Harris JE, Connolly GN, Brooks D, et al. Cigarette smoking before and after an excise tax increase and an antismoking media campaign: Massachusetts, 1990–1996. *Morbidity and Mortality Weekly Report* 1996;45:966–970.

Henningfield JE, Cohen C, Pickworth WB. Psychopharmacology of nicotine. In: Orleans CT, Slade J, eds. *Nicotine Addiction: Principles and Management.* New York: Oxford University Press, 1993.

Jacobson PD, Warner KE. Litigation and public health policy making: The case of tobacco control. *Journal on Health Politics, Policy and Law* 1999;24:769–804.

Jason LA, Ji PY, Anes MD, et al. Active enforcement of cigarette control laws in the prevention of cigarette sales to minors. *Journal of the American Medical Association* 1991;266:3159–3161.

Kennedy M. Smoking hazards to be depicted on cigarette packs. Government set to force warnings that show graphic cancer photos. *Ottawa Citizen* January 6, 2000.

Lancaster T, Stead LF. Interventions for preventing tobacco sales to minors. *Cochrane Database of Systematic Reviews* 1999;4.

Lantz PM, Jacobson PD, Warner KE, et al. Investing in youth tobacco control: A review of smoking prevention strategies. *Tobacco Control* 2000; 9:47–63.

Levy DT, Friend K, Coggeshall M. *A simulation model of tobacco youth access policies.* Working paper. Rockville, MD: National Center for the Advancement of Prevention, December 1998.

Lynch BS, Bonnie RJ, eds. Growing Up Tobacco Free: *Preventing Nicotine Addiction in Children and Youths.* Washington, DC: National Academy Press, 1994.

Marsh A, Matheson J. *Smoking attitudes and behavior.* An enquiry carried out on behalf of the Department of Health and Social Security, Office of Population Census and Surveys. London: Her Majesty's Stationary Office, 1983.

McGinnis JM. Foege WH. Actual causes of death in the United States. *Journal of the American Medical Association* 1993, 270:2207–2212.

Mendez D, Warner KE. Has smoking cessation ceased? Expected trends in the prevalence of smoking in the United States. *American Journal of Epidemiology* 1998;148: 249–258.

Monardi F, Glantz SA. Are tobacco industry campaign contributions influencing state legislative behavior? *American Journal of Public Health* 1998;88:918–923.

Monitoring the Future. http://monitoringthefuture.org/, 2000.

Murray CJL, Lopez AD. Evidence-based public health policy—lessons from the Global Burden of Disease study. *Science* 1996;274:740–743.

Napier K. Cigarettes: *What the Warning Label Doesn't Tell You. The First Comprehensive Guide to the Health Consequences of Smoking.* New York: American Council on Science and Health, 1996.

National Association of Attorneys General. http://www.naag.org/tob2.htm, 2000.

National Cancer Institute. *The impact of cigarette excise taxes on smoking among children and adults*: summary report of a National Cancer institute expert panel. Bethesda, MD: Division of Cancer Prevention and Control, NCI, August 1993.

National Cancer Policy Board. *State Tobacco Programs Can Reduce Tobacco Use.* Washington, DC: National Academy Press, 2000.

Nelson DE, Giovino GA, Emont SL, et al. Trends in cigarette smoking among US physicians and nurses. *Journal of the American Medical Association* 1994;271:1273–1275.

Ohsfeldt RL, Boyle RG, Capilouto EI. *Tobacco taxes, smoking restrictions, and tobacco use.* Cambridge, MA: National Bureau of Economic Research Working Paper No. 6486, 1998.

Philip Morris, Inc. http://www.philipmorris.com/tobacco_bus/tobacco_issues/youth_smoking_prevention.html. 2000.

Pierce JP, Gilpin EA, Emery SL, et al. Has the California tobacco control program reduced smoking? *Journal of the American Medical Association* 1998;280:893–899.

Pomerleau OF. Individual differences in sensitivity to nicotine: Implications for genetic research on nicotine dependence. *Behavior Genetics* 1995;25:161–177.

Popham WJ, Potter LD, Hetrick MA, et al. Effectiveness of the California 1990–1991 tobacco education media campaign. *American Journal of Preventive Medicine* 1994; 10:319–326.

Prochaska JO, DiClemente CC, Velicer WF, et al. Standardized, individualized, interactive and personalized self-help programs for smoking cessation. *Health Psychology* 1993;12:399–405.

Ramirez AG, Gallion KJ. Nicotine dependence among blacks and Hispanics. In: Orleans CT, Slade J, eds. *Nicotine Addiction: Principles and Management.* New York: Oxford University Press, 1993.

Rigotti NA, DiFranza JR, Chang Y, et al. The effect of enforcing tobacco-sales laws on adolescents' access to tobacco and smoking behavior. *New England Journal of Medicine* 1997;337:1044–1051.

R.J. Reynolds Tobacco Co., Inc. http://www.rjrt.com/TI/Pages/TIcover.asp. 2000.

Roper. A *Study of Public Attitudes toward Cigarette Smoking and the Tobacco Industry in 1978.* Vol. 1. Roper Organization, May 1978.

Saffer H, Chaloupka FJ. *Tobacco Advertising: Economic Theory and International Evidence.* Cambridge, MA: National Bureau of Economic Research, Working Paper No. 6958, February 1999.

Samuels B. Glantz SA. The politics of local tobacco control. *Journal of the American Medical Association* 1991;266:2110–2117.

Siegel M, Carol J, Jordan J, et al. Preemption in tobacco control. Review of an emerging
public health problem. *Journal of the American Medical Association* 1997;278:858–
863.

Tax Treatment of Organizations Providing Health Care Services, and Excise Taxes on
Tobacco, Guns and Ammunition. Hearing before the Committee on Finance, United
States Senate, 103rd Congress, 2nd Session, April 28, 1994. Washington, DC: U.S.
Government Printing Office, 1994.

Taylor P. *The Smoke Ring: Tobacco, Money, and Multi-National Politics.* New York:
Pantheon, 1984.

Tilley NM. *The RJ Reynolds Tobacco Company.* Chapel Hill, NC: University of North
Carolina Press, 1985.

Tobacco Dependence: Innovative regulatory approaches to reduce death and disease. *Food
and Drug Law Journal* 1998;53(suppl).

Tobacco Institute. The Tax Burden on Tobacco. *Historical Compilation* 1995. Vol. 30.
Washington, DC: Tobacco Institute, 1998.

Townsend JL, Roderick P, Cooper J. Cigarette smoking by socioeconomic group, sex, and
age: effects of price, income, and health publicity. *British Medical Journal* 1994;309:
923–926.

U.S. Department of Health, Education, and Welfare. *Smoking and Health.* Report of the
Advisory Committee to the Surgeon General of the Public Health Service. Washing-
ton, DC: U.S. Department of Health, Education, and Welfare, Public Health Service,
Center for Disease Control. Public Health Service Publication No. 1103, 1964.

U.S. Department of Health and Human Services. *The Health Consequences of Smoking:
Nicotine Addiction. A Report of the Surgeon General.* Rockville, MD: U.S. Department of Health and Human Services, Public Health Service, Centers for Disease Control, Center for Health Promotion and Education, Office on Smoking and Health. Department of Health and Human Services Publication No. (CDC) 88-8406, 1988.

U.S. Department of Health and Human Services. *Reducing the Health Consequences of
Smoking: 25 Years of Progress. A Report of the Surgeon General.* Atlanta, GA: U.S.
Department of Health and Human Services, Public Health Service, Centers for Disease
Control, National Center for Chronic Disease Prevention and Health Promotion, Office
of Smoking and Health. Department of Health and Human Services Publication No.
(CDC) 89-8411, 1989.

U.S. Department of Health and Human Services, 1991. *Strategies to Control Tobacco
Use in the United States: A Blueprint for Public Health Action in the 1990's.*
Smoking and Tobacco Control Monographs No. 1. Department of Health and Hu-
man Services, Public Health Service, National Institutes of Health. NIH Publication
No. 92-3316. Bethesda, MD: National Cancer Institute, 1991.

U.S. Department of Health and Human Services. *Smoking and Health in the Americas.* A
1992 Report of the Surgeon General in Collaboration with the Pan American Health
Organization. Atlanta, GA: U.S. Department of Health and Human Services, Public
Health Service, Centers for Disease Control, National Center for Chronic Disease
Prevention and Health Promotion, Office on Smoking and Health. Department of
Health and Human Services Publication No. (CDC) 92-8419, 1992.

U.S. Department of Health and Human Services. *Preventing Tobacco Use Among Young
People: A Report of the Surgeon General.* U.S. Department of Health and Human
Services, Public Health Service, Centers for Disease Control, National Center for
Chronic Disease Prevention and Health Promotion, Office on Smoking and Health.
Washington, DC: U.S. Government Printing Office, 1994.

U.S. Department of Health and Human Services. *Smoking Cessation*. Clinical Practice Guideline Number 18. Public Health Service, Agency for Health Care Policy and Research, Centers for Disease Control and Prevention. AHCPR Publication No. 96-0692. Rockville, MD: AHCPR, 1996.

U.S. Department of Health and Human Services. *Tobacco Use Among U.S. Racial/Ethnic Minority Groups—African Americans, American Indians and Alaska Natives, Asian Americans and Pacific Islanders, and Hispanics: A Report of the Surgeon General*. Atlanta, GA: U.S. Department of Health and Human Services, Centers for Disease Control and Prevention, National Center for Chronic Disease Prevention and Health Promotion, Office on Smoking and Health, 1998.

Wagner S. *Cigarette Country: Tobacco in American History and Politics*. New York: Praeger, 1971.

Walsh DC. Gordon NP. Legal approaches to smoking deterrence. *Annual Review of Public Health* 1986;7:127–149.

Warner KE. Clearing the airwaves: the cigarette ad ban revisited. *Policy Analysis* 1979;5:435–450.

Warner KE. *Selling Smoke: Cigarette Advertising and Public Health*. Washington, DC: American Public Health Association, 1986.

Warner KE. Effects of the antismoking campaign: an update. *American Journal of Public Health* 1989;79:144–151.

Warner KE. Reducing harms to smokers: methods, their effectiveness, and the role of policy. In: Rabin RL, Sugarman SD, eds. *Regulating Tobacco: Premises and Policy Options*. New York: Oxford University Press, in press.

Warner KE. Cost-effectiveness of smoking cessation therapies: interpretation of the evidence and implications for coverage. *PharmacoEconomics* 1997;11:538–549.

Warner KE, Murt HA. Impact of the antismoking campaign on smoking prevalence: a cohort analysis. *Journal of Public Health Policy* 1982;3:374–389.

Warner KE, Murt HA. Economic incentives for health. *Annual Review of Public Health* 1984;5:107–133.

Warner KE, Chaloupka FJ, Cook PJ, et al. Criteria for determining an optimal cigarette tax: the economist's perspective. *Tobacco Control* 1995;4:380–386.

Warner KE, Citrin T, Pickett G, et al. Licit and illicit drug policies: a typology. *British Journal of Addiction* 1990;85:255–262.

Warner KE, Goldenhar LM, McLaughlin CG. Cigarette advertising and magazine coverage of the hazards of smoking: a statistical analysis. *New England Journal of Medicine* 1992;326:305–309.

Warner KE, Slade J, Sweanor DT. The emerging market for long-term nicotine maintenance. *Journal of the American Medical Association* 1997;278:1087–1092.

Wasserman J, Manning WG, Newhouse JP, et al. The effects of excise taxes and regulations on cigarette smoking. *Journal of Health Economics* 1991;10:43–64.

Whelan EM, Sheridan MJ, Meister KA, et al. Analysis of coverage of tobacco hazards in women's magazines. *Journal of Public Health Policy* 1981;2:28–35.

World Bank. *Curbing the Epidemic: Governments and the Economics of Tobacco Control*. Washington, DC: World Bank, 1999.

Behavioral and Psychosocial Intervention to Modify Pathophysiology and Disease Course

Andrew Baum

BEHAVIOR, STRESS, AND DISEASE

Evidence of behavioral influences in disease outcomes is growing and comes from many diverse sources. This paper considers summaries of this rapidly growing literature focusing on studies of cardiovascular disease, cancer, and HIV disease/AIDS (Figure 1). Other diseases and serious medical conditions are also considered briefly.

Stress and Cardiovascular Disease

The effects of stress on the pathophysiology of heart disease, hypertension, stroke, and other cardiovascular disorders are broad and increasingly well documented. Stress appears to contribute directly to atherosclerotic processes by which blood vessels become increasingly narrow and unable to adapt to changing circulatory demands (e.g., Smith and Gallo, 1994; Kopp, 1999). Among the effects of stress on the circulatory system are increases in damage to vessel walls and lining, increases in fat deposits in injured intimal areas and lipid pro-

Dr. Baum is director, Behavioral Medicine and Oncology and professor of psychiatry and psychology, University of Pittsburgh Cancer Institute, Pittsburgh Mind-Body Center, Departments of Psychiatry and Psychology, University of Pittsburgh. This paper was prepared for the symposium on "Capitalizing on Social Science and Behavioral Research to Improve the Public's Health," the Institute of Medicine and the Commission on Behavioral and Social Sciences and Education of the National Research Council, Atlanta, GA, February 2-3, 2000.

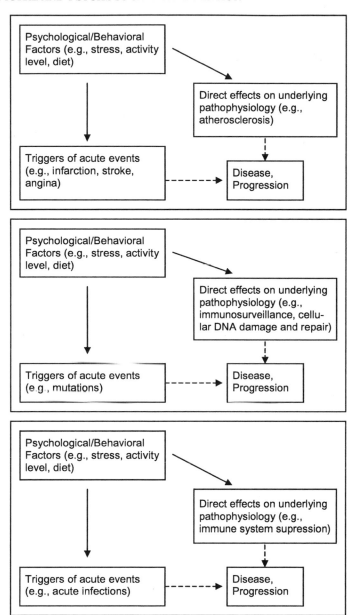

FIGURE 1 Schematic drawings of the basic relationships between stress or behaviors and diseases discussed in this chapter. The first describes simple relationships between behavioral variables and cardiovascular disease, the second considers behavioral influence and cancer, and the third depicts simple relationships between behavior and HIV disease.

files in general, and increases in plaque associated with repair and overgrowth of these injury sites in blood vessels (Schneiderman, 1983; Foreyt and Poston, 1996). Though far more complex than can be portrayed here, atherosclerosis is a lifelong process of gradual narrowing of arteries and veins, in part because of this repeated pattern of vessel damage, repair, and growth of plaque.

In coronary heart disease, factors such as diet, tobacco use, and stress modify the vessels that provide nutrients to the heart and periphery and demand for delivery of nutrients. Sharp increases in demand in an organism with occluded coronary arteries can precipitate cardiovascular events such as infarction, angina, or arrhythmias (e.g., Kamarck and Jennings, 1991). Stress also affects platelets and other clotting factors in the blood that can increase the likelihood of troublesome or dangerous clot formation, pulmonary embolism, or other untoward events (Markovitz and Matthews, 1991; Allen and Patterson, 1995). Finally, these factors can increase blood pressure in several different ways (e.g., Barnes et al., 1997). Some influences on blood pressure are directly related to stress, as is the case, for example, for beta-adrenergic receptor density (Dimsdale et al., 1994). Other effects are more broadly caused by a number of biobehavioral processes, and differences in the magnitude of acute blood pressure and heart rate changes associated with stress appear to be a risk factor for hypertension and coronary heart disease (e.g., Manuck and Krantz, 1984; Manuck et al., 1997). However, evidence is mixed, with some studies suggesting that acute stress-related effects on blood pressure are related to hypertension and some finding little or no evidence of such a relationship (Fredrikson and Matthews, 1990; Pickering and Gerin, 1990). Overall increases in blood pressure associated with chronic stress may also contribute to hypertension (Blumenthal et al., 1995).

Direct evidence that stress and other behavioral factors cause cardiovascular dysfunction or disease is increasingly conclusive, but the data are not complete. This is due in part to the nature of these diseases and their development over one's lifetime. Because the development of disease is a very long term process, it is difficult if not impossible to monitor all potential contributors to pathophysiologic disease processes or to pinpoint specific instances of stress-related plaque formation or blood pressure adjustment. However, general patterns are very clear and intermediate events or changes in a bodily system that are highly correlated with disease outcomes (such as elevated blood pressure or intimal narrowing of coronary arteries) are reliably observed as a function of stress. Animal studies, in which investigators can observe or control major stressors and can exert greater experimental control (including the possibility of genetic comparability or manipulation), offer some of the best evidence of stress effects on cardiovascular diseases (e.g., Manuck et al., 1983). Animal studies clearly suggest that stress can accelerate pathogenesis of coronary heart disease and hypertension and can evoke cardiac events (Smith and Gallo, 1994). Although not all studies agree that stress can cause cardiovascular problems, there is certainly enough evidence to warrant further study and intervention (e.g., Elliott, 1995).

As an example, consider a series of experimental and observational studies of cynomolgous monkeys by Manuck and colleagues. This species shares many characteristic cardiovascular properties with humans, and many aspects of their behavior also resemble or parallel human social activity (e.g., Kaplan et al., 1982). When these animals have been exposed repeatedly to disruption of their social environments, they have exhibited greater evidence of coronary heart disease (Manuck et al., 1986). When unfamiliar animals are introduced into a stable group of monkeys, the result is a destabilization of the social hierarchy that had been established. This destabilizing influence is a powerful social stressor for the monkeys, and they respond to it by becoming more aggressive and more prone to cardiovascular disease (Manuck et al., 1986). Periodic reorganization of social groups has been used to generate chronic stress as animals repeatedly experience unstable social conditions, and this manipulation has permitted detailed observation of the impact of social dominance, diet, and stress on the development of cardiovascular disease (Kaplan et al., 1984). Dominant monkeys in unstable conditions exhibited the most extensive signs of heart disease, but these effects were dramatically increased by high-cholesterol diets (Manuck et al., 1986).

Interestingly, when females were studied, dominant animals showed few signs of atherosclerosis but subordinate females showed more evidence of atherosclerosis and elevated cortisol as well as ovarian dysfunction (Kaplan et al., 1996). Further stress was associated with endothelial injury through sympathetic activation (the effect was reduced by beta-adrenergic blockage), suggesting that stress-related central nervous system arousal can initiate as well as exacerbate arterial damage (Skantze et al., 1998).

Epidemiological studies of large samples of people who were thought to vary in level of chronic stress provide the most general evidence of stress effects on cardiovascular disease. For example, longitudinal studies of civil servants in the United Kingdom found that lower-status occupations thought to be more stressful were associated with higher rates of cardiovascular disease (Marmot, 1994). Several other explanations for such an effect are possible, but stress remains a viable explanation for many effects attributed to socioeconomic status (SES) (e.g., Baum et al., 1999). Other large-scale studies have found robust correlations between stress and cardiovascular outcomes, although these relationships are frequently complicated by moderating variables such as SES, social support or social integration, and personality variables (e.g., Mellors et al., 1994). For example, hostility and Type A behavior have been associated with cardiovascular disease or related intermediate outcomes in several studies (e.g., Suarez and Williams, 1990; Bennett and Carroll, 1990a; Rosenman, 1991; Houston et al., 1992), presumably because of the effects of these personality or behavioral styles on biological processes regulating atherosclerosis or other aspects of cardiovascular pathophysiology. Depression also appears to be related to some cardiovascular outcomes (Freedland et al., 1992; Musselman et al., 1998), and several studies have related low social support or poor social integration to disease (e.g., Uchino et al., 1996; Knox and Uvnaes-Moberg, 1998). All of these studies suggest that stress, together with a number of other psychosocial or behavioral variables, affects cardiovascular disease enough to represent targetable variance in disease risk management (Niaura and Goldstein, 1992).

Another complicating factor in studies of stress and cardiovascular risk is the fact that many other behavioral influences on cardiovascular disease, such as diet, active versus sedentary life-style, tobacco use, and coronary-proven behaviors are correlated with stress (e.g., Eysenk, 1990, 1991; Shekelle et al., 1991; Krantz et al., 1996). Smoking, consumption of high-fat diets, sedentary behavior, and hostile, competitive behaviors are independently correlated with cardiovascular outcomes but are also reliably influenced by stress. Smoking contributes to a range of outcomes and appears to be influenced by stress, as is exercise or other behavioral factors that may affect cardiovascular health (e.g. Krantz et al., 1996). Separating direct effects of stress on physiological activity from those effects of stress-induced smoking, sleep problems, or other potential behavioral pathogens is difficult but necessary if we are to most effectively target disease processes for intervention (Matarrazo, 1980).

Most of these studies look at one or more conditions thought to be stressful and statistically isolate relationships between these conditions and cardiovascular disease. For example, among women, stress associated with having several roles (e.g., employment, educational attainment) appears to increase risk for cardiovascular disease (Baum and Grunberg, 1991; Brezinka and Kittel, 1996). Job stress, particularly when demand is high and control is low, has also been linked to cardiovascular disease (e.g., Johnson et al., 1996; Kasl, 1996; Theorell and Karasek 1996; Peter and Siegrist, 1997; Weidner et al., 1997). Several studies find associations between mood or distress and hypertension, coronary artery disease, or other disorders (e.g., Carney et al., 1995; Kubzansky et al., 1998; Everson et al., 1998; Barrick, 1999; Jacob et al., 1999). Personality variables related to hostility, optimism, and coping and social variables such as support that typically buffer the effects of stress are also associated with the development of disease, disease events, and recovery outcomes (e.g., Eaker, 1989; Fontana et al., 1989; Johnson et al., 1989; Orth-Gomer and Unden, 1990). In general, research shows a broadly characterized effect of life-style behaviors and stress on cardiovascular disease and health (Kringlen, 1986; Krantz et al., 1988).

Stress and Cancer

Like heart disease, cancer is a slowly developing disease that features gradual pathophysiological activity and disease events that may have specific triggers. Also like cardiovascular disease, cancer may be influenced by behavioral factors at several different stages. However, cancer is also different from cardiovascular disease in several ways. First, the underlying pathophysiology is difficult to identify or measure, so detection and intervention during this long recruitment stage are difficult or impossible. In addition, the immune system appears to have direct surveillance responsibilities in cancer defense and some of the most important medical advances in treatment are those that boost immunological defenses or help the immune system identify and target malignant or premalignant cells. Adding to this is the fact that cancer is not a single disease nor does it attack only one or a few systems. Cancer is best thought of as a group of more than 100 diseases that all feature dysfunctional controls on cell proliferation.

Cancer begins with mutations that occur in a cell or small cluster of cells, and progresses and becomes malignant through several other mutations in these same cells. These mutations are a function of increasing genomic instability due to age, exposure to mutagenic agents, or other factors, and are reflected in greater and greater relaxation of inhibitions on cell proliferation. In other words, each mutation makes the likelihood of uncontrolled cell growth and proliferation more likely and affected cells begin to grow in uncontrolled fashion. This instability is also related to repair rates or capabilities of cells throughout the body to repair mutations or flush them out. Mutations or more basic damage to DNA that could contribute to further mutation or instability is ordinarily repaired through a variety of cellular repair processes or eliminated through apoptotic activity (which leads cells to destroy themselves). In some cases, repair mechanisms are inhibited, damage is increased, and/or apoptotic controls are reduced, allowing mutations to be reproduced and further increasing proliferation of abnormal cells. Recent theory in immunology posits several mechanisms for immune system surveillance and defense against developing tumors; natural killer (NK) cells, for example, can conjugate or bind with tumor cells, create pores in the tumor cell membrane, and inject substances that can initiate apoptosis in tumor cells. Immune defenses against tumor cells depend on accurate identification of tumor cells and rapid elimination of them. Anything that interferes with these processes may inhibit overall tumor rejection and enhance cancer development.

There is some evidence that stress can contribute to the onset of cancer, including a considerable amount of circumstantial evidence of such links, mostly in the form of correlations between stressors and cancer diagnosis. Most studies that address stress or other behavioral factors in the etiology of cancer do not find large effects of these variables, for many reasons. The most important, perhaps, is the issue of timing and matching disease-related events to stressful episodes or other life experiences. If one is interested in the relationship between stress and cancer etiology, it is necessary to identify stressors characterizing a fairly long, extended period during which the disease develops. Unfortunately, we cannot detect early development of most cancers and cannot specify the length of the recruitment period. In some cases, a nascent breast cancer, for example, may be detectable after 5 years of development, in other cases, this developing tumor may grow for 10 years before it is detected. Correlating stressful life events or other stressors with possible disease processes that cannot be identified readily over such long periods of time is a difficult task and is likely to yield moderate to weak correlations due to "noise" or nuisance variance associated with other events or other illnesses generated during these extended periods. Large, long term prospective studies in high-risk populations involving collection of bio-markers of disease development are needed, to accomplish this in a meaningful and interpretable manner; such studies would be very expensive, and time con-suming, and are presently not feasible given the state of biomarker research and scientific funding. As a result, we are left with suggestive studies indicating that psychosocial variables are related to cancer incidence and progression (Spiegel et al., 1996). For example, loss experienced within a 7-year period preceding diag-nosis of cancer was associated with this diagnosis (e.g., Ramirez et al., 1989). Cancer is a stressful disease and treatments for it are stressful as well. Increasing stress, together with economic costs and loss of self-esteem, confer a substantial burden for many patients (Schulz et al., 1995). There are also many animal stud-ies that suggest a link between stress and tumor growth or rejection of neoplasms (e.g., Sklar and Anisman, 1981; Kerr et al., 1999).

A meta-analysis of 46 studies linking mood and anxiety disorders, child-hood environment, personality, coping, and stress with the development of breast cancer yielded small but significant effects for denial or repressive cop-ing, separation and loss experiences, and stressful life events (McKenna et al., 1999). The authors concluded that there was evidence of a moderate association between these psychological variables and breast cancer, but the size of these relationships was interpreted as equivocal support for the notion that stress con-tributes to development of the disease (McKenna et al., 1999). However, a more limited review and meta-analysis of research on breast cancer and stressful life events did not find evidence of an association between negative events and the onset of breast cancer (Pettigrew et al., 1999). Given the considerations dis-cussed briefly above, however, it is possible or likely that methodological limi-tations made it unlikely that stronger effects could be found. The observed mod-est effect sizes provide some evidence of a connection between stress and coping on the one hand and cancer development on the other and may actually underestimate one's risk.

There is some evidence that stress or other behaviors affect damage and re-pair processes in individual cells. As noted earlier, cells can experience damage from any number of sources, including radiation, some toxins, sun exposure, tobacco and tobacco smoke, and some chemicals. The extent to which damage is experienced and the rate at which damage is repaired are critical in early events characterizing the development of cancer and would appear to be a viable mechanism underlying the effects of behavioral processes on cancer patho-physiology. An early study (Kiecolt-Glaser et al., 1985) found that stress was associated with slower repair of x-ray-induced DNA damage, and subsequent studies found evidence of stress-related suppression of DNA repair enzymes in rats (Glaser et al., 1985). Studies of medical students comparing high-stress examination periods with lower-stress periods also yielded evidence of inhibited apoptotic activity following cell damage and decreased RNA expression of genetic tumor regulation in stressed medical students (Tomei et al., 1990; Glaser et al., 1993). Although not extensive, these data suggest that stress can interfere with basic cellular processes that could constitute a pathway to the development of new cancers or the enhancement of existing tumor growth.

Investigators have reported considerably more evidence that stress, coping, and other behavioral or psychosocial variables affect the course of cancer. Stress has been associated with relapse and recurrence of cancer in several studies (e.g., Spiegel et al., 1998). The extent to which the original diagnosis of cancer was stressful did not predict recurrence of breast cancer in one study but chronic stress assessed before cancer diagnosis was made was a strong predictor of relapse (e.g., De Brabander and Gertis, 1999). Other studies have also shown associations between stress or other biobehavioral factors and cancer recurrence or progression (e.g., Levy et al., 1985, 1989, 1990; Ramirez et al., 1989). Animal studies show this relationship even more clearly and suggest immunological mediation of some of these effects (e.g., Ben-Eliyahu et al., 1991, 1999). Because of the central role of immune system activity in defense against tumors, studies showing relationships between stress and immune system activity among cancer patients are particularly important, suggesting that stress-related immune system changes and tumor growth or metastasis of tumor cells are related (Tejwani et al., 1991; Ishihara et al., 1999). Moreover, investigation of immune system variables that might be modifiable should have an important impact on the course of cancer.

There is growing evidence of stress effects on immune system activity mediated principally by central and sympathetic nervous system activity and neuroendocrine systems (e.g., O'Leary, 1990; Felten and Felten, 1991). As noted, the immune system plays several roles in cancer defense, including immunosurveillance functions that involve immune system activity directed at locating and eliminating new or developing tumors and controlling metastases (e.g., Herberman, 1991). Natural killer cells, cytotoxic T lymphocytes, and other effectors in the system can detect tumor cells and in most cases conjugate or adhere to them to produce killing. These processes are mediated by a number of other activities, factors, and cells, suggesting that a broad look at immune system mediation of stress effects on cancer course is necessary. Evidence suggests that behavioral intervention in healthy populations or in groups with other immune system-related diseases are useful in supporting or boosting a number of aspects of immune function (e.g., Hall and O'Grady, 1991; McGrady et al., 1992).

There is also evidence that these relationships hold in studies of people who have cancer. For example, anticipating surgery shortly after the diagnosis of cancer or other stressors associated with cancer or cancer treatment may sup-

press natural killer cell activity and thereby inhibit defense against micrometas-
tases or spread of cancer cells (e.g., Van der Pompe et al., 1998). A good deal of
evidence of stress-related effects on NK cells has been reported (e.g., McKinnon
et al., 1989; Kiecolt-Glaser and Glaser, 1992; Cohen et al., 1993; Schedlowski et
al., 1993; Delahanty et al., 1996; Ironson et al., 1997;) and many of these effects
are also apparent in cancer patient populations (e.g., Levy et al., 1985; Van der
Pompe et al., 1998; Gerits and De Brabander, 1999). Cancer surgery has also
been associated with suppressed NK cell lysis of tumor cells, interferon production, and lymphocyte proliferation to mitogen challenge (Andersen et al., 1998).
Studies have found endocrine sequelae of stress in cancer patients that are associated with immune system regulation in healthy populations, including elevated
resting levels of cortisol and attenuated hypothalamic-pituitary-adrenal reactivity to acute stressors (e.g., Van der Pompe et al., 1996). To make a long and
growing story short, evidence strongly suggests that stress and other behaviors
or biobehavioral processes can affect cancer course and likely do so through
effects on cellular repair mechanisms and on immune system surveillance.

Stress and HIV Disease

HIV disease and AIDS are also different from cardiovascular disease in
many ways. They refer to the chronic disease established by infection with the
human immunodeficiency virus, a relatively new retrovirus that lives in and
destroys components of the immune system. Earlier we noted that advances in
sanitation, public health, and drug development had greatly limited the dangers
of infectious illnesses and had eradicated most of them as major sources of disease and disability. HIV disease and AIDS are an exception to this trend, having
emerged in the past 25 years as a major threat to life and well being. The virus is
resistant to traditional antiviral therapies. It is spread through intimate sexual
contact or in blood or blood products and is therefore commonly contracted as a
result of sexual activity or intravenous drug use. It is lymphotropic, being drawn
to and living in lymphocytes that are integral components of the immune system. Once established, it replicates itself many times over and destroys its host
cell, releasing new viral particles to search for additional host cells. Historically,
we have gauged the disease's progress by monitoring helper T lymphocytes,
which appear to be a preferred and/or primary host for the HIV. Advancing disease ordinarily causes a precipitous decline in the numbers of helper cells and a
corresponding inhibition of immunocompetence.

While HIV disease is initiated when the virus is introduced into the body
and infection established, it can pass through many stages before reaching its
end stage, AIDS. Often it passes through a period of latency or greatly reduced
activity. Several viruses similarly become latent once establishing infection, and
herpes viruses are reactivated periodically when immune or neural control of
them is reduced or eliminated. Unlike these viruses, however, latency and

reactivation of HIV do not appear to be recurrent, episodic phenomena. Once the HIV is activated or is able to overcome immune system defenses that hold it in check, it systematically compromises the immune system and affects a range of other functions. Criteria for AIDS have varied as classification schemes for the disease have been proposed and revised, but generally AIDS refers to the point at which the immune system has been so compromised that the patient becomes susceptible to opportunistic infections—diseases or disorders that are not as prevalent or dangerous when the immune system is intact.

Behavioral issues have been particularly important in studying and dealing with the HIV/AIDS epidemic. First, HIV infection is associated with behaviors such as sexual activity and drug use, and infection can generally be prevented through a combination of abstinence, monogamy, contraception, and use of clean, uninfected needles. Most attention from the behavioral science community has been in this area of prevention, with program development in teaching people to use "safer sex," distribution of bleach and/or clean needles to intravenous (IV) drug users, and so on. Less attention has been paid to whether behavioral factors affect the HIV and progression of disease once infection has been established. However, there are now sufficient data to establish a plausible case for such influences.

Like cardiovascular disease and cancer, HIV disease has a variable course and progresses through latency or as it overwhelms immune defenses at widely variable rates. Some people who have been infected with HIV may remain healthy and free from opportunistic infection for many years, but others decline more rapidly and become symptomatic soon after infection (e.g., Munoz et al., 1989; Phair et al., 1992). This variable course has been attributed to differences in viral strains, host immune resistance, and psychosocial variables such as stress (e.g., Levy, 1991; Kemeny, 1994; Cole et al., 1996). Early in the study of HIV disease and AIDS, scientists interested in the effects of stress or behavior on immune status and function began to theorize about application of this work to HIV progression (Soloman, 1987; Solomon et al., 1991). Noting that HIV disease could be discussed in the context of interactions between the central nervous system and the immune system, these theorists argued that anything that perturbed or altered the ability of the immune system to defend the organism could affect the speed of spread of HIV and hasten the development of AIDS.

Early data suggested that several variables might be involved, most notably stress, coping, social support, and emotional or autonomic reactivity (Solomon et al., 1991). Since then data have accumulated suggesting that stress and coping are significant predictors of progression of HIV disease (e.g., Goodkind et al., 1992; Remiea et al., 1992; Reed, 1994; Schlebush and Cassidy, 1995; Mulder et al., 1999). Coping and self-efficacy appear to mediate stressful effects of being HIV seropositive, reducing distress and stress-related immune system fluctuations (e.g., Antoni et al., 1995; Benight et al., 1997). Major stressors may cause exacerbations or intensification of disease processes or symptoms in several diseases (e.g., Lutgendorf et al., 1995), and variation in stress hormones appears to be related to differences in rates of HIV infection (e.g., Antoni et al., 1991). Depression is also known to affect immune status and function but is not necessarily associated with progression of HIV disease (Lyketsos et al., 1996; Miller et al., 1997). Finally, there is some evidence that psychological inhibition confers negative effects on several basic bodily processes and that gay man with HIV infection appear to progress more rapidly when they report concealing their sexual orientation (Cole et al., 1996).

Interpretation of these studies is complicated by their correlational nature and the complexities of the disease and its social context. For example, social or stress-related changes associated with HIV disease may be both a cause and an effect of disease progression. In a study of 925 Australians living with HIV disease or AIDS, disease progression predicted employment status (Ezzy et al., 1999). Half of those leaving work reported that declining health was the reason, and since unemployment appears to be stressful one could expect that losing work might further contribute to disease progression. This same reasoning complicates the appropriate interpretation of studies of depression and HIV/AIDS. For example, Siegel and her colleagues found that gay and bisexual men with HIV or AIDS were at greater risk for psychological distress than would be expected if they did not have the disease and that risk increased as their disease progressed (Siegel et al., 1996). The results of this clearly indicated that adjustment problems associated with HIV disease were an important source of distress but could not specify whether these adjustment problems were a product of disease progression or fed back to affect disease course.

An interesting avenue of investigation has been studies of inhibition and stress as predictors of disease course. As noted earlier, psychological inhibition, defined as either voluntary or involuntary constraint of discussion or disclosure about a stressful or important event or fact, can also affect well being (e.g., Pennebaker et al., 1987). Many people living with HIV are gay or bisexual, and some of these people may be reluctant to disclose their sexual identities or lifestyles. It is possible, then, that the concealment of one's sexual preferences is stressful and that men who do not disclose such information are at risk for more serious disease. This is similar to the findings of a study by Cole and his associates (Cole et al., 1996) that followed HIV-seropositive but asymptomatic men for 9 years. Time to critical levels of helper lymphocytes, AIDS, and AIDS-related mortality were related to the degree to which homosexual activities were concealed (Cole et al., 1996). These effects may have been due to coping style differences associated with disclosure rather than to the effects of psychological inhibition (e.g., Ostrow, 1996), but the importance of these findings is broader than the specific mechanisms involved.

There are not many studies that specifically measure the mediating effects of immune system activity when evaluating effects of stress on HIV disease progression. There is evidence that changes in several immune parameters that are affected by behavioral variables predict disease progression, including numbers of helper lymphocytes, loss of antibody response, and other immune system variables (Fernandex-Cruz et al., 1990). Bereavement is a significant stressor for people living with HIV since intimate partners or close friends may also have HIV disease and may die of AIDS-related complications. In a study of 78 bereaved and nonbereaved people with HIV, there was a significant increase in immune system activation but a decrease in T cell proliferation after the death of an intimate friend (Kemeny et al., 1995). Studies like this are rare but no matter how daunting the complexities underlying psychosocial moderation of HIV disease may be, definitive studies of stress or other behavioral factors as factors in the progression of HIV and AIDS should be possible. Data suggest, for example, that stress predicts physical symptoms of AIDS but does not predict progression of HIV disease or related immunological changes (e.g., Rabkin et al., 1991; Perry et al., 1992). Complicated characteristics of the virus and of different "strains" of the HIV are important and not well understood, as are long term effects of new treatment regimens for HIV and AIDS (e.g., Hall, 1988; Levy, 1993). Because HIV disease and AIDS are diseases that are centrally immunological and involve suppression of immune responses that are also suppressed by stress, it remains likely that behavioral influences on immune status constitute modifiable variance in disease progression.

CONCEPTUAL BASES FOR BEHAVIORAL INTERVENTIONS

Simply stated, theories underlying behavioral intervention to modify disease course are based on the assumptions that behavioral or psychosocial influences on disease course are modifiable and that reducing negative influences will slow disease progression or minimize recurrence of disease following treatment. The simplest forms of this theory are inherent in prevention-oriented campaigns that urge people to quit smoking, eat healthy foods, or exercise. Tobacco use, poor diets, and sedentary life-styles all appear to contribute directly to development and persistence of cardiovascular disorders, cancers, and other chronic illnesses. These behaviors as well as stress and other factors (e.g., alcohol use, drug abuse, and obesity) affect basic biological processes, including lipid profiles, insulin resistance, immune function, and sympathetic or hemodynamic tone. These basic processes mediate a number of important pathophysiological outcomes and affect tumor rejection, atherosclerosis, resistance to viral infection, and blood pressure (e.g., Baum and Posluszny, 1999). Modifying behavioral input at the start of these causal sequences is thought to reduce disease outcomes by altering mediating biological conditions.

The logic for this kind of approach is appealing and has received at least circumstantial support. The studies reviewed in the first section of this chapter provide a considerable empirical base for these efforts. A number of behaviors and biobehavioral processes appear to affect key events in the etiology of cardiovascular disease and cancer and in the development and progression of HIV disease. How these behaviors or processes can best be modified and the extent to which one or another system or condition mediates disease risk or outcome is less clearly specified by the literature. Cessation or prevention of smoking or other tobacco use is unarguably an important public health objective, but how best to accomplish this or how its negative effects are conveyed has not been addressed convincingly. Further, how these behaviors are influenced by stress, or how stress reduction affects them; is often not part of basic prevention or behavior change interventions nor is this clearly delineated. Stress interferes with early detection and surveillance, appears to affect diet and exercise, is a cause of smoking or drug use relapse after cessation, and is a factor in other instances of health-related behavior modification (e.g., Baum and Posluszny, 1999). The best ways to intervene and help people reduce stress, cope with uncertainty, manage side effects, comply with difficult treatments, and the like are not yet established. What has become clear is that modification of these "health-impairing" behaviors and processes is an important goal, that comprehensive programs appear to be well suited for this effort, and that an emphasis on substituting "health-enhancing" behaviors for less healthy activities is important as well.

As suggested by this, interventions remain eclectic and loosely centered on one or another basic approach to stress management, psychoeducation, support provision, and/or behavior change. Many are considered cognitive-behavioral approaches and share emphasis on relaxation training, coping, and appraisal. These approaches work to (1) reduce negative mood and "excess" arousal associated with stress, (2) enhance knowledge of coping so that people can deal with stress more effectively, and (3) modify appraisals of stressors and/or their environmental contexts to reduce the extent to which stress is experienced. These objectives are derived directly from research and theory on cognitive-behavioral therapy, the efficacy of reducing arousal or teaching relaxation, and theories of stress and coping (e.g., Mason, 1975; Leventhal, 1980; Turk et al., 1983; Lazarus and Folkman, 1984). Broader or more comprehensive approaches add one or more other components or focal points, with some success. Some, for example, add aerobic exercise as an adjunct to relaxation (to help disperse arousal and ameliorate mood) which also has a direct benefit (e.g., enhanced cardiovascular or metabolic tone, and fitness). Other interventions may focus instruction in coping or problem solving on a particular problem or problem behavior, using it to illustrate appraisal and coping issues and providing basic knowledge about disease processes.

Many overarching models of health and behavior are relevant to this effort, including those describing three basic pathways between psychosocial or behavioral variables and health or treatment outcomes (e.g., Krantz et al., 1985; Baum and Posluszny, 1999). Behavioral variables or stressors may have direct effects on biological systems involved in pathobiology and may affect other behaviors that in turn have direct effects on these same biological systems or may affect "sick" behavior or how people behave when they are ill. Andersen et al. (1994) proposed a biobehavioral model that included these general pathways and specifically focused on adjustment to cancer, citing "ample evidence . . . that adults experiencing other long term stressors experience . . . important biological effects, such as persistent down regulation of elements of the immune system and adverse health outcomes" (p. 389). Their model summarizes and organizes a great deal of research and proposes several mechanisms linking psychosocial and behavioral variables with biological processes and treatment outcomes.

Arguing that cancer itself poses a great many sources of stress and that this burden can affect disease course, Andersen and her colleagues suggest that behavioral systems such as compliance and health behaviors are affected by and contribute to direct effects of stressors on central and peripheral nervous system activity, endocrine activity, and immune system functions. Many of these sources of stress are persistent and last well beyond the completion of treatment, including social stigmatization, irrevocable changes in sexual or reproductive function, loss of stamina, economic loss, and diminished cognitive capabilities (e.g., Cella and Tross, 1986; Wingard et al., 1991; Kaplan, 1992; Yellen et al., 1993). These sources of stress, working with other stressors and psychological trauma associated with cancer diagnoses, can affect local and metastatic disease by influencing a range of behavioral and biological variables (e.g., Baum and Posluszny, in press).

The model proposes specific behavioral pathways that may affect disease course, citing evidence that stress can contribute to appetitive disturbances common in cancer patients, sleep disturbances, self-medication with alcohol and other drugs, tobacco use, and sedentary behaviors (Andersen et al., 1994). Nearly 40% of cancer patients report problems with loss of appetite or inability to eat, and cancer patients or survivors appear more likely than healthy people or people who have never had cancer to report sleep difficulties (e.g., Cella and Tross, 1986; Wellisch et al., 1989). The detailed analysis of these and other health behaviors as well as direct effects of cancer treatments on these behaviors describes a compelling framework within which to view psychosocial and biobehavioral mediation of disease course. Importantly, it also specifies a range of intervention targets for stress reduction and enhancement of treatment outcomes.

Theories underlying intervention for medical populations are far more complex and extensive than can be considered here (see Figure 2 for an example). Disease-specific models for other syndromes have been developed, research on mechanisms underlying hypothesized effects has continued to expand, and we are learning more about modifiable behavioral variance in disease course as these developments continue. For now, it is sufficient to note that these models offer a number of intervention targets and suggest a range of approaches and strategies. Evaluation of existing knowledge about intervention effects can be

464

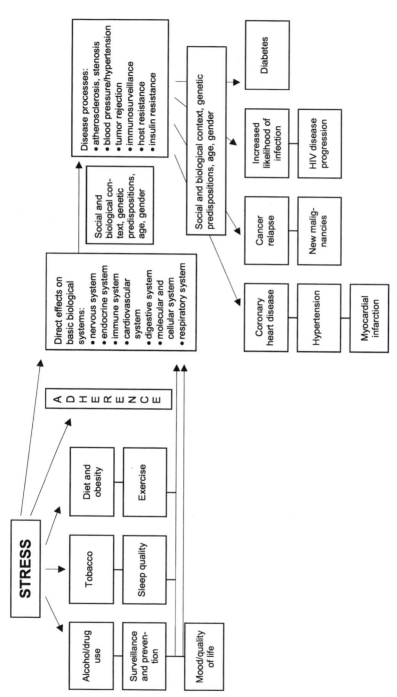

FIGURE 2 A model of processes underlying efforts to intervene to modify disease course. Stress and a wide range of health-impairing or health-protective behaviors interact to produce effects on basic bodily systems that can contribute to pathophysiology. Stress also exerts direct effects on those systems, on mood and quality of life, and on attempts to modify health-impairing or protective behaviors to prevent or detect early disease. These, in turn, also affect pathophysioloical processes. Stress affects adherence and success of behavior change efforts, which also affect biological processes. Effects of these bodily changes are translated into variable disease processes by differences in initial fitness or systemic state, use of chemopreventive regimens, age, and other factors, affecting a number of important disease outcomes.

viewed in the context of these models, and they serve an important organizing function as well.

INTERVENTIONS AND STRESS REDUCTION FOR CHRONIC ILLNESSES

Based on these data and developing theoretical models of health and behavior, a number of interventions for disease prevention and control have been implemented and evaluated. Clearly, intervention can occur at several different points in the process; early on, healthy behaviors can be established and reinforced and the earliest development of disease slowed or stopped. Early detection and surveillance efforts are important in identifying risk profiles and more readily treated early manifestations of disease. Interventions for patients and families designed to reduce stress, buffer immune and endocrine activity from effects of stress or treatment, and otherwise reduce or eliminate behavioral contributions to advancing disease are all warranted by the emerging literatures on these topics. Intervention across the entire course of illnesses, from early asymptomatic stages through more complex advanced stages and need for palliation, seems justified. At the same time, behavioral and psychosocial factors that predict participation in and adherence to interventions add another important dimension to this effort (e.g., Naeslund et al., 1993). The present discussion focuses primarily on comprehensive stress management interventions as they affect cardiovascular disease, cancer course, and the development of AIDS.

STRESS MANAGEMENT AND CARDIOVASCULAR DISEASE

Although there would seem to be numerous avenues of approach to intervention to reduce behavioral effects on the development of cardiovascular disease, there have not been extensive investigations of these interventions beyond smoking cessation, nutrition management, and fitness programs. As we have suggested, interventions directed at smoking or other tobacco use would go a long way to reducing morbidity and mortality from cardiovascular disease, cancer, and many other illnesses. However, interventions to reduce or deflect stress and/or alter life-style have been less frequent. Stress management interventions should, if our reasoning holds, reduce or deflect some of the conditions that regulate or contribute to the pathophysiology of heart disease, stroke, hypertension, and other cardiovascular disorders.

Some studies find evidence supporting the notion that behavioral interventions can reduce risk for cardiovascular disease by reducing physiological developments that predispose or trigger these disorders. For example, stress management interventions can reduce the hostility, competitiveness, and time urgency associated with Type A behavior; can lower serum cholesterol; and can reduce blood pressure (Bennett and Carroll, 1990b).

A meta-analysis of studies of intervention to modify Type A behavior suggested that after intervention, participants reduced Type A behavior scores by about half a standard deviation and the probability of 3-year mortality or heart attack corresponded to a 50% reduction in risk (Nunes et al., 1987). Distress and psychiatric disorders associated with the diagnosis of cardiovascular disease, including hostility, are reduced by regular clinic visits, again suggesting personality-based dynamics in risk for cardiovascular disease (Mann, 1984). Type A behavior may also influence the efficacy of intervention designed to enhance relaxation responses independent of hostility or time urgency. Progressive muscle relaxation training was evaluated among Type A men with borderline hypertension (Haaga et al., 1994). The intervention was intended to modify acute reactivity to challenges rather than hostility or anger. The relaxation training was effective in reducing reactivity and had mild effects on anger or hostility (Haaga et al., 1994).

As late as 1985, Type A behavior was considered to be a major source of risk for heart disease and other cardiovascular disorders (e.g., Matthews and Haynes, 1986). Since then, a focus on the more toxic components of this behavior pattern, most notably hostility (e.g., Dembrosky et al., 1989), has redefined this literature and retargeted some intervention efforts. However, evidence remains that Type A behavior has some predictive value in estimating risk for coronary heart disease, that interventions can reduce biological underpinnings of this behavioral style, and that modification of these and related behaviors still has potential for reducing postinfarction morbidity and mortality (Bennett, 1994).

Stress management programs often focus on relaxation but can be broader in scope. Programs involving both relaxation and more cognitive elements can reduce risk and intermediate outcomes that predict disease progression or contribute to atherosclerosis (e.g., Steptoe, 1989). More intensive interventions appear to be more effective than less involving ones, as was the case in a study of stress management among police recruits (McNulty et al., 1984). An intervention consisting of ten 90-minute sessions dealing with stress management was associated with lower catecholamine levels than was a loosely-organized program of occasional lectures (McNulty et al., 1984). Relaxation training has been associated with lower levels of cortisol, prolactin, and urinary catecholamines (Gallois et al., 1984). Behavioral procedures that are effective in treating circulatory disorders such as Raynaud's disease also provide evidence of the value of these efforts in modifying basic underlying biological causes of disease, in this case beta-adrenergic stimulation in the peripheral circulatory system (Freedman, 1987). Biofeedback-assisted stress management can also reduce muscle tension and cortisol responses that contribute to high blood pressure (McGrady et al., 1987).

The most frequent target of interventions to reduce cardiovascular disease have been directed at hypertension. Primary management of hypertension has typically been pharmacological, administering drugs to reduce heart rate, preserve blood volume, or otherwise alter activity by the heart and vasculature. However, nonpharmacological, behavioral approaches to reducing blood pressure and risk for stroke or other disorders have increased dramatically since 1975 (e.g., Shapiro, 1983). Several studies suggest that stress management interventions that effectively reduce blood pressure or blood pressure responsiveness to challenge are useful in treating hypertension (e.g., Jacob et al., 1987; Irvine and Logan, 1991). One, combining education about stress and hypertension with relaxation training and problem solving, showed that those receiving the intervention were more likely to achieve a significant reduction in resting blood pressure and to maintain normotensive readings (Garcia-Vera et al., 1997). Increases in problem-solving skills were correlated with reductions in blood pressure among intervention participants but not among waiting list control participants (Garcia-Vera et al., 1998). Enhanced problem solving partially mediated the effects of the intervention on blood pressure, swamping effects associated with relaxation training or education. Similarly, a study of 41 hypertensive, African American men suggested that coping skills training reduced blood pressure and distress (Bosley and Allen, 1989). Participants in the skill-building group exhibited larger decreases in systolic blood pressure and in state anxiety than did control participants.

The efficacy of relaxation training in reducing blood pressure has been shown as well (e.g., Irvine et al., 1986; Albright et al., 1991; Broota et al., 1995). A 4-year study of relaxation and behavior change to reduce cardiovascular disease risk found poor long term adherence to the program (only 17% of the intervention group reported that they still engaged in regular relaxation after 4 years), but blood pressure reductions were greater among this group than among participants who had never practiced regular relaxation or had stopped using relaxation exercises within 30 months of the intervention sessions (Steptoe et al., 1987). Other studies also suggest that continued practice of relaxation exercises is important in blood pressure control (Hoelscher, 1987). The effects of these relaxation-oriented interventions are broad and include effects on blood pressure, cortisol, aldosterone, and plasma catecholamines (McGrady et al., 1987).

They are also manifest when applied to hypertensive patients for whom pharmacologic interventions have not been effective (Jacob et al., 1992) or as a sole treatment for hypertension (Irvine and Logan, 1991). In the latter study, relaxation decreased blood pressure and also reduced alcohol consumption (which was associated with high blood pressure) (Irvine and Logan, 1991).

Efforts to intervene with hypertensives have also focused on modifying acute blood pressure reactivity to challenge or stressful stimuli (e.g., Haaga et al., 1994). These efforts often combine modification of personality, behavior patterns, and/or emotional reactions to stress and challenge. One study found that relaxation training significantly lowered blood pressure reactivity to a laboratory stressor and that this effect was dependent on endogenous opioid activity (McCubbin et al., 1996). When opioid activity was blocked with naltrexone, effects of relaxation training were reversed. Other interventions address emotional reactivity or style, as did a successful application of relaxation therapies to borderline hypertension and heart rate (Davison et al., 1991). A comprehensive evaluation of stress management training and Type A management training designed to reduce anger, hostility, and acute blood pressure reactivity found that both interventions reduced resting blood pressure and reactivity to the Type A assessment interview (Bennett et al., 1991). The Type A management intervention was better at modifying anger, hostility, and blood pressure reactivity, suggesting that the emotions that accompany this behavior pattern are a key component of heightened reactivity.

Although large-scale prospective evaluations of comprehensive cardiovascular risk reduction interventions using biological markers of disease progression have generally not been reported, several studies using broad interventions to slow disease progress or otherwise reduce the likelihood of disorders or cardiovascular events have been done. For example, cardiovascular risk reduction programs that are aimed at simultaneous alteration of several risk-enhancing behaviors are associated with beneficial changes in several intermediate outcomes linked with coronary heart disease (Lovibond et al., 1986). Intervention-based changes were maintained for a year and included weight loss of about 20 pounds (on average), 5–10% reductions in blood pressure, 33% reductions in serum cholesterol, and an overall decrease in risk for coronary heart disease.

Psychoeducational programs for coronary heart disease patients (combining education with stress management and general risk behavior reduction) also appear to be important adjuncts to conventional medical care. A study of a behavioral intervention for life-style change among angioplasty patients achieved significant reductions in smoking, exercise, diet, weight reduction, chest pain, and aerobic capacity (King et al., 1999). Meta-analysis of intervention programs, including 37 studies, suggests that there are impressive benefits from these interventions, with reductions of overall cardiac mortality of more than a third and a 29% decrease in recurrent myocardial infarction (Dusseldorp et al., 1999). Significant reductions in blood pressure, cholesterol, body weight, and smoking as well as changes in exercise and diet were also noted. These interventions did not reliably affect anxiety or depression, suggesting that they were not operating through mood enhancement. Finally, and perhaps most importantly, those interventions that had the largest effects on mediating or intervening conditions such as blood pressure, smoking, or exercise also had the most substantial effects on mortality and morbidity (Dusseldorp et al., 1999).

This growing literature strongly suggests that behavioral management of cardiovascular disease processes is an important way to reduce risk of heart attack, hypertension, stroke, or other disorders. Clearly, broad approaches that emphasize education, reduction in behaviors that confer risk, and reduction in stress or stress reactivity are called for to combat the nation's number one cause of death. Education is not sufficient by itself (Suminski et al., 1999), and programs that provide education, skill training, risk behavior intervention, problem-solving experiences, and relaxation appear best suited to the task. The major behavioral interventions for hypertension, including relaxation, biofeedback, weight loss, diet modification, exercise, and reduction of alcohol use, can reduce risk of cardiovascular disease or events such as infarction or stroke (Dusseldorp et al., 1999). Treatment of depression may enhance conditions ranging from myocardial ischemia, platelet activation, and hyperactivity and improves survival and quality of life (Musselman et al., 1998). The promise of these interventions and the health and cost benefits of behavioral management of chronic illness strongly suggest that investigation and use of such approaches to public health problems like cardiovascular disease are warranted (e.g., Johnston, 1987; Sobel, 1995; Lorig et al., 1999).

Stress Reduction and Cancer

There are now a number of studies of interventions for cancer patients directed at reducing stress and providing context for coping with cancer. Only a few have examined putative mechanisms by which stress might affect cancer course or outcomes, and only a handful have been able to examine effects on recurrence or survival. However, the results of several of these early efforts and intermediate outcome data from ongoing trials are encouraging and suggest that behavioral or psychosocial interventions are an effective means of reducing modifiable variance in cancer mortality.

As noted earlier, the idea that stress affects the nature and course of cancer and/or response to treatment has been popular for some time, and a variety of early efforts at intervention were reported (e.g., Richardson et al., 1990; Andersen, 1992). However, it was the publication of the results of an intervention with advanced-stage breast cancer patients by Spiegel and his associates (e.g., Spiegel et al., 1989) and of an intervention with melanoma patients by Fawzy and his colleagues (Fawzy et al., 1990, 1993) that sparked the current storm of interest in this approach to cancer care. The Spiegel study found evidence of dramatic gains in survival due to an intensive, year-long psychosocial intervention that addressed social support needs as well as existential stressors and other aspects of advanced-stage breast cancer (Spiegel et al., 1989). Fawzy and colleagues found smaller but equally robust gains in survival for melanoma patients with a different but related intervention focusing on stress, coping, and problem solving (Fawzy et al., 1990, 1993). The study included immunological measures and found predicted changes in some indices of immunity, but did not find that these immune system changes mediated survival gains. These findings caught some by surprise, and the clear demonstration of prolonged survival and enhanced quality of life was encouraging and strongly suggested an impact of different intervention approaches on aspects of cancer progression and patient well-being.

Since the appearance of these studies, several investigators have initiated intervention studies. Many are with breast cancer patients (e.g., Helgeson et al., 1999), but this approach is being broadened to include other cancers at a variety of stages (e.g., Baum et al., 1995). Meta-analyses and critical reviews of this growing literature suggest that psychosocial or psychotherapeutic interventions and differences in social support or social integration can contribute to psychological adjustment and well-being as well as disease course and immune status (Frischenschlayer et al., 1992; Meyer and Mark, 1995; Helgeson and Cohen 1996). For example, Helgeson and her colleagues have compared a psychoeducational intervention for primary-stage breast cancer patients with an intervention concentrating on social support and one dealing with both approaches simultaneously (Helgeson et al., in press). These three interventions were also compared with a control group, and both the psychoeducational and the combined interventions were associated with better adjustment and less distress than the social support intervention or control condition. This major trial produced convincing evidence of the value of these interventions (Helgeson et al., in press). Interestingly, the social support intervention was not associated with better life quality and functioning over the first 6 months after the intervention was complete, raising the strong possibility that different stages of disease with different prognoses are best met with different intervention approaches (Helgeson et al., in press). These possibilities are currently being evaluated in a newly initiated trial at the Pittsburgh Mind-Body Center of Carnegie-Mellon University and the University of Pittsburgh.

Other ongoing trials in Pittsburgh and at Ohio State University, as well as several other sites, are evaluating the generality of interventions to other cancers, some of the immunologic and endocrine mediators of intervention effects on disease, and relative impacts of group and individually delivered interventions. Data from these studies are not yet available, but preliminary evaluations of some of the data are encouraging (e.g., Andersen et al., 1998; Andersen, personal communication, 1999; Helgeson, personal communication, 1999). The further development and study of these interventions as well as interventions, to reduce stress and facilitate psychological adjustment among people at high risk for cancer, seem warranted (e.g., Glanz and Lerman, 1992; Baum and Andersen, in press).

Of particular interest in this literature are studies of interventions that include measures of putative psychological and biological mechanisms underlying observed benefits of these programs (Levy and Wise, 1989). Several ongoing studies have included endocrine and immune measures in their evaluation phases (e.g., Cruess et al., in press), and data are being collected to determine, for example, whether gains in survival and well-being are related to immune system activity, better cell repair and tumor rejection, enhanced adherence to and tolerability of medical treatments, or other phenomena that may be altered or enhanced by psychotherapeutic interventions. Initial reports of intervention for melanoma patients (Fawzy et al., 1990) indicated that six 90-minute intervention sessions were associated with enhanced mood and acute increases in numbers of CD8 T lymphocytes and in numbers and cytotoxicity of natural killer cells 6 months after the intervention. Later reports indicated the same general pattern of result over a longer period of time, with immune system gains correlated with the magnitude of decreases in anxiety and depression (Fawzy et al., 1993). Greater NK cell cytotoxicity was associated with less recurrence (Fawzy, 1994). Other investigations have also found evidence of immune system change that is associated with psychosocial or behavioral interventions. Cancer patients receiving biofeedback training and psychoeducation exhibited lower levels of arousal, lower cortisol levels, and better immune status than did untrained controls (Gruber et al., 1993). Relaxation training, education, and coping skills training also reduced levels of stress hormones and increased overall numbers of lymphocytes among breast cancer patients (Schedlowski et al., 1984). Two months of relaxation training for ovarian cancer patients who were receiving chemotherapy were associated with more lymphocytes and higher white blood cell counts (Lekander et al., 1997). These promising data offer evidence of the impact of behavioral interventions on potential immune mediators of disease course. More focused work on the effects of these interventions on regulatory functions and specific antitumor activities is in progress.

Increased interest and commitment to prevention and surveillance for new or recurrent cancer may also be associated with better adjustment (e.g., Schulz et al., 1995; Charles et al., 1996; Moyer and Salovey, 1996). Interventions focusing on intact families and/or spouses of cancer patients have also been described (e.g., Keller et al., 1996). Other mechanisms by which these interventions may help to achieve better cancer control are related to mental health and associated behaviors, to life-style changes that minimize nonstress conditions contributing to cancer course, and to more effective risk management and reduction (e.g., Gritz, 1991; Glanz and Lerman, 1992; Ganz et al., 1993; Spiegel, 1995; Miller et al., 1996; Spiegel and Kato, 1996, Van der Pompe et al., 1996; Redd, 1997).

To summarize, psychosocial intervention has been an active adjunct to medical care for cancer patients, particularly over the past 10–15 years. Some evidence of enhanced survival and of immune system effects of these interventions suggests that they accrue benefits, in part, by deflecting pathophysiological processes and either slowing or delaying disease progression or contributing to remission of the illness (e.g., Spiegel et al., 1989; Richardson et al., 1990; Fawzy et al., 1993; Garssen and Goodkind, 1999). Although we will know much more in the next 5 years about how these interventions work and how well they deflect disease course or bolster well-being, available data are sufficient to support widespread, broad-based application of interventions for early- and later-stage cancer patients and their families (e.g., Dreher, 1997; Spiegel et al., 1998).

Psychosocial Intervention and HIV/AIDS

One reason for the lack of large, definitive natural history studies of stress, immunity, and HIV disease is that interventions directed at sources of variance in stress and immune status have already returned encouraging results. Understandably, investigators and funding agencies may be less interested in conducting careful, large-scale, prospective investigations of unintervened subjects and reluctant to propose studies that do not include an intervention component. However, data from these interventions are far from definitive, and the rush to intervene may still be premature.

Early studies of stress management interventions yielded mixed results. One attempt to intervene featured stress management training and efforts to enhance safer sex practices in asymptomatic HIV-seropositive men (Coates et al., 1989). The intervention was successful in reducing some risky sexual behaviors but did not affect immune system status. On the other hand, 10-week stress management and aerobic exercise interventions for men at risk for HIV and AIDS was effective in buffering effects of stress associated with notification of HIV serostatus (LaPerriere et al., 1990; Schneiderman et al., 1992). Notification that they were HIV seropositive was associated with stress and suppression of natural killer cell activity and cell proliferation. The intervention reduced some of these effects.

Several interventions have been shown to affect quality of life and psychological distress (Lutgendorf et al., 1995; Vaughan and Kinnier, 1996; Pomeroy et al., 1997; Belcher et al., 1998; Kelly, 1998). The vast majority of interventions, as noted earlier, were more prevention-oriented and aimed at reducing risk for infection (Baum and Nesselhof, 1988; Fisher et al., 1996; Ford et al., 1996). For the most part, however, these interventions have not addressed mechanistic components, nor have they been broadly conceived to cover the long-range progression of disease. One, designed to improve coping following AIDS-related bereavement is a case in point. The intervention, which provided social support, permitted and encouraged emotional expression, and identified and reviewed AIDS-related problems and coping strategies, was associated with reduced distress (Sikkema et al., 1995). Presumably this reduction in distress could affect immune status and/or disease progression, but these measures were not targets of the study.

There are other behavioral factors that affect immunity in ways that could contribute to HIV disease progression, but evidence is insufficient to draw firm conclusions. Many of these factors are also affected by stress: alcohol use, for instance, is affected by stress (Breslin et al., 1995) and may be linked to HIV disease, but evidence is too inconsistent to permit us to conclude that alcohol is a cofactor in infection or a modulator of progression (e.g., Dingle and Oei, 1997).

A series of studies conducted at the University of Miami provides the most comprehensive picture of psychosocial intervention for people with HIV infection or AIDS. These studies consider a broad application of cognitive behavioral stress management techniques to populations of HIV-seropositive men. The interventions were typically evaluated in randomized, wait list control trials, and a range of outcomes tapping mood, psychological adjustment, mental health, and stress were assessed. Findings have been consistent and dramatic, suggesting that this intervention approach is associated with enhanced mood (less anxiety, anger, or depression), less perceived stress, lower production or excretion of stress hormones (norepinephrine, cortisol) and testosterone, and "better" immune function (more cytotoxic T cells, lower latent viral antibody titers) when compared with wait list controls (e.g., Lutgendorf et al., 1995; Antoni et al., 2000; Cruess et al., in press). These effects appear to be relatively stable over time and provide compelling evidence of the pervasive influences of biobehavioral processes on HIV disease and of the ameliorative impact of intervention in this population.

An important issue that requires at least brief consideration reflects recent developments in treatment of HIV with protease inhibitors and combination therapies. These treatment modalities have had good success and a substantial impact on the treatment and toll of HIV and AIDS. They represent real progress in medical efforts to stop HIV and its spread through the body. These new therapies were introduced in the mid-1990s and appear to be effective in inhibiting viral replication and disease progression. However, even with the availability of effective treatments, the prevention of infection remains the most effective approach. Further, as Schneiderman and Antoni (in press) have suggested, these drugs have unpleasant side effects, often involve complex regimens that make adherence difficult, and may not be available to everyone who needs them. Interventions that address these issues as well as more conventional targets such as stress and psychological adjustment are of greater significance than those that target only systemic resistance. Since issues such as adherence will ultimately influence the effectiveness of therapy and whether desired treatment outcomes are achieved, they key targets for behavior modification, shaping, and support (e.g., Schneiderman and Antoni, in press).

CONCLUSIONS

Research clearly suggests that behavioral and social phenomena contribute to health and illness and that interventions designed to modify these factors can improve overall health and well-being. Although we have focused on stress as a general source of variability in disease course and as an influence on health-impairing and health-enhancing behaviors, there are many important influences on these processes, ranging from SES and cultural variables to behavioral inhibition and coping styles. There are also many intervention approaches that may be effective in modifying adverse outcomes, including ways to alter disclosure and inhibition profiles, modify consequences of lower SES, and "legislate" behavioral changes that can enhance health. The most important conclusions that one can reach at this juncture suggest that behavioral and social influences on disease and disease course are pervasive, that these influences represent modifiable variance that can be altered to reduce overall morbidity and mortality, and that interventions directed at these relationships between behavior and disease can sharply reduce health care costs and improve quality of life and well-being.

These conclusions are consistent with those reached in the Healthy People 2010 document recently released by the U.S. Department of Health and Human

Services (DHHS). The latest in a series of initiatives released periodically by DHHS and the Surgeon General, this report continues a trend that has seen behavioral and life-style factors and disease prevention play an increasingly important role in setting and achieving national health objectives. These goals must address the complexities introduced by changing population demographics such as age and cultural diversity, changing health care economics, and the revolutions in technology and informatics that have characterized the past 20 years and will likely dominate the next 20 years. These issues clearly affect the value and yield of interventions such as those described in this paper, and the broad sources of influence that are often targets of these interventions will advance our knowledge and health practices toward the 2010 objectives. The realistic promise of dramatic decreases in morbidity and mortality that can be achieved through modification of behavioral contributions to disease processes is increasingly within reach.

The importance of cultural diversity, SES, and other population variables cannot be overlooked in discussing these interventions. However, the differences in effectiveness, acceptability, or dynamics of interventions to affect disease-related behavior and stress have generally not varied or examined gender, ethnicity, or age of target participants. One would expect that factors such as gender, age, national origin, and ethnicity could influence receptivity to and appropriateness of psychotherapeutic interventions. In general, gender-, age-, and culturally appropriate intervention programs are best-suited to modifying behavioral variance in disease course, and it is likely that inappropriately generalized approaches could fail to effect positive changes or add to patients' burden of stress. Yet, there are few studies evaluating these issues and none that compare approaches directly across population groups. It has been assumed, for example, that women respond more positively to group interventions and social support than do men, and a variety of theoretical justifications can support such predictions. Comparisons are sparse, in part because the majority of these studies are for breast cancer, and early results from prostate cancer interventions suggest that men also respond well to these approaches. Similarly, there are now data suggesting that women find individual psychoeducational interventions effective and beneficial as well. Age and ethnicity are also important potential mediators but have not received direct attention, and issues related to discrimination, prejudice, and the burdens of minority status in the United States have not been directly addressed either. Extension of this research and clinical literature to systematically evaluate possible differences across population groups will be an important addition over the next decade.

The significance of evolving research on and implementation of interventions that are designed to modify behavioral contributions to disease processes is not limited to its enormous potential for disease control. It is also important as a means of advancing basic research on stress and other biobehavioral aspects of health and illness. Research in these areas is usually correlational or quasiexperimental, and this has imposed limits on how conclusive or applicable findings have been. To some extent, interventions offer the possibility of conducting experimental in addition to correlational studies of disease progression. Under normal circumstances, one has no control over who is exposed to stress, when exposure occurs, or who develops diseases or progresses more rapidly. As a result, most human studies of psychological or behavioral mediation of cancer course are essentially prospective or retrospective correlations between reported experiences and measures of disease outcomes. Interventions to reduce stress or alter other behavioral conditions or characteristics, when randomized and appropriately applied, constitute a manipulation that permits stronger evaluation of the contribution of stress to disease outcomes. Not surprisingly, evidence of psychosocial mediation of cancer course has been more convincing in studies of psychotherapeutic interventions than in natural history studies that rely on observed associations between psychological variables and disease outcomes (Garssen and Goodkin, 1999). Extending this effort will provide greater insight into disease etiology and progression as well as help to identify promising methods of intervention to reduce these pathophysiologic processes.

REFERENCES

Albright, G.L., Andreassi, J.L., and Brockwell, A.L. (1991). Effects of stress management on blood pressure and other cardiovascular variables. *International Journal of Psychophysiology*, 11(2), 213–217.

Allen, M.T., and Patterson, S.M. (1995). Hemoconcentration and stress: A review of physiological mechanisms and relevance for cardiovascular disease risk. *Biological Psychology*, 31(1), 1–27.

Andersen, B.L. (1992). Psychological interventions for cancer patients to enhance the quality of life. *Journal of Consulting and Clinical Psychology*, 60(4), 552–568.

Andersen, B.L., Farrar, W.B., Golden-Kreutz, D., Kutz, L.A., MacCallum, R., Courtney, M.E. and Glaser, R. (1998). Stress and immune responses after surgical treatment for regional breast cancer. *Journal of the National Cancer Institute*, 90(1), 30–36.

Andersen, B.L., Kiecolt-Glaser, J.K., and Glaser, R. (1994). A biobehavioral model of cancer stress and disease course. *American Psychologist*, 49(5) 389–404.

Antoni, M.H., LaPerriere, A., Schneiderman, N., and Fletcher, M.A. (1991). Stress and immunity in individuals at risk for AIDS. *Stress Medicine*, 7(1), 35–44.

Antoni, M.H., Esterling, B.A., Lutgendorf, S., Fletcher, M., Schneiderman, N. (1995). Psychosocial stressors, herpesvirus reactivation and HIV-1 infection. Stein, M., Baum, A., et al. (Eds). *Chronic diseases. Perspectives in behavioral medicine* (pp. 135–168). Mahwah, NJ, USA: Lawrence Erlbaum Assoc., Inc.

Barrick, C.B. (1999). Sad, glad, or mad hearts? Epidemiological evidence for a causal relationship between mood disorders and coronary artery disease. *Journal of Affective Disorders*, 53(2), 193–201.

Barnes, V., Schneider, R., Alexander, C., Staggers, F. (1997). Stress, stress reduction, and hypertension in African Americans: An updated review. *Journal of the National Medical Association*, 89(7) 464–476.

Baum, A and Andersen, B (eds) Psychosocial interventions for cancer. Washington DC: *APA Books* (in press).

Baum, A., Garofalo, J.P., and Yali, A.M. (1999). Socioeconomic status and chronic stress: Does stress account for SES effects on health? *Annals of the New York Academy of Sciences*, 896, 131–144.

Baum, A., and Grunberg, N.E. (1991). Gender, stress, and health. *Health Psychology*, 10(2), 80–85.

Baum, A., Herberman, H., and Cohen, L. (1995). Managing stress and managing illness: Survival and quality of life in chronic disease. *Journal of Clinical Psychology in Medical Settings*, 2(4), 309–333

Baum, A., and Nesselhof, S. E. (1988), Psychological research and the prevention, etiology, and treatment of AIDS. *American Psychologist*, 43(11), 900–906.

Baum, A. and Posluszny, D.M. (1999). Health Psychology: Mapping the biobehavioral contributions to health and illness. *Annual Review of Psychology*, 50, 137–163.

Baum, A. and Posluszny, D.M. (In press). Cancer and traumatic stress. In A. Baum and B. Andersen (Eds.). *Psychosocial Interventions for Cancer*. Washington, DC: APA Books.

Belcher, L., Kalichman, S., Topping, M., Smith, S., Emshoff, J., Norris, F., and Nurss, J. (1998). Randomized trail of a brief HIV risk reduction counseling intervention for women. *Journal of Consulting and Clinical Psychology*, 66(5), 856–861.

Ben-Eliyahu, S., Yirmiya, R., Liebeskind, J.C., Taylor, A.N., and Gale, R.P. (1991). Stress increases metastatic spread of a mammary tumor in rats: evidence for mediation by the immune system. *Brain, Behavior, and Immunity*, 5(2), 193–205.

Ben-Eliyahu, S., Page, G.G., Yirmiya, R., and Shakhar, G. (1999). Evidence that stress and surgical interventions promote tumor development by suppressing natural killer cell activity. *International Journal of Cancer*, 80(6), 880–888.

Bennett, P. (1994). Should we intervene to modify Type A behaviors in patients with manifest heart disease? *Behavioral and Cognitive Psychotherapy*, 22(2), 125–145.

Bennett, P., and Carroll, D. (1990a). Type A behaviors and heart disease: Epidemiological and experimental foundations. *Behavioral Neurology,* 3(4), 261–277.

Bennett, P., and Carroll, D. (1990b). Stress management approaches to the prevention of coronary heart disease. *British Journal of Clinical Psychology*. 29(1), 1–12.

Bennett, P., Wallace, L., Carroll, D., and Smith, N. (1991). Treating Type A behaviors and mild hypertension in middle-aged men. *Journal of Psychosomatic Research* 35(2–3), 209–223.

Benight, C.C., Antoni, M.H., Kilbourn, K., Ironson, G., Kumar, M.A., Fletcher, M.A., Redwine, L., and Baum, A. (1997). Coping self-efficacy buffers psychological and physiological disturbances in HIV-infected men following a natural disaster. *Health Psychology*, 16(3), 248–255.

Bennett, P. (1994). Should we intervene to modify Type A behaviors in patients with manifest heart disease? *Behavioral and Cognitive Psychotherapy*, 22(2), 125–145.

Blumenthal, J.A., Thyrum, E.T., and Siegel, W.C. (1995). Contribution of job strain, job status and marital status to laboratory and ambulatory blood pressure in patients with mild hypertension. *Journal of Psychosomatic Research,* 39(2), 133–144.

Bosley, F., and Allen, T.W. (1989) Stress Management training for hypertensives: Cognitive and physiological effects. *Journal of Behavioral Medicine* 12(1), 77–89.

Breslin, F.C., O'Keeffe, Burrell, L., Ratliff-Crain, J., and Baum, A. (1995). The effects of stress and coping on daily alcohol use in women. *Addictive Behaviors*, 20(2), 141–147.

Brezinka, V., and Kittel, F. (1996). Psychosocial factors of coronary heart disease in women: A review. *Social Science and Medicine,* 42(10), 1351–1365.

Broota, A., Varma, R., and Singh, A. (1995). Role of relaxation in hypertension. *Journal of the Indian Academy of Applied Psychology,* 21(1), 29–36.

Carney, R.M., Rich, M.W., and Jaffe, A.S. (1995). Depression as a risk factor for cardiac events in established coronary heart disease: A review of possible mechanisms. *Annals of Behavioral Medicine,* 17(2), 142–149.

Cella, D.F., and Tross, S. (1986). Psychological adjustment to survival from Hodgkin's disease. *Journal of Consulting and Clinical Psychology,* 54(5), 616–622.

Charles, K., Sellick, S.M., Montesanto, B., and Mohide, E.A. (1996). Priorities of cancer survivors regarding Psychosocial needs source. *Journal of Psychosoical Oncology,* 14(2), 57–72.

Coates, T.J., McKusick, L., Kuno, R., and Stites, D.P. (1989). Stress reduction for men with HIV. *Advances,* 6(3), 7–8.

Cohen, L., Delahanty, D., Schmitz, J. B., Jenkins, F. J., and Baum, A. (1993). The effects of stress on natural killer cell activity in healthy men. *Journal of Applied Biobehavioral Research,* 1(2), 120–132.

Cole, S.W., Kemeny, M.E., Taylor, S.E., Visscher, B.R., and Fahey, J.L. (1996). Accelerated course of human immunodeficiency virus infection in gay men who conceal their homosexual identity. *Psychosomatic Medicine,* 58(3), 219–231.

Cruess, D.G., Antoni, M.H., McGregor, M..S., Kilbourn, K.M., Boyers, A.E., Alferi, S.M., Carver, C.S., and Kumar, M. (In press). *Cognitive Behavioral Stress Management Reduces Serum Cortisol by Enhancing Positive Contributions among Women Being Treated for Early-Stage Breast Cancer.*

Davison, G.C., Williams, M.E., Nezami, E., Bice, Traci, L., et al. (1991). Relaxation, reduction in angry articulated thoughts, and improvements in borderline hypertension and heart rate. *Journal of Behavioral Medicine,* 14(5), 453–468.

De Brabander, B., and Gertis, P. (1999). Chronic and acute stress as predictors of relapse in primary breast cancer patients. *Patient Education and Counseling,* 37(3), 265–272.

Delahanty, D.L., Dougall, A.L., Craig, K.L., Jenkins, F.J., and Baum, A. (1997). Chronic stress and natural killer cell activity after exposure to traumatic death. *Psychosomatic Medicine,* 59(5), 467–476.

Dembroski, T.M., MacDougall, J.M., Costa, P.T.,and Grandits, J.A. (1989). Components of hostility as predictors of sudden death and myocardial infarction in the Multiple Risk Factor Intervention Trail. *Psychosomatic Medicine,* 51, 514–522.

Dimsdale, J.E., Mills, P., Patterson, T., Ziegler, M., et al., (1994). Effects of chronic stress on beta-adrenergic receptors in the homeless. *Psychosomatic Medicine* 56(4), 290–295.

Dingle, G.A. and Oei, T.P. (1997). Is alcohol a cofactor of HIV and AIDS? Evidence from immunological and behavioral studies. *Psychological Bulletin,* 122(1), 56–71.

Dreher, H. (1997). The scientific and moral imperative for broad-based psychological interventions for cancer. *Advances,* 13(3), 38–49.

Dusseldorp, E., van Elderen, T., Maes, S., Meulman, J., and Kraaij, V. (1999). A meta-analysis of psychoeducational programs for coronary heart disease. *Health Psychology,* 18(5), 506–519.

Eaker, E.D., (1989). Psychosocial factors in the epidemiology of coronary heart disease in women. *Psychiatric Clinics of North America,* 12(1), 167–173.

Elliott, S.J. (1995). Psychosocial stress, women and heart health: A critical review. *Social Science and Medicine,* 40(1), 105–115.

Everson, S.A., Goldberg, D.E., Kaplan, G.A., Julkunen, J., and Salonen, J.T. (1998). Anger expression and incident hypertension. *Psychosomatic Medicine,* 60(6), 730–735.

Eysenck, H.J. (1990) Type A behavior and coronary heart disease: The third stage. *Journal of Social Behavior and Personality,* 5(1), 25–44

Ezzy, D., deVisser, R., and Bartos, M. (1999). Poverty, disease progression and employment among people living with HIV/AIDS in Australia. *AIDS Care,* 11(4), 405–414.

Fawzy, F.I. (1994). Immune effects of a short-term intervention for cancer patients. *Advances,* 10(4), 32–33.

Fawzy, F.I., Cousins, N., Fawzy, N.W., Kemeny, M.E., et al (1990). A structured psychiatric intervention for cancer patients: I. Changes over time in methods of coping and affective disturbance. *Archives of General Psychiatry,* 47(8), 720–725.

Fawzy, F.I., Kemeny, M.E., Fawzy, N.W., Elashoff, R., et al. (1990). A structured psychiatric intervention for cancer patients: II. Changes over time in immunological measures. *Archives of General Psychiatry,* 47(8), 729–735.

Fawzy, F.I., Fawzy, N.W., Hyun, C.S., Elashoff, R., Guthrie, D., Fahey, J.L., and Morton, D.L. (1993). Malignant melanoma: Effects of an early structured psychiatric intervention, coping, and affective state on recurrence and survival 6 years later. *Archives of General Psychiatry,* 50(9), 681–689.

Felten, D.L., and Felten, S.Y. (1991). Brain-immune signaling: Substrate for reciprocal immunological signaling of the nervous system. Frederickson, R.C., McGaugh, J.L., et al. (Eds). Peripheral signaling of the brain: Role in neural-immune interactions and learning and memory. *Neuronal control of bodily function: Basic and clinical aspects,* Vol 6 (pp 3–17). Lewiston, NY, USA: Hogrefe and Huber Publishers.

Fernandez-Cruz, E., Desco, M., Garcia Montes, M., Longo, N, et al. (1990). Immunological and serological markers predictive to progression to AIDS in a cohort of HIV-infected drug users. *AIDS,* 4(10), 987–994.

Fisher, J.D., Fisher, W.A., Misovich, S.J., Kimble, D.L., and Malloy, T.E. (1996). Changing AIDS risk behavior: Effects of an intervention emphasizing AIDS risk reduction information, motivation, and behavioral skills in a college student population. *Health Psychology,* 15(2), 114–123.

Fontana, A.F., Kerns, R.D., Rosenberg, R.L., and Colonese, K.L. (1989). Support, stress, and recovery from coronary heart disease: A longitudinal causal model. *Health Psychology,* 8(2), 175–193.

Ford, K., Wirawan, D.N., Fajans, P., Meliawan, P., et al. (1996). Behavioral interventions for reduction of sexually transmitted disease/HIV transmission among female commercial sex workers and clients in Bali, Indonesia. *AIDS,* 10(2), 213–22.

Foreyt, J.P., and Poston, W.S. (1996) Reducing risk for cardiovascular disease. *Psychotherapy,* 33(4), 576–586.

Freedland, K.E., Carney, R.M., Lustman, P.J., Rich, M.W., et al. (1992). Major depression in coronary artery disease patients with versus without a prior history of depression. *Psychosomatic Medicine,* 54(4), 416–421.

Freedman, R.R. (1987) Long term effectiveness of behavioral treatments for Raynaud's disease. *Behavior Therapy*, 18(4), 387–399.

Fredrikson, M., and Matthews, K.A. (1990). Cardiovascular responses to behavioral stress and hypertension: A meta-analytic review. *Annals of Behavioral Medicine*, 12(1), 30–39.

Frischenschlager, O., Broemmel, B., and Russinger, U. (1992). The effectivity of psychosocial care of cancer patients: A critical review of empirical studies. *Psychotherapie Psychosomatik Medizinische Psychologie*, 42(6), 206–213.

Gallois, P., Forzy, G., and Dhont, J.L. (1984). Hormonal changes induced by relaxation. *Encephale*, 10(2), 79–82.

Ganz, P.M., Hirji, K., Sim, M., Schag, C.A., et al. (1993). Predicting psychosocial risk in patients with breast cancer. *Medical Care*, 31(5), 419–431.

Garcia-Vera, M.P., Labrador, F.J., and Sanz, J. (1997). Stress-management training for essential hypertension: A controlled study. *Applied Psychophysiology and Biofeedback*, 22(4), 261–283.

Garcia-Vera, M.P., Labrador, F.J., and Sanz, J. (1998). Psychological changes accompanying and mediating stress-management training for essential hypertension. *Applied Psychophysiology and Biofeedback*, 23(3), 159–178.

Garssen, B., and Goodkin, K. (1999). On the role of immunological factors as mediators between psychosocial factors and cancer progression. *Psychiatry Research*, 85(1), 51–61.

Gerits, P., and De Brabander, B (1999). Psychosocial predictors of psychological, neurochemical and immunological symptoms of acute stress among breast cancer patients. *Psychiatry Research*, 85(1), 95–103.

Glanz, K., and Lerman, C. (1992). Psychosoical impact of breast cancer: a critical review. *Annals of Behavioral Medicine*,14(3), 204–212.

Glaser, R., Kennedy, S., Lafuse, W.P., Bonneau, R.H., Speicher, C., Hillhouse, J., and Kiecolt-Glaser, J.K. (1990). Psychological stress-induced modulation of interleukin 2 receptor gene expression and interleukin 2 production in peripheral blood leukocytes. *Archives of General Psychiatry*, 47(8), 707–712.

Glaser, R., Thorn, B.E., Tarr, K.L., Kiecolt-Glaser, J.K., and D'Ambrosio, S.M. (1985). Effects of stress on methyltransferase synthesis: an important DNA repair enzyme. *Health Psychology*, 4(5), 403–412.

Goodkin, K., Fuchs, I., Feaster, D, Leeka, J., et al. (1992). Life stressors and coping style are associated with immune measures in HIV-1 infection: A preliminary report. *International Journal of Psychiatry in Medicine*, 22(2), 155–172.

Gritz, E.R. (1991). Smoking and smoking cessation in cancer patients. *British Journal of Addiction*, 86(5), 549–554.

Gruber, G.L., Hersch, S.P., Hall, N.R., Waletzky, L.R., Kunz, J.F., Carpenter, J.K., Kverno, K.S., and Weiss, S.M. (1993). Immunological responses of breast cancer patients to behavioral interventions. *Biofeedback and Self-Regulation*, 18(1), 1–22.

Gulick, R.M., (1998). HIV Treatment strategies: Planning for the long term. *Journal of the American Medical Association*, 279(12), 957–959.

Haaga, D.A., Davison, G.C., Williams, M.E., Dolezal, S.L., et al. (1994). Mode-specific impact of relaxation training for hypertensive men with Type A behavior pattern. *Behavior Therapy*, 25(2), 209–223.

Hall, N.R. (1988). The virology of AIDS. *American Psychologist*, 43(11), 907–913.

Hall, N.R.S., and O'Grady, M.P. (1991). Psychological interventions and immune function. Ader R., Felten, D.L., and Cohen N. (Eds): *Psychoneuroimmunology*, ed 2, (pp 1067–1080) New York, Academic Press.

Helgeson, V., and Cohen, S. (1996). Social support and adjustment to cancer: reconciling descriptive, correlational, and intervention research. *Health Psychology*, 15(2), 135–148.

Helgeson, V., Cohen, S., Schulz, R., and Yasko, J. (1999). Education and peer discussion group interventions and adjustment to breast cancer. *Archives of General Psychiatry*, 56(4), 340–347.

Helgeson, V.S., Cohen, S., Schulz, R., and Yasko, J. (In press). Group support interventions for people with cancer: Benefits and hazards. Baum, A., and Andersen B. (Eds). *Psychosocial Intervention for Cancer*. Washington, D.C. APA Books.

Helgeson, V.S., Cohen, S., Schulz, R., and Yasko, J. (In press*). Group support interventions for women with cancer: Who benefits from what?*

Herberman, R.B. (1991). Sources of confounding in immunologic data. *Reviews of Infectious Diseases*, 13, 84–86.

Hoelscher, T.J. (1987). Maintenance of relaxation-induced blood pressure reductions: The importance of continued relaxation practice. *Biofeedback and Self Regulation*, 12(1), 3–12.

Houston, B.K., Chesney, M.A., Black, G.W., Cates, D.S., et al. (1992). Behavioral clusters and coronary heart disease risk. *Psychosomatic Medicine*, 54(4), 447–461.

Ironson, G., Wynings, C., Schneiderman, N., Baum, A., Rodriguez, M., Greenwood, D., Benight, C., Antoni, M., LaPerriere, A., Hui-Sheng, H., Klimas, N., and Fletcher, M.A. (1997) Posttraumatic stress symptoms, intrusive thoughts, loss, and immune function after Hurricane Andrew. *Psychosomatic Medicine*, 59, 128–141.

Irvine, M.J., Johnston, D.W., Jenner, D.A., and Marie, G.V. (1986). Relaxation and stress management in the treatment of essential hypertension. *Journal of Psychosomatic Research*, 30(4), 437–450.

Irvin, M.J., and Logan, A.G., (1991). Relaxation behavior therapy as sole treatment for mild hypertension. *Psychosomatic Medicine*, 53(6), 587–597.

Ishihara, Y., Matsunaga, K., Iijima, H., Fujii, T., Oguchi, Y., and Kagawa, J. (1999). Time-dependent effects of stressor application on metastasis of tumor cells in the lung and its regulation by an immunomodulator in mice. *Psychoneuroendocrinology*, 24(7), 713–726.

Jacob, R.G., Thayer, J.F., Manuck, S.B., Muldoon, M.F., Tamres, L.K., Williams, D.M., Ding, Y., and Gatsonis, C. (1999). Ambulatory blood pressure responses and the circumplex model of mood: A 4-day study. *Psychosomatic Medicine*, 61(3), 319–333.

Jacob, R.G., Shapiro, A.P., O'Hara, P., Portser, S., et al. (1992). Relaxation therapy for Hypertension: Setting-specific effects. *Psychosomatic Medicine*, 54(1), 87–101.

Jacob, R.G., Wing, R.R., and Shapiro, A.P. (1987). The behavioral treatment of hypertension: Long term effects. *Behavior Therapy*, 18(4), 325–352.

Johnson, J.V., Hall, E.M., and Theorell, T. (1989). Combined effects of job strain and social isolation on cardiovascular disease morbidity and mortality in a random sample of the Swedish male working population. *Scandinavian Journal of Work, Environment and Health*, 15(4), 271–279.

Johnson, J.V., Stewart, W., Hall, E.M., Fredlunc, P., et al. (1996). Long term psychosocial work environment and cardiovascular mortality among Swedish men. *American Journal of Public Health*, 86(3), 324–331.

Johnston, M., Wakeling, A., Graham, N., and Stokes, F. (1987). Cognitive impairment, emotional disorder and length of stay of elderly patients in a district general hospital. *British Journal of Medical Psychology*, 60(2), 133–139.

Kamarck, T.W., and Jennings, J.R. (1991). Biobehavioral factors in sudden cardiac death. *Psychological Bulletin*, 109(1), 42–75.

Kaplan, G.A. (1992). Health and aging in the Alameda County Study. Schaie, K.W., Blazer, D.G., et al (Eds). Aging, health behaviors, and health outcomes. *Social structure and aging*. (pp 69–88). Hillsdale, NJ, USA: Lawrence Erlbaum Assoc., Inc.

Kaplan, J.R., Manuck, S.B., Clarkson, T.B., Lusso, F.M., and Taub, D.B. (1982). Social status, environment and atherosclerosis in cynomolgus monkeys. *Arteriosclerosis*, 2, 359–368.

Kaplan, J.R., Adams, M.R., Clarkson, T.B., Koritnick, D.R. (1984). Psychosocial influences on female "protection" among cynomolgus macaques. *Atherosclerosis*, 53, 283–295.

Kaplan, J.R., Adams, M.R., Clarkson, T.B., Manuck, S.B., Shively, C.A., and Williams, J.K. (1996). Psychological factors, sex differences, and atherosclerosis: Lessons from animal models. *Psychosomatic Medicine*, 58, 598–611.

Kasl, S.V. (1996). The influence of the work environment on cardiovascular health: A historical, conceptual, and methodological perspective. *Journal of Occupational Health Psychology*, 1(1), 42–56.

Kiecolt-Glaser, J.K., Stephens, R.E., Lipetz, P.D., Speicher, C.E., and Glaser, R. (1985). Distress and DNA repair in human lymphocytes. *Journal of Behavioral Medicine*, 8(4), 311–320.

Keller, M., Henrich, G., Sellschopp, A., and Beutel, M. (1996). Between distress and support: Spouses of cancer patients. Baider, L., Cooper, C.L., et al (Eds). *Cancer and the family* (pp 187–223). Chichester, England UK: John Wiley and Sons.

Kelly, J.A. (1998). Group psychotherapy for persons with HIV and AIDS-related illnesses. *International Journal of Group Psychotherapy*, 48(2), 143–162.

Kemeny, M.E. (1994). Psychoneuroimmunology of HIV infection. *Psychiatric Clinics of North America*, 71(1), 55–68.

Kemeny, M.E., Weiner, H., Duran, R., Taylor, S.E., et al. (1995). Immune system changes after the death of a partner in HIV-positive gay men. *Psychosomatic Medicine*, 57(6), 547–554.

Kerr, L.R., Wilkinson, D.A., Emerman, J.T., and Weinberg, J. (1999). Interactive effects of psychosocial stressors and gender on mouse mammary tumor growth. *Physiology and Behavior*, 66(2), 277–281.

Kiecolt-Glaser, J.K., and Glaser, R. (1992). Psychoneuroimmunology: can psychological interventions modulate immunity? *Journal of Consulting and Clinical Psychology*, 60(4), 569–575.

King, M., Speck, P., Thomas, A. (1999). The effect of spiritual beliefs on outcome from illness. *Social Science and Medicine*, 48(9), 1291–1299.

Knox, S.S., and Uvnaes-Moberg, K. (1998). Social isolation and cardiovascular disease: An atherosclerotic pathway? *Psychoneuroendocrinology*, 23(8), 877–890.

Kop, W.J. (1999). Chronic and acute psychological risk factors for clinical manifestations of coronary artery disease. *Psychosomatic Medicine*, 61(4), 476–487.

Krantz, D.S., Contrada, R.J., Hill, D.R., and Friedler, E. (1988). Environmental stress and biobehavioral antecedents of coronary heart disease. *Journal of Consulting and Clinical Psychology*, 56(3), 333–341.

Krantz, D.S., Grunberg, N.E, and Baum, A. (1985). Health psychology. In: Annual review of psychology. Vol. 36. Palo Alto, CA: *Annual Reviews, Inc.* (p. 349–383).

Krantz, D.S., Kop, W.J., Antiago, H.T., and Gottdiener, J.S. (1996). Mental stress as a trigger of myocardial ischemia and infarction. *Cardiology Clinics*, 14(2), 271–287.

Krantz, D.S., Schneiderman, N., Chesney, M.A., McCann, B.S., et al. (1989). Biobehavioral research on cardiovascular disorders. *Health Psychology*, 8(6), 737–746.

Kringlen, E. (1986). Psychosocial aspects of coronary heart disease. *Acta Psychiatrica Scandinavica*, 74(3), 225–237.

Kubzansky, L.D., Kawachi, I., Weiss, S.T., and Sparrow, D. (1998). Anxiety and coronary heart disease: A synthesis of epidemiological, psychological, and experimental evidence. *Annals of Behavioral Medicine*, 20(2), 47–58.

LaPerriere, A., Schneiderman, N., Antoni, M.H., and Fletcher, M.A. (1990). Aerobic exercise training and psychoneuroimmunology in AIDS research. Temoshok, L, Baum, A., et al (Eds). *Psychosocial perspectives on AIDS: Etiology, prevention, and treatment,* (pp. 259–286). Hillsdale, NJ, USA: Lawrence Erlbaum Associates, Inc.

Lazarus, R.S. and S. Folkman. (1984). *Stress, appraisal, and coping.* Springer. New York

Lekander, M., Furst, C.J., Rotstein, S., Hursti, T.J., and Fredrikson, M. (1997). Immune effects of relaxation during chemotherapy for ovarian cancer. *Psychotherapy and Psychosomatics*, 66, 185–191.

Leventhal, H. (1980). Toward a comprehensive theory of emotion. Berkowitz, L. (Ed): *Advances in Experimental Social Psychology* (pp 140–208). Academic Press.

Levy, S.M. (1991). Behavioral and immunological host factors in cancer risk. McCabe, P.M., and Schneiderman, N., et al (Eds). *Stress, coping, and disease. Stress and coping.* Hillsdale, NJ, USA. Lawrence Erlbaum Associates, Inc.

Levy, S.M., Cottrell, M.C., and Black, P.H. (1990). Psychological and immunological associations in men with AIDS pursuing a macrobiotic regimen as an alternative therapy: A pilot study. *Brain, Behavior and Immunity*, 3(2), 175–182.

Levy, S.M., Herberman, R.B., Maluish, A.M., Schlien, V., and Lippman, M. (1985). Prognostic risk assessment in primary breast cancer by behavioral and immunological parameters. *Health Psychology*, 4(2), 99–113.

Levy, S.M. (1990). Psychosocial risk factors and cancer progression: Mediating pathways linking behavior and disease. Craig, K.D., Weiss, S.M., et al (Eds). Health enhancement, disease prevention, and early intervention: *Biobehavioral perspectives* (pp. 348–369). New York, NY, USA: Springer Publishing Co., Inc.

Levy, S.M., and Wise, B.D. (1989). Psychosocial risk factors, natural immunity, and cancer progression: Implications for intervention. Johnston, M., and Marteau, T., et al. (Eds). *Applications in health psychology* (pp. 141–155). New Brunswick, NJ, USA: Transaction Publishers.

Lorig, K.R., Sobel, D.S., Stewart, A.L., Brown, B.W., Bandura, A., Ritter, P., Gonzalez, V.M., Laurent, D.D., and Holman, H.R. (1999). Evidence suggesting that a chronic disease self-management program can improve health status while reducing hospitalization. *Medical Care*, 37(1), 5–14.

Lovibond, S.H., Birrell, P.C., and Langeluddecke, P. (1986). Changing coronary heart disease risk-factor status: The effects of three behavioral programs. *Journal of Behavioral Medicine* 9(5), 415–437.

Lutgendorf, S., Antoni, M.H., Schneiderman, N., Ironson, G., Fletcher, M.A. (1995). Psychosocial interventions and quality of life changes across the HIV spectrum. Dimsdale, J.E., and Baum, A. (Eds). Quality of life in behavioral medicine research. *Perspectives in behavioral medicine* (pp. 205–239). Hillsdale, NJ, USA: Lawrence Erlbaum Associates, Inc.

Lyketsos, C.G., Hoover, D.R., and Guccione, M. (1996). Depression and survival among HIV-infected persons. *Journal of the American Medical Association,* 275(1), 35–36.

Mann, A.H. (1984). Hypertension: Psychological aspects and diagnostic impact in a clinical trial. *Psychological Medicine,* Mono Suppl 5, 35.

Manuck, S.B., Kaplan, J.R., and Clarkson, T.B. (1983). Social instability and coronary artery atherosclerosis in cynomolgus monkeys. *Neuroscience and Biobehavioral Reviews,* 74(4), 485–491.

Manuck, S.B., and Krantz, D.S. (1984). Psychophysiologic reactivity in coronary heart disease. *Behavioral Medicine Update,* 6(3), 11–15.

Manuck, S.B., Adams, M.R., McCaffery, J.M., and Kaplan, J.R. (1997) *Behaviorally elicited heart rate reactivity and atherosclerosis in ovariectomized cynomolgus monkeys (Macaca fascicularis).* American Heart Association, Inc.

Manuck, S.B., Kaplan, J.R., and Matthews, K.A. (1986). Behavioral antecedents of coronary heart disease and atherosclerosis. *Arteriosclerosis,* 6, 2–14

Markovitz, J.H. and Matthews, K.A. (1991). Platelets and coronary heart disease: Potential psychophysiologic mechanisms. *Psychosomatic Medicine,* 53(6), 643–668.

Marmot, M. (1994). Work and other factors influencing coronary health and sickness absence. *Work and Stress,* 8(2), 191–201.

Mason, J.W., (1975). A historical view of the stress field. *Journal of Human Stress,* 1, 22–36.

Matarazzo, J.D. (1980). Behavioral health and behavioral medicine: Frontiers for a new health psychology. *American Psychologist,* 35(9), 807–817.

Matthews, K.A., and Haynes, S.G. (1986). Type A behavior patterns and coronary disease risk: Update and critical evaluation. *American Journal of Epidemiology,* 123(6), 923–960.

McCubbin, J.A., Wilson, J.F., Bruehl, S., Ibarra, P., et al. (1996). Relaxation training and opioid inhibition of blood pressure response to stress. *Journal of Consulting and Clinical Psychology,* 64(3), 593–601.

McGrady, A., Conran, P., Dickey, D., Garman, D., Farris, E., and Schumann-Brezezinski, C. (1992). The effects of biofeedback-assisted relaxation on cell-mediated immunity, cortisol, and white blood cell count in healthy adult subjects. *Journal of Behavioral Medicine,* 15, 343–354.

McGrady, A.V., Woerner, M., Bernal, G.A., and Higgins, J.T. (1987). Effect of biofeedback-assisted relaxation on blood pressure and cortisol levels in normotensives and hypertensives. *Journal of Behavioral Medicine,* 10(3), 301–310.

McGrady, A., Turner, J.W., Fine, T.H., and Higgins, J.T. (1987). Effects of biobehaviorally-assisted relaxation training on blood pressure, plasma renin, cortisol, and aldosterone levels in borderline hypertension. *Clinical Biofeedback and Health: An International Journal,* 10(1), 16–25.

McKenna, M.C., Zevon, M.A., Corn, B., and Rounds, J. (1999). Psychosocial factors and the development of breast cancer: A meta-analysis. *Health Psychology,* 18(5), 520–531.

McKinnon, W., Weisse, C.S., Reynolds, C.P., Bowles, C.A. and Baum, A. (1989). Chronic stress, leukocyte subpopulations, and humoral response to latent viruses. *Health Psychology*, 8(4), 389–402.

McNulty, S., Jefferys, D., Singer, G., and Singer, L. (1984). Use of hormone analysis in the assessment of the efficacy of stress management training in police recruits. *Journal of Police Science and Administration,* 12(2), 130–132.

Mellors, V., Boyle, G.J., and Roberts L. (1994). Effects of personality, stress and lifestyle on hypertension: An Australian twin study. *Personality and Individual Differences,* 16(6), 967–974.

Meyer, T.J., Mark, M.M., (1995). Effects of psychological interventions with adult cancer patients: A meta-analysis of randomized experiments. *Health Psychology,* 14(2),101–108.

Miller, G.E., Kemeny, M.E., Taylor, S.E., Cole, S.W., and Visscher, B.R. (1997). Social relationships and immune processes in HIV seropositive gay and bisexual men. *Annals of Behavioral Medicine,* 19(2), 139–151.

Miller, S.M., Mischel, W., O'Leary, A., and Mills, M. (1996). From human papilloma virus (HPV) to cervical cancer: Psychosocial processes in infection, detection, and control. *Annals of Behavioral Medicine,* 18(4), 219–228.

Moyer, A., and Salovey, P. (1996). Psychosocial sequelae of breast cancer and its treatment. *Annals of Behavioral Medicine,* 18(2), 110–125.

Mulder, C.L., deVroome, E.M., van Griensven, G.J., Antoni, M.H., and Sandfort, T.G. (1999). Avoidance as a predictor of the biological course of HIV infection over a 7-year period in gay men. *Health Psychology*, 18(2), 107–113.

Munoz, A., Wang, M.C., Bass, S., Taylor, J.M., Kingsley, L.A., Chmiel, J.S., and Polk, B.F. (1989). Acquired immunodeficiency syndrome (AIDS)-free time after human immunodeficiency virus type 1 (HIV-1) seroconversion in homosexual men. Multicenter AIDS Cohort Study Group. *American Journal of Epidemiology*, 130(3), 530–539.

Musselman, D.L., Evans, D.L., and Nemeroff, Charles B. (1998). The relationship of depression to cardiovascular disease: epidemiology, biology, and treatment. *Archives of General Psychiatry*, 55(7), 580–592.

Naeslund, G.K., Fredrikson, M., and Holm, L. (1993). Psychosocial factors associated with participation and nonparticipation in a diet intervention program. *Journal of Psychosocial Oncology,* 19(4), 93–107.

Niaura, R., and Goldstein, M.G. (1992). Psychological factors affecting physical condition: Cardiovascular disease literature review: II. Coronary artery disease and sudden death and hypertension. *Psychosomatics* 33(2), 146–155.

Nunes, E.V., Frank, K.A., and Kornfeld, D.S. (1987). Psychologic treatment for the Type A behavior pattern and for coronary heart disease: A meta-analysis of the literature. *Psychosomatic Medicine*, 49(2), 159–173.

O'Leary, A. (1990). Stress, emotion, and human immune function. *Psychological Bulletin*, 108, 363–382.

Orth-Gomer, K., and Unden, A. (1990). Type A behavior, social support, and coronary risk: Interaction and significance for mortality in cardiac patients. *Psychosomatic Medicine,* 52(1), 59–72.

Ostrow, D.G. (1996). The search for the elusive psychosocial modulators of human immunodeficiency virus disease progression. *Psychosomatic Medicine,* 58(3), 232–233.

Pennebaker, J.W., Hughes, C.F., and O'Heeron, R.C. (1987). The psychophysiology of confession: Linking inhibitory and psychosomatic processes. *Journal of Personality and Social Psychology,* 52(4), 781–793.

Perry, S.W., Fishman, B., Jacobsberg, L., Frances, A.J. (1992) Relationships over 1 year between lymphocyte subsets and psychosocial variables among adults with infection by human immunodeficiency virus. *Archives of General Psychiatry,* 49(5), 396–401.

Peter, R., and Siegrist, J. (1997). Chronic work stress, sickness absence and hypertension in middle managers: General or specific sociological explanations? *Social Science and Medicine,* 45(7), 1111–1120.

Petticrew, M., Fraser, J.M. and Regan, M.F. (1999). Adverse life-events and risk of breast cancer: A meta-analysis. *British Journal of Health Psychology,* 4(1), 1–17.

Phair, J.P., Farzadegan, H., Chmiel, J., Munoz, A., Detels, R., Saah, A. and Kaslow, R. Progression of HIV-infection: markers or determinants. *Transactions of the American Clinical and Climatoloigcal Association,* 104, 123–128, discussion 129–129.

Pickering, T.G., and Gerin, W. (1990). Cardiovascular reactivity in the laboratory and the role of behavioral factors in hypertension: A critical review. *Annals of Behavioral Medicine,* 12(1), 3–16.

Pomeroy, E.C., Rubin, A., Van Laningham, L., and Walker, R.J. (1997). "Straight talk": The effectiveness of a psychoeducational group intervention for heterosexuals with HIV/AIDS. *Research on Social Work Practice,* 7(2), 149–164.

Rabkin, J.G., Williams, J.B., Remien, R.H., Goetz, R., et al. (1991). Depression, distress, lymphocyte subsets, and human immunodeficiency virus symptoms on two occasions in HIV-positive homosexual men. *Achieves of General Psychiatry,* 48(2), 111–119.

Ramirez, A.J., Craig, T.K., Watson, J.P., Fentiman, I.S., North, W.R., and Rubens, R.D. (1989). Stress and the relapse of breast cancer. *British Medical Journal,* 298, 291–293.

Reed, G.M., Kemeny, M.E., Taylor, S.E., Wang, H.J., et al. (1994). Realistic acceptance as a predictor of decreased survival time in gay men with AIDS. *Health Psychology,* 13(4), 299–307.

Redd, W.H. (1997). Behavioral intervention in cancer treatment. Baer, D.M., Elsie, M., et al. (Eds). *Environment and behavior* (Pp. 155–162). Boulder, CO, USA: Westview Press.

Remien, R.H., Rabkin, J.G., Williams, J.B., and Katoff, L. (1992). Coping strategies and health beliefs of AIDS longterm surivors. *Psychology and Health,* 6(4), 335–345.

Richardson, J.L., Zarnegar, Z., Bisno, B., and Levine, A. (1990). Psychosocial status at initiation of cancer treatment and survival. *Journal of Psychosomatic Research,* 34(2), 189–201.

Roscnman, R.H. (1991). Type A behavior pattern and coronary heart disease: The hostility factor? *Stress Medicine,* 7(4), 245–253.

Schedlowski, M., Jacobs, R., Alker, J., Proehl, F., et al. (1993). Psychophysiological, neuroendocrine and cellular immune reactions under psychological stress. *Neuropsychobiology*, 28(1–2), 87–90.

Schulz, R., Williamson, G.M., Knapp, J.E., Bookwala, J., et al. (1995). The psychological, social, and economic impact of illness among patients with recurrent cancer. *Journal of Psychosocial Oncology*, 13(3), 21–45.

Schlebusch, L., and Cassidy, M.J. (1995). Stress, social support and biopsychosocial dynamics in HIV-AIDS. *South African Journal of Psychology*, 25(1), 27–30.

Schneiderman, N., (1983). Animal Behavior Models of Coronary Heart Disease. Krantz, D.S., Baum, A., and Singer, J.E. (Eds) *Handbook of Psychology and Health Vol. III Cardiovascular Disorders and Behavior*. (pp. 19–56). Hillsdale, N.J.: Lawrence Erlbaum Assoc., Inc

Schneiderman, N., Antoni, M.H., Ironson, G., LaPeriere, A., et al. (1992). Applied psychological science and HIV-1 spectrum disease. *Applied and Preventive Psychology*, 1(2), 67–82.

Shapiro, A.P. (1983). Krantz, D.S., Baum, A., Singer, J.E. (Eds) The Non-Pharmacologic Treatment of Hypertension. *Handbook of Psychology and Health Vol. III Cardiovascular Disorders and Behavior*. (pp 277–294). Hillsdale, N.J.: Lawrence Erlbaum Assoc., Inc.

Shedlowski, M., Jung, C., Shimanski, G., Tewes, V., and Schmoll, H.J. (1994). Effects of behavioral intervention on plasma cortisol and lymphocytes in breast cancer patients: an exploratory study. *Psycho Oncology*, 3, 181–187.

Shekelle, R.B., Vernon, S.W., Ostfeld, A.M. (1991). Personality and coronary heart disease. *Psychosomatic Medicine* 53(2), 176–184.

Siegel, K., Karus, D., Epstein, J., and Raveis, V.H. (1996). Psychological and psychosocial adjustment of HIV-infected gay/bisexual men: Diseases stage comparisons. *Journal of Community Psychology*, 24(3), 229–243.

Sikkema, K.J., Kalichman, S.C., Kelly, J.A., and Koob, J.J. (1995). Group intervention to improve coping with AIDS-related bereavement: model development and an illustrative clinical example. *AIDS Care*, 7(4), 463–475.

Skantze, H.B., Kaplan, J., Pettersson, K., Manuck, S., Blomqvist, N., Kyes, R., Williams, K., and Bondjers, G. (1998). Psychosocial stress causes endothelial injury in cynomolgus monkeys via • beta-adrenoceptor activation. *Atherosclerosis*, 136, 153–161.

Sklar, L.S., and Anisman, H. (1981). Stress and Cancer. *Psychological Bulletin*, 89(3), 369–406.

Sobel, D.S. (1995). Rethinking medicine: Improving health outcomes with cost-effective psychosocial interventions. *Psychosomatic Medicine*, 57(3), 234–244.

Solomon, G.F., (1987). Psychoneuroimmunologic approaches to research on AIDS. *Annals of the New York Academy of Sciences*, 496, 628–636.

Solomon, G.F., Kemeny, M.E., and Temoshok, L. (1991). Psychoneuroimmunologic aspects of human immunodeficiency virus infection. Ader, R., Felten, D.L. et al (Eds). *Psychoneuroimmunology* (2nd Ed) (pp. 1081–1113). San Diego, CA, USA: Academic Press, Inc.

Suarez, E.W., and Williams, R.B. (1990). The relationships between dimensions of hostility and cardiovascular reactivity as a function of task characteristics. *Psychosomatic Medicine*, 52(5), 558–570.

Smith, T.W., and Gallo, L.C. (1994). Psychosocial influences on coronary heart disease. *Irish Journal of Psychology*, 15(1), 2–26.

Spiegel, D. (1995) Psychosocial influences on cancer survival. Stein, M., and Baum, A. (Eds). Chronic diseases. *Perspectives in behavioral medicine* (pp 223–223). Mahwah, NJ, USA: Lawrence Erlbaum Associates, Inc.

Spiegel, D. (1996). Cancer and depression. British Journal of Psychiatry—Supplement, 30, 109–116.

Spiegel, D., Bloom, J.R., Kraemer, H.C., and Gottheil E. (1989). Effect of psychosocial treatment on survival of patients with metastatic breast cancer. *Lancet*, 2(8668), 888–891.

Spiegel, D., and Kato, P.M. (1996). Psychosocial influences on cancer incidence and progression. *Harvard Review of Psychiatry* 4(1), 10–26.

Spiegel, D., Sephton, S.E., and Sites, D.P. (1998). Effects of psychosocial treatment in prolonging cancer survival may be mediated by neuroimmune pathways. McCann, S.M., and Lipton, J.M. (Eds) *Annals of the New York Academy of Sciences*, Vol. 840: Neuroimmunomodualtion: Molecular aspects, integrative systems, and clinical advances. *Annals of the New York Academy of Sciences*, Vol. 840. (pp 674–683). New York, NY USA: New York Academy of Sciences.

Steptoe, A.(1989). Psychophysiological interventions in behavioral medicine. Turpin, G. (Ed.). *Handbook of Clinical Psychophysiology*. Chi Chester: John Wiley.

Steptoe, A., Patel, C., Marmot, M., and Hunt, B. (1987). Frequency of relaxation practice, blood pressure reduciton and the general effects of relaxation following a controlled trial of behavior modification for reducing coronary risk. *Stress Medicine*, 3(2), 101–107.

Suminski, R.R., Anding, J., Smith, D.W., Zhang, J.J., Utter, A.C., and Kang, J. (1999). Risk and reality: The association between cardiovascular disease risk factor knowledge and selected risk-reducing behaviors. *Family and Community Health* 21(4), 51–62.

Tejwani, G.A., Gudehithlu, K.P., Hanissian, S.H., Gienapp, I.E., Whitacre, C.C., and Malarkey, W.B. (1991). Facilitation of dimethylbenz [a] anthracene-induced rat mammary tumorigenesis by restraint stress: role of beta-endorphin, prolactin and naltrexone. *Carcinogenesis*, 12(4), 637–641.

Theorell, T., and Karasek, R.A. (1996). Current issues relating to psychosocial job strain and cardiovascular disease research. *Journal of Occupational Health Psychology* 1(1), 9–26.

Tomei, L.D., Kiecolt-Glaser, J.K., Kennedy, S., and Glaser, R. (1990). Psychological stress and phorbol ester inhibition of radiation-induced apoptosis in human peripheral blood leukocytes. *Psychiatry Resource*, 33, 59–71.

Turk, D.C., Meichenbau, D., and Genest, M.(Eds) (1983). *Pain and Behavioral Medicine A Cognitive-Behavioral Perspective*. New York: The Guilford Press.

Uchino, B.N., Cacioppo, J.T., and Keicolt-Glaser, J.K. (1996). The relationship between social support and physiological processes: A review with emphasis on underlying mechanisms and implications for health. *Psychological Bulletin*, 119(3), 488–531.

Van der Pompe, G, Antoni, M., Visser, A., and Garssen, B. (1996). Adjustment to breast cancer: The psychobiological effects of psychosocial interventions. *Patient Education and Counseling*, 28(2), 209–219.

Van der Pompe, G., Antoni, M.H., and Heijnen, C.J. (1996). Elevated basal cortisol levels and attenuated ACTH and cortisol responses to a behavioral challenge in women with metastatic breast cancer. *Psychoneuroendocrinology*, 21(4), 361–374.

Van der Pompe, G., Antoni, M.H., and Heijnen, C.J. (1998). The effects of surgical stress and psychological stress on the immune function of operative cancer patients. *Psychology and Health*, 13(6), 1015–1026.

Van der Pompe, G., Antoni, M.H., Visser, A., and Heijnen, C.J.(1998). Effect of mild acute stress on immune cell distribution and natural killer cell activity in breast cancer patients. *Biological Psychology*, 48(1), 21–36.

Vaughn, S.M., and Kinnier, R.T. (1996). Psychological effects of a life review intervention for persons with HIV disease. *Journal of Counseling and Development*, 75(2), 115–123.

Weidner, G., Boughal, T., Connor, S.L., Pieper, C., et al., (1997). Relationship of job strain to standard coronary risk factors and psychological characteristics in women and men of the Family Heart Study. *Health Psychology*, 16(3), 239–247.

Wellisch, D.K., Wolcott, D.L. Pasnau, R.O., Fawzy, F., et al., (1989). An evaluation of the psychosocial problems of the homebound cancer patient: Relationship of patient adjustment to family problems. *Journal of Psychosocial Oncology*, 71, 55–76.

Wingard, J.R., Curbow, B., Baker, F., Zabora, J., and Piantadosi, S. (1992). Sexual satisfaction in survivors of bone marrow transplantation. *Bone Marrow Transplantation*, 9(3), 185–190.

Yellen, S.B., Cella, D.F., and Bonomi, A. (1993). Quality of life in people with Hodgkin's disease. *Oncology* (Huntington), 7(8), 41–45.

Committee Biographies

S. Leonard Syme, Ph.D., is emeritus Professor of Epidemiology at the University of California at Berkeley. Dr. Syme's research focuses on risk factors for coronary heart disease. His major interest has been psychosocial risk factors such as job stress, social support and poverty. Since his retirement in 1993, Dr. Syme has devoted most of his time to the development of interventions to prevent disease and promote health. He currently is the Director of the Center for Community Wellness, which provides useful health information to people and their communities. Dr. Syme was elected to the Institute of Medicine of the National Academy of Sciences and received the Berkeley Citation for Distinguished Achievement, the Lilienfeld Award for Excellence in Teaching, the California Senate Commendation for Illustrious Record of Accomplishment, and the American College of Physicians Award for Distinguished Contributions in Preventive Medicine.

Hortensia Amaro, Ph.D., is Professor of Social and Behavioral Sciences at the Boston University School of Public Health and board member of the Boston Public Health Commission. Her research career over the last 20 years has focused on the public health issues of substance abuse, adolescent pregnancy, HIV prevention, and mental health among Hispanic and African American communities. Dr. Amaro's professional contributions have been recognized by numerous organizations including the American Psychological Association, the Association of Women in Psychology, the Massachusetts Public Health Association, the U.S. Department of Health and Human Services, and Simmons College, who conferred upon her an honorary doctorate degree in humane letters. At the national level, Dr. Amaro has served on numerous committees including the National Committee on Vital and Health Statistics and the Advisory Board to the National Institute on Drug Abuse. She serves as Associate Editor of the *Psychology of Women Quarterly* and on the editorial board of the *American Journal of Public Health*.

Eugene Emory, Ph.D., is Professor of Psychology at Emory University. Dr. Emory's clinical and research interests are in developmental psychophysiology and neuropsychology, psychobiological approaches to high risk research, perinatal brain trauma and early stress, neuropsychological assessment of developmental disorders, differential diagnosis and court testimony, cognitive-behavior therapy, and parent training. His current research projects include studies in behavioral perinatology, psychosocial stress in women of reproductive age, and cerebral blood flow during pregnancy. Dr. Emory was a recipient of the Research Scientist Development Award from the National Institute of Mental Health. An editorial board member of the *International Journal of Psychophysiology* since 1984, and *Child Development*, Dr. Emory has published numerous research materials including Psychophysiological Responses to Stress during Pregnancy and Salivary Caffeine and Neonatal Behavior.

Arthur Kellermann, M.D., M.P.H., is Professor and Director, Center for Injury Control, Rollins School of Public Health, Emory University, and Professor and Chairman, Department of Emergency Medicine, School of Medicine, Emory University. Dr. Kellermann has served as Principal Investigator or Co-Investigator on several research grants, including federally funded studies of handgun related violence and injury, emergency cardiac care, and the use of emergency room services. Among his many awards and distinctions, he is a Fellow of the American College of Emergency Physicians (1992), and is the recipient of a meritorious service award from the Tennessee State Legislature (1993) and the Hal Jayne Academic Excellence Award from the Society for Academic Emergency Medicine (1997), and was elected to the membership of the Institute of Medicine (1999). In addition, Dr. Kellermann is a member of the Editorial Board of the journal *Annals of Emergency Medicine*, and has served as a reviewer for the *New England Journal of Medicine*, the *Journal of the American Medical Association*, and the *American Journal of Public Health*.

Janice Kiecolt-Glaser, Ph.D., is Professor of Psychiatry and Psychology in the Ohio State University College of Medicine, as well as Director of the Division of Health Psychology in the Department of Psychiatry. Working in the area of stress and immune function, she has authored more than 140 articles and chapters (most in collaboration with Ronald Glaser), and together they coedited the *Handbook of Human Stress and Immunity* (Academic Press, 1994). She has served on the

NIMH Mental Health and AIDS study section, as well as the editorial boards of 10 professional journals including the *Journal of Consulting and Clinical Psychology*, *Psychosomatic Medicine*, and *Health Psychology*. Her research is supported by several grants from the National Institutes of Health, including a MERIT award from NIMH on which she is the Principal Investigator, and a Research Career Development Award. A Fellow of the American Psychological Association, she received an Award for Outstanding Contributions to Health Psychology from the American Psychological Association's Division of Health Psychology, and she is the Past President of the Division of Health Psychology.

Marie C. McCormick, M.D., Sc.D., is the Sumner and Ester Feldberg Professor and Chair of the Department of Maternal and Child Health, Harvard School of Public Health, and Professor of Pediatrics at the Harvard Medical School. Her research interests are in the epidemiology of infant mortality and low birth weight, the measurement of and factors associated with child health status, especially among very low birth weight infants, and evaluation of maternal and child health services, especially those focused on infant mortality reduction and early childhood development. Dr. McCormick is a member of the Institute of Medicine and the Board on Health Promotion and Disease Prevention. In addition, she is a member of the editorial board of the *Journal of Developmental and Behavioral Pediatrics*. Among her many awards and distinctions, Dr. McCormick is a recipient of the Ambulatory Pediatric Association Research Award, is a member of Delta Omega (Alpha Chapter), and is a Fellow of the Association for Health Services Research.

David Mechanic, Ph.D., is the René Dubos University Professor of Behavioral Sciences and Director of the Institute for Health, Health Care Policy, and Aging Research at Rutgers University. He also directs the NIMH Center at Rutgers for Research on the Organization and Financing of Care for the Severely Mentally Ill. Dr. Mechanic's research and writing deal with social aspects of health and health care. He has written or edited 24 books and more than 400 research articles, chapters and other publications in medical sociology, health policy, health services research, and the social and behavioral sciences. Dr. Mechanic is a member of the National Academy of Sciences, the American Academy of Arts and Sciences, and the Institute of Medicine. He has received many awards, including the Health Services Research Prize from the Association of University Programs in Health Administration and the Baxter Allegiance Foundation, the Distinguished Investigator Award from the Association for Health Services Research, the First Carl Taube Award for Distinguished Contributions to Mental Health Services Research from the American Public Health Association, and the Distinguished Medical Sociologist Award and Lifetime Contributions Award in Mental Health from the American Sociological Association.

Paul G. Shekelle, M.D., Ph.D., is a consultant in health sciences at RAND, Associate Professor of Medicine at the UCLA School of Medicine, a staff physician at the VA Medical Center in West Los Angeles, and a Senior Research Associate of the VA Health Services Research and Development Service. He has been the principal investigator for 10 studies that have examined such questions as the reliability of expert panel processes at setting quality criteria; the effects of differing practice guidelines on the likelihood of physician behavior change; the usefulness of the RAND appropriateness method in the AHCPR clinical practice guideline development process; the current measurement of the quality of back care, diabetes care, and hypertension care; and the effect of practice guidelines on patient outcomes in the emergency department. Since 1997, Dr. Shekelle has been the Director of the Southern California Evidence-Based Practice Center.

Glorian Sorensen, Ph.D., M.P.H., Director, Center for Community-Based Research, Dana-Farber Cancer Institute, and Professor of Health and Social Behavior, at the Harvard School of Public Health, Boston. The core of Dr. Sorensen's research is randomized worksite- and community-based studies that test the effectiveness of theory-driven interventions targeting individual and organizational change. Dr. Sorensen conducted the first randomized controlled worksite intervention trials to integrate messages on occupational health and health behaviors. She is currently the Principal Investigator of the National Cancer Institute-funded Harvard Cancer Prevention Program Project focusing on "Cancer Control in Working Class, Multi-Ethnic Populations." Dr. Sorensen is a member of the NCI's National 5-a-Day for Better Health External Advisory Group, and was a member of the NIH study section on Community Prevention and Control. In addition, Dr. Sorensen is a member of the Editorial Board for the journal *Cancer Epidemiology, Biomarkers, and Prevention*, and formerly served on the Editorial Boards of the *American Journal of Health Behavior*, the *American Journal of Health Promotion*, and the *Journal of Health and Social Behavior*.

Claire E. Sterk, Ph.D., is Professor and Chair of the Department of Behavioral Sciences and Health Education at the Rollins School of Public Health of Emory University. In addition, she has adjunct appointments in the Departments of Anthropology, Sociology and Women's Studies, and a joined appointment in the Department of Family and Preventive Medicine. Dr. Sterk's research interests include women's health, community-based health prevention and intervention, substance abuse, HIV/AIDS, and access to health care. Dr. Sterk is the Atlanta representative on the Community Epidemiology Working Group of the National Institute on Drug Abuse, and is a member of the Atlanta/Fulton County Commission on Children and Youth. In addition, she is a member of the National Institutes of Health Behavioral AIDS Review group and serves as an ad hoc reviewer on several other panels. Dr. Sterk also serves as a member of an expert committee reviewing the anti-drug media campaign targeting adolescents and launched by the National Institute on Drug Abuse. Dr. Sterk is a Fellow of the Society for Applied Anthropology, and is a member of the editorial board of the journal *AIDS and Anthropology Bulletin*.

John A. Swets, Ph.D., is Chief Scientist, Emeritus at BBN Technologies; Senior Research Associate in Radiology, Brigham and Women's Hospital, Boston; and Lecturer on Health Care Policy, Harvard Medical School, Boston. Dr. Swets's research centers on the psychological processes of sensation, perception, attention, thinking, learning, and decision making; computer-aided instruction; enhancement of human performance; information retrieval; evaluation of diagnostic systems; and enhancement of diagnostic performance. He has been a member of several national panels and committees, recently serving as chair of the National Research Council's Commission on Behavioral and Social Sciences and Education and as senior consultant to the Federal Interagency Coordinating Committee on the Human Brain Project. He is a member of the National Academy of Sciences, the American Academy of Arts and Sciences, and is a fellow of the Society of Experimental Psychologists, the American Psychological Association, the American Psychological Society, the Acoustical Society of America, and the American Association for the Advancement of Science.